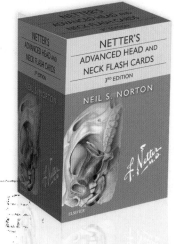
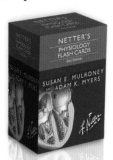
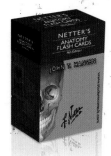
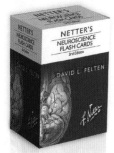

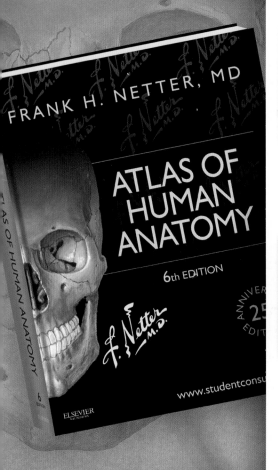
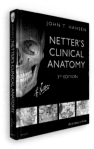
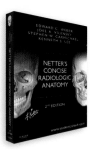
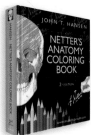

NEIL S. NORTON

# NETTER'S HEAD AND NECK ANATOMY FOR DENTISTRY

## 3RD EDITION

**NEIL S. NORTON, PhD**
Associate Dean for Admissions
Professor of Oral Biology
School of Dentistry
Creighton University
Omaha, Nebraska

Illustrations by Frank H. Netter, MD

Contributing Illustrators
Carlos A.G. Machado, MD
Kip Carter, MS, CMI
Andrew E. B. Swift, MS, CMI
William M. Winn, MS, FAMI
Tiffany S. DaVanzo, MA, CMI
James A. Perkins, MS, MFA
John A. Craig, MD

**ELSEVIER**

# ELSEVIER

1600 John F. Kennedy Blvd.
Ste 1800
Philadelphia, PA 19103-2899

Netter's Head and Neck Anatomy for Dentistry                    ISBN: 978-0-323-39228-0

---

### Notices

---

Previous editions copyrighted 2012 and 2007 by Saunders, an imprint of Elsevier Inc.

**Library of Congress Cataloging-in-Publication Data**

Names: Norton, Neil Scott, author. | Netter, Frank H. (Frank Henry),
   1906-1991, illustrator.
Title: Netter's head and neck anatomy for dentistry / Neil S. Norton ;
   illustrations by Frank H. Netter ; contributing illustrators, Carlos A.G.
   Machado [and 6 others].
Other titles: Head and neck anatomy for dentistry
Description: 3rd edition. | Philadelphia, PA : Elsevier, [2017] | Includes
   index.
Identifiers: LCCN 2016012134 | ISBN 9780323392280 (pbk. : alk. paper)
Subjects: | MESH: Dentistry | Head–anatomy & histology | Neck–anatomy &
   histology | Atlases
Classification: LCC RK280 | NLM WU 17 | DDC 611/.91–dc23 LC record available at
   http://lccn.loc.gov/2016012134

*Executive Content Strategist:* Elyse O'Grady
*Senior Content Developmental Specialist:* Marybeth Thiel
*Publishing Services Manager:* Patricia Tannian
*Project Manager:* Stephanie Turza
*Design Direction:* Julia Dummit

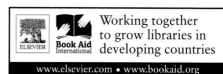

Working together
to grow libraries in
developing countries

www.elsevier.com • www.bookaid.org

Printed in China
Last digit is the print number:   9   8   7   6   5   4   3   2   1

*I dedicate this book to the following influential people in my life,*

*To my late mother Chari, who worked tirelessly*
*and sacrificed everything throughout her life*
*so that her children would not be without.*

*To Elizabeth, who made me a better man.*
*I owe you everything for all that you have done for me.*

*To my brother John, who helped raise me.*

*And to my mentors, the late Frs. John G. Holbrook,*
*S.J., and John P. Schlegel, S.J., who helped me appreciate the importance*
*of service to others. They taught me the dedicated ways of cura personalis,*
*or care for the individual. I have tried to live by those words every day of my life.*

# About the Author

**Neil S. Norton, PhD,** joined Creighton University in 1996 and is currently the Associate Dean for Admissions and Professor of Oral Biology in the School of Dentistry. After graduating Phi Beta Kappa from Randolph-Macon College with a BA in Biology, he went on to receive his PhD training in Anatomy from the University of Nebraska Medical Center. Dr. Norton has been the recipient of over 25 teaching awards, including multiple Outstanding Instructor of the Year Awards from Freshman classes and Dr. Theodore J. Urban Pre-Clinical Awards, presented by graduating Senior classes for outstanding Basic Science instruction. Dr. Norton is the third professor in the history of the School of Dentistry to receive the prestigious Robert F. Kennedy Memorial Award for Teaching Achievement, the highest teaching recognition offered by the University. In 2007 Dr. Norton received the GlaxoSmithKline Sensodyne Teaching Award, the highest national teaching award given by the American Dental Education Association (ADEA). An active member of the School of Dentistry faculty, he was elected by colleagues to honorary membership in Omicron Kappa Upsilon, the National Dental Honor Society whose regular membership is reserved for dentists. His teaching responsibilities include Head and Neck Anatomy, General Anatomy, Neuroscience, and Pain Control. Dr. Norton served four years as President of the University Faculty and chaired many committees, including the University Committee on Rank and Tenure and the University Committee on Academic Freedom and Responsibility. Currently he serves as the Faculty Athletic Representative for Creighton to the BIG EAST Conference. He continues to actively publish on a variety of anatomical topics in addition to his administrative duties. He is an active member of the American Association of Clinical Anatomists (AACA), having served as the Treasurer for seven years and as President from 2015–2017.

# About the Artists

## Frank H. Netter, MD

Frank H. Netter was born in 1906, in New York City. He studied art at the Art Student's League and the National Academy of Design before entering medical school at New York University, where he received his MD in 1931. During his student years, Dr. Netter's notebook sketches attracted the attention of the medical faculty and other physicians, allowing him to augment his income by illustrating articles and textbooks. He continued illustrating as a sideline after establishing a surgical practice in 1933, but he ultimately opted to give up his practice in favor of a full-time commitment to art. After service in the United States Army during World War II, Dr. Netter began his long collaboration with the CIBA Pharmaceutical Company (now Novartis Pharmaceuticals). This 45-year partnership resulted in the production of the extraordinary collection of medical art so familiar to physicians and other medical professionals worldwide.

In 2005, Elsevier, Inc., purchased the Netter Collection and all publications from Icon Learning Systems. There are now over 50 publications featuring the art of Dr. Netter available through Elsevier, Inc. (in the United States: www.us.elsevierhealth.com/Netter and outside the United States: www.elsevierhealth.com).

Dr. Netter's works are among the finest examples of the use of illustration in the teaching of medical concepts. The 13-book *Netter Collection of Medical Illustrations,* which includes the greater part of the more than 20,000 paintings created by Dr. Netter, became and remains one of the most famous medical works ever published. *The Netter Atlas of Human Anatomy,* first published in 1989, presents the anatomical paintings from the Netter Collection. Now translated into 16 languages, it is the anatomy atlas of choice among medical and health professions students the world over.

The Netter illustrations are appreciated not only for their aesthetic qualities, but, more important, for their intellectual content. As Dr. Netter wrote in 1949, "… clarification of a subject is the aim and goal of illustration. No matter how beautifully painted, how delicately and subtly rendered a subject may be, it is of little value as a *medical illustration* if it does not serve to make clear some medical point." Dr. Netter's planning, conception, point of view, and approach are what inform his paintings and what make them so intellectually valuable.

Frank H. Netter, MD, physician and artist, died in 1991.

Learn more about the physician-artist whose work has inspired the Netter Reference collection at www.netterimages.com/artist/netter.htm.

## Carlos Machado, MD

Carlos Machado was chosen by Novartis to be Dr. Netter's successor. He continues to be the main artist who contributes to the Netter collection of medical illustrations.

Self-taught in medical illustration, cardiologist Carlos Machado has contributed meticulous updates to some of Dr. Netter's original plates and has created many paintings of his own in the style of Netter as an extension of the Netter collection. Dr. Machado's photorealistic expertise and his keen insight into the physician/patient relationship inform his vivid and unforgettable visual style. His dedication to researching each topic and subject he paints places him among the premier medical illustrators at work today.

Learn more about his background and see more of his art at www.netterimages.com/artist/machado.htm.

# Acknowledgments

It is hard to believe that it has been over a decade since the seeds of *Netter's Head & Neck Anatomy for Dentistry* were planted. The 3rd edition, like the previous editions, is the result of many long hours of work. I would not have been able to accomplish such a task without the help of many talented and dedicated individuals.

Beginning my academic career at the Creighton University School of Dentistry in 1996, I was overwhelmed by the comradery that existed at both the School and University level. Twenty years later – it still exists. I am grateful every day to be part of such a fine institution that is committed to the education of students. The support and assistance my fellow colleagues have provided to help in the creation of each edition have been immeasurable. I would especially like to thank for their review of chapters, suggestions, and willingness to provide materials the following members of the Creighton School of Dentistry family (past and present): Drs. David Blaha, W. Thomas Cavel, Paul Edwards, James Howard, Terry Lanphier, John McCabe, Kirstin McCarville, Timothy McVaney, Takanari Miyamoto, Barbara O'Kane, Cyndi Russell, and Tarjit Saini. I owe a very special thanks to my former Dean, Dr. Wayne W. Barkmeier. He was the person willing to give a young anatomist an opportunity at Creighton, and I owe my career to Dr. Barkmeier. It was he and Dr. Frank J. Ayers who pushed me and provided me the opportunity in Admissions and Student Affairs. For that, I'll always be grateful. Since the publication of the 2nd edition, I would not have been able to continue to develop this book without the support of my current Dean, Dr. Mark A. Latta.

Additionally, I am extremely grateful to Dr. Laura C. Barritt who provided excellent suggestions and reviews that were instrumental in the creation of the Development section of the book, as well as providing various suggestions in many other chapters. Special thanks go to Dr. Margaret A. Jergenson, chair of the Department of Oral Biology. Since 1996, Dr. Jergenson and I have taught general anatomy and head and neck anatomy to freshman dental students. Her clinical background as a dentist has been invaluable in helping me appreciate head and neck anatomy from a dental perspective. Along with Dr. Barbara O'Kane, we have enjoyed working together as the anatomical team in the School of Dentistry. I could not ask for better colleagues with whom to teach anatomy.

My sincere appreciation to my Creighton colleagues outside of the School of Dentistry. Creighton is a family, and I have been fortunate to spend my career at such a fine university. Over the years there have been a few individuals who have helped me immensely. In particular, I owe a special acknowledgment of gratitude to Frs. Richard Hauser, S.J., and Thomas Shanahan, S.J. My sincere appreciation goes to my friend and colleague Dr. Thomas Quinn, who offered helpful comments and words of encouragement throughout the textual writing and development of the art.

My thanks to the reviewers who examined the chapters in the first edition and provided excellent feedback: Drs. Robert Spears, Kathleen M. Klueber, and Brian R. MacPherson, and Professor Cindy Evans. A very special thanks to my friend and colleague Dr. Vidhya (Vid) Persaud for his helpful comments regarding the Development section of the text.

Over the years, I have enlisted the help of my dental students to make *Netter's Head and Neck Anatomy for Dentistry* more student-friendly. Special thanks go to Drs. Joseph Opack, Ryan Dobbs, Steve Midstokke, Paul Mendes, Kyle D. Smith, and Thomas Spellman for their invaluable assistance.

This book would not be possible if not for the beautiful new artwork created by the incredible medical illustrators at Elsevier. A very special thanks to Carlos Machado, MD, who created new artwork specifically for this atlas. Quite simply, Dr. Machado is one of the greatest medical illustrators of our time and it has been a distinct honor and privilege to have worked with him. A sincere thanks to Tiffany DaVanzo, who was instrumental in the creation of the new pieces in both the 2nd and 3rd editions. I am very grateful for the work of Kip Carter, William Winn, and

Andrew Swift in the 1st edition. All of these illustrators helped put my vision into art. Their artistic interpretations are simply magnificent.

I can never thank the amazing Elsevier team enough! Two people in particular have always been there to help: Elyse O'Grady and Marybeth Thiel. Elyse has been a constant source of support and fantastic ideas for all editions. Marybeth has been there since I submitted the first chapter of the 1st edition, always keeping me on track. This book would not be possible without them. The Elsevier team has been an absolute pleasure! In particular, I sincerely thank my Project Manager, Stephanie Turza, for her attention to detail and keeping everything on time for this book. Additionally, I would like to acknowledge the work of those who helped me complete the first edition of the book: Jennifer Surich, Carolyn Kruse, and Jonathan Dimes.

Very special thanks go to Paul Kelly. I have had the great honor and privilege of knowing Paul for nearly 20 years. Paul encouraged me to put together an anatomical project for dentistry. I presented him with the rough outline and prospectus for a text/atlas that evolved into the first edition of this book.

Lastly, I thank all of the students whom I have instructed over my career. You have always served as a great inspiration to me. It has been an honor and privilege to be a part of your education. *Netter's Head and Neck Anatomy for Dentistry* is for you.

# Preface

*Netter's Head and Neck Anatomy for Dentistry* is a text/atlas written to help dental students and professionals learn and review head and neck anatomy. Designed for first-year dental students, it also serves to teach anatomy to students of dental hygiene as well as a review for the practicing clinician. The head and neck comprise the foundation for dental anatomical study. The many small, interrelated structures are not easily observable, which makes head and neck anatomy one of the most difficult disciplines for students to master.

This 3rd edition has received a bit of a facelift. Elsevier has redesigned the look of the book, and I hope you are as pleased with the outcome as I am. There are numerous additions and revisions to the book. First is the appendix on the lymphatics — with emphasis on the head and neck. Second, more than 30 radiographic images have been added to the existing image catalog to complement the anatomy illustrations throughout the text. Radiology is an important part of the education of every dental student, and it is a natural addition to any anatomy text. Third, more clinical correlates have been added to provide real world scenarios for the student. Fourth, many of the tables and artwork have been revised following the suggestions of many of our readers of the previous editions. In the 3rd edition, there are 50 new questions that cover the chapters in the text. However, to give our readers more, Elsevier has created a test bank of questions on Student Consult. Thus, students can access all of the questions from previous editions as well as other review questions on Student Consult for a more robust review of the material. Another perk of Student Consult includes the addition of short anatomical video clips using the imaging from the 3rd edition.

To understand the clinical significance of an anatomical concept is to understand the anatomy. It is with that in mind that a series of clinical correlates that relate specifically to dentistry are provided at the end of the chapters. There are many anatomical topics covered in traditional head and neck courses that have been expanded especially for this text. A chapter has been dedicated to the temporomandibular joint. In the chapter on the oral cavity, more information has been provided for the reader on such topics as dentition. Chapters on the development of the head and neck and basic neuroscience are included to help connect with other related anatomical areas. A chapter on intraoral injections is included to help teach and reinforce an area often overlooked. The intent of these chapters is to provide the reader with a brief overview of important concepts related to head and neck anatomy.

A superb team of medical illustrators created new art to complement the anatomical illustrations of Dr. Frank H. Netter, which resulted in a more complete learning tool. In particular, the new illustrations of Dr. Carlos Machado demonstrate why he continues to be the preeminent medical illustrator in his field. The Temporomandibular Joint chapter features 6 new figures by Dr. Machado, and I know you will find them as spectacular as I do. Essential information is presented in tables and brief text that are integrated with the Netter art to help bridge gaps and augment the readers' knowledge of head and neck anatomy.

*Netter's Head and Neck Anatomy for Dentistry* is for those in all stages of the dental profession. My hope is that this book will provide an essential resource to readers in helping them to learn and appreciate the complex anatomy of the head and neck.

# Contents

# DEVELOPMENT OF THE HEAD AND NECK

- 3 major germ layers form the initial developing embryo:
  - Ectoderm
  - Mesoderm
  - Endoderm
- Mesoderm differentiates into:
  - Paraxial mesoderm
  - Intermediate mesoderm
  - Lateral plate mesoderm
- Ectoderm gives rise to 3 layers:
  - Neuroectoderm
  - Neural crest
  - Epidermis
- The head and neck are formed by:
  - Paraxial mesoderm
  - Lateral plate mesoderm
  - Neural crest
  - Ectodermal placodes
- Most of the head and neck is formed from the pharyngeal region of the embryo

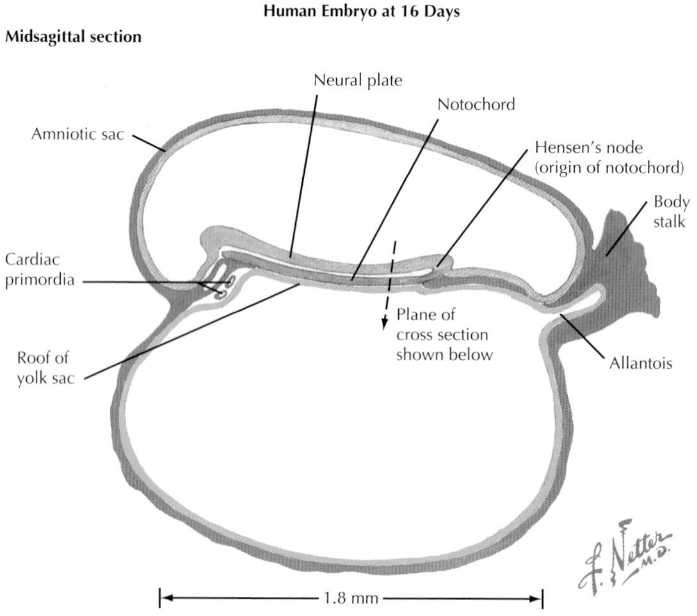

**Human Embryo at 16 Days**

**Midsagittal section**

Neural plate

Notochord

Amniotic sac

Hensen's node
(origin of notochord)

Body
stalk

Cardiac
primordia

Plane of
cross section
shown below

Roof of
yolk sac

Allantois

|◄——————— 1.8 mm ———————►|

**Figure 1-1**

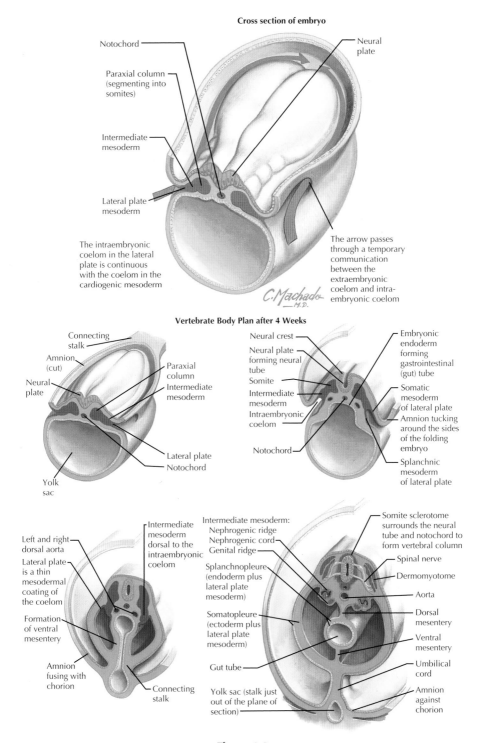

**Cross section of embryo**

Notochord

Neural plate

Paraxial column (segmenting into somites)

Intermediate mesoderm

Lateral plate mesoderm

The intraembryonic coelom in the lateral plate is continuous with the coelom in the cardiogenic mesoderm

The arrow passes through a temporary communication between the extraembryonic coelom and intraembryonic coelom

C. Machado —M.D.

**Vertebrate Body Plan after 4 Weeks**

Connecting stalk

Amnion (cut)

Neural plate

Paraxial column

Intermediate mesoderm

Lateral plate

Notochord

Yolk sac

Neural crest

Neural plate forming neural tube

Somite

Intermediate mesoderm

Intraembryonic coelom

Notochord

Embryonic endoderm forming gastrointestinal (gut) tube

Somatic mesoderm of lateral plate

Amnion tucking around the sides of the folding embryo

Splanchnic mesoderm of lateral plate

Left and right dorsal aorta

Lateral plate is a thin mesodermal coating of the coelom

Formation of ventral mesentery

Amnion fusing with chorion

Intermediate mesoderm dorsal to the intraembryonic coelom

Connecting stalk

Intermediate mesoderm: Nephrogenic ridge Nephrogenic cord Genital ridge

Splanchnopleure (endoderm plus lateral plate mesoderm)

Somatopleure (ectoderm plus lateral plate mesoderm)

Gut tube

Yolk sac (stalk just out of the plane of section)

Somite sclerotome surrounds the neural tube and notochord to form vertebral column

Spinal nerve

Dermomyotome

Aorta

Dorsal mesentery

Ventral mesentery

Umbilical cord

Amnion against chorion

**Figure 1-2**

- Start forming in the 4th week of development
- Develop as blocks separated by pharyngeal clefts (formed by ectoderm)
- Initially, 6 pharyngeal arches develop, but the 5th regresses
- Arising from the endoderm are compartments called pharyngeal pouches that extend toward the pharyngeal clefts, separated by pharyngeal membranes
- Help form 4 of the 5 swellings (embryonic primordia) of the face:
  - 2 mandibular processes (pharyngeal arch)
  - 2 maxillary processes (pharyngeal arch)
  - 1 frontonasal prominence
- Composed of:
  - External surface–ectoderm
  - Internal surface–endoderm
  - Central part–lateral plate mesoderm, paraxial mesoderm, neural crest
- Skeletal components and associated connective tissue develop from the neural crest cells
- Muscular structures develop collectively from the mesoderm
- Each arch is innervated by a cranial nerve that migrates with the muscles

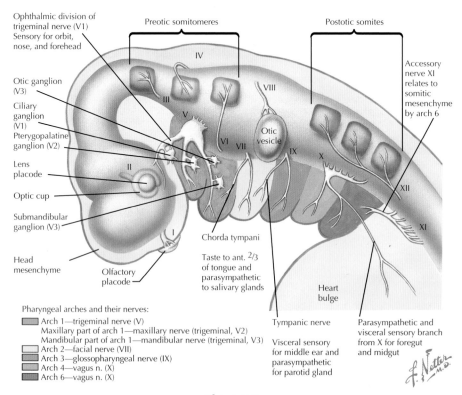

Ophthalmic division of trigeminal nerve (V1) Sensory for orbit, nose, and forehead

Preotic somitomeres

Postotic somites

IV

VIII

Accessory nerve XI relates to somitic mesenchyme by arch 6

Otic ganglion (V3)

III

Ciliary ganglion (V1)

V

Pterygopalatine ganglion (V2)

VI  VII

Otic vesicle

IX

X

Lens placode

II

XII

Optic cup

Submandibular ganglion (V3)

XI

I

Chorda tympani

Head mesenchyme

Olfactory placode

Taste to ant. 2/3 of tongue and parasympathetic to salivary glands

Heart bulge

Pharyngeal arches and their nerves:

Arch 1—trigeminal nerve (V)
Maxillary part of arch 1—maxillary nerve (trigeminal, V2)
Mandibular part of arch 1—mandibular nerve (trigeminal, V3)
Arch 2—facial nerve (VII)
Arch 3—glossopharyngeal nerve (IX)
Arch 4—vagus n. (X)
Arch 6—vagus n. (X)

Tympanic nerve

Visceral sensory for middle ear and parasympathetic for parotid gland

Parasympathetic and visceral sensory branch from X for foregut and midgut

**Figure 1-3**

| Arch | Muscle(s) from Mesoderm | Cartilage Structure(s) from Neural Crest | Cartilage Structure(s) from Mesoderm | Connective Tissue Structure(s) from Neural Crest | Nerve |
|------|-------------------------|------------------------------------------|--------------------------------------|--------------------------------------------------|-------|
| 1 (also called the Mandibular arch)<br>Develops into:<br>• Maxillary process<br>• Mandibular process | Masseter<br>Temporalis<br>Lateral pterygoid<br>Medial pterygoid<br>Mylohyoid<br>Anterior digastric<br>Tensor tympani<br>Tensor veli palatini | Malleus<br>Incus (both from Meckel's cartilage, which degenerates in adulthood) | | Sphenomandibular ligament<br>Anterior ligament of the malleus (both from Meckel's cartilage, which degenerates in adulthood) | Trigeminal |
| 2 (also called the Hyoid arch) | Muscles of facial expression<br>Posterior digastric<br>Stylohyoid<br>Stapedius | Lesser cornu of the hyoid<br>Superior part of the hyoid body<br>Styloid process<br>Stapes (all from Reichert's cartilage) | | Stylohyoid ligament<br>Connective tissue of the tonsil | Facial |
| 3 | Stylopharyngeus | Greater cornu of the hyoid<br>Inferior part of the hyoid body | | Connective tissue of the thymus and inferior parathyroid | Glossopha-ryngeal |
| 4 | Musculus uvulae<br>Levator veli palatini<br>Palatopharyngeus<br>Palatoglossus<br>Superior constrictor<br>Middle constrictor<br>Inferior constrictor<br>Salpingopharyn-geus<br>Cricothyroid | | Epiglottis<br>Thyroid (both from lateral plate mesoderm) | Connective tissue of the superior parathyroid and the thyroid | Vagus |
| 6 | Thyroarytenoid<br>Vocalis<br>Lateral cricoarytenoid<br>Oblique arytenoids<br>Transverse arytenoids<br>Posterior cricoarytenoid<br>Aryepiglottis<br>Thyroepiglottis | | Arytenoid<br>Cricoid<br>Cuneiform<br>Corniculate (all from lateral plate mesoderm) | | Vagus |

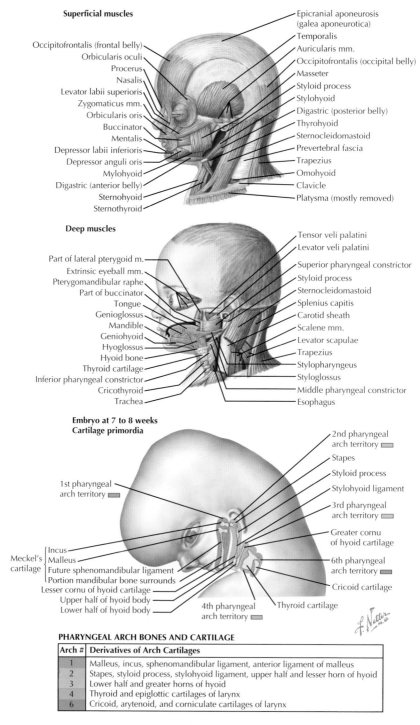

**Superficial muscles**

Occipitofrontalis (frontal belly)
Orbicularis oculi
Procerus
Nasalis
Levator labii superioris
Zygomaticus mm.
Orbicularis oris
Buccinator
Mentalis
Depressor labii inferioris
Depressor anguli oris
Mylohyoid
Digastric (anterior belly)
Sternohyoid
Sternothyroid

Epicranial aponeurosis (galea aponeurotica)
Temporalis
Auricularis mm.
Occipitofrontalis (occipital belly)
Masseter
Styloid process
Stylohyoid
Digastric (posterior belly)
Thyrohyoid
Sternocleidomastoid
Prevertebral fascia
Trapezius
Omohyoid
Clavicle
Platysma (mostly removed)

**Deep muscles**

Part of lateral pterygoid m.
Extrinsic eyeball mm.
Pterygomandibular raphe
Part of buccinator
Tongue
Genioglossus
Mandible
Geniohyoid
Hyoglossus
Hyoid bone
Thyroid cartilage
Inferior pharyngeal constrictor
Cricothyroid
Trachea

Tensor veli palatini
Levator veli palatini
Superior pharyngeal constrictor
Styloid process
Sternocleidomastoid
Splenius capitis
Carotid sheath
Scalene mm.
Levator scapulae
Trapezius
Stylopharyngeus
Styloglossus
Middle pharyngeal constrictor
Esophagus

**Embryo at 7 to 8 weeks**
**Cartilage primordia**

1st pharyngeal arch territory

2nd pharyngeal arch territory
Stapes
Styloid process
Stylohyoid ligament
3rd pharyngeal arch territory
Greater cornu of hyoid cartilage
6th pharyngeal arch territory
Cricoid cartilage

Meckel's cartilage
Incus
Malleus
Future sphenomandibular ligament
Portion mandibular bone surrounds
Lesser cornu of hyoid cartilage
Upper half of hyoid body
Lower half of hyoid body

4th pharyngeal arch territory
Thyroid cartilage

*f. Netter M.D.*

**PHARYNGEAL ARCH BONES AND CARTILAGE**

| Arch # | Derivatives of Arch Cartilages |
|---|---|
| 1 | Malleus, incus, sphenomandibular ligament, anterior ligament of malleus |
| 2 | Stapes, styloid process, stylohyoid ligament, upper half and lesser horn of hyoid |
| 3 | Lower half and greater horns of hyoid |
| 4 | Thyroid and epiglottic cartilages of larynx |
| 6 | Cricoid, arytenoid, and corniculate cartilages of larynx |

**Figure 1-4**

- Pharyngeal pouches–4 develop from endoderm
- Pharyngeal clefts–each is a groove formed from ectoderm
- Pharyngeal membranes–each is composed of tissue located between a pharyngeal pouch and a pharyngeal cleft; composed of external ectoderm, mesoderm and neural crest in the core, and an internal endoderm lining

### Pharyngeal Pouches

| Pouch | Location | Embryonic Structure | Adult Structure |
|---|---|---|---|
| 1 | Opposite the 1st pharyngeal cleft, separated by the 1st pharyngeal membrane | Tubotympanic recess | Epithelium of the (pharyngotympanic auditory) tube<br><br>Tympanic cavity |
| 2 | Opposite the 2nd pharyngeal cleft, separated by the 2nd pharyngeal membrane | Primordial palatine tonsils | Tonsillar (sinus fossa)<br><br>Epithelium of the palatine tonsil |
| 3 | Opposite the 3rd pharyngeal cleft, separated by the 3rd pharyngeal membrane | Divides into a dorsal and a ventral part<br><br>Dorsal part migrates inferiorly toward the thorax | Inferior parathyroid gland (from the dorsal part)<br><br>Thymus (from the ventral part) |
| 4 | Opposite the 4th pharyngeal cleft, separated by the 4th pharyngeal membrane | Divides into a dorsal and a ventral part<br><br>Ventral part is invaded by neural crest to form the parafollicular or C cells | Superior parathyroid gland (from the dorsal part)<br><br>Ultimobranchial body (from the ventral part) |

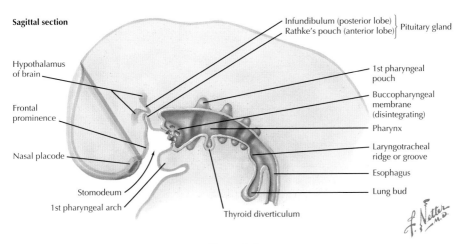

**Figure 1-5**

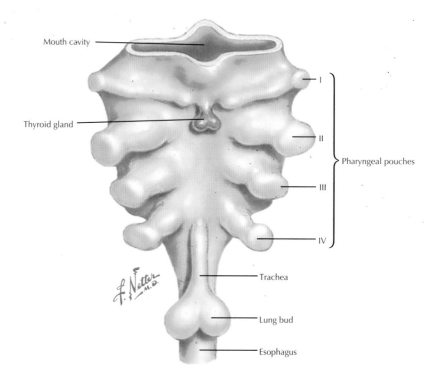

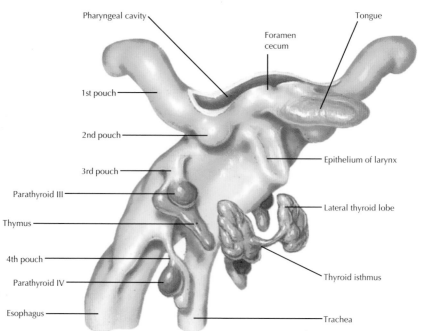

**Figure 1-6**

| Membrane | Location | Adult Structure |
|---|---|---|
| 1 | Between the 1st pharyngeal cleft and the 1st pharyngeal pouch | Tympanic membrane |
| 2 | Between the 2nd pharyngeal cleft and the 2nd pharyngeal pouch | |
| 3 | Between the 3rd pharyngeal cleft and the 3rd pharyngeal pouch | |
| 4 | Between the 4th pharyngeal cleft and the 4th pharyngeal pouch | |

## Pharyngeal Clefts

| Cleft | Location | Adult Structure |
|---|---|---|
| 1 | A groove between the 1st and 2nd pharyngeal arches | External acoustic meatus |
| 2 | A groove between the 2nd and 3rd pharyngeal arches | Obliterated cervical sinus by the 2nd pharyngeal arch, which grows over the clefts |
| 3 | A groove between the 3rd and 4th pharyngeal arches | |
| 4 | A groove between the 4th and 6th pharyngeal arches | |

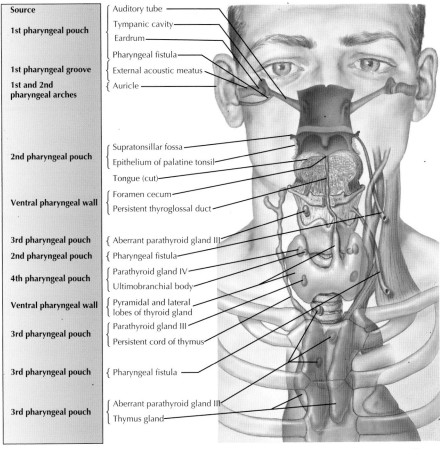

| Source | |
|---|---|
| 1st pharyngeal pouch | Auditory tube |
| | Tympanic cavity |
| | Eardrum |
| 1st pharyngeal groove | Pharyngeal fistula |
| | External acoustic meatus |
| 1st and 2nd pharyngeal arches | Auricle |
| 2nd pharyngeal pouch | Supratonsillar fossa |
| | Epithelium of palatine tonsil |
| | Tongue (cut) |
| Ventral pharyngeal wall | Foramen cecum |
| | Persistent thyroglossal duct |
| 3rd pharyngeal pouch | Aberrant parathyroid gland III |
| 2nd pharyngeal pouch | Pharyngeal fistula |
| 4th pharyngeal pouch | Parathyroid gland IV |
| | Ultimobranchial body |
| Ventral pharyngeal wall | Pyramidal and lateral lobes of thyroid gland |
| 3rd pharyngeal pouch | Parathyroid gland III |
| | Persistent cord of thymus |
| 3rd pharyngeal pouch | Pharyngeal fistula |
| 3rd pharyngeal pouch | Aberrant parathyroid gland III |
| | Thymus gland |

Figure 1-7

- Cranium (skull) is formed from:
  - Lateral plate mesoderm (neck region)
  - Paraxial mesoderm
  - Neural crest
- Cranium development is divided into 2 parts:
  - Viscerocranium–forms the bones of the face (from the pharyngeal arches)
  - Forms completely from neural crest
  - Neurocranium–forms the bones of the cranial base and cranial vault, and the function is to protect and surround the brain and organs of special sense (olfaction, vision, auditory, and equilibrium). It can be divided into:
    - Membranous neurocranium (forms from neural crest and paraxial mesoderm)
    - Cartilaginous neurocranium (forms from neural crest and paraxial mesoderm)
- Bony skull is formed by either of 2 mechanisms:
  - Intramembranous ossification
  - Endochondral ossification

### Viscerocranium

| Germ Layers | Origins | Adult Structure(s) | Ossification |
|---|---|---|---|
| Neural crest | 1st pharyngeal arch *Maxillary process* | Maxilla | Intramembranous |
| | | Temporal bone | |
| | | Zygoma | |
| | | Palatine | |
| | | Lacrimal | |
| | | Vomer | |
| | | Nasal | |
| | | Inferior nasal concha | Endochondral |
| | 1st pharyngeal arch *Mandibular process* | Mandible | Intramembranous (body) Endochondral (coronoid and condylar process) |
| | | Malleus | Endochondral |
| | | Incus | |
| | 2nd pharyngeal arch | Styloid process | Endochondral |
| | | Stapes | |
| | | Hyoid | |

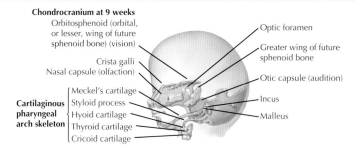

**Chondrocranium at 9 weeks**

Orbitosphenoid (orbital, or lesser, wing of future sphenoid bone) (vision)

Optic foramen

Greater wing of future sphenoid bone

Crista galli
Nasal capsule (olfaction)

Otic capsule (audition)

Cartilaginous pharyngeal arch skeleton
{
Meckel's cartilage
Styloid process
Hyoid cartilage
Thyroid cartilage
Cricoid cartilage
}

Incus

Malleus

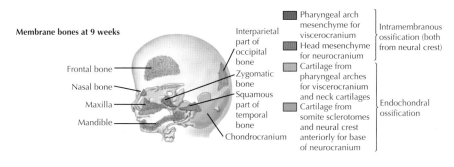

**Membrane bones at 9 weeks**

Frontal bone

Nasal bone

Maxilla

Mandible

Interparietal part of occipital bone

Zygomatic bone

Squamous part of temporal bone

Chondrocranium

Pharyngeal arch mesenchyme for viscerocranium

Head mesenchyme for neurocranium

Cartilage from pharyngeal arches for viscerocranium and neck cartilages

Cartilage from somite sclerotomes and neural crest anteriorly for base of neurocranium

Intramembranous ossification (both from neural crest)

Endochondral ossification

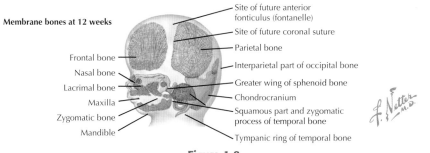

**Membrane bones at 12 weeks**

Frontal bone
Nasal bone
Lacrimal bone
Maxilla
Zygomatic bone
Mandible

Site of future anterior fonticulus (fontanelle)

Site of future coronal suture

Parietal bone

Interparietal part of occipital bone

Greater wing of sphenoid bone

Chondrocranium

Squamous part and zygomatic process of temporal bone

Tympanic ring of temporal bone

**Figure 1-8**

## Cranial Fontanelles

| Fontanelle | Time of Closure |
|---|---|
| Anterior fontanelle (bregma) | 4–26 months |
| Posterior fontanelle (lambda) | 1–2 months |
| Sphenoidal fontanelle (pterion) | 2–3 months |
| Mastoid fontanelle (asterion) | 12–18 months |

| Germ Layer | Portions of Neurocranium | Adult Structure | Ossification |
|---|---|---|---|
| Neural crest | Main portion of the roof and lateral sides of the cranial vault | Frontal bone<br>Squamous portion of the temporal bone | Intramembranous |
| Paraxial mesoderm | | Parietal bone<br>Occipital bone (intraparietal portion) | |

## Cartilaginous Neurocranium

| Germ Layer | Portions of Neurocranium | Adult Structure | Ossification |
|---|---|---|---|
| Neural crest | Prechordal<br>Anterior to the sella turcica | Ethmoid<br>Sphenoid | Endochondral |
| Paraxial mesoderm | Chordal<br>Posterior to the sella turcica | Petrous portion of the temporal bone<br>Mastoid process of the temporal bone<br>Occipital bone | |

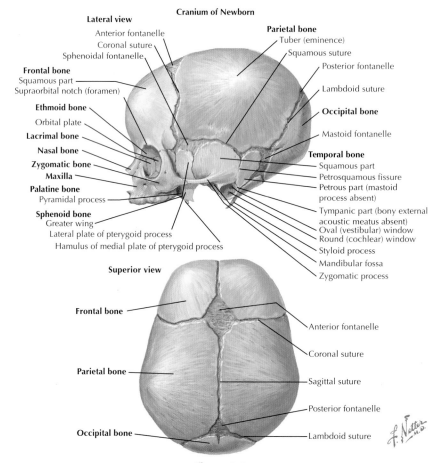

**Cranium of Newborn**

**Lateral view**

Anterior fontanelle
Coronal suture
Sphenoidal fontanelle

**Frontal bone**
Squamous part
Supraorbital notch (foramen)

**Ethmoid bone**
Orbital plate
**Lacrimal bone**
**Nasal bone**
**Zygomatic bone**
**Maxilla**
**Palatine bone**
Pyramidal process
**Sphenoid bone**
Greater wing
Lateral plate of pterygoid process
Hamulus of medial plate of pterygoid process

**Parietal bone**
Tuber (eminence)
Squamous suture
Posterior fontanelle

Lambdoid suture

**Occipital bone**

Mastoid fontanelle

**Temporal bone**
Squamous part
Petrosquamous fissure
Petrous part (mastoid process absent)
Tympanic part (bony external acoustic meatus absent)
Oval (vestibular) window
Round (cochlear) window
Styloid process
Mandibular fossa
Zygomatic process

**Superior view**

**Frontal bone**

Anterior fontanelle

Coronal suture

**Parietal bone**

Sagittal suture

Posterior fontanelle

**Occipital bone**

Lambdoid suture

**Figure 1-9**

- The face is formed mainly from neural crest, which makes 3 swellings (prominences) that surround the stomodeum:
  - Frontonasal prominence
  - Maxillary prominence (from the 1st pharyngeal arch)
  - Mandibular prominence (from the 1st pharyngeal arch)
- Lateral to the frontonasal prominence, 2 additional areas of ectoderm form the 2 nasal placodes that invaginate in the center to form nasal pits, creating ridges of tissue on either side of the pits:
  - Lateral nasal prominence
  - Medial nasal prominence
- Fusion of the medial nasal prominences at the midline results in formation of the intermaxillary segment

| ADULT STRUCTURES OF THE FACE | |
|---|---|
| **Structure** | **Develop(s) from** |
| Forehead | Frontonasal prominence |
| Upper lip | Maxillary prominence (lateral part of upper lip)<br>Medial nasal prominence (middle part of upper lip) |
| Lower lip | Mandibular prominence |
| Lacrimal sac<br>Nasolacrimal duct | A nasolacrimal groove that separates the lateral nasal prominence and the maxillary prominence |
| Nose | Frontonasal prominence (bridge of nose)<br>Medial nasal prominence (nose attaching at philtrum)<br>Lateral nasal prominence (alae of nose) |
| Cheeks | Maxillary prominence |
| Philtrum | Medial nasal prominence |
| Primary palate<br>Upper jaw containing the central and lateral incisors | Intermaxillary segment (fusion of medial nasal prominences) |

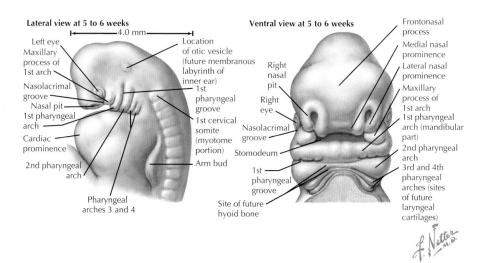

**Lateral view at 5 to 6 weeks**

|←———4.0 mm———→|

Left eye
Maxillary process of 1st arch
Nasolacrimal groove
Nasal pit
1st pharyngeal arch
Cardiac prominence
2nd pharyngeal arch
Pharyngeal arches 3 and 4

Location of otic vesicle (future membranous labyrinth of inner ear)
1st pharyngeal groove
1st cervical somite (myotome portion)
Arm bud

**Ventral view at 5 to 6 weeks**

Right nasal pit
Right eye
Nasolacrimal groove
Stomodeum
1st pharyngeal groove
Site of future hyoid bone

Frontonasal process
Medial nasal prominence
Lateral nasal prominence
Maxillary process of 1st arch
1st pharyngeal arch (mandibular part)
2nd pharyngeal arch
3rd and 4th pharyngeal arches (sites of future laryngeal cartilages)

**Figure 1-10**

**Lateral view at 6 to 7 weeks**

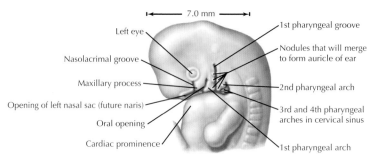

←——— 7.0 mm ———→

Left eye

Nasolacrimal groove

Maxillary process

Opening of left nasal sac (future naris)

Oral opening

Cardiac prominence

1st pharyngeal groove

Nodules that will merge to form auricle of ear

2nd pharyngeal arch

3rd and 4th pharyngeal arches in cervical sinus

1st pharyngeal arch

**Ventral view at 6 to 7 weeks**

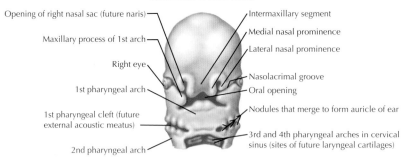

Opening of right nasal sac (future naris)

Maxillary process of 1st arch

Right eye

1st pharyngeal arch

1st pharyngeal cleft (future external acoustic meatus)

2nd pharyngeal arch

Intermaxillary segment

Medial nasal prominence

Lateral nasal prominence

Nasolacrimal groove

Oral opening

Nodules that merge to form auricle of ear

3rd and 4th pharyngeal arches in cervical sinus (sites of future laryngeal cartilages)

**Ventral view at 7 to 8 weeks**

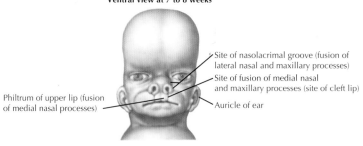

Site of nasolacrimal groove (fusion of lateral nasal and maxillary processes)

Site of fusion of medial nasal and maxillary processes (site of cleft lip)

Philtrum of upper lip (fusion of medial nasal processes)

Auricle of ear

**Lateral view at 7 to 8 weeks**

**Lateral view at 8 to 10 weeks**

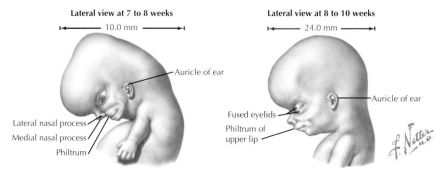

←——— 10.0 mm ———→

Auricle of ear

Lateral nasal process

Medial nasal process

Philtrum

←——— 24.0 mm ———→

Auricle of ear

Fused eyelids

Philtrum of upper lip

**Figure 1-11**

- Formed by the:
  - Primary palate (intermaxillary segment)
  - Secondary palate (protrusions from the maxillary prominences)
- Intermaxillary segment: the initial portion of the palate in development; contains the central and lateral incisors
- Swellings of the maxillary prominence form shelves (lateral palatine processes) that project medially and are separated by the tongue
- When the tongue no longer occupies the space between the palatal shelves, these lateral palatine processes fuse together to form the secondary palate
- The primary and secondary palatal tissues all meet at the *incisive foramen*
- Primary and secondary palates and the nasal septum fuse to form the definitive palate

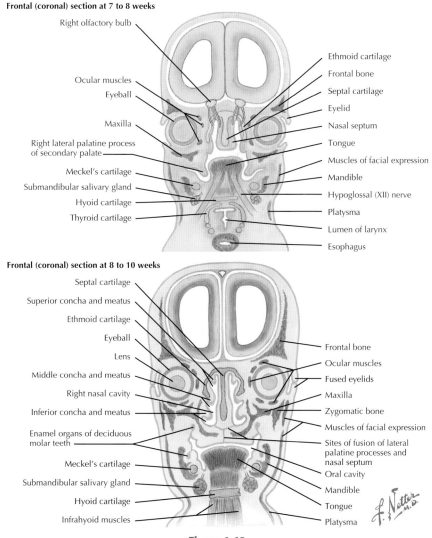

Frontal (coronal) section at 7 to 8 weeks

Right olfactory bulb

Ocular muscles
Eyeball

Maxilla

Right lateral palatine process of secondary palate

Meckel's cartilage
Submandibular salivary gland
Hyoid cartilage
Thyroid cartilage

Ethmoid cartilage
Frontal bone
Septal cartilage
Eyelid
Nasal septum
Tongue
Muscles of facial expression
Mandible
Hypoglossal (XII) nerve
Platysma
Lumen of larynx
Esophagus

Frontal (coronal) section at 8 to 10 weeks

Septal cartilage
Superior concha and meatus
Ethmoid cartilage
Eyeball
Lens
Middle concha and meatus
Right nasal cavity
Inferior concha and meatus
Enamel organs of deciduous molar teeth
Meckel's cartilage
Submandibular salivary gland
Hyoid cartilage
Infrahyoid muscles

Frontal bone
Ocular muscles
Fused eyelids
Maxilla
Zygomatic bone
Muscles of facial expression
Sites of fusion of lateral palatine processes and nasal septum
Oral cavity
Mandible
Tongue
Platysma

**Figure 1-12**

Roof of stomodeum (inferior view; 6 to 7 weeks)

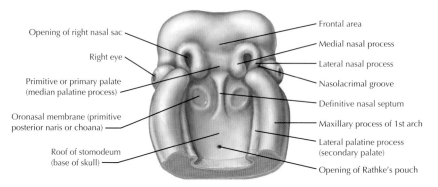

Opening of right nasal sac

Right eye

Primitive or primary palate
(median palatine process)

Oronasal membrane (primitive
posterior naris or choana)

Roof of stomodeum
(base of skull)

Frontal area

Medial nasal process

Lateral nasal process

Nasolacrimal groove

Definitive nasal septum

Maxillary process of 1st arch

Lateral palatine process
(secondary palate)

Opening of Rathke's pouch

Palate formation (inferior view; 7 to 8 weeks)

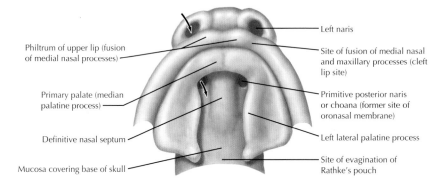

Philtrum of upper lip (fusion
of medial nasal processes)

Primary palate (median
palatine process)

Definitive nasal septum

Mucosa covering base of skull

Left naris

Site of fusion of medial nasal
and maxillary processes (cleft
lip site)

Primitive posterior naris
or choana (former site of
oronasal membrane)

Left lateral palatine process

Site of evagination of
Rathke's pouch

Roof of oral cavity (inferior view; 8 to 10 weeks)

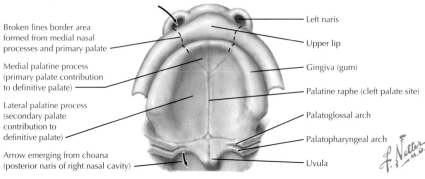

Broken lines border area
formed from medial nasal
processes and primary palate

Medial palatine process
(primary palate contribution
to definitive palate)

Lateral palatine process
(secondary palate
contribution to
definitive palate)

Arrow emerging from choana
(posterior naris of right nasal cavity)

Left naris

Upper lip

Gingiva (gum)

Palatine raphe (cleft palate site)

Palatoglossal arch

Palatopharyngeal arch

Uvula

**Figure 1-13**

- The GSA fibers that supply the epithelium of the tongue mirror the development of the tongue by the pharyngeal arches (arches 1, 3, and 4)
- Although the 2nd pharyngeal arch does not contribute to the tongue, the SVA fibers (taste) that travel to the anterior two-thirds of the tongue come from the chorda tympani (a branch of the facial n.), which joins the lingual n. in the infratemporal fossa, allowing the SVA fibers to be distributed to the anterior two-thirds of the tongue

| Pharyngeal Arch | Embryonic Structure(s) | Adult Structure | Innervation |
|---|---|---|---|
| 1 | 2 lateral lingual swellings<br>Tuberculum impar | Anterior 2/3 of the tongue | *GSA:* Lingual branch of the mandibular division of the trigeminal n. |
| 2 | Is overgrown by the 3rd arch; does not contribute to the adult tongue<br>Very little contributes to the hypopharyngeal eminence | Does not contribute to the adult tongue | |
| 3 | Hypopharyngeal eminence | Posterior 1/3 of the tongue | *GSA:* Glossopharyngeal n.<br>*SVA:* Glossopharyngeal n. |
| 4 | Hypopharyngeal eminence<br>Epiglottic swelling<br>Arytenoid swelling<br>Laryngotracheal groove | Root of the tongue | *GSA:* Internal laryngeal branch of the vagus n.<br>*SVA:* Internal laryngeal branch of the vagus n. |

**Muscles**

- Mesoderm from the occipital somites migrates anteriorly with the hypoglossal nerve to give rise to the extrinsic and intrinsic muscles of the tongue, except the palatoglossus, which is from mesoderm from the 4th pharyngeal arch (and thus is innervated by the vagus nerve)

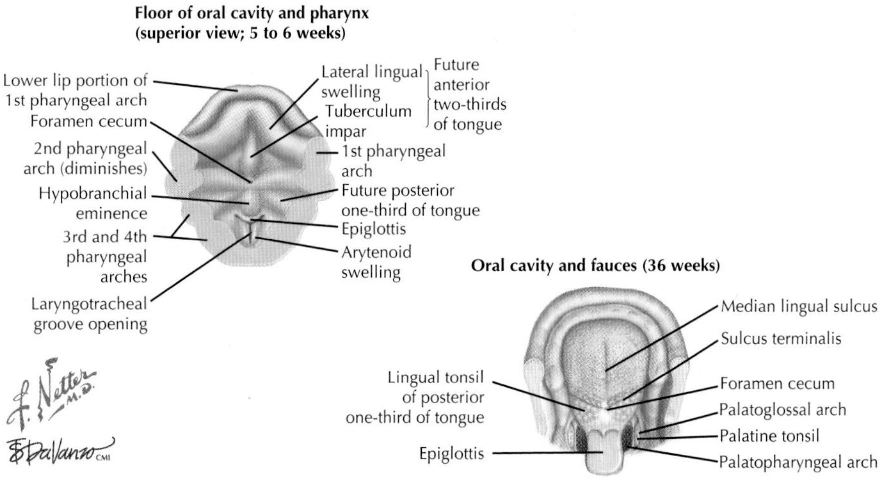

**Floor of oral cavity and pharynx
(superior view; 5 to 6 weeks)**

Lower lip portion of 1st pharyngeal arch
Foramen cecum
2nd pharyngeal arch (diminishes)
Hypobranchial eminence
3rd and 4th pharyngeal arches
Laryngotracheal groove opening

Lateral lingual swelling
Tuberculum impar
} Future anterior two-thirds of tongue
1st pharyngeal arch
Future posterior one-third of tongue
Epiglottis
Arytenoid swelling

**Oral cavity and fauces (36 weeks)**

Lingual tonsil of posterior one-third of tongue
Epiglottis

Median lingual sulcus
Sulcus terminalis
Foramen cecum
Palatoglossal arch
Palatine tonsil
Palatopharyngeal arch

**Figure 1-14**

- Begins in the floor of the pharynx as an invagination at the foramen cecum
- Descends inferiorly to its final position alongside the larynx
- May be connected to the foramen cecum by the thyroglossal duct (which normally atrophies and disappears; remnants may persist and form cysts)
- Divided into 2 lateral lobes connected by an isthmus, from which a pyramidal lobe sometimes develops
- Follicular cells are derived from the endoderm; parafollicular cells are derived from the ultimobranchial body

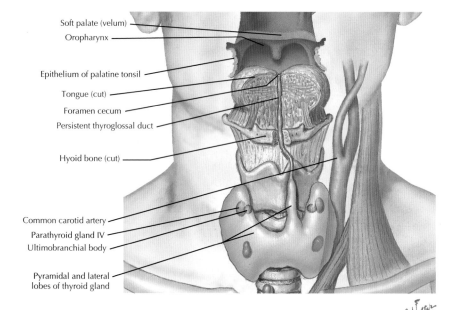

Soft palate (velum)
Oropharynx
Epithelium of palatine tonsil
Tongue (cut)
Foramen cecum
Persistent thyroglossal duct
Hyoid bone (cut)
Common carotid artery
Parathyroid gland IV
Ultimobranchial body
Pyramidal and lateral lobes of thyroid gland

**Figure 1-15**

## ECTOPIC THYROID

- Thyroid tissue in an aberrant location
- Often the only thyroid tissue in the affected person
- Susceptible to thyroid diseases like normal thyroid tissue
- May occur anywhere along the migratory pathway of the thyroid gland beginning at the foramen cecum
- Usually located at the base of the tongue (lingual thyroid)
- Common locations include:
  - Lingual thyroid
  - Sublingual thyroid
  - Thyroglossal duct remnant
  - Anterior mediastinum
  - Prelaryngeal
  - Intralingual
  - Intratracheal

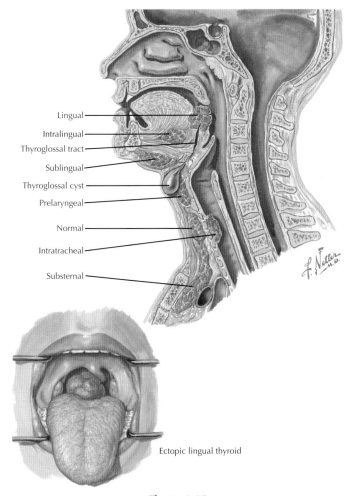

Lingual
Intralingual
Thyroglossal tract
Sublingual
Thyroglossal cyst
Prelaryngeal
Normal
Intratracheal
Substernal

Ectopic lingual thyroid

**Figure 1-16**

## PIERRE ROBIN

- First reported as a condition characterized by micrognathia, cleft palate, and glossoptosis
- Now includes any condition with a series of anomalies caused by events initiated by a single malformation
- In this micrognathia, the inferior dental arch is posterior to the superior arch
- The clefting may affect the hard and the soft palate
- Glossoptosis (posterior displacement of the tongue) may cause airway obstruction or apnea
- The mandible usually grows fairly quickly during childhood
- Multiple surgeries typically needed to correct the cleft palate and to aid speech development in children

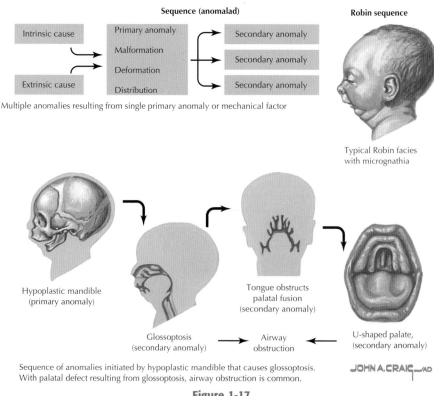

Sequence (anomalad)

Robin sequence

Intrinsic cause

Primary anomaly

Malformation

Deformation

Distribution

Extrinsic cause

Secondary anomaly

Secondary anomaly

Secondary anomaly

Multiple anomalies resulting from single primary anomaly or mechanical factor

Typical Robin facies with micrognathia

Hypoplastic mandible (primary anomaly)

Glossoptosis (secondary anomaly) → Airway obstruction

Tongue obstructs palatal fusion (secondary anomaly)

U-shaped palate, (secondary anomaly)

Sequence of anomalies initiated by hypoplastic mandible that causes glossoptosis. With palatal defect resulting from glossoptosis, airway obstruction is common.

JOHN A.CRAIG—AD

**Figure 1-17**

TREACHER COLLINS

- A hereditary condition affecting the head and neck
- Caused by haploinsufficiency of the gene *TCOF1* (Treacher Collins–Franceschetti syndrome 1) which is officially known as Treacle Ribosome Biogenesis Factor 1.
- The gene product is the treacle protein, which contributes to development of cartilage and bone of the face
- Children of an affected parent have a 50% risk of having the syndrome
- Clinical manifestations include:
  - Downslanting eyes
  - Incomplete orbits
  - Notching of the lower eyelids
  - Hypoplastic mandible
  - Hypoplastic zygomatic bones (malar hypoplasia)
  - Underdeveloped or malformed ears or "sideburns," or both, are prominent
- Common associated problems include:
  - Hearing loss
  - Eating/breathing difficulties
  - Cleft palate

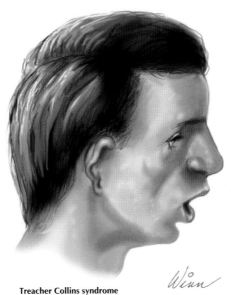

Treacher Collins syndrome

**Figure 1-18**

DIGEORGE SYNDROME

- A rare condition caused by a deletion on chromosome 22, characterized by a wide array of clinical manifestations
- Possible explanation: Proper development is dependent on migration of neural crest cells to the area of the pharyngeal pouches
- Although researchers described the syndrome as abnormal development of the 3rd and 4th pharyngeal pouches, defects involving the 1st to the 6th pouches have been observed
- Thus, the affected individual is born without a thymus and parathyroid glands
- Possible associated problems include:
  - Congenital heart defects (such as tetralogy of Fallot, right infundibular stenosis, truncus arteriosus, aberrant left subclavian artery, and ventricular septal defect)
  - Facial defects (such as cleft palate, microstomia, downslanting eyes, low-set ears, or hypertelorism)
  - Increased vulnerability to infections (due to impaired immune system from the loss of T cells associated with absence or hypoplasia of the thymus)

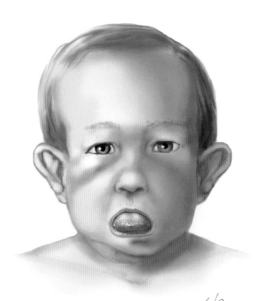

DiGeorge syndrome

Figure 1-19

- **Cleft lip:** a gap in the upper lip
- **Cleft palate:** a gap in the palate
- Classification of the developmental defect is with reference to the incisive foramen:
  - Primary cleft
  - Secondary cleft
  - Complete cleft
- Both cleft lip and cleft palate often cause difficulty with feeding and eventually speech
- Surgery is the most common form of treatment for both

## PRIMARY

- Occurs anterior to the incisive foramen and results from a failure of the mesenchyme in the lateral palatine process (derived from maxillary prominence) to fuse with the intermaxillary segment (or primary palate, which is derived from the fusion of the right and left medial nasal prominences)
- Common types of primary cleft:
  - Unilateral cleft lip
  - Unilateral cleft alveolus
  - Unilateral cleft lip and primary palate
  - Bilateral cleft lip and primary palate

## SECONDARY

- Occurs posterior to the incisive foramen; results from failure of the lateral palatine process (derived from maxillary prominence) to fuse together
- Common types of secondary cleft:
  - Cleft in soft palate
  - Unilateral cleft in hard and soft palate
  - Bilateral cleft of hard and soft palate

## COMPLETE

- Extends through the lip, the primary palate, and the lateral palatine process; results from a failure of the lateral palatine process (derived from maxillary prominence) to fuse with each other, as well as with the nasal septum and primary palate (derived from intermaxillary segment)
- Common types of complete cleft:
  - Unilateral cleft lip and cleft palate
  - Bilateral cleft lip and cleft palate

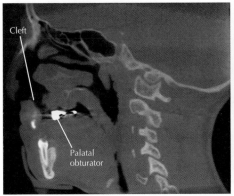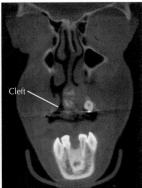

Note the communication between nasal cavity and oral cavity.

**Figure 1-20**

*See next page.*

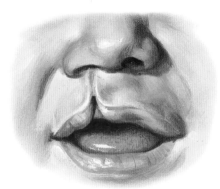

Unilateral cleft lip—partial

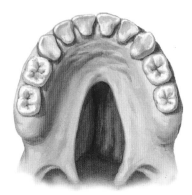

Partial cleft of palate

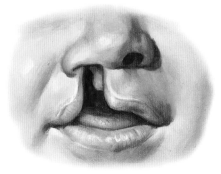

Unilateral cleft of primary palate—
complete, involving lip and alveolar ridge

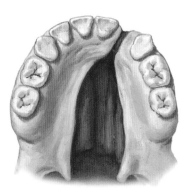

Complete cleft of secondary palate
and unilateral cleft of primary palate

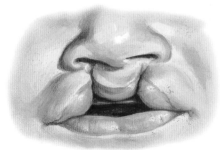

Bilateral cleft lip

**Figure 1-21**

# OSTEOLOGY

- Most complicated bony structure in the human body
- The complete bony framework of the head; includes the mandible
- 28 individual bones make up the skull:
  - 11 are paired
  - 6 are single
- Wormian bones, or sutural bones, are irregularly shaped small bones found along sutures that occur naturally

## FUNCTIONS

- Most important function: to protect the brain
- Also protects the 5 organs of special sense:
  - Olfaction
  - Vision
  - Taste
  - Vestibular function
  - Auditory function

## DIVISIONS

- 2 major ways to divide the bones of the skull:
  - Regional
  - Developmental
- **Regionally**, the skull is divided into the mandible (lower jaw) and cranium (skull without the mandible)
- Cranium is further divided into:
  - Cranial vault–upper portion of the skull
  - Cranial base–inferior portion of the skull
  - Cranial cavity–interior of the skull
  - Facial skeleton–bones that make up the face
  - Acoustic skeleton–ear ossicles
- **Developmentally**, the skull is divided into:
  - Viscerocranium–the portion of the skull related to the digestive and respiratory systems
  - Neurocranium–the portion of the skull that protects the brain and the 5 organs of special sense
- Cranial cavity divisions:
  - Anterior cranial fossa–contains the frontal lobe of the brain
  - Middle cranial fossa–contains the temporal lobe of the brain
  - Posterior cranial fossa–contains the cerebellum
- Skull is depicted by observing it from 5 views:
  - Norma frontalis–the anterior view
  - Norma lateralis–the lateral view
  - Norma occipitalis–the posterior view
  - Norma basalis–the inferior view
  - Norma verticalis–the superior view

| Bone | Single | Paired | Articulates With |
|------|--------|--------|------------------|
| Frontal | X | | Parietal, sphenoid, zygomatic, maxilla, ethmoid, nasal, lacrimal |
| Parietal | | X | Frontal, parietal, temporal, occipital, sphenoid |
| Temporal | | X | Parietal, occipital, sphenoid, zygomatic, mandible |
| Occipital | X | | Parietal, temporal, sphenoid, and atlas (C1) |
| Sphenoid | X | | Frontal, parietal, temporal, occipital, zygomatic, maxilla, ethmoid, palatine, vomer |
| Zygomatic | | X | Frontal, temporal, maxilla |
| Maxilla | | X | Frontal, sphenoid, zygomatic, maxilla, ethmoid, palatine, vomer, nasal, lacrimal, inferior nasal concha |
| Ethmoid | X | | Frontal, sphenoid, maxilla, palatine, vomer, nasal, lacrimal, inferior nasal concha |
| Palatine | | X | Sphenoid, maxilla, ethmoid, palatine, vomer, inferior nasal concha |
| Vomer | X | | Sphenoid, maxilla, ethmoid, palatine |
| Nasal | | X | Frontal, maxilla, nasal |
| Lacrimal | | X | Frontal, maxilla, ethmoid, inferior nasal concha |
| Inferior nasal concha | | X | Maxilla, ethmoid, palatine, lacrimal |
| Mandible | X | | Temporal |

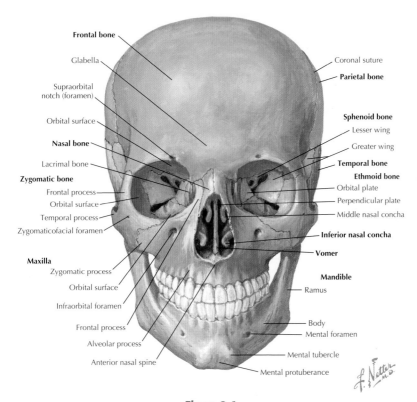

**Figure 2-1**

| Characteristics | Parts | Ossification | Comments |
|---|---|---|---|
| Contains the frontal paranasal sinuses<br><br>Has 2 primary centers that ossify along the frontal suture (metopic) in the 2nd year<br><br>Helps form the foramen cecum, which allows passage of an emissary vein that connects to the superior sagittal sinus<br><br>There is 1 frontal bone | Squamous portion | Intramembranous (for all 3 parts) | The largest part of the frontal bone<br>Forms the majority of the forehead<br>Forms the supraorbital margin and the superciliary arch<br>The zygomatic process of the frontal bone extends from the posterior part of the supraorbital margin<br>*Arachnoid foveae*—depressions caused by arachnoid granulations that push on the dura mater, causing bone resorption on the endocranial surface |
| | Orbital portion | | Forms the roof of the orbit and the floor of the anterior cranial fossa |
| | Nasal portion | | The trochlea of the orbit articulates with the orbital portion<br>Articulates with the nasal bones and the frontal process of the maxilla to form the root of the nose |

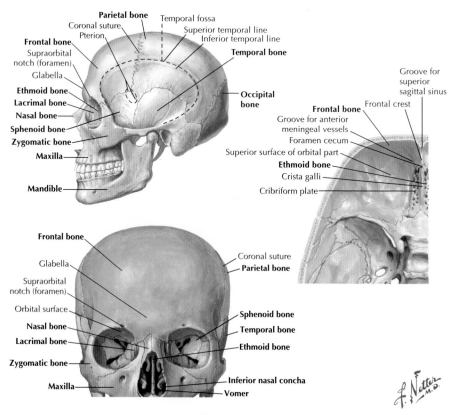

**Figure 2-2**

| Characteristics | Parts | Ossification | Comments |
|---|---|---|---|
| Forms the majority of the cranial vault<br>Provides for the attachment of the temporalis muscle<br>The 4 corners of the parietal are not ossified at birth and give rise to the fontanelles<br>There are 2 parietal bones | The 4 corners:<br>• Frontal–located at bregma<br>• Sphenoid–located at pterion<br>• Occipital–located at lambda<br>• Mastoid–located at asterion | Intramembranous | Relatively square, forming the roof and sides of the cranial vault<br>Endocranial surface is filled with grooves made by branches of the middle meningeal a.<br>Sigmoid sulcus is a groove caused by the beginning of the transverse sinus, located at the mastoid angle |

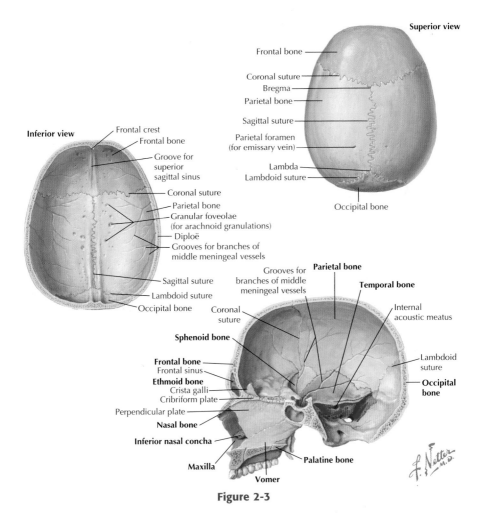

**Figure 2-3**

| Characteristics | Parts | Ossification | Comments |
|---|---|---|---|
| Forms the posterior part of the cranial vault<br><br>Articulates with the atlas<br><br>The squamous and lateral portions normally ossify together by year 4<br><br>The basilar portion unites to this section at year 6<br><br>There is 1 occipital bone | Squamous portion | Intramembranous | Articulates with the temporal and parietal bones<br><br>The largest portion of the occipital bone<br><br>Located posterior and superior to the foramen magnum<br><br>Has the external occipital protuberance (more pronounced in males)<br><br>Has the superior and the inferior nuchal lines<br><br>Has grooves on the internal surface for 3 of the sinuses forming the confluence of the sinuses (the superior sagittal and the right and left transverse sinuses)<br><br>The depression superior to the transverse sinus is for the occipital lobes of the brain<br><br>The depression inferior to the transverse sinus is for the cerebellum |
| | Lateral portion | Endochondral | Articulates with the temporal bone<br><br>Is the portion lateral to the foramen magnum<br><br>Has the occipital condyles that articulate with the atlas<br><br>Contains the hypoglossal canal<br><br>Forms a portion of the jugular foramen |
| | Basilar portion | Endochondral | Articulates with the petrous part of the temporal and the sphenoid bones<br><br>Is the portion immediately anterior to the foramen magnum<br><br>Pharyngeal tubercle is part of the basilar portion that provides attachment for the superior constrictor<br><br>Internal surface of the basilar portion is called the clivus, and part of the brainstem lies against it |

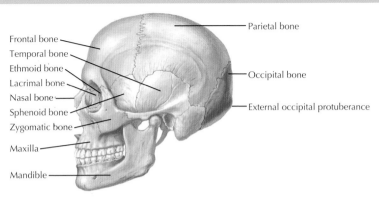

Frontal bone
Temporal bone
Ethmoid bone
Lacrimal bone
Nasal bone
Sphenoid bone
Zygomatic bone
Maxilla
Mandible

Parietal bone
Occipital bone
External occipital protuberance

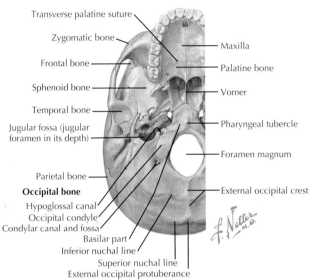

Transverse palatine suture
Zygomatic bone
Frontal bone
Sphenoid bone
Temporal bone
Jugular fossa (jugular foramen in its depth)
Parietal bone
**Occipital bone**
Hypoglossal canal
Occipital condyle
Condylar canal and fossa
Basilar part
Inferior nuchal line
Superior nuchal line
External occipital protuberance

Maxilla
Palatine bone
Vomer
Pharyngeal tubercle
Foramen magnum
External occipital crest

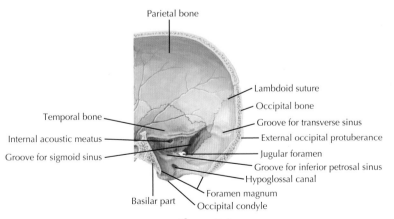

Parietal bone

Temporal bone
Internal acoustic meatus
Groove for sigmoid sinus

Basilar part

Lambdoid suture
Occipital bone
Groove for transverse sinus
External occipital protuberance
Jugular foramen
Groove for inferior petrosal sinus
Hypoglossal canal
Foramen magnum
Occipital condyle

**Figure 2-4**

| Characteristics | Parts | Ossification | Comments |
|---|---|---|---|
| The paired temporal bones:<br><br>  Help form the base and the lateral walls of the skull<br>  House the auditory and vestibular apparatuses<br>  Contain mastoid air cells<br><br>Each bone has 8 centers of ossification that give rise to the 3 major centers observed before birth<br><br>There are 2 temporal bones | Squamous part | Intramembranous<br>Endochondral | The largest portion of the bone<br>3 portions to the squamous part:<br>• Temporal<br>• Zygomatic process<br>• Glenoid fossa<br>*Temporal portion* is the thin large area on the squamous part of the temporal<br>On the internal surface of the temporal portion lies a groove for the middle meningeal a.<br>The *zygomatic process* extends laterally and anteriorly from the squamous portion; it articulates with the temporal process of the zygomatic bone to make the zygomatic arch<br>*Glenoid fossa* is inferior and medial to the zygomatic process; it articulates with the mandibular condyle, forming the temporomandibular joint |
| | Petrous part | | Forms the solid portion of bone<br>The auditory and vestibular apparatuses are located within the petrous part<br>Helps separate the temporal and the occipital lobes of the brain; it extends anteriorly and medially<br>The medial part articulates with the sphenoid bone to form the foramen lacerum<br>Internal acoustic meatus is observed on the medial side of the petrous part<br>Carotid canal lies on the inferior part of the petrous part<br>Petrotympanic fissure lies between the petrous part of the temporal bone and the tympanic part of the temporal bone<br>On the medial portion of the petrous part lie grooves for the superior and inferior petrosal sinuses<br>On the posterior inferior surface of the petrous part lies the jugular fossa<br>Between the jugular fossa and the carotid canal is the tympanic canaliculus<br>The mastoid process extends posteriorly and has large mastoid air cells |
| | Tympanic part | Intramembranous | A plate of bone forming the anterior, posterior, and inferior portions of the external acoustic meatus<br>Anterior part forms the posterior portion of the glenoid fossa |
| | Styloid process | Endochondral | A projection from the temporal bone<br>The stylomastoid foramen lies posterior to this process |

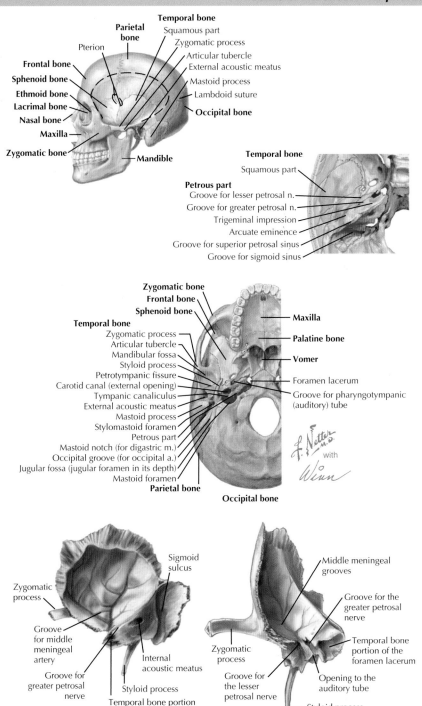

**Temporal bone**
Squamous part
Zygomatic process
Articular tubercle
External acoustic meatus
Mastoid process
Lambdoid suture

**Parietal bone**

Pterion

**Frontal bone**
**Sphenoid bone**
**Ethmoid bone**
**Lacrimal bone**
**Nasal bone**
**Maxilla**
**Zygomatic bone**

**Occipital bone**

**Mandible**

**Temporal bone**
Squamous part

**Petrous part**
Groove for lesser petrosal n.
Groove for greater petrosal n.
Trigeminal impression
Arcuate eminence
Groove for superior petrosal sinus
Groove for sigmoid sinus

**Zygomatic bone**
**Frontal bone**
**Sphenoid bone**
**Temporal bone**
Zygomatic process
Articular tubercle
Mandibular fossa
Styloid process
Petrotympanic fissure
Carotid canal (external opening)
Tympanic canaliculus
External acoustic meatus
Mastoid process
Stylomastoid foramen
Petrous part
Mastoid notch (for digastric m.)
Occipital groove (for occipital a.)
Jugular fossa (jugular foramen in its depth)
Mastoid foramen
**Parietal bone**

**Maxilla**
**Palatine bone**
**Vomer**
Foramen lacerum
Groove for pharyngotympanic (auditory) tube

*F. Netter M.D.*
with
*Winn*

**Occipital bone**

Sigmoid sulcus

Zygomatic process

Groove for middle meningeal artery

Groove for greater petrosal nerve

Internal acoustic meatus

Styloid process

Temporal bone portion of the foramen lacerum

Middle meningeal grooves

Groove for the greater petrosal nerve

Temporal bone portion of the foramen lacerum

Zygomatic process

Groove for the lesser petrosal nerve

Opening to the auditory tube

Styloid process

**Figure 2-5**

| Characteristics | Parts | Ossification | Comments |
|---|---|---|---|
| Forms the majority of the middle portion of the cranial base<br><br>Forms the majority of the middle cranial fossa<br><br>Contains the sphenoid paranasal sinus<br><br>There is 1 sphenoid bone | Body | Endochondral | The center of the sphenoid<br><br>Anterior portion of the body helps form part of the nasal cavity<br><br>Superior part of the body, known as the sella turcica, is saddle-shaped and possesses the anterior and posterior clinoid processes<br><br>Hypophyseal fossa, the deepest part of the sella turcica, houses the pituitary gland<br><br>Dorsum sellae is a square-shaped part of the bone that lies posterior to the sella turcica<br><br>Clivus is the portion that slopes posterior to the body<br><br>Body contains the sphenoid paranasal sinuses<br><br>Lateral portion of the body is covered by the cavernous sinus<br><br>Optic canal is found in the body of the sphenoid |
| | Greater wing | Endochondral and intramembranous | Extends laterally and anteriorly from the posterior portion of the body of the sphenoid<br><br>Endocranial portion helps form a large part of the middle cranial fossa<br><br>Lateral portion is the infratemporal surface<br><br>Anterior portion lies in the orbit<br><br>Contains 3 foramina:<br>• Foramen spinosum<br>• Foramen rotundum<br>• Foramen ovale |
| | Lesser wing | Endochondral | Extends laterally and anteriorly from the superior portion of the sphenoid body<br><br>Separated from the greater wing by the superior orbital fissure |
| | Pterygoid process | Intramembranous | Arises from the inferior surface of the body<br><br>There are 2 pterygoid processes<br><br>Each has a:<br>• Lateral pterygoid plate<br>• Medial pterygoid plate<br>Pterygoid hamulus extends from the medial pterygoid plate<br><br>2 canals are associated with the pterygoid process:<br>• Pterygoid canal<br>• Pharyngeal canal |

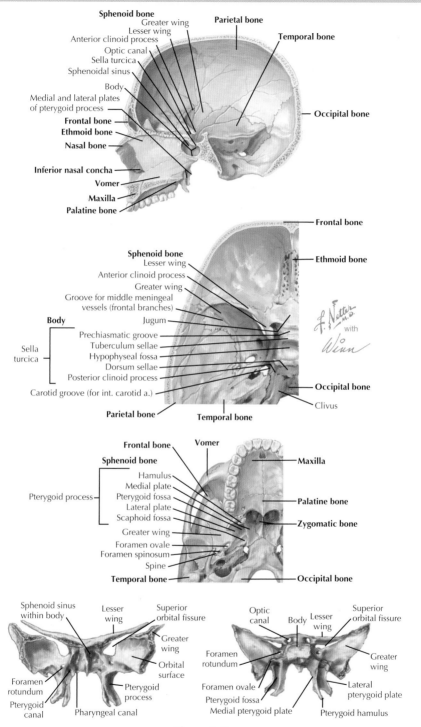

**Figure 2-6**

| Characteristics | Parts | Ossification | Comments |
|---|---|---|---|
| Lacrimal bone is small and rectangular in shape and very thin and fragile<br><br>There are 2 lacrimal bones | | Intramembranous | Forms a small portion of the medial wall of the orbit<br><br>Articulates with the frontal process of the maxilla, orbital plate of the ethmoid bone, the frontal bone, and the inferior nasal concha<br><br>The region that articulates with the frontal process of the maxilla forms the lacrimal fossa, the location of the lacrimal sac<br><br>The inferior part of the lacrimal forms a small portion of the lateral wall of the nasal cavity |

## Nasal Bone

| Characteristics | Parts | Ossification | Comments |
|---|---|---|---|
| Inferior portion forms the superior margin of the nasal aperture<br><br>Forms the bridge of the nose<br><br>There are 2 nasal bones | | Intramembranous | Articulates with the nasal bone of the opposite side, the nasal portion of the frontal bone, the frontal process of the maxilla, and the perpendicular plate of the ethmoid<br><br>Inferior portion of the nasal bones attaches with the lateral nasal cartilages and septal cartilage |

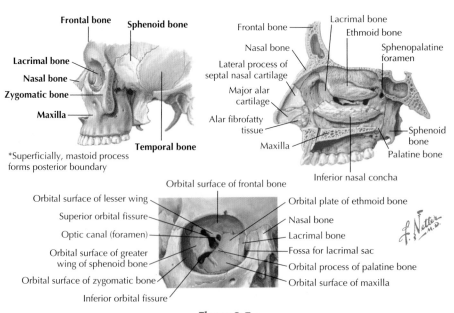

**Figure 2-7**

| Characteristics | Parts | Ossification | Comments |
|---|---|---|---|
| Forms the majority of the skeleton of the cheek | Frontal process | Intramembranous | Articulates with the frontal bone to help form the orbit |
| Provides for attachment of the masseter<br>3 foramina in the zygoma:<br>• Zygomatico-orbital foramen<br>• Zygomaticofacial foramen<br>• Zygomaticotemporal foramen<br>There are 2 zygomatic bones | Temporal process | | Articulates with the zygomatic process of the temporal bone to form the zygomatic arch |
| | Maxillary process | | Articulates with the zygomatic process of the maxillary bone to help form the orbit |

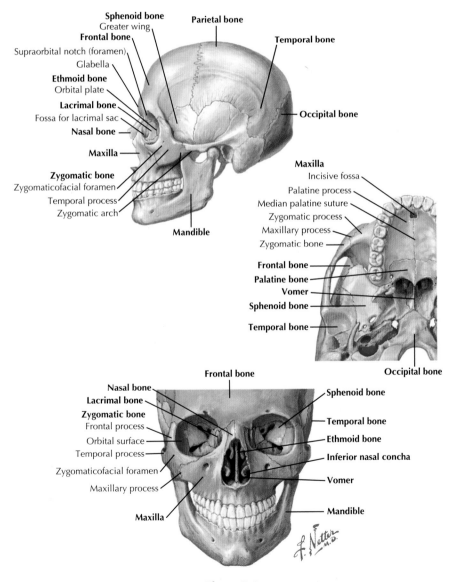

**Figure 2-8**

| Characteristics | Parts | Ossification | Comments |
|---|---|---|---|
| A porous bone that forms the major portion of the middle part of the face between the orbits<br><br>Helps form the orbit, nasal cavity, nasal septum, and anterior cranial fossa<br><br>There is 1 ethmoid bone | Perpendicular plate | Endochondral | A flat plate that descends from the cribriform plate to form part of the nasal septum<br><br>Articulates with the vomer inferiorly |
| | Cribriform plate | | A horizontal bone that forms the superior surface of the ethmoid<br><br>Contains numerous foramina for the olfactory n.<br><br>Crista galli is a vertical plate that extends superiorly from the cribriform plate, providing attachment for the falx cerebri of the meninges<br><br>Associated with a small foramen cecum |
| | Ethmoid labyrinth | | The largest part of the ethmoid bone<br><br>Descends inferiorly from the cribriform plate<br><br>Ethmoid paranasal sinuses are located within the ethmoid labyrinth<br><br>Ethmoid labyrinth forms 2 major structures within the nasal cavity:<br>• Superior nasal concha<br>• Middle nasal concha<br><br>Ethmoid bulla is the large elevation of bone located by the middle ethmoid paranasal sinuses<br><br>Uncinate process is a curved piece of bone<br><br>Between the uncinate process and the ethmoid bulla is the hiatus semilunaris |

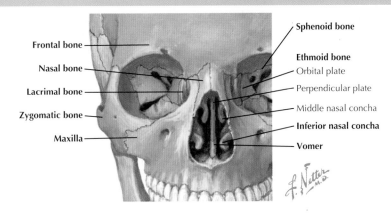

Frontal bone

Nasal bone

Lacrimal bone

Zygomatic bone

Maxilla

Sphenoid bone

**Ethmoid bone**
Orbital plate

Perpendicular plate

Middle nasal concha

**Inferior nasal concha**

**Vomer**

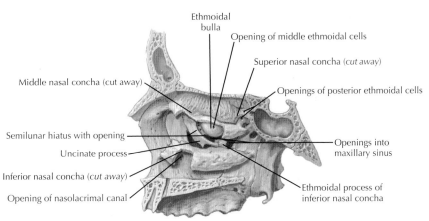

Ethmoidal bulla

Opening of middle ethmoidal cells

Superior nasal concha (*cut away*)

Middle nasal concha (cut away)

Openings of posterior ethmoidal cells

Semilunar hiatus with opening

Uncinate process

Inferior nasal concha (*cut away*)

Opening of nasolacrimal canal

Openings into maxillary sinus

Ethmoidal process of inferior nasal concha

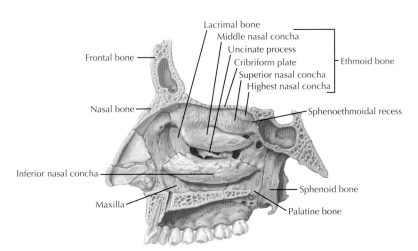

Lacrimal bone
Middle nasal concha
Uncinate process
Cribriform plate
Superior nasal concha
Highest nasal concha

Frontal bone

Ethmoid bone

Nasal bone

Sphenoethmoidal recess

Inferior nasal concha

Maxilla

Sphenoid bone

Palatine bone

**Figure 2-9**

| Characteristics | Parts | Ossification | Comments |
|---|---|---|---|
| Shaped like a plow<br>Forms the posterior inferior part of the nasal septum<br>There is 1 vomer bone | | Intramembranous | Articulates with the perpendicular plate of the ethmoid, maxilla, palatine, and sphenoid bones and septal cartilage<br>Posterior border does not articulate with any other bone |

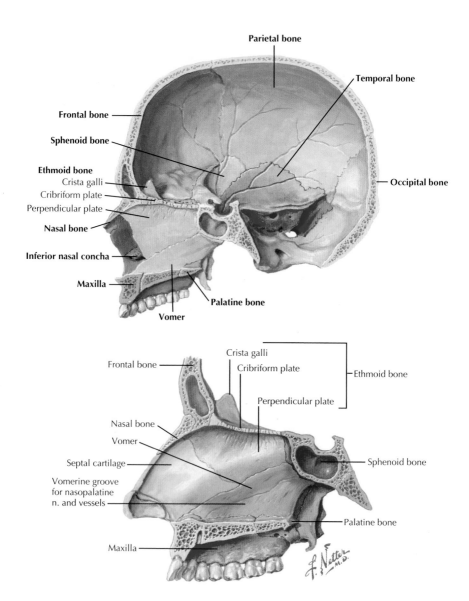

Figure 2-10

| Characteristics | Parts | Ossification | Comments |
|---|---|---|---|
| Is described as a curved bone that forms part of the lateral wall of the nasal cavity<br>There are 2 inferior nasal conchae | | Endochondral | Lies within a curve in the lateral wall of the nasal cavity<br>Articulates with the maxilla and perpendicular plate of the palatine, lacrimal, and ethmoid bones |

## Palatine Bone

| Characteristics | Parts | Ossification | Comments |
|---|---|---|---|
| Forms part of the nasal cavity and the hard palate<br>Is L-shaped<br>There are 2 palatine bones | Perpendicular plate | Intramembranous | Is in the shape of a vertical rectangle<br>On the superior border is a notch that articulates with the sphenoid bone, forming the sphenopalatine foramen<br>A small orbital process helps form part of the orbit<br>Forms part of the wall of the pterygopalatine fossa and the lateral wall of the nasal cavity<br>Lateral wall articulates with the maxilla to form the palatine canal |
| | Horizontal plate | | Forms the posterior portion of the hard palate<br>Superior to the horizontal plate is the nasal cavity<br>On the medial part, formed by both of the horizontal plates, is the posterior nasal spine<br>Greater palatine foramen is on this plate |
| | Pyramidal process | | Extends posteriorly and inferiorly from the junction of the perpendicular and horizontal plates of the palatine<br>Lesser palatine foramina are located here |

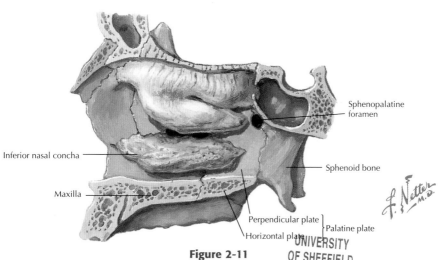

Sphenopalatine foramen

Inferior nasal concha

Sphenoid bone

Maxilla

Perpendicular plate ⎤
Horizontal plate ⎦ Palatine plate

**Figure 2-11**

| Characteristics | Parts | Ossification | Comments |
|---|---|---|---|
| Forms the majority of the skeleton of the face and the upper jaw<br>Contains the maxillary paranasal sinus<br>Articulates with the opposite maxilla and the frontal, sphenoid, nasal, vomer, and ethmoid bones; inferior nasal concha; palatine, lacrimal, and zygomatic bones; and the septal and nasal cartilages<br>There are 2 maxilla bones (maxillae) | Body | Intramembranous | Major part of the bone<br>Shaped like a pyramid<br>Contains the maxillary paranasal sinus<br>Gives rise to 4 different regions:<br>• Orbit<br>• Nasal cavity<br>• Infratemporal fossa<br>• Face<br>Infraorbital canal and foramen pass from the orbit region to the face region |
| | Frontal process | | Extends superiorly to articulate with the nasal, frontal, ethmoid, and lacrimal bones<br>Forms the posterior boundary of the lacrimal fossa |
| | Zygomatic process | | Extends laterally to articulate with the maxillary process of the zygomatic bone |
| | Palatine process | | Extends medially to form the majority of the hard palate<br>Articulates with the palatine process of the opposite side and the horizontal plate of the palatine bone<br>Incisive foramen is located in the anterior portion |
| | Alveolar process | | The part of the maxilla that supports all of the maxillary teeth<br>Extends inferiorly from the maxilla<br>Each maxilla contains 5 primary and 8 permanent teeth<br>Alveolar bone is resorbed when a tooth is lost |

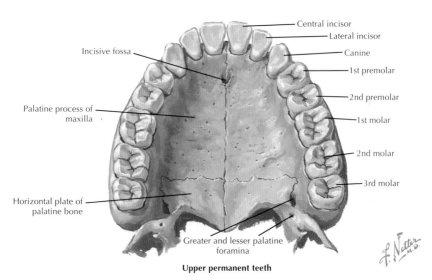

Central incisor
Lateral incisor
Canine
1st premolar
2nd premolar
1st molar
2nd molar
3rd molar
Incisive fossa
Palatine process of maxilla
Horizontal plate of palatine bone
Greater and lesser palatine foramina

**Upper permanent teeth**

**Figure 2-12**

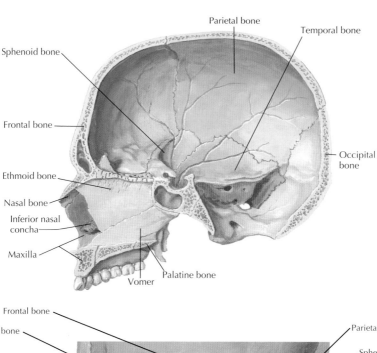

Parietal bone

Temporal bone

Sphenoid bone

Frontal bone

Occipital
bone

Ethmoid bone

Nasal bone

Inferior nasal
concha

Maxilla

Vomer

Palatine bone

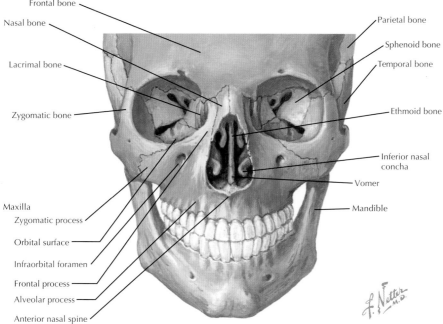

Frontal bone

Nasal bone

Lacrimal bone

Zygomatic bone

Maxilla
Zygomatic process

Orbital surface

Infraorbital foramen

Frontal process

Alveolar process

Anterior nasal spine

Parietal bone

Sphenoid bone

Temporal bone

Ethmoid bone

Inferior nasal
concha

Vomer

Mandible

**Figure 2-13**

| Characteristics | Parts | Ossification | Comments |
|---|---|---|---|
| Forms the lower jaw<br>Described as horseshoe-shaped<br>All muscles of mastication attach to the mandible<br>There is 1 mandible | Body | Intramembranous (ossifies around Meckel's cartilage) | Mental foramen lies on the anterior part of the lateral surface of the body<br>External oblique line is observed on the lateral side of the mandible<br>On the medial side of the body lies the mylohyoid line<br>Mylohyoid line helps divide a sublingual from a submandibular fossa<br>Posterior border of the mylohyoid line provides for attachment of the pterygomandibular raphe<br>At the midline on the medial side are the superior and inferior genial tubercles, as well as the digastric fossa<br>A small lingual foramen (or foramina) is located by the genial tubercles |
| | Ramus | | Meets the body of the mandible at the angle of the mandible on each side<br>Masseter m. attaches to the lateral side<br>Medial pterygoid m. and sphenomandibular lig. attach to the medial aspect<br>Mandibular foramen is located on the medial aspect of the ramus<br>Superior part divides into a coronoid process anteriorly and a condylar process posteriorly, separated by a mandibular notch |
| | Coronoid process | | The anteriormost superior extension of each ramus<br>Temporalis m. attaches to the coronoid process |
| | Condylar process | | Articulates with the temporal bone in the temporomandibular joint<br>Has a neck that forms a condyle superiorly<br>Lateral pterygoid muscle attaches to pterygoid fovea on the neck |
| | Alveolar process | | Extends superiorly from the body<br>Created by a thick buccal and a thin lingual plate of bone<br>The part of the mandible that supports the mandibular teeth<br>Each side of the mandible contains 5 primary and 8 permanent teeth<br>Alveolar bone is resorbed when a tooth is lost |

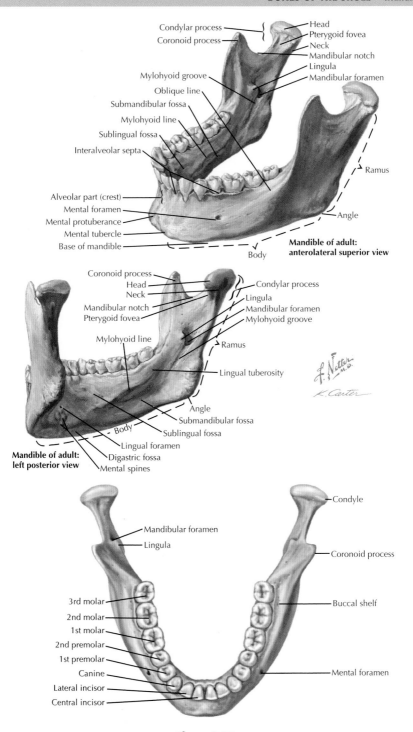

Condylar process
Coronoid process
Head
Pterygoid fovea
Neck
Mandibular notch
Lingula
Mandibular foramen
Mylohyoid groove
Oblique line
Submandibular fossa
Mylohyoid line
Sublingual fossa
Interalveolar septa
Ramus
Alveolar part (crest)
Mental foramen
Mental protuberance
Mental tubercle
Base of mandible
Angle
Body

**Mandible of adult: anterolateral superior view**

Coronoid process
Head
Neck
Mandibular notch
Pterygoid fovea
Condylar process
Lingula
Mandibular foramen
Mylohyoid groove
Mylohyoid line
Ramus
Lingual tuberosity
Angle
Submandibular fossa
Sublingual fossa
Body
Lingual foramen
Digastric fossa
Mental spines

**Mandible of adult: left posterior view**

Condyle
Mandibular foramen
Lingula
Coronoid process
3rd molar
2nd molar
1st molar
2nd premolar
1st premolar
Canine
Lateral incisor
Central incisor
Buccal shelf
Mental foramen

**Figure 2-14**

| Bones | Major Sutures |
|---|---|
| Frontal | Frontonasal |
| Nasal | Frontozygomatic |
| Maxilla | Zygomaticomaxillary |
| Zygomatic | Metopic |
| Mandible | |
| Vomer | |
| Ethmoid | |
| Sphenoid | |
| Palatine | |
| Lacrimal | |

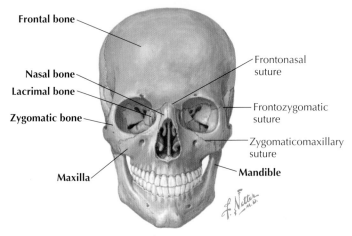

**Figure 2-15**

*Norma Occipitalis*

| Bones | Major Sutures |
|---|---|
| Parietal | Sagittal |
| Occipital | Lambdoid |
| Temporal | |

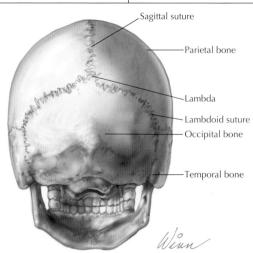

**Figure 2-16**

| Bones | Major Sutures |
|---|---|
| Frontal | Coronal |
| Parietal | Sagittal |
| Occipital | Lambdoid |

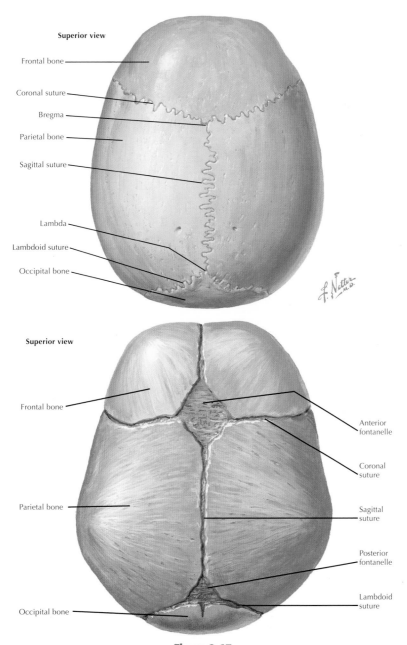

Figure 2-17

| Bones | Major Sutures |
|-------|---------------|
| Frontal | Coronal |
| Parietal | Squamosal |
| Temporal | Sphenofrontal |
| Zygomatic | Sphenoparietal |
| Maxilla | Lambdoid |
| Nasal | Occipitomastoid |
| Occipital | Temporozygomatic |
| Greater wing of the sphenoid | Frontozygomatic |
| Mandible | |

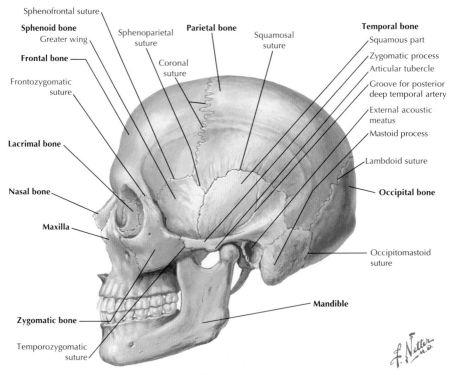

**Figure 2-18**

| Bones | Major Sutures |
|---|---|
| Maxilla (Palatine process) | Intermaxillary |
| Occipital | Transverse palatine |
| Temporal | Petro-occipital |
| Palatine (Horizontal plate) | Spheno-occipital |
| Vomer | Petrosquamous |
| Zygomatic | Petrotympanic |
| Sphenoid: | Squamotympanic |
|    Greater wing | |
|    Medial pterygoid plate | |
|    Lateral pterygoid plate | |

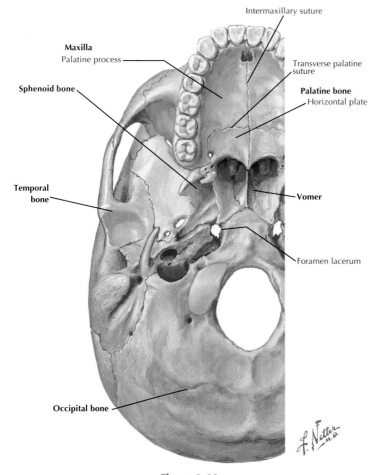

**Figure 2-19**

| Foramen/Fissure/Opening | Located in or Formed by | Vessels Passing Through | Nerves Passing Through |
|---|---|---|---|
| Supraorbital foramen | Frontal | Supraorbital a. & v. | Supraorbital n. |
| Optic canal | Sphenoid | Ophthalmic a. | Optic n. |
| Superior orbital fissure | Between the:<br>• Greater wing of the sphenoid and<br>• Lesser wing of the sphenoid | Superior ophthalmic v.<br>Inferior ophthalmic v. | Nasociliary, frontal, and lacrimal branches of the ophthalmic division of the trigeminal n.<br>Oculomotor n.<br>Trochlear n.<br>Abducens n. |
| Inferior orbital fissure | Between the:<br>• Greater wing of the sphenoid and<br>• Maxilla and orbital portion of the palatine bones | Infraorbital a. & v.<br>Inferior ophthalmic v. (portion communicating to pterygoid plexus) | Infraorbital n.<br>Zygomatic n. |
| Anterior ethmoid foramen | Between the:<br>• Frontal and<br>• Ethmoid | Anterior ethmoid a. & v. | Anterior ethmoid n. |
| Posterior ethmoid foramen | | Posterior ethmoid a. & v. | Posterior ethmoid n. |
| Zygomaticofacial foramen | Zygomatic | Zygomaticotemporal a. & v. | Zygomaticofacial n. |
| Infraorbital foramen | Maxilla | Infraorbital a. & v. | Infraorbital n. |
| Mental foramen | Mandible | Mental a. & v. | Mental n. |

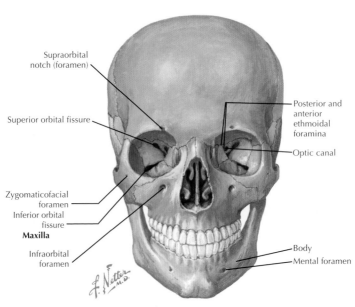

**Figure 2-20**

| Foramen/Fissure | Located in or Formed by | Vessels Passing Through | Nerves Passing Through |
|---|---|---|---|
| Mandibular foramen | Mandible | Inferior alveolar a. & v. | Inferior alveolar n. |
| Mental foramen | | Mental a. & v. | Mental n. |
| Lingual foramen | | Arterial branch from the anastomosis of the sublingual aa. | Branches of the mylohyoid n. have been observed to enter the foramen occasionally |

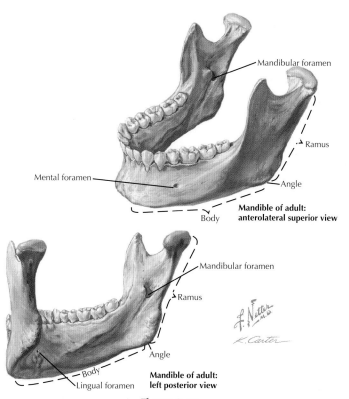

Mandibular foramen

Ramus

Mental foramen

Angle

**Mandible of adult:**
**anterolateral superior view**

Body

Mandibular foramen

Ramus

Angle

Body

Lingual foramen

**Mandible of adult:**
**left posterior view**

**Figure 2-21**

## Superior View of the Cranial Base

| Foramen/Fissure | Located in or Formed by | Vessels Passing Through | Nerves Passing Through |
|---|---|---|---|
| Cribriform plate foramina | Ethmoid | | Olfactory nn. from the olfactory bulb |
| Foramen cecum | Between the:<br>• Frontal and<br>• Ethmoid | Emissary v. from nasal cavity to the superior sagittal sinus | |
| Anterior ethmoid foramen | | Anterior ethmoid a. & v. | Anterior ethmoid n. |
| Posterior ethmoid foramen | | Posterior ethmoid a. & v. | Posterior ethmoid n. |

*Continued on next page*

| Foramen/Fissure | Located in or Formed by | Vessels Passing Through | Nerves Passing Through |
|---|---|---|---|
| Optic canal | Sphenoid | Ophthalmic a. | Optic n. |
| Superior orbital fissure | Between the:<br>• Greater wing of the sphenoid and<br>• Lesser wing of the sphenoid | Superior ophthalmic v.<br>Inferior ophthalmic v. | Nasociliary, frontal, and lacrimal branches of the ophthalmic division of the trigeminal n.<br>Oculomotor n.<br>Trochlear n.<br>Abducens n. |
| Foramen rotundum | Sphenoid | | Maxillary division of the trigeminal n. |
| Foramen ovale | | Accessory meningeal a.<br>Emissary v. | Mandibular division of the trigeminal n.<br>Lesser petrosal n. |
| Foramen spinosum | | Middle meningeal a. & v. | Meningeal branch of the mandibular division of the trigeminal n. |
| Sphenoid foramen | | Emissary v. | |
| Foramen lacerum | Articulation of the:<br>• Sphenoid (greater wing and body)<br>• Temporal (petrous portion)<br>• Occipital (basilar portion) bones | | *Nothing passes through it–but within the foramen, the greater petrosal n. joins the deep petrosal n.<br>Filled with fibrocartilage during life (although the anterior wall of the foramen has an opening for the pterygoid canal and the posterior wall has an opening for the carotid canal) |
| Carotid canal | Temporal (petrous portion) | Internal carotid a. | Internal carotid n. plexus (sympathetics) |
| Hiatus for the lesser petrosal n. | | | Lesser petrosal n. |
| Hiatus for the greater petrosal n. | | | Greater petrosal n. |
| Internal acoustic meatus | | Labyrinthine a. | Facial n.<br>Vestibulocochlear n., |
| Opening of the vestibular aqueduct | | *(No nerves or vessels–transmits the Endolymphatic duct) | |
| Mastoid foramen | Temporal (mastoid portion) | Mastoid emissary v<br>Posterior meningeal a. from the occipital a. | |
| Jugular foramen | Temporal (petrous portion) and occipital | Inferior petrosal sinus<br>Sigmoid sinus<br>Posterior meningeal a. | Glossopharyngeal n.<br>Vagus n.<br>Accessory n. |
| Condylar canal | Occipital | Emissary v.<br>Meningeal branch of ascending pharyngeal a. | |
| Hypoglossal canal | | | Hypoglossal n. |
| Foramen magnum | | Vertebral aa.<br>Venous plexus | Medulla oblongata<br>Accessory n. (Spinal roots) |

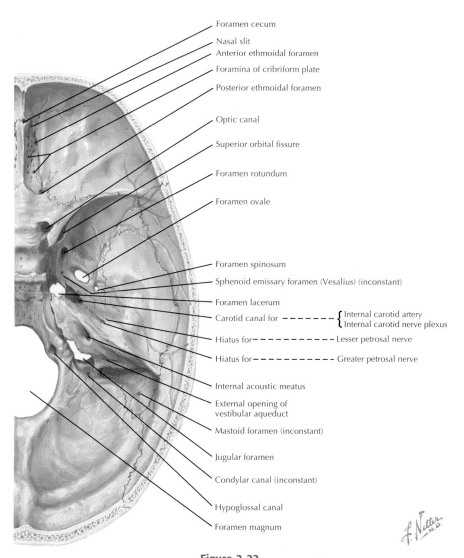

Foramen cecum

Nasal slit
Anterior ethmoidal foramen

Foramina of cribriform plate

Posterior ethmoidal foramen

Optic canal

Superior orbital fissure

Foramen rotundum

Foramen ovale

Foramen spinosum

Sphenoid emissary foramen (Vesalius) (inconstant)

Foramen lacerum

Carotid canal for ‒ ‒ ‒ ‒ ‒ ‒ ‒ { Internal carotid artery
                                         { Internal carotid nerve plexus

Hiatus for‒ ‒ ‒ ‒ ‒ ‒ ‒ ‒ ‒ ‒ Lesser petrosal nerve

Hiatus for‒ ‒ ‒ ‒ ‒ ‒ ‒ ‒ ‒ ‒ Greater petrosal nerve

Internal acoustic meatus

External opening of
vestibular aqueduct

Mastoid foramen (inconstant)

Jugular foramen

Condylar canal (inconstant)

Hypoglossal canal

Foramen magnum

**Figure 2-22**

| Foramen/Fissure | Located in or Formed by | Vessels Passing Through | Nerves Passing Through |
|---|---|---|---|
| Incisive foramen | Maxilla (palatine process) | Sphenopalatine a. & v. | Nasopalatine n. |
| Greater palatine foramen | Palatine | Greater palatine a. & v. | Greater palatine n. |
| Lesser palatine foramina | Palatine | Lesser palatine a. & v. | Lesser palatine n. |
| Foramen ovale | Sphenoid | Accessory meningeal a. Emissary v. | Mandibular division of the trigeminal n. Lesser petrosal n. |
| Foramen spinosum | Sphenoid | Middle meningeal a. & v. | Meningeal branch of the mandibular division of the trigeminal n. |
| Foramen lacerum | Articulation of the: <br>• Sphenoid (greater wing and body) <br>• Temporal (petrous portion) <br>• Occipital (basilar portion) bones | | *Nothing passes through it—but within the foramen, the greater petrosal n. joins the deep petrosal n. <br>Filled with fibrocartilage during life (although the anterior wall of the foramen has an opening for the pterygoid canal and the posterior wall has an opening for the carotid canal) |
| Opening for auditory tube | Temporal and sphenoid | *(No nerves or vessels—transmits the cartilaginous portion of the auditory tube) ||
| Carotid canal | Temporal (petrous portion) | Internal carotid a. | Internal carotid n. plexus (sympathetics) |
| Tympanic canaliculus | Temporal | | Tympanic branch of the glossopharyngeal n. |
| Jugular foramen | Temporal (petrous portion) and occipital | Inferior petrosal sinus Sigmoid sinus Posterior meningeal a. | Glossopharyngeal n. Vagus n. Accessory n. |
| Mastoid canaliculus | Temporal (within the jugular fossa) | | Auricular branch of the vagus n. |
| Petrotympanic fissure | Temporal | Anterior tympanic a. | Chorda tympani n. |
| Stylomastoid foramen | | Stylomastoid a. | Facial n. |
| Mastoid foramen | | Mastoid emissary v. Posterior meningeal a. from the occipital a. | |
| Hypoglossal canal | Occipital | | Hypoglossal n. |
| Condylar canal | | Emissary v. Meningeal branch of ascending pharyngeal a. | |
| Foramen magnum | | Vertebral aa. Venous plexus | Medulla oblongata Accessory n. (Spinal roots) |

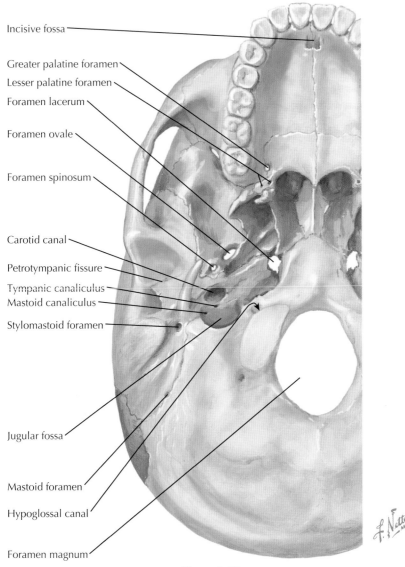

Incisive fossa

Greater palatine foramen
Lesser palatine foramen
Foramen lacerum

Foramen ovale

Foramen spinosum

Carotid canal

Petrotympanic fissure
Tympanic canaliculus
Mastoid canaliculus

Stylomastoid foramen

Jugular fossa

Mastoid foramen

Hypoglossal canal

Foramen magnum

**Figure 2-23**

- 7 cervical vertebrae (C1 to C7)
- The smallest vertebrae in the body
- The 1st, 2nd, and 7th cervical vertebrae are unique in their shape; the 3rd to the 6th are similarly shaped

| Vertebra | Characteristics |
|---|---|
| Atlas (C1) | Supports the skull<br>No body<br>No spinous process<br>Has an anterior arch and a posterior arch<br>Large lateral masses support the occipital condyles of the skull superiorly and articulate with the axis inferiorly<br>Foramen transversarium located in the large transverse process |
| Axis (C2) | Dens (odontoid process) located on the body's superior surface<br>Foramen transversarium located in the small transverse process<br>Spinous process is large and bifid |
| C3–C6 | Cervical vertebrae have small bodies<br>Pedicles project posteriorly and laterally<br>Spinous processes are short and bifid<br>Vertebral foramina are large and triangular<br>Each foramen transversarium is located in the transverse process<br>Vertebral a. enters the foramen transversarium at C6<br>Transverse processes each have an anterior and a posterior portion called the anterior tubercle and the posterior tubercle |
| C7 | Also called "vertebra prominens" because its long spinous process makes it visible under the skin<br>Long spinous process is not bifid<br>Foramen transversarium located in the large transverse process<br>Normally, the vertebral vessels do not pass through the foramen transversarium of C7 (the veins pass through more frequently than the arteries) |

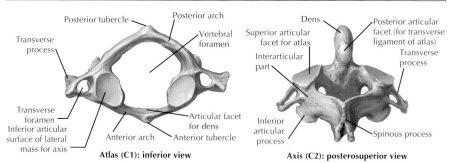

Atlas (C1): inferior view

Axis (C2): posterosuperior view

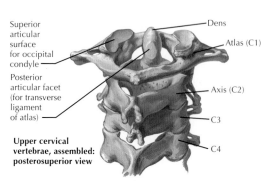

Upper cervical vertebrae, assembled: posterosuperior view

**Figure 2-24**

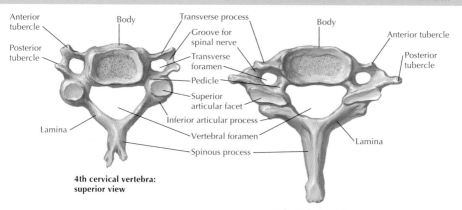

Anterior tubercle

Body

Transverse process

Groove for spinal nerve

Transverse foramen

Posterior tubercle

Pedicle

Superior articular facet

Inferior articular process

Lamina

Vertebral foramen

Spinous process

**4th cervical vertebra: superior view**

Body

Anterior tubercle

Posterior tubercle

Lamina

**7th cervical vertebra: superior view**

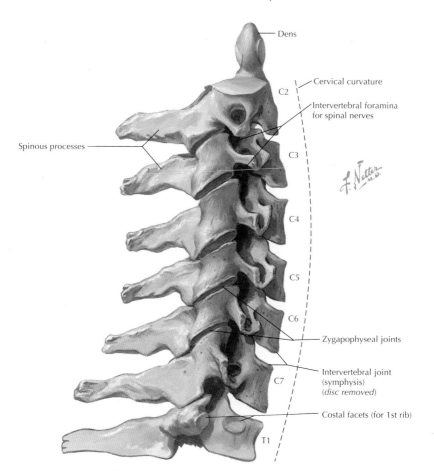

Dens

Cervical curvature

C2

Intervertebral foramina for spinal nerves

Spinous processes

C3

C4

C5

C6

Zygapophyseal joints

Intervertebral joint (symphysis) (*disc removed*)

C7

Costal facets (for 1st rib)

T1

**2nd cervical to 1st thoracic vertebrae: right lateral view**

**Figure 2-25**

| Ligament(s)/Membrane(s) | Comments |
|---|---|
| Anterior longitudinal ligament | Attached to the anterior surfaces of the vertebral bodies, extending from the axis to the sacrum<br>Superior to the axis, it is continuous with the anterior atlantoaxial lig. |
| Ligamenta flava | Attached to the anterior surfaces of the lamina within the vertebral foramen, extending from the axis to the 1st sacral vertebra |
| Ligamentum nuchae | Extends from the external occipital protuberance and median nuchal line to the spinous process of C7<br>Between these attachments, it attaches to the posterior tubercle of the atlas and the spinous processes of the axis and C3–C6 |
| Anterior atlanto-occipital membrane | Extends from the anterior margin of the foramen magnum superiorly and the anterior arch of the atlas inferiorly<br>Continuous with the capsule of the atlanto-occipital joint laterally |
| Posterior atlanto-occipital membrane | Extends from the posterior margin of the foramen magnum superiorly to the posterior arch of the atlas inferiorly<br>Allows passage of the vertebral a. on the lateral margin |

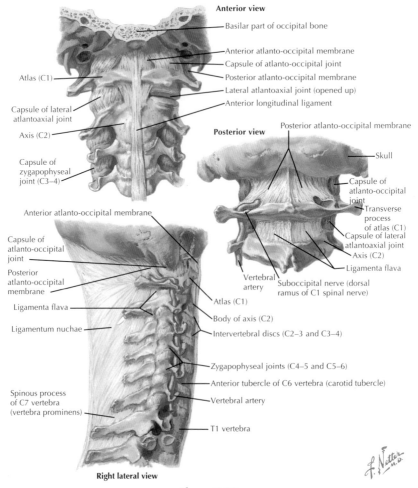

**Figure 2-26**

| Ligament(s)/Membrane(s) | Comments |
|---|---|
| **DEEP LIGAMENTS/MEMBRANES** | |
| Alar ligament | Extends from the dens to the medial portions of the occipital condyles<br>Also known as "check ligaments" because they limit skull rotation |
| Apical ligament of the dens | Extends from the dens to the anterior margin of the foramen magnum |
| Cruciate ligament | |
| *Superior longitudinal band* | Part of the transverse lig. of the atlas, which extends superiorly to attach to the basilar portion of the occipital bone |
| *Transverse ligament of atlas* | Thick ligament extending from one side of the internal surface of the anterior arch of the atlas to the other side, holding the dens in contact with the anterior arch |
| *Inferior longitudinal band* | Part of the transverse lig. of the atlas that extends inferiorly, attaching to the posterior body of the axis |
| **SUPERFICIAL LIGAMENTS/MEMBRANES** | |
| Tectorial membrane | Extends from the basilar portion of the occipital bone, where it blends with the dura mater, to the posterior portion of the body of the axis<br>Continuous inferiorly with the posterior longitudinal lig. |
| Posterior longitudinal ligament | Attached to the posterior surfaces of the bodies of the vertebrae extending within the vertebral foramen from the axis to the sacrum<br>Superior to the axis, it is continuous with the tectorial membrane |

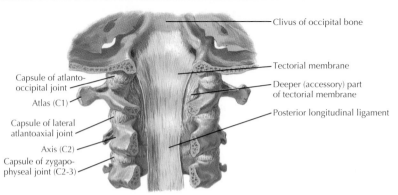

Clivus of occipital bone

Tectorial membrane

Deeper (accessory) part of tectorial membrane

Posterior longitudinal ligament

Capsule of atlanto-occipital joint

Atlas (C1)

Capsule of lateral atlantoaxial joint

Axis (C2)

Capsule of zygapo-physeal joint (C2-3)

**Upper part of vertebral canal with spinous processes and parts of vertebral arches removed to expose ligaments of posterior vertebral bodies: posterior view**

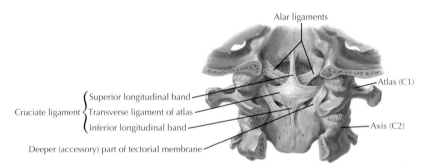

Alar ligaments

Atlas (C1)

Superior longitudinal band

Cruciate ligament {  Transverse ligament of atlas

Inferior longitudinal band

Axis (C2)

Deeper (accessory) part of tectorial membrane

**Principal part of tectorial membrane removed to expose deeper ligaments: posterior view**

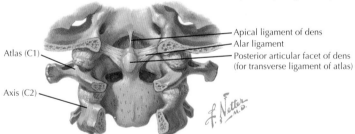

Apical ligament of dens

Alar ligament

Posterior articular facet of dens (for transverse ligament of atlas)

Atlas (C1)

Axis (C2)

**Cruciate ligament removed to show deepest ligaments: posterior view**

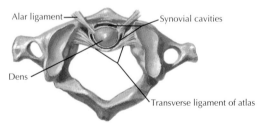

Alar ligament

Synovial cavities

Dens

Transverse ligament of atlas

**Median atlantoaxial joint: superior view**

**Figure 2-27**

- Zygoma is the 2nd most commonly fractured bone of the face after the nasal bone
- Susceptible to fracture, usually due to a facial blow from a fist or trauma incurred in a motor vehicle crash
- In fractures due to blows from a fist, the left zygomatic bone is more frequently fractured than the right
- Most fractures are unilateral
- May displace the zygomatic bone along the sutures, or more severe displacement in a posterior, medial, or inferior direction may occur
- Common clinical manifestations include:
  - Pain
  - Swelling
  - Diplopia
  - Paresthesia
  - Depressed cheek

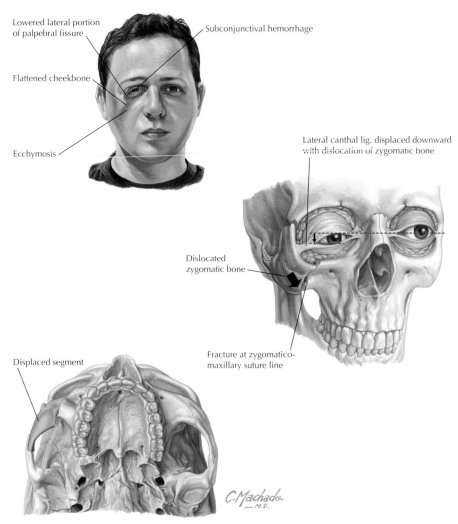

Lowered lateral portion of palpebral fissure

Subconjunctival hemorrhage

Flattened cheekbone

Ecchymosis

Lateral canthal lig. displaced downward with dislocation of zygomatic bone

Dislocated zygomatic bone

Fracture at zygomatico-maxillary suture line

Displaced segment

C.Machado
—M.D.

**Figure 2-28**

- Trauma to the midface usually follows 1 of 3 patterns of fracture:
  - Le Fort I
  - Le Fort II
  - Le Fort III

## LE FORT I

- Horizontal, extending from the lateral margin of the piriform aperture to the pterygoid plates just superior to the apices of the teeth
- Gives rise to a detached upper jaw relative to the rest of the maxillofacial skeleton

## LE FORT II

- Pyramidal in outline, extending from the bridge of the nose at or inferior to the nasofrontal suture or maxilla, then inferiorly and laterally through the inferior orbital floor near the infraorbital foramen, through the anterior wall of the maxillary sinus, to the pterygoid plates

## LE FORT III

- Transverse, extending from the nasofrontal suture and frontomaxillary suture and passing posteriorly along the medial wall of the orbit through the nasolacrimal groove and ethmoid, then following the inferior orbital fissure to the lateral wall of the orbit, and extending through the frontozygomatic suture
- Within the nose, the fracture extends along the perpendicular plate, vomer, and pterygoid plates
- In a Le Fort III fracture, the facial skeleton is detached from the base of the skull

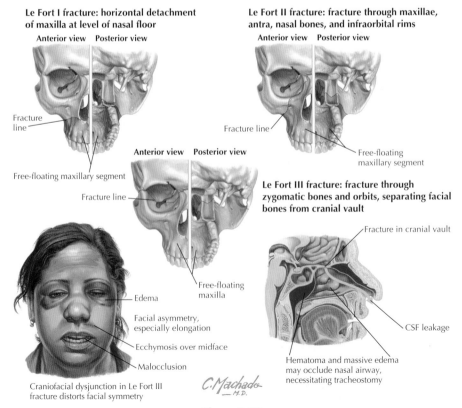

Le Fort I fracture: horizontal detachment of maxilla at level of nasal floor

Anterior view   Posterior view

Fracture line

Free-floating maxillary segment

Le Fort II fracture: fracture through maxillae, antra, nasal bones, and infraorbital rims

Anterior view   Posterior view

Fracture line

Free-floating maxillary segment

Anterior view   Posterior view

Fracture line

Free-floating maxilla

Le Fort III fracture: fracture through zygomatic bones and orbits, separating facial bones from cranial vault

Fracture in cranial vault

CSF leakage

Hematoma and massive edema may occlude nasal airway, necessitating tracheostomy

Edema

Facial asymmetry, especially elongation

Ecchymosis over midface

Malocclusion

Craniofacial dysjunction in Le Fort III fracture distorts facial symmetry

C. Machado — M.D.

**Figure 2-29**

- Mandible is a frequently fractured bone
- Fractures result from blow from a fist or trauma incurred in motor vehicle crash
- Common sites (in decreasing order of frequency):
  - Condyle
  - Angle
  - Body
  - Symphysis
  - Ramus
  - Alveolus
  - Coronoid process
- With double mandibular fractures, the 2nd usually is contralateral

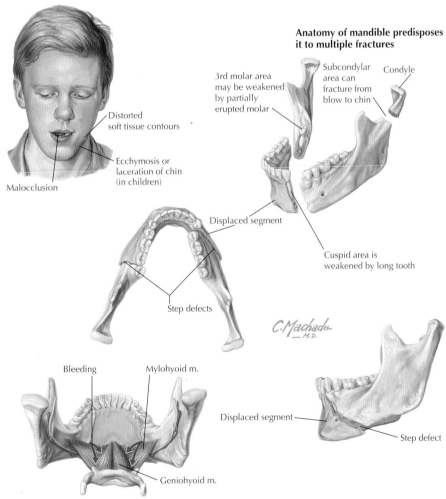

**Anatomy of mandible predisposes it to multiple fractures**

Subcondylar area can fracture from blow to chin

Condyle

3rd molar area may be weakened by partially erupted molar

Distorted soft tissue contours

Ecchymosis or laceration of chin (in children)

Malocclusion

Displaced segment

Cuspid area is weakened by long tooth

Step defects

C. Machado
—M.D.

Bleeding    Mylohyoid m.

Displaced segment

Step defect

Geniohyoid m.

Bleeding caused by fracture is trapped by fanlike attachment of mylohyoid musculature to mandible, and presents clinically as ecchymosis in floor of mouth

**Figure 2-30**

- 2 common types of cervical fractures:
  - Jefferson fracture (at C1)
  - Hangman's fracture (at C2)

### JEFFERSON FRACTURE

- Involves the atlas
- Results from skull compression due to axial loading, causing the atlas to burst
- Most patients are neurologically intact but have severe neck pain
- Vertebral artery can be compromised
- Classified as stable or unstable according to whether the transverse ligament of the atlas is intact:
  - *Stable fractures* can be treated with an orthosis such as a soft collar
  - *Unstable fractures* are more problematic; may require cranial traction applied with use of a halo, as well as cervical fusion

### HANGMAN'S FRACTURE

- Occurs through the vertebral arch of the axis between the superior and the inferior articulating facets
- A traumatic spondylolisthesis often is caused by extension of the neck with axial compression, common in car accidents
- The historical hangman's fracture is caused by extension and distraction of the neck

### ODONTOID FRACTURE

- Involves the axis
- Classification into 3 types:
  - Type I–fracture at the tip of the odontoid process
  - Type II–fracture along the base or the neck of the odontoid
  - Type III–fracture that passes through the body of the axis

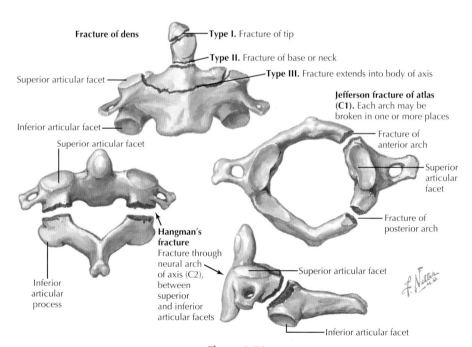

**Fracture of dens**

**Type I.** Fracture of tip

**Type II.** Fracture of base or neck

**Type III.** Fracture extends into body of axis

Superior articular facet

Inferior articular facet

Superior articular facet

**Jefferson fracture of atlas (C1).** Each arch may be broken in one or more places

Fracture of anterior arch

Superior articular facet

Fracture of posterior arch

**Hangman's fracture** Fracture through neural arch of axis (C2), between superior and inferior articular facets

Superior articular facet

Inferior articular process

Inferior articular facet

**Figure 2-31**

# CHAPTER 3

# BASIC NEUROANATOMY AND CRANIAL NERVES

- Nervous tissue is divided into 2 major cell types:
  - Neurons
  - Neuroglial cells (the neuroglia)

## NEURONS

- The structural and functional cells in the nervous system
- Respond to a nervous stimulus and conduct the stimulus along the length of the cell
- A neuron's cell body is called the perikaryon, or soma
- Cell bodies are classified by their location:
  - Ganglion: a collection of nerve cell bodies located in the peripheral nervous system (e.g., dorsal root ganglion, trigeminal ganglion, ciliary ganglion)
  - Nucleus: a collection of nerve cell bodies located in the central nervous system (e.g., Edinger-Westphal nucleus, chief sensory nucleus of cranial nerve [CN] V, motor nucleus of CN VII)
- Neuron's cell bodies contain typical cellular organelles within their cytoplasm:
  - Mitochondria
  - Nucleus
  - Nucleolus
  - Ribosomes
  - Rough endoplasmic reticulum (Nissl substance)
  - Neurotubules
  - Golgi apparatus
  - Lysosomes
- Neurons have 2 types of processes that extend from the nerve cell body:
  - Dendrite: process that carries nerve impulses toward the nerve cell body; neurons may have multiple dendrites
  - Axon: process that carries nerve impulses away from the nerve cell body; neurons can have *only 1* axon
- 3 major types of neurons:
  - Unipolar: has only 1 process from the cell body (sensory neurons)
  - Bipolar: has 2 processes from the cell body: 1 dendrite and 1 axon (sensory neurons; located only in the retina, olfactory epithelium, and the vestibular and cochlear ganglia)
  - Multipolar: has 3 or more processes from the cell body: 2 or more dendrites and 1 axon (motor neurons and interneurons)

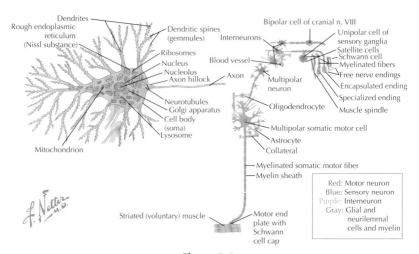

**Figure 3-1**

- Neuroglia is the supporting nervous tissue for neurons, although neuroglial cells also have assistive roles in neuron function
- Neuroglial cells have only 1 type of process
- Classification:
    - Astrocytes: located in the central nervous system; help keep neurons in place, provide nutritional support, regulate the extracellular matrix, form part of the blood-brain barrier
    - Oligodendrocytes: located in the central nervous system; responsible for axon myelination in the central nervous system; 1 oligodendrocyte can myelinate 1 segment of multiple axons
    - Microglial cells: located in the central nervous system; responsible for phagocytosis to remove waste
    - Schwann cells: located in the peripheral nervous system; responsible for axon myelination in the peripheral nervous system; 1 Schwann cell can myelinate 1 segment of 1 axon
    - Satellite cells: located in the peripheral nervous system; surround the nerve cell bodies of ganglia

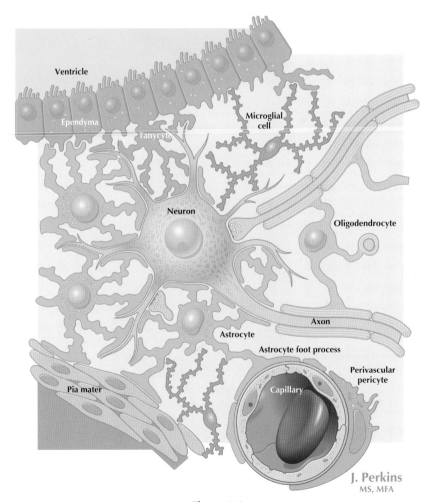

Figure 3-2

- The central nervous system is composed of the:
  - Brain
  - Spinal cord

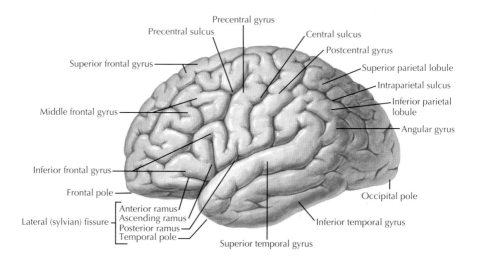

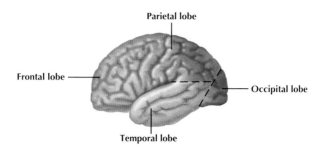

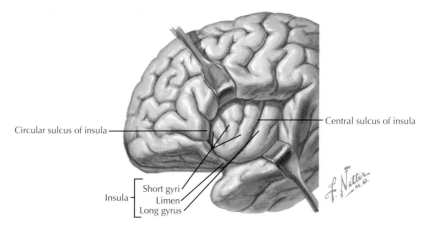

**Figure 3-3**

## CEREBRUM

- The surface of the cerebral cortex of the brain is divided by:
  - Gyri (singular *gyrus*): the elevations of brain tissue on the surface
  - Sulci (singular *sulcus*): the grooves or fissures located between the gyri
- There are 3 large sulci that help divide the cerebral hemispheres into 4 of its lobes:
  - Central sulcus (of Rolando): divides frontal lobe from parietal lobe
  - Lateral sulcus (of Sylvius): divides the frontal and parietal lobes from the temporal lobe
  - Parieto-occipital sulcus: divides the parietal lobe from the occipital lobe
- The brain is divided into 5 lobes:
  - Frontal: motor movement, motor aspect of speech (Broca's area), reasoning, emotions, personality, and problem solving
  - Parietal: sensory perceptions related to pain, temperature, touch and pressure, spatial orientation and perception, sensory aspect of language (Wernicke's area)
  - Temporal: auditory perceptions, learning, and memory
  - Occipital: vision
  - Insula: associated with visceral functions including taste

## DIENCEPHALON

- Composed of 4 parts:
  - Thalamus: major relay center of the somatosensory system and parts of the motor system
  - Hypothalamus: controls the autonomic nervous system and endocrine system
  - Epithalamus: major structures include the pineal gland (circadian rhythms) and the habenula
  - Subthalamus: an extrapyramidal nucleus of the motor system; lesions of this nucleus will result in a contralateral hemiballismus

## BRAINSTEM

- Composed of 3 parts:
  - Midbrain
  - Pons
  - Medulla

## CEREBELLUM

- Part of the motor system
- Receives sensory input of all forms that use the deep cerebellar nuclei
- Associated with:
  - Equilibrium
  - Posture
  - Tone of axial muscles
  - Gait

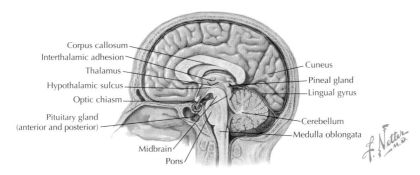

Corpus callosum
Interthalamic adhesion
Thalamus
Hypothalamic sulcus
Optic chiasm
Pituitary gland (anterior and posterior)
Midbrain
Pons
Cuneus
Pineal gland
Lingual gyrus
Cerebellum
Medulla oblongata

**Figure 3-4**

- The caudal continuation of the central nervous system
- Begins at the caudal end of the medulla and ends at vertebral level L1–2, tapering into the conus medullaris
- Has 2 enlargements associated with the limbs:
  - Cervical—associated with the upper limb and found between the spinal cord at levels C4 to T1
  - Lumbosacral—associated with the lower limb and found between the spinal cord at levels L1 to S2
- Composed of:
  - Gray matter—location of nerve cell bodies and neuroglial cells
  - White matter—location of the axons and neuroglial cells
- Has 5 levels:
  - Cervical—8 spinal nerves
  - Thoracic—12 spinal nerves
  - Lumbar—5 spinal nerves
  - Sacral—5 spinal nerves
  - Coccygeal—1 spinal nerve

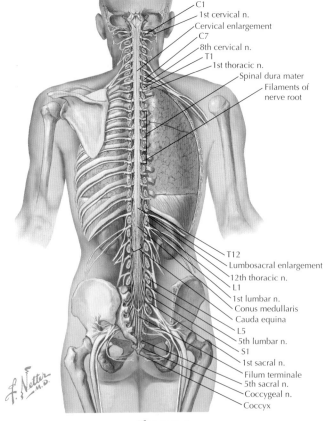

**Figure 3-5**

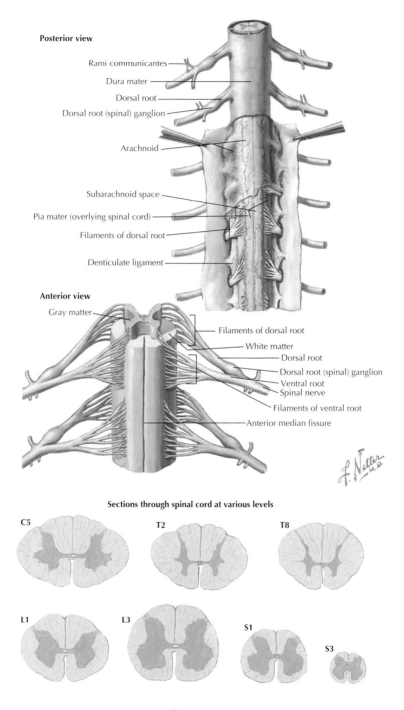

**Posterior view**

Rami communicantes

Dura mater

Dorsal root

Dorsal root (spinal) ganglion

Arachnoid

Subarachnoid space

Pia mater (overlying spinal cord)

Filaments of dorsal root

Denticulate ligament

**Anterior view**

Gray matter

Filaments of dorsal root

White matter

Dorsal root

Dorsal root (spinal) ganglion

Ventral root

Spinal nerve

Filaments of ventral root

Anterior median fissure

**Sections through spinal cord at various levels**

C5    T2    T8

L1    L3    S1    S3

**Figure 3-6**

- Peripheral nervous system is the portion of the nervous system located external to the central nervous system
- Consists of:
  - Cranial nerves—12 pairs
  - Spinal nerves—31 pairs
- Can be subdivided into:
  - Somatic nervous system—voluntary system associated with afferent (sensory) and efferent (motor) fibers
  - Autonomic nervous system—involuntary system associated with homeostasis of the body

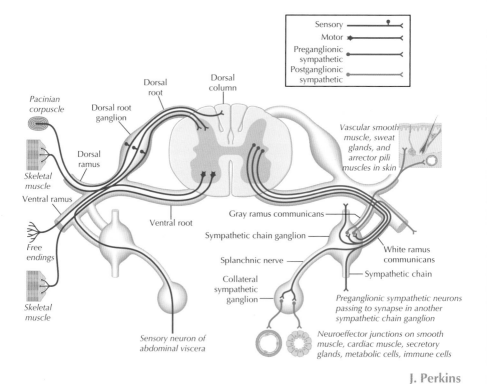

Figure 3-7

J. Perkins
MS, MFA

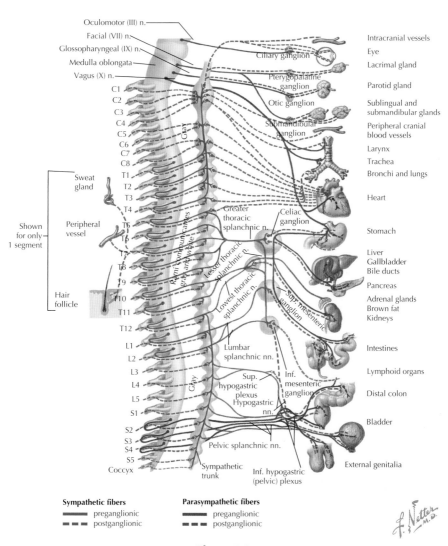

**Figure 3-8**

- Cranial nerves or cerebral nerves are peripheral nerves that leave the brain or brainstem
- The cranial nerves customarily are subdivided into 12 pairs:

  I: Olfactory nerve      VII: Facial nerve
  II: Optic nerve      VIII: Vestibulocochlear nerve
  III: Oculomotor nerve      IX: Glossopharyngeal nerve
  IV: Trochlear nerve      X: Vagus nerve
  V: Trigeminal nerve      XI: Accessory nerve
  VI: Abducens nerve      XII: Hypoglossal nerve

- Because of the high degree of differentiation in the brain of humans, cranial nerves are more complex in structure and function than spinal nerves

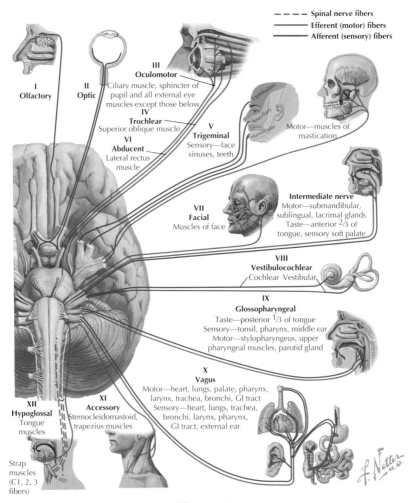

Figure 3-9

- 7 functional components (or functional columns) of the cranial nerves are recognized
  - Concept of functional columns comes from studies of spinal nerves—functions associated with different neurologic pathways along spinal column are assigned corresponding "columns"
- A given cranial nerve may have 1 to 5 functional columns
- The functional columns are classified as *general* or *special*:
  - General—these functional columns have the same functions as those for spinal nerves
  - Special—these functional columns are specific only to cranial nerves
- General and special functional columns each are subdivided into 2 additional categories:
  - *Afferent* (sensory) and *efferent* (motor)
  - *Somatic* (body-related) and *visceral* (organ-related)

## SUMMARY OF FUNCTIONS*

**GSA**: Exteroceptors and proprioceptors (e.g., for pain, touch, and temperature, or within tendons and joints). These are the same as in spinal nerves.

**SSA**: Special senses in eye and ear (vision; hearing and equilibrium)

**GVA**: Sensory from viscera (e.g., gut). These are the same as in spinal nerves.

**SVA**: Olfaction and taste

**GVE**: Autonomic nervous system (innervates cardiac muscle, smooth muscle, and glands). These are the same as in spinal nerves.

**GSE**: Skeletal (somatic) muscle. These are the same as in spinal nerves.

**SVE**: Skeletal muscle, which develops from the pharyngeal (branchial) arches (homologous to GSE)

*Within each designation: G or S, general or special; S or V, somatic or visceral; A or E, afferent or efferent.*

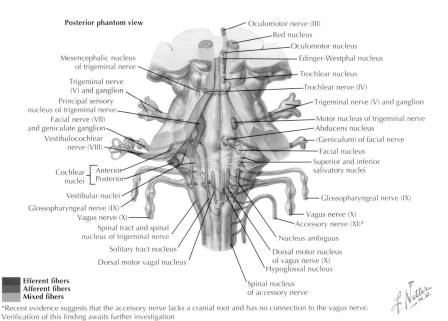

Posterior phantom view

Oculomotor nerve (III)
Red nucleus
Oculomotor nucleus
Edinger-Westphal nucleus
Mesencephalic nucleus of trigeminal nerve
Trochlear nucleus
Trigeminal nerve (V) and ganglion
Trochlear nerve (IV)
Principal sensory nucleus of trigeminal nerve
Trigeminal nerve (V) and ganglion
Facial nerve (VII) and geniculate ganglion
Motor nucleus of trigeminal nerve
Abducens nucleus
Vestibulocochlear nerve (VIII)
(Geniculum) of facial nerve
Facial nucleus
Superior and inferior salivatory nuclei
Cochlear nuclei — Anterior / Posterior
Vestibular nuclei
Glossopharyngeal nerve (IX)
Glossopharyngeal nerve (IX)
Vagus nerve (X)
Vagus nerve (X)
Accessory nerve (XI)*
Spinal tract and spinal nucleus of trigeminal nerve
Nucleus ambiguus
Solitary tract nucleus
Dorsal motor nucleus of vagus nerve (X)
Dorsal motor vagal nucleus
Hypoglossal nucleus
Spinal nucleus of accessory nerve

Efferent fibers
Afferent fibers
Mixed fibers

*Recent evidence suggests that the accessory nerve lacks a cranial root and has no connection to the vagus nerve. Verification of this finding awaits further investigation

**Figure 3-10**

| Functional Column | Origin of Fibers | Termination of Fibers | Summary | Comment |
|---|---|---|---|---|
| SVA | Fibers originate in the neurosensory cells of the olfactory epithelium<br><br>The primary fibers (which are bipolar neurons) travel through the cribriform plate to synapse on the secondary fibers within the olfactory bulb<br><br>These fibers continue posteriorly as the olfactory tract that carries the fibers to the olfactory areas | The secondary fibers continue to synapse in the olfactory areas:<br>• Lateral olfactory area<br>• Anterior olfactory nucleus<br>• Intermediate olfactory area<br>• Medial olfactory area<br>• Amygdala<br>• Entorhinal cortex<br>• Piriform cortex | The SVA fibers are responsible for the sense of smell | Tumors of the olfactory lobe can affect the olfactory system<br><br>Trauma to the head can cause a shearing of the primary fibers as they pass through the cribriform plate |

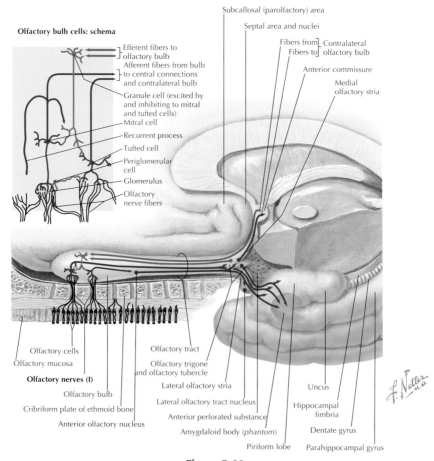

**Figure 3-11**

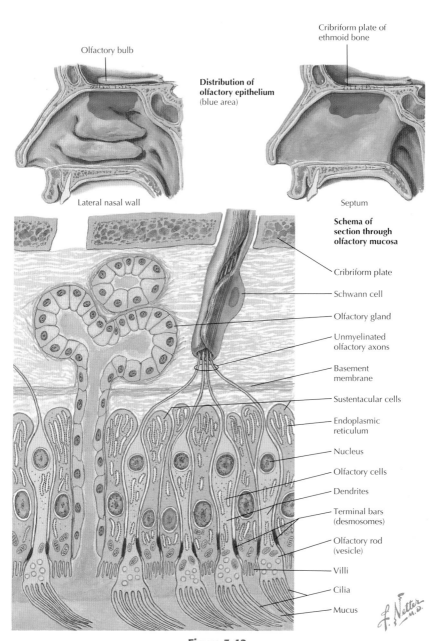

Olfactory bulb

**Distribution of olfactory epithelium** (blue area)

Cribriform plate of ethmoid bone

Lateral nasal wall

Septum

**Schema of section through olfactory mucosa**

Cribriform plate

Schwann cell

Olfactory gland

Unmyelinated olfactory axons

Basement membrane

Sustentacular cells

Endoplasmic reticulum

Nucleus

Olfactory cells

Dendrites

Terminal bars (desmosomes)

Olfactory rod (vesicle)

Villi

Cilia

Mucus

**Figure 3-12**

| Functional Column | Origin of Fibers | Termination of Fibers | Summary | Comment |
|---|---|---|---|---|
| SSA | Begins in the retina with the receptors of rods and cones that synapse on bipolar cells, which synapse with ganglion cells | Ganglionic axons form the optic nerve that meets in an incomplete crossing at the optic chiasm where:<br>• Nasal retinal fibers decussate to the opposite side<br>• Temporal retinal fibers remain on the ipsilateral side<br>These form an optic tract that terminates on the lateral geniculate nucleus<br>Fibers from the lateral geniculate travel to synapse in the occipital lobe | The SSA fibers are responsible for vision | Lesions of the optic nerve lead to blindness<br>Lesions of the optic chiasm lead to bitemporal hemianopsia<br>Lesions of the optic tract lead to homonymous hemianopsia |

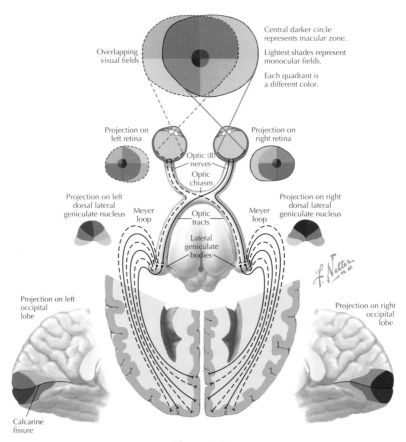

Overlapping visual fields

Central darker circle represents macular zone.

Lightest shades represent monocular fields.

Each quadrant is a different color.

Projection on left retina

Projection on right retina

Optic (II) nerves

Optic chiasm

Projection on left dorsal lateral geniculate nucleus

Meyer loop

Optic tracts

Meyer loop

Projection on right dorsal lateral geniculate nucleus

Lateral geniculate bodies

Projection on left occipital lobe

Projection on right occipital lobe

Calcarine fissure

**Figure 3-13**

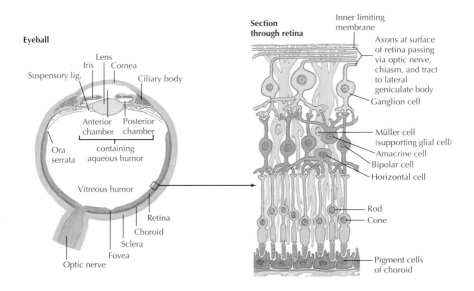

**Eyeball**

Lens
Iris   Cornea
Suspensory lig.
Ciliary body

Anterior   Posterior
chamber   chamber

Ora
serrata   containing
aqueous humor

Vitreous humor

Retina
Choroid
Sclera
Fovea
Optic nerve

**Section through retina**

Inner limiting membrane
Axons at surface of retina passing via optic nerve, chiasm, and tract to lateral geniculate body
Ganglion cell

Müller cell (supporting glial cell)
Amacrine cell
Bipolar cell
Horizontal cell

Rod
Cone

Pigment cells of choroid

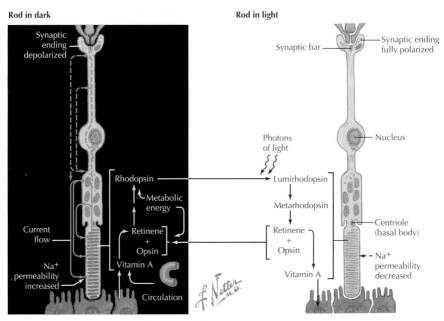

**Rod in dark**

Synaptic ending depolarized

Rhodopsin

Metabolic energy

Current flow

Retinene + Opsin

Na⁺ permeability increased

Vitamin A

Circulation

**Rod in light**

Synaptic bar

Synaptic ending fully polarized

Nucleus

Photons of light

Lumirhodopsin

Metarhodopsin

Retinene + Opsin

Vitamin A

Centriole (basal body)

Na⁺ permeability decreased

**Figure 3-14**

| Functional Column | Origin of Fibers | Termination of Fibers | Summary | Comment |
|---|---|---|---|---|
| **OCULOMOTOR NERVE** | | | | |
| GSE | Begins in the oculomotor nucleus (of the midbrain) | Enters orbit through superior orbital fissure and divides into:<br>• Superior division, which innervates the superior rectus and levator palpebrae superioris mm.<br>• Inferior division, which innervates the inferior rectus, medial rectus, and inferior oblique mm. | GSE fibers are responsible for innervating the majority of the extraocular eye muscles | Lesions of the oculomotor nerve result in diplopia (GSE), lateral strabismus (GSE), ptosis (GVE), and mydriasis (GVE) |
| GVE | Preganglionic parasympathetic fibers begin in the Edinger-Westphal nucleus (of the midbrain) | Preganglionic parasympathetic fibers synapse with postganglionic parasympathetic fibers at the ciliary ganglion<br>Postganglionic fibers travel through the short ciliary nn. to innervate the sphincter pupillae and ciliary mm. | GVE fibers are responsible for providing the parasympathetic innervation to the intrinsic eye muscles:<br>• Ciliary muscle<br>• Sphincter pupillae | GVE fibers utilize 1 ganglion:<br>• Ciliary ganglion |
| **TROCHLEAR NERVE** | | | | |
| GSE | Begins in the trochlear nucleus (of the midbrain) | Enters orbit through superior orbital fissure and innervates the superior oblique m. | GSE fibers are responsible for innervating 1 extraocular muscle of the eye: the superior oblique | The trochlear nerve exits the brainstem dorsally<br>Lesions of the trochlear n. result in diplopia<br>In trochlear n. lesions, the eye is adducted and elevated |
| **ABDUCENS NERVE** | | | | |
| GSE | Begins in the abducens nucleus (of the pons) | Enters orbit through superior orbital fissure and innervates the lateral rectus m. | GSE fibers are responsible for innervating 1 extraocular muscle of the eye: the lateral rectus | Lesions of the abducens nerve result in diplopia and medial strabismus |

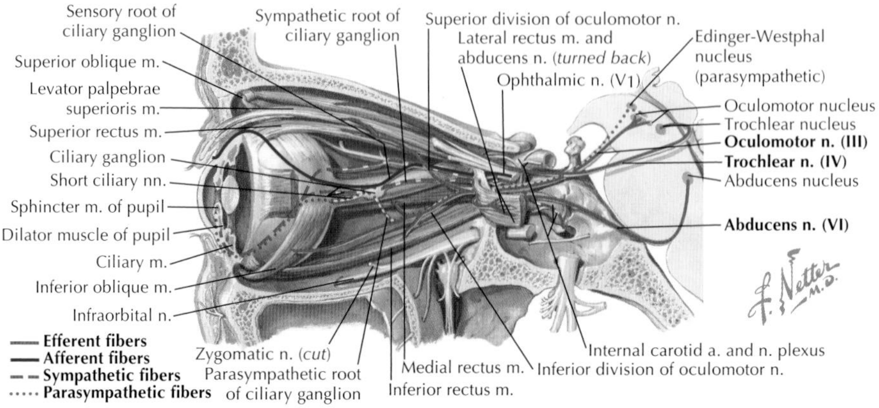

**Figure 3-15**

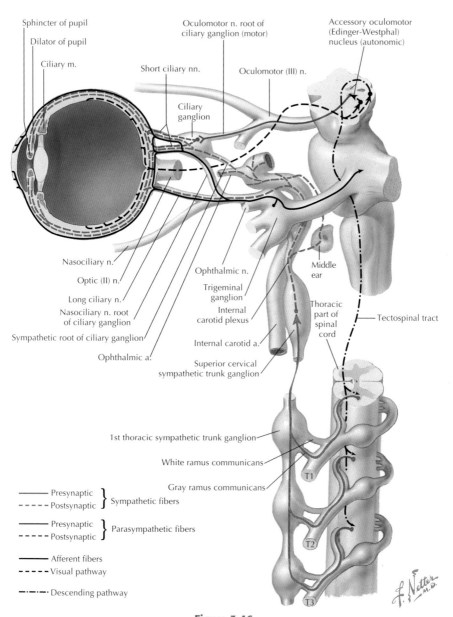

Sphincter of pupil

Dilator of pupil

Ciliary m.

Short ciliary nn.

Oculomotor n. root of
ciliary ganglion (motor)

Oculomotor (III) n.

Accessory oculomotor
(Edinger-Westphal)
nucleus (autonomic)

Ciliary
ganglion

Nasociliary n.

Optic (II) n.

Long ciliary n.

Nasociliary n. root
of ciliary ganglion

Sympathetic root of ciliary ganglion

Ophthalmic a.

Ophthalmic n.

Trigeminal
ganglion

Internal
carotid plexus

Internal carotid a.

Superior cervical
sympathetic trunk ganglion

Middle
ear

Thoracic
part of
spinal
cord

Tectospinal tract

1st thoracic sympathetic trunk ganglion

White ramus communicans

Gray ramus communicans

———— Presynaptic ⎫
- - - - Postsynaptic ⎬ Sympathetic fibers

———— Presynaptic ⎫
- - - - Postsynaptic ⎬ Parasympathetic fibers

———— Afferent fibers
- - - - Visual pathway
—·—·— Descending pathway

T1

T2

T3

**Figure 3-16**

OVERVIEW

- Consists of a large sensory root and a small motor root which joins the mandibular division at the level of the foramen ovale
- The sensory root is created by 3 divisions that come together at the trigeminal ganglion within the middle cranial fossa:
  - Ophthalmic division of the trigeminal, which passes through the superior orbital fissure (connects to orbit)
  - Maxillary division of the trigeminal, which passes through the foramen rotundum (connects to pterygopalatine fossa)
  - Mandibular division of the trigeminal, which passes through the foramen ovale (connects to infratemporal fossa)
- Each division carries the primary neurons for:
  - Pain and temperature (the cell body of the primary neuron is located in the trigeminal ganglion)
  - Discriminative touch (the cell body of the primary neuron is located in the trigeminal ganglion)
  - Proprioception (the cell body of the primary neuron is located in the mesencephalic nucleus of V)
- Parasympathetics use all of the divisions of the trigeminal nerve to distribute their fibers throughout the head and neck

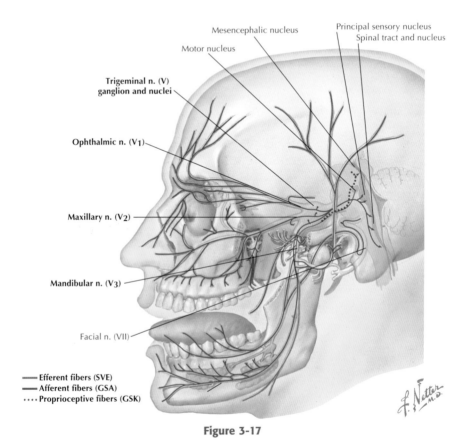

**Figure 3-17**

| Functional Column | Origin of Fibers | Termination of Fibers | Summary | Comment |
|---|---|---|---|---|
| GSA | Afferent fibers begin in the various receptors (nociceptors, mechanoceptors, proprioceptors) of the skin and deep tissues of the head | Pain and temperature and light touch fibers terminate in the spinal nucleus of V<br><br>Discriminative touch fibers terminate in the main sensory nucleus of V<br><br>Proprioception fibers have their cell bodies in the mesencephalic nucleus of V | GSA fibers are responsible for providing sensory innervation to the major part of the head<br><br>GSA fibers utilize the trigeminothalamic lemniscus to carry their sensory impulses to consciousness | Provides sensory innervation through 3 main divisions:<br>• Ophthalmic<br>• Maxillary<br>• Mandibular<br>The nerve cell bodies for the primary fibers for pain and temperature and touch are located in the trigeminal ganglion<br>The nerve cell bodies for the primary fibers for proprioception are located in the mesencephalic nucleus |
| SVE | Begins in the motor nucleus of the trigeminal (located in the pons) | Innervates the muscles of mastication:<br>• Masseter<br>• Temporalis<br>• Medial pterygoid<br>• Lateral pterygoid<br>Also innervates:<br>• Mylohyoid<br>• Anterior digastric<br>• Tensor tympani<br>• Tensor veli palatini | The SVE fibers are responsible for innervating the muscles of the 1st pharyngeal arch | |

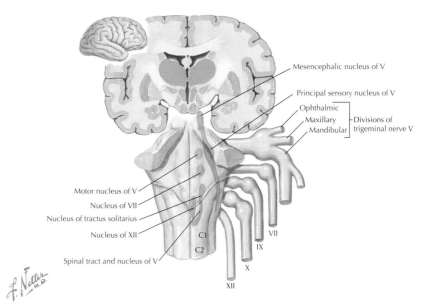

**Figure 3-18**

| OPHTHALMIC DIVISION OF THE TRIGEMINAL NERVE |
|---|
| • The ophthalmic division (V₁), being a branch of the trigeminal n., is sensory in function |

- The ophthalmic division ($V_1$), being a branch of the trigeminal n., is sensory in function
- Arises from the main nerve in the middle cranial fossa
- Passes anterior on the lateral wall of the cavernous sinus immediately inferior to the oculomotor and trochlear nn., but superior to the maxillary division of the trigeminal n.
- Before entering the orbit, it gives rise to a small tentorial branch
- Immediately before entering the orbit, through the superior orbital fissure, it divides into 3 major branches:
  - Lacrimal
  - Frontal
  - Nasociliary

| Branches Within the Middle Cranial Fossa | | |
|---|---|---|
| **Nerve** | **Source** | **Course** |
| Tentorial (meningeal) | Ophthalmic division of the trigeminal | Is recurrent in nature and passes posteriorly to provide innervation to small parts of the dura mater:<br>• Falx cerebri<br>• Tentorium cerebelli |
| Lacrimal | 1 of the 3 major branches of the ophthalmic division of the trigeminal n. | Smallest of the major branches of the ophthalmic division of the trigeminal n.<br>Passes anteriorly to enter the orbit through the superior orbital fissure<br>In the orbit it travels superolaterally on the superior border of the lateral rectus with the lacrimal a.<br>Before reaching the lacrimal gland, it communicates with the zygomatic branch of the maxillary division of the trigeminal n. to receive autonomic nervous fibers<br>Enters the lacrimal gland and supplies it and the conjunctiva before piercing the orbital septum to supply the skin of the upper eyelid |
| Frontal | 1 of the 3 major branches of the ophthalmic division of the trigeminal n. | Largest branch of the ophthalmic division of the trigeminal n.<br>Passes anteriorly to enter the orbit through the superior orbital fissure<br>In the orbit it passes anteriorly between the periosteum of the orbit and the levator palpebrae superioris m.<br>About halfway in the orbit, it divides into its 2 terminal nerves:<br>• Supraorbital n.<br>• Supratrochlear n. |
| *Supraorbital* | Frontal n. | 1 of the 2 terminal branches of the frontal n. in the orbit<br>Passes between the levator palpebrae superioris m. and periosteum of the orbit<br>Continues anteriorly to the supraorbital foramen (notch)<br>At the level of the supraorbital margin, it sends nerve supply to the frontal sinus, skin, and conjunctiva of the upper eyelid<br>Continues to ascend superiorly along the scalp<br>Divides into medial and lateral branches, which travel up to the vertex of the scalp |
| *Supratrochlear* | | 1 of the 2 terminal branches of the frontal n. in the orbit<br>Once the supratrochlear a. joins it within the orbit, it continues to pass anteriorly toward the trochlear n.<br>In the trochlear region, it exits the orbit at the frontal notch<br>Ascends along the scalp, at first deep to the musculature in the region, before piercing these muscles to reach the cutaneous innervation along the scalp |
| Nasociliary | 1 of the 3 major branches of the ophthalmic division of the trigeminal n. | Passes anteriorly to enter the orbit through the superior orbital fissure<br>Enters the orbit lateral to the optic n.<br>Travels across the optic n. anteriorly and medially to lie between the medial rectus m. and the superior oblique m. along the medial wall of the orbit<br>All along its path, it gives rise to other nerves, including the sensory root of the ciliary ganglion and the long ciliary and posterior ethmoid nn., until terminating into the anterior ethmoid and infratrochlear nn. near the anterior ethmoid foramen |

*Continued on next page*

| Nerve | Source | Course |
|---|---|---|
| *Sensory root of the ciliary ganglion* | Nasociliary n. | Travels anteriorly on the lateral side of the optic n. to enter the ciliary ganglion<br>Carries general sensory fibers, which are distributed by the short ciliary nn. |
| • *Short ciliary* | Ciliary ganglion | Arises from the ciliary ganglion to travel to the posterior surface of the eye<br>Supplies the sensory fibers to the eye and helps carry the postganglionic parasympathetic fibers to the sphincter pupillae and the ciliary muscle |
| *Long ciliary* | Nasociliary n. | Has 2 to 4 branches that travel anteriorly to enter the posterior part of the sclera of the eye<br>Postganglionic sympathetics traveling to the dilator pupillae will join the long ciliary to get to the eye |
| *Posterior ethmoid* | | Travels deep to the superior oblique m. to pass through the posterior ethmoid foramen<br>Supplies the sphenoid sinus and the posterior ethmoid sinus |
| *Anterior ethmoid* | | Arises on the medial wall of the orbit<br>Enters the anterior ethmoid foramen and travels through the canal to enter the anterior cranial fossa<br>Supplies the anterior and middle ethmoid sinus before entering and supplying the nasal cavity via internal nasal n. (medial and lateral branches)<br>Terminates as the external nasal n. on the nose |
| • *External nasal* | A terminal branch of the anterior ethmoid n. | Exits between the lateral nasal cartilage and the inferior border of the nasal bone<br>Supplies the skin of the ala and apex of the nose around the nares |
| • *Internal nasal* | | Upon entering the nasal cavity, it divides into medial (septal) and lateral branches, which supplies the skin on the internal surface of the vestibule |
| *Infratrochlear* | Nasociliary n. | 1 of the terminal branches of the nasociliary branch of the ophthalmic division of the trigeminal n.<br>Passes anteriorly on the superior border of the medial rectus m.<br>Passes inferior to the trochlea toward the medial angle of the eye<br>Supplies the skin of the eyelids and the bridge of the nose, the conjunctiva, and all of the lacrimal structures |

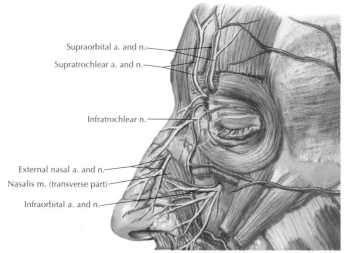

Supraorbital a. and n.
Supratrochlear a. and n.
Infratrochlear n.
External nasal a. and n.
Nasalis m. (transverse part)
Infraorbital a. and n.

**Figure 3-19**

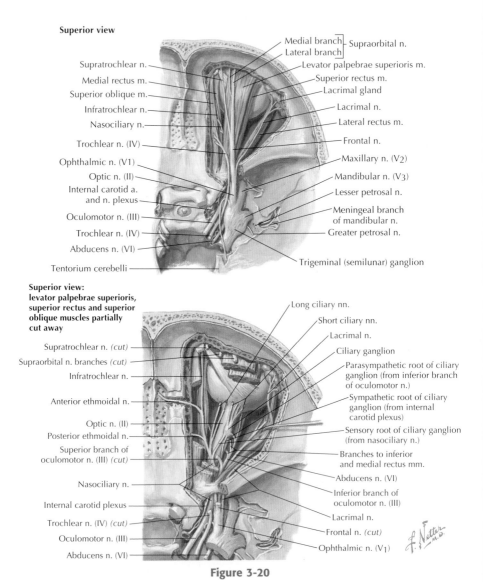

**Superior view**

Supratrochlear n.
Medial rectus m.
Superior oblique m.
Infratrochlear n.
Nasociliary n.
Trochlear n. (IV)
Ophthalmic n. (V1)
Optic n. (II)
Internal carotid a. and n. plexus
Oculomotor n. (III)
Trochlear n. (IV)
Abducens n. (VI)
Tentorium cerebelli

Medial branch ⎱ Supraorbital n.
Lateral branch ⎰
Levator palpebrae superioris m.
Superior rectus m.
Lacrimal gland
Lacrimal n.
Lateral rectus m.
Frontal n.
Maxillary n. (V2)
Mandibular n. (V3)
Lesser petrosal n.
Meningeal branch of mandibular n.
Greater petrosal n.
Trigeminal (semilunar) ganglion

**Superior view: levator palpebrae superioris, superior rectus and superior oblique muscles partially cut away**

Supratrochlear n. *(cut)*
Supraorbital n. branches *(cut)*
Infratrochlear n.
Anterior ethmoidal n.
Optic n. (II)
Posterior ethmoidal n.
Superior branch of oculomotor n. (III) *(cut)*
Nasociliary n.
Internal carotid plexus
Trochlear n. (IV) *(cut)*
Oculomotor n. (III)
Abducens n. (VI)

Long ciliary nn.
Short ciliary nn.
Lacrimal n.
Ciliary ganglion
Parasympathetic root of ciliary ganglion (from inferior branch of oculomotor n.)
Sympathetic root of ciliary ganglion (from internal carotid plexus)
Sensory root of ciliary ganglion (from nasociliary n.)
Branches to inferior and medial rectus mm.
Abducens n. (VI)
Inferior branch of oculomotor n. (III)
Lacrimal n.
Frontal n. *(cut)*
Ophthalmic n. (V1)

**Figure 3-20**

| MAXILLARY DIVISION OF THE TRIGEMINAL NERVE |
|---|
| • The maxillary division ($V_2$), being a branch of the trigeminal n., is sensory in function |
| • Branches from the trigeminal n. and travels along the lateral wall of the cavernous sinus |
| • Passes from the middle cranial fossa into the pterygopalatine fossa via the foramen rotundum |
| • Within the pterygopalatine fossa, it gives rise to 4 branches |
| • 1 of those nerves, the infraorbital n., is considered the continuation of the maxillary division of the trigeminal n. |

| Nerve | Course |
|---|---|
| Branches Within the Middle Cranial Fossa | |
| Meningeal | A small meningeal branch is given off within the middle cranial fossa |
| | The nerve supplies the meninges |
| Branches Within the Pterygopalatine Fossa | |
| Posterior superior alveolar | Passes through the pterygomaxillary fissure to enter the infratemporal fossa |
| | In the infratemporal fossa, it passes on the posterior surface of the maxilla along the region of the maxillary tuberosity |
| | Gives rise to a gingival branch alongside the maxillary molars |
| | Enters the posterior surface of the maxilla and supplies the maxillary sinus and the maxillary molars, with the possible exception of the mesiobuccal root of the 1st maxillary molar, and the gingiva and mucosa alongside the same teeth |
| Zygomatic | Passes through the inferior orbital fissure to enter the orbit |
| | Passes on the lateral wall of the orbit and branches into the zygomaticotemporal (supplies sensory to skin of the temple) and zygomaticofacial branches (supplies sensory to skin over the cheek) |
| | A communicating branch from it joins the lacrimal n. from the ophthalmic division of the trigeminal n. to carry autonomics to the lacrimal gland |
| Ganglionic branches | Usually 2 ganglionic branches that connect the maxillary division of the trigeminal n. to the pterygopalatine ganglion |
| | Contain sensory fibers that pass through the pterygopalatine ganglion (without synapsing) to be distributed with the nerves that arise from the pterygopalatine ganglion |
| | Also contain postganglionic autonomic fibers to the lacrimal gland that pass through the pterygopalatine ganglion (parasympathetic fibers form a synapse here between the preganglionic fibers from the vidian n. and the postganglionic fibers) |
| Infraorbital | Considered the continuation of the maxillary division of the trigeminal n. |
| | Passes through the inferior orbital fissure to enter the orbit |
| | Passes anteriorly through the infraorbital groove and infraorbital canal and exits onto the face via the infraorbital foramen |
| | While in the infraorbital canal it gives rise to 2 branches: |
| | • Anterior superior alveolar n |
| | • Middle superior alveolar n. |
| Branches Associated With the Pterygopalatine Ganglion | |
| Pharyngeal | Passes through the palatovaginal (pharyngeal) canal to enter and supply the nasopharynx |
| Orbital | Small branches that enter the orbit through the inferior orbital fissure |
| | Provide sensory to the orbital periosteum and send branches that supply the sphenoid sinus |
| Posterior superior nasal | A branch of the maxillary division of the trigeminal n. |
| | Arises from the pterygopalatine ganglion in the pterygopalatine fossa |
| | Passes through the sphenopalatine foramen to enter the nasal cavity and branches into the: |
| | • Posterior superior medial nasal n. |
| | • Posterior superior lateral nasal n. |

*Continued on next page*

| Nerve | Course |
|---|---|
| Branches Associated With the Pterygopalatine Ganglion *Continued* | |
| Posterior superior lateral nasal | A branch of the posterior superior nasal n. that supplies the posterosuperior portion of the lateral wall of the nasal cavity in the region of the superior and middle concha and the posterior ethmoid air cells |
| Posterior superior medial nasal | Arises from the posterior superior nasal n. from the maxillary division of the trigeminal n.<br>This nerve supplies the posterior portion of the nasal septum and nasal roof |
| Greater palatine | Passes through the palatine canal to enter the hard palate via the greater palatine foramen<br>Supplies the palatal gingiva and mucosa from the area in the premolar region to the posterior border of the hard palate to the midline |
| Posterior inferior nasal branch of the greater palatine | While descending in the palatine canal, the greater palatine n. gives rise to a posterior inferior nasal branch<br>Supplies the posterior part of the lateral wall of the nasal cavity in the region of the middle meatus |
| Lesser palatine | Passes through the palatine canal to enter and supply the soft palate via the lesser palatine foramen |
| Nasopalatine | Branches from the pterygopalatine ganglion in the pterygopalatine fossa<br>Passes through the sphenopalatine foramen to enter the nasal cavity<br>Passes along the superior portion of the nasal cavity to the nasal septum, where it travels anteroinferiorly to the incisive canal, supplying the septum<br>Passes through the incisive canal to supply the gingiva and mucosa of the hard palate from central incisor to canine |
| Branches Within the Infraorbital Canal | |
| Middle superior alveolar | A variable nerve, present in about 30% of individuals<br>When present, it branches off the infraorbital n. as it travels in the infraorbital canal<br>As the nerve descends to form the superior dental plexus, it innervates part of the maxillary sinus; the premolars and possibly the mesiobuccal root of the 1st molar; and the gingiva and mucosa alongside the same teeth |
| Anterior superior alveolar | While in the infraorbital canal, it gives rise to the anterior superior alveolar n., which has a small branch that supplies the nasal cavity in the region of the inferior meatus and inferior corresponding portion of the nasal septum, the maxillary sinus<br>As the nerve descends to form the superior dental plexus, it innervates part of the maxillary sinus; maxillary central incisor, lateral incisor, and canine teeth; and the gingiva and mucosa alongside the same teeth |
| Branches After Infraorbital Nerve Emerges From the Infraorbital Foramen | |
| Superior labial branch of the infraorbital | Supplies the skin of the upper lip |
| Nasal branch of the infraorbital | Supplies the skin along the ala of the nose |
| Inferior palpebral branch of the infraorbital | Supplies the skin of the lower eyelid |

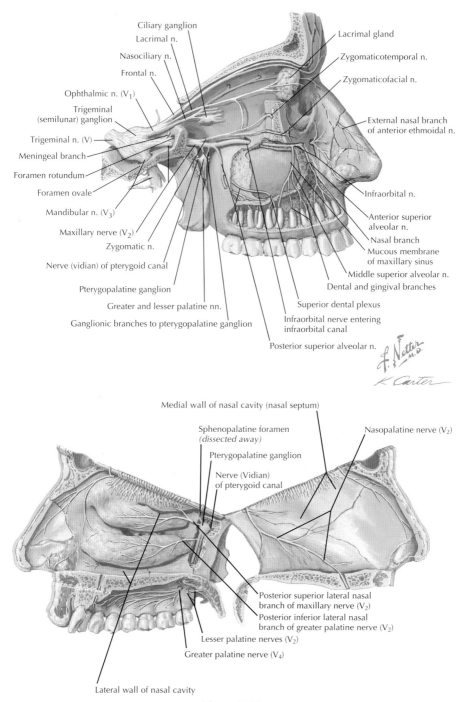

Ciliary ganglion
Lacrimal n.
Nasociliary n.
Frontal n.
Ophthalmic n. (V₁)
Trigeminal (semilunar) ganglion
Trigeminal n. (V)
Meningeal branch
Foramen rotundum
Foramen ovale
Mandibular n. (V₃)
Maxillary nerve (V₂)
Zygomatic n.
Nerve (vidian) of pterygoid canal
Pterygopalatine ganglion
Greater and lesser palatine nn.
Ganglionic branches to pterygopalatine ganglion

Lacrimal gland
Zygomaticotemporal n.
Zygomaticofacial n.
External nasal branch of anterior ethmoidal n.
Infraorbital n.
Anterior superior alveolar n.
Nasal branch
Mucous membrane of maxillary sinus
Middle superior alveolar n.
Dental and gingival branches
Superior dental plexus
Infraorbital nerve entering infraorbital canal
Posterior superior alveolar n.

Medial wall of nasal cavity (nasal septum)
Sphenopalatine foramen *(dissected away)*
Pterygopalatine ganglion
Nerve (Vidian) of pterygoid canal
Nasopalatine nerve (V₂)
Posterior superior lateral nasal branch of maxillary nerve (V₂)
Posterior inferior lateral nasal branch of greater palatine nerve (V₂)
Lesser palatine nerves (V₂)
Greater palatine nerve (V₄)
Lateral wall of nasal cavity

**Figure 3-21**

| MANDIBULAR DIVISION OF THE TRIGEMINAL NERVE | | | | |
|---|---|---|---|---|
| | | | **Divisions** | |
| **Description** | **Source** | **Course** | **Anterior** | **Posterior** |
| Mandibular division (V₃) is the largest of the 3 divisions of the trigeminal n.<br><br>Has motor *and* sensory functions | Created by a large sensory root and a small motor root that unite just after passing through the foramen ovale to enter the infratemporal fossa | Immediately gives rise to a meningeal branch and a medial pterygoid branch before dividing into anterior and posterior divisions | Smaller; mainly motor, with 1 sensory branch (buccal):<br>• Masseteric<br>• Anterior and posterior deep temporal<br>• Lateral pterygoid<br>• Buccal | Larger; mainly sensory, with 1 motor branch (nerve to the mylohyoid):<br>• Auriculotemporal<br>• Lingual<br>• Inferior alveolar<br>• Mylohyoid nerve |

| BRANCHES FROM THE UNDIVIDED TRUNK | |
|---|---|
| **Branch** | **Course** |
| Meningeal (nervus spinosum) | After passing through the foramen ovale, the undivided trigeminal trunk is located between the tensor veli palatini and the lateral pterygoid<br>The undivided trunk then gives rise to a lateral branch called the meningeal nerve<br>The branch travels through the foramen spinosum to enter the middle cranial fossa and innervate the dura mater |
| Medial pterygoid | After passing through the foramen ovale, the undivided trigeminal trunk is located between the tensor veli palatini and the lateral pterygoid<br>The undivided trunk then gives rise to a medial branch to the medial pterygoid<br>This branch continues to supply the tensor veli palatini and the tensor tympani |

| Anterior Division of the Mandibular Division | |
|---|---|
| **Branch** | **Course** |
| Masseteric | Passes laterally superior to the lateral pterygoid m.<br>Lies anterior to the temporomandibular joint and posterior to the tendon of the temporalis m.<br>Crosses the mandibular notch with the masseteric a. to innervate the masseter m.<br>Also provides a small branch to the temporomandibular joint |
| Anterior and posterior deep temporal | Pass superior to the lateral pterygoid m. between the skull and the temporalis m. while passing deep to the muscle to innervate it<br>Provides a small branch to the temporomandibular joint |
| Lateral pterygoid | Passes into the deep surface of the muscle<br>Often arises from the buccal n. |
| Buccal | Passes anteriorly between the 2 heads of the lateral pterygoid m.<br>Descends inferiorly along the lower part of the temporalis m. to appear from deep to the anterior border of the masseter m.<br>Supplies the skin over the buccinator m. before passing through it to supply the mucous membrane lining its inner surface and the gingiva along the mandibular molars |

*Continued on next page*

| Posterior Division of the Mandibular Division | |
|---|---|
| **Branch** | **Course** |
| Auriculotemporal | Normally arises by 2 roots, between which the middle meningeal a. passes |
| | Runs posteriorly just inferior to the lateral pterygoid and continues to the medial side of the neck of the mandible |
| | Then it turns superiorly with the superficial temporal vessels between the auricle and condyle of the mandible deep to the parotid gland |
| | On exiting the parotid gland, it ascends over the zygomatic arch and divides into superficial temporal branches |
| Lingual | Lies inferior to the lateral pterygoid and medial and anterior to the inferior alveolar n. |
| | The chorda tympani n. also joins the posterior part |
| | The lingual n. passes between the medial pterygoid and the ramus of the mandible, then passes obliquely to enter the oral cavity bounded by the superior pharyngeal constrictor m., medial pterygoid, and the mandible |
| | Supplies the mucous membrane of the anterior 2/3 of the tongue and gingiva on the lingual aspect of the mandibular teeth |
| Inferior alveolar | The largest branch of the mandibular division |
| | Descends following the inferior alveolar a. inferior to the lateral pterygoid and finally between the sphenomandibular lig. and the ramus of the mandible until it enters the mandibular foramen |
| | After entering the mandibular foramen, it travels in the mandibular canal until it terminates as the mental and incisive nn. in the area of the 2nd premolar |
| | Innervates all mandibular teeth (via inferior alveolar and incisive nn.), periodontal ligaments (via inferior alveolar and incisive nn.), and the gingiva from the premolars anteriorly to the midline (via the mental n.) |
| Mylohyoid | Branches from the inferior alveolar n. immediately before it enters the mandibular foramen |
| | Descends in a groove on the deep side of the ramus of the mandible until it reaches the superficial surface of the mylohyoid |
| | Supplies the mylohyoid and the anterior belly of the digastric m. |

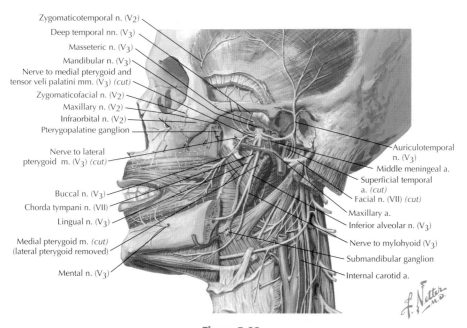

**Figure 3-22**

## TRIGEMINAL NERVE PATHWAYS

- Responsible for carrying to conscious level:
  - Pain and temperature
  - Light touch
  - Discriminative touch
  - Pressure
- Utilizes a 3-neuron sensory system:
  - Primary neuron
  - Secondary neuron
  - Tertiary neuron
- Utilizes the contralateral ventral trigeminothalamic tract
- Some discriminative touch and pressure fibers utilize the ipsilateral dorsal trigeminothalamic tract, but this contribution is very minor
- Proprioception fibers are unique in that the cell body for the sensory nerve fiber is located in the central nervous system (mesencephalic nucleus)

| Types of Fibers | Trigeminal Sensory Nucleus | Ascending Pathway |
|---|---|---|
| Pain and temperature<br>Light touch | Spinal (descending) nucleus | Ventral trigeminothalamic tract |
| Discriminative touch<br>Pressure | Principal (main) sensory nucleus | Ventral trigeminothalamic tract (dorsal trigeminothalamic tract subserves discriminative touch and pressure) |
| Proprioception | Mesencephalic nucleus | Projects to motor nucleus of V to control the jaw jerk reflex and force of bite |

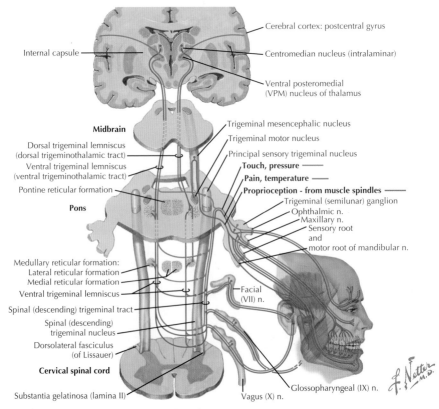

**Figure 3-23**

| MAJOR ASCENDING PATHWAYS OF THE TRIGEMINAL NERVE | | | |
|---|---|---|---|
| Types of Neurons | Path of Pain and Temperature | Path of Light Touch | Path of Discriminative Touch and Pressure |
| Primary neuron | Fibers (Aδ or C) travel from the receptor from the ophthalmic, maxillary, and mandibular divisions of the trigeminal n. <br><br> The nerve cell body of the primary neuron is located in the trigeminal ganglion <br><br> Fibers enter the pons <br><br> Fibers descend in the spinal (descending) tract located from the pons to the upper cervical spinal cord <br><br> Fibers synapse on the nerve cell body of the secondary neuron | Fibers (Aβ) travel from the receptor from the ophthalmic, maxillary, and mandibular divisions of the trigeminal n. <br><br> The nerve cell body of the primary neuron is located in the trigeminal ganglion <br><br> Fibers enter the pons <br><br> Fibers may have either of 2 courses: <br> • May descend in the spinal (descending) tract located from the pons to the upper cervical spinal cord <br> • May ascend to synapse on the nerve cell body of the secondary neuron <br><br> Fibers synapse on the nerve cell body of the secondary neuron | Fibers (Aβ) travel from the receptor from the ophthalmic, maxillary, and mandibular divisions of the trigeminal n. <br><br> The nerve cell body of the primary neuron is located in the trigeminal ganglion <br><br> Fibers enter the pons <br><br> Fibers ascend to synapse on the nerve cell body of the secondary neuron |
| Secondary neuron | Secondary nerve cell bodies begin in the spinal (descending) nucleus located from the pons to the upper cervical spinal cord (pars caudalis) <br><br> Fibers decussate and ascend in the ventral trigeminothalamic tract (lemniscus) to the thalamus <br><br> Fibers synapse on the nerve cell body of the tertiary neuron | Secondary nerve cell bodies may reach the thalamus along either of 2 courses: <br> • May begin in the spinal (descending) nucleus (pars interpolaris and pars oralis) and decussate and ascend in the ventral trigeminothalamic tract (lemniscus) to the thalamus <br> • May begin in the principal (main) sensory nucleus and decussate and ascend in the ventral trigeminothalamic tract (lemniscus) to the thalamus (*Note*: some fibers ascend in the ipsilateral dorsal trigeminothalamic tract) <br><br> Fibers synapse on the nerve cell body of the tertiary neuron | Secondary nerve cell bodies begin in the principal (main) sensory nucleus located in the pons <br><br> Fibers decussate and ascend in the ventral trigeminothalamic tract (lemniscus) to the thalamus (*Note*: some fibers ascend in the ipsilateral dorsal trigeminothalamic tract) <br><br> Fibers synapse on the nerve cell body of the tertiary neuron |
| Tertiary neuron | Tertiary nerve cell bodies begin in the ventral posteromedial nucleus of the thalamus (VPM) <br><br> Fibers ascend through the posterior limb of the internal capsule to terminate in the postcentral gyrus | Tertiary nerve cell bodies begin in the VPM <br><br> Fibers ascend through the posterior limb of the internal capsule to terminate in the postcentral gyrus | Tertiary nerve cell bodies begin in the VPM <br><br> Fibers ascend through the posterior limb of the internal capsule to terminate in the postcentral gyrus |
| PROPRIOCEPTION OF THE TRIGEMINAL NERVE | | | |

- Sensory fibers carry input from the neuromuscular spindles along the mandibular division of the trigeminal n.
- The nerve cell bodies of these sensory neurons are located in the mesencephalic nucleus of the midbrain
- These fibers project to the motor nucleus of the trigeminal n. and innervate the muscles of mastication, to control the jaw jerk reflex and force of bite

| Functional Column | Origin of Fibers | Termination of Fibers | Summary | Comment |
|---|---|---|---|---|
| GSA | Afferent fibers begin in the various receptors (nociceptors, mechanoceptors, proprioceptors) of the skin of the external ear and tympanic membrane | Pain and temperature fibers terminate in the spinal nucleus of V | GSA fibers are carried in the nervus intermedius portion of the facial n.<br><br>GSA fibers are responsible for providing sensory innervation to a portion of the external ear and tympanic membrane<br><br>GSA fibers of the facial n. utilize the trigeminothalamic lemniscus to carry their sensory impulses to consciousness | Facial nerve provides a very small area of GSA distribution<br><br>Nerve cell bodies for the primary fibers are located in the geniculate ganglion |
| SVA | Afferent fibers begin in the taste receptors of the anterior 2/3 of the tongue | Primary afferent fibers travel in the tractus solitarius and terminate in the nucleus solitarius | SVA fibers are carried in the nervus intermedius portion of the facial n.<br><br>SVA fibers are responsible for carrying the taste fibers from the taste buds on the anterior 2/3 of the tongue | Nerve cell bodies for the primary fibers are located in the geniculate ganglion |
| GVA | Afferent fibers begin in the various receptors (such as nociceptors) of the mucous membranes of the nasopharynx | Primary afferent fibers travel in the tractus solitarius and terminate in the nucleus solitarius | GVA fibers are carried in the nervus intermedius portion of the facial n.<br><br>GVA fibers utilize the same pathway as the SVA fibers | Nerve cell bodies for the primary fibers are located in the geniculate ganglion |
| GVE | Preganglionic parasympathetic fibers begin in the superior salivatory nucleus | Postganglionic parasympathetic fibers innervate the lacrimal, nasal, submandibular, and sublingual glands | GVE fibers are carried in the nervus intermedius portion of the facial n. | GVE fibers utilize 2 ganglia:<br>• Pterygopalatine<br>• Submandibular |
| SVE | Begins in the motor nucleus of the facial n. | Innervates the muscles of facial expression, stylohyoid, posterior digastric, and stapedius mm. | SVE fibers are carried in the motor root of the facial n.<br><br>SVE fibers are responsible for innervating the muscles of the 2nd pharyngeal arch | In Bell's palsy, the easiest symptom to observe is that the muscles innervated by the SVE fibers are paralyzed |

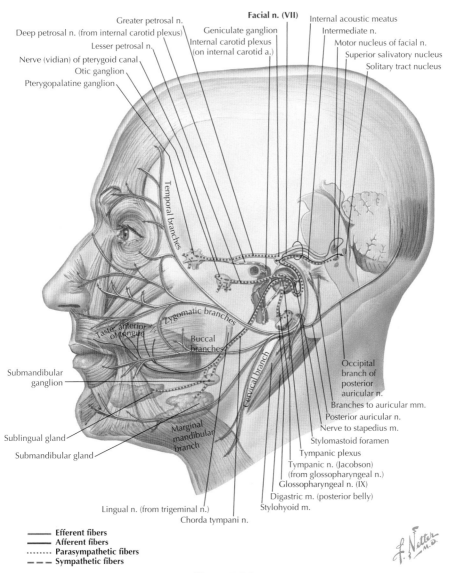

Greater petrosal n.

Deep petrosal n. (from internal carotid plexus)

Lesser petrosal n.

Nerve (vidian) of pterygoid canal

Otic ganglion

Pterygopalatine ganglion

**Facial n. (VII)**

Geniculate ganglion

Internal carotid plexus (on internal carotid a.)

Internal acoustic meatus

Intermediate n.

Motor nucleus of facial n.

Superior salivatory nucleus

Solitary tract nucleus

Temporal branches

Zygomatic branches

Taste: anterior ⅔ of tongue

Buccal branches

Cervical branch

Submandibular ganglion

Sublingual gland

Submandibular gland

Marginal mandibular branch

Occipital branch of posterior auricular n.

Branches to auricular mm.

Posterior auricular n.

Nerve to stapedius m.

Stylomastoid foramen

Tympanic plexus

Tympanic n. (Jacobson) (from glossopharyngeal n.)

Glossopharyngeal n. (IX)

Digastric m. (posterior belly)

Stylohyoid m.

Lingual n. (from trigeminal n.)

Chorda tympani n.

——— Efferent fibers
——— Afferent fibers
········ Parasympathetic fibers
— — — Sympathetic fibers

**Figure 3-24**

| Functional Column | Origin of Fibers | Termination of Fibers | Summary | Comment |
|---|---|---|---|---|
| SSA | Organ of Corti<br>Cristae of semicircular canals<br>Maculae of utricle and saccule | Cochlear and vestibular nuclei | SSA fibers travel from the various vestibulocochlear receptors to their respective nuclei in the brainstem | Vestibulocochlear and facial nn. both enter the internal acoustic meatus and can be affected by tumors in the region |

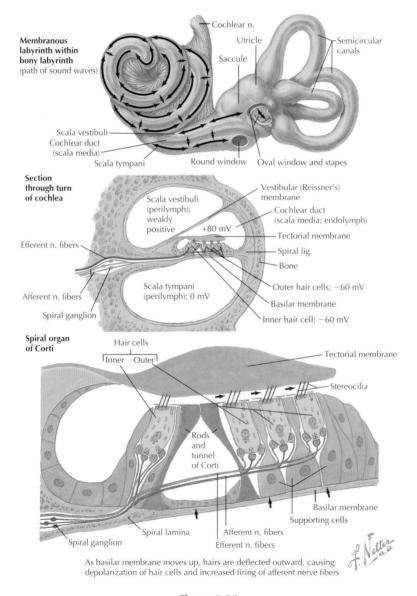

As basilar membrane moves up, hairs are deflected outward, causing depolarization of hair cells and increased firing of afferent nerve fibers

**Figure 3-25**

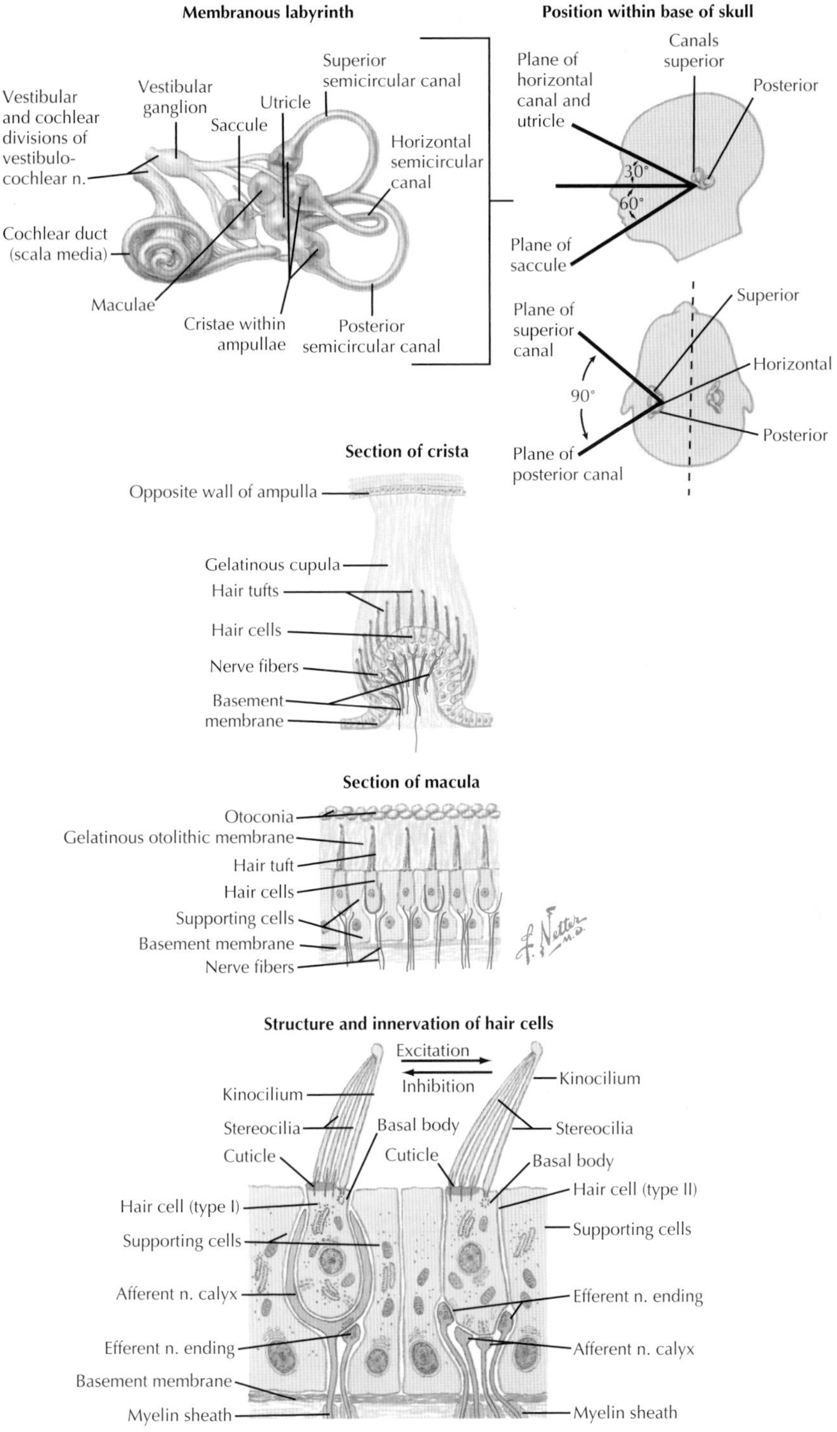

**Membranous labyrinth**

Vestibular and cochlear divisions of vestibulo-cochlear n.

Vestibular ganglion

Saccule

Utricle

Superior semicircular canal

Horizontal semicircular canal

Cochlear duct (scala media)

Maculae

Cristae within ampullae

Posterior semicircular canal

**Position within base of skull**

Canals superior

Plane of horizontal canal and utricle

Posterior

30°

60°

Plane of saccule

Plane of superior canal

Superior

Horizontal

90°

Posterior

Plane of posterior canal

**Section of crista**

Opposite wall of ampulla

Gelatinous cupula

Hair tufts

Hair cells

Nerve fibers

Basement membrane

**Section of macula**

Otoconia

Gelatinous otolithic membrane

Hair tuft

Hair cells

Supporting cells

Basement membrane

Nerve fibers

**Structure and innervation of hair cells**

Excitation

Inhibition

Kinocilium

Stereocilia

Cuticle

Basal body

Cuticle

Kinocilium

Stereocilia

Basal body

Hair cell (type I)

Supporting cells

Afferent n. calyx

Efferent n. ending

Basement membrane

Myelin sheath

Hair cell (type II)

Supporting cells

Efferent n. ending

Afferent n. calyx

Myelin sheath

**Figure 3-26**

| Functional Column | Origin of Fibers | Termination of Fibers | Summary | Comment |
|---|---|---|---|---|
| GSA | Afferent fibers begin in the various receptors of the skin of the external ear and the posterior 1/3 of the tongue | Pain and temperature fibers terminate in the spinal nucleus of V | GSA fibers are responsible for providing sensory innervation to a small portion of the external ear and posterior 1/3 of the tongue<br><br>GSA fibers of the glossopharyngeal n. utilize the trigeminothalamic lemniscus to carry their sensory impulses to consciousness | Nerve cell bodies for the primary fibers are located in the superior ganglion of IX |
| SVA | Afferent fibers begin in the taste receptors of the posterior 1/3 of the tongue | Primary afferent fibers travel in the tractus solitarius and terminate in the nucleus solitarius | SVA fibers are responsible for carrying the taste fibers from the circumvallate papillae and the taste buds on the posterior 1/3 of the tongue | Nerve cell bodies for the primary fibers are located in the inferior ganglion of IX |
| GVA | Afferent fibers begin in the various receptors of the mucous membranes of the nasopharynx, oropharynx, middle ear, carotid body, and carotid sinus | Primary afferent fibers travel in the tractus solitarius and terminate in the nucleus solitarius | GVA fibers utilize the same pathway as the SVA fibers | The nerve cell bodies for the primary fibers are located in the inferior ganglion of IX<br><br>GVA fibers are predominantly the sensory portion of the pharyngeal plexus |
| GVE | Preganglionic parasympathetic fibers begin in the inferior salivatory nucleus | Postganglionic parasympathetic fibers innervate parotid gland | The GVE fibers are responsible for providing the parasympathetic innervation to the parotid gland | GVE fibers utilize 1 ganglion:<br>• Otic |
| SVE | Begins in the nucleus ambiguus | Innervates the stylopharyngeus m. | SVE fibers are responsible for innervating the muscles of the 3rd pharyngeal arch | Stylopharyngeus is the only muscle innervated by the glossopharyngeal n. |

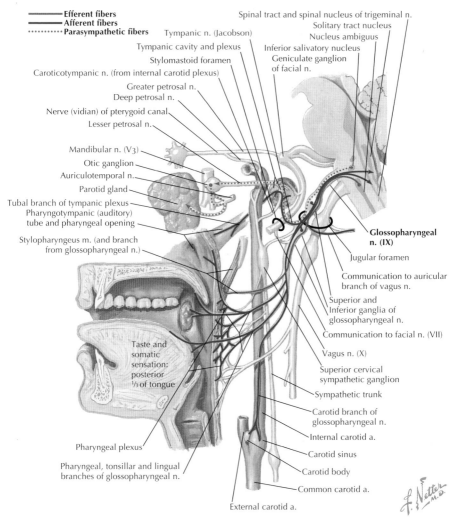

Efferent fibers
Afferent fibers
Parasympathetic fibers

Tympanic n. (Jacobson)
Tympanic cavity and plexus
Stylomastoid foramen
Caroticotympanic n. (from internal carotid plexus)
Greater petrosal n.
Deep petrosal n.
Nerve (vidian) of pterygoid canal
Lesser petrosal n.

Mandibular n. (V3)
Otic ganglion
Auriculotemporal n.
Parotid gland
Tubal branch of tympanic plexus
Pharyngotympanic (auditory) tube and pharyngeal opening
Stylopharyngeus m. (and branch from glossopharyngeal n.)

Taste and somatic sensation: posterior 1/3 of tongue

Pharyngeal plexus
Pharyngeal, tonsillar and lingual branches of glossopharyngeal n.

Spinal tract and spinal nucleus of trigeminal n.
Solitary tract nucleus
Nucleus ambiguus
Inferior salivatory nucleus
Geniculate ganglion of facial n.

Glossopharyngeal n. (IX)
Jugular foramen
Communication to auricular branch of vagus n.
Superior and Inferior ganglia of glossopharyngeal n.
Communication to facial n. (VII)
Vagus n. (X)
Superior cervical sympathetic ganglion
Sympathetic trunk
Carotid branch of glossopharyngeal n.
Internal carotid a.
Carotid sinus
Carotid body
Common carotid a.
External carotid a.

**Figure 3-27**

| Functional Column | Origin of Fibers | Termination of Fibers | Summary | Comment |
|---|---|---|---|---|
| GSA | Afferent fibers begin in the various receptors on a small part of the skin of the external ear | Pain and temperature fibers terminate in the spinal nucleus of V | The GSA fibers are responsible for providing sensory innervation to a very small portion of the external ear<br><br>The GSA fibers of the glossopharyngeal n. utilize the trigeminothalamic lemniscus to carry their sensory impulses to consciousness | The nerve cell bodies for the primary fibers are located in the superior ganglion of X |
| SVA | Afferent fibers begin in the taste receptors of the epiglottic region and are scattered on the palate | Primary afferent fibers travel in the tractus solitarius and terminate in the nucleus solitarius | The SVA fibers are responsible for carrying the taste fibers from the epiglottic region and are scattered on the palate | The nerve cell bodies for the primary fibers are located in the inferior ganglion of X |
| GVA | Afferent fibers begin in the various receptors of the mucous membranes of the laryngopharynx, larynx, thorax, and abdomen | Primary afferent fibers travel in the tractus solitarius and terminate in the nucleus solitarius | The GVA fibers utilize the same pathway as the SVA fibers | The nerve cell bodies for the primary fibers are located in the inferior ganglion of X |
| GVE | Preganglionic parasympathetic fibers begin in the dorsal motor nucleus of the vagus n. | Postganglionic parasympathetic fibers innervate thoracic and abdominal viscera | The GVE fibers are responsible for providing the parasympathetic innervation to the thoracic and abdominal viscera | The GVE fibers utilize:<br>• Intramural ganglia |
| SVE | Begins in the nucleus ambiguus | Innervates the muscles of the pharynx (via the pharyngeal plexus) and the larynx | The SVE fibers are responsible for innervating the muscles of the 4th and 6th pharyngeal arches | The SVE fibers are the motor component to the pharyngeal plexus (muscles of pharynx) and muscles of the larynx<br><br>Lesions of the vagus paralyze the muscles of the larynx on the affected side |

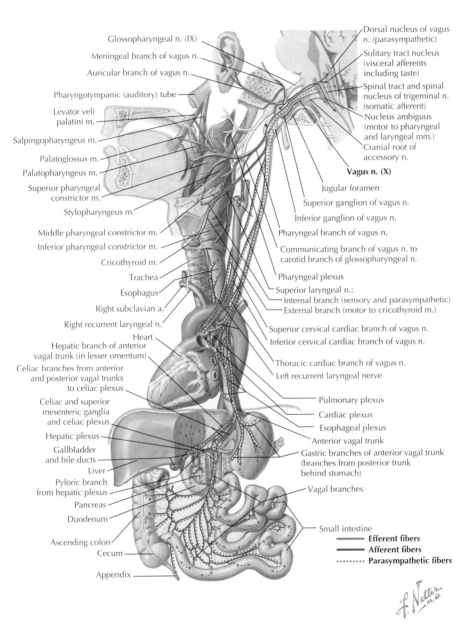

Glossopharyngeal n. (IX)

Meningeal branch of vagus n.

Auricular branch of vagus n.

Pharyngotympanic (auditory) tube

Levator veli palatini m.

Salpingopharyngeus m.

Palatoglossus m.

Palatopharyngeus m.

Superior pharyngeal constrictor m.

Stylopharyngeus m.

Middle pharyngeal constrictor m.

Inferior pharyngeal constrictor m.

Cricothyroid m.

Trachea

Esophagus

Right subclavian a.

Right recurrent laryngeal n.

Heart

Hepatic branch of anterior vagal trunk (in lesser omentum)

Celiac branches from anterior and posterior vagal trunks to celiac plexus

Celiac and superior mesenteric ganglia and celiac plexus

Hepatic plexus

Gallbladder and bile ducts

Liver

Pyloric branch from hepatic plexus

Pancreas

Duodenum

Ascending colon

Cecum

Appendix

Dorsal nucleus of vagus n. (parasympathetic)

Solitary tract nucleus (visceral afferents including taste)

Spinal tract and spinal nucleus of trigeminal n. (somatic afferent)

Nucleus ambiguus (motor to pharyngeal and laryngeal mm.)

Cranial root of accessory n.

**Vagus n. (X)**

Jugular foramen

Superior ganglion of vagus n.

Inferior ganglion of vagus n.

Pharyngeal branch of vagus n.

Communicating branch of vagus n. to carotid branch of glossopharyngeal n.

Pharyngeal plexus

Superior laryngeal n.:
Internal branch (sensory and parasympathetic)
External branch (motor to cricothyroid m.)

Superior cervical cardiac branch of vagus n.

Inferior cervical cardiac branch of vagus n.

Thoracic cardiac branch of vagus n.

Left recurrent laryngeal nerve

Pulmonary plexus

Cardiac plexus

Esophageal plexus

Anterior vagal trunk

Gastric branches of anterior vagal trunk (branches from posterior trunk behind stomach)

Vagal branches

Small intestine

Efferent fibers
Afferent fibers
Parasympathetic fibers

**Figure 3-28**

OVERVIEW

- The anatomy of the accessory nerve is controversial in the literature
- It is traditionally described as having a cranial root and a spinal root
- The cranial fibers are argued to be part of the vagus nerve and not the accessory nerve
- The traditional description is noted in the table

| Functional Column | Origin of Fibers | Termination of Fibers | Summary | Comment |
|---|---|---|---|---|
| SVE/GSE* | *Cranial part*: Begins in the nucleus ambiguus <br> *Spinal part*: Begins in the upper cervical levels of the spinal cord | Innervates the trapezius and sternocleidomastoid mm. | These fibers of the cranial part travel with the vagus n. <br> The spinal part begins in the cervical levels of the spinal cord and enters the skull via the foramen magnum <br> Once inside the cranium, the accessory n. exits the jugular foramen with the glossopharyngeal and vagus nn. | The cranial and spinal parts are described as separating so that the cranial part can follow the vagus nerve and the spinal part can pass into the sternocleidomastoid m. and travel through the posterior triangle until reaching the trapezius m. |

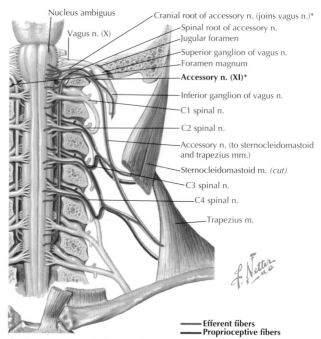

Nucleus ambiguus

Vagus n. (X)

Cranial root of accessory n. (joins vagus n.)*
Spinal root of accessory n.
Jugular foramen
Superior ganglion of vagus n.
Foramen magnum
**Accessory n. (XI)***
Inferior ganglion of vagus n.
C1 spinal n.
C2 spinal n.
Accessory n. (to sternocleidomastoid and trapezius mm.)
Sternocleidomastoid m. *(cut)*
C3 spinal n.
C4 spinal n.
Trapezius m.

——— Efferent fibers
——— Proprioceptive fibers

*Recent evidence suggests that the accessory nerve lacks a cranial root and has no connection to the vagus nerve. There is disagreement whether the branchiomeric innervation to the trapezius and sternocleidomastoid is from SVE or GSE fibers.

**Figure 3-29**

| Functional Column | Origin of Fibers | Termination of Fibers | Summary | Comment |
|---|---|---|---|---|
| GSE | Begins in the hypoglossal nucleus | Innervates the genioglossus, hyoglossus, and styloglossus mm. and the intrinsic mm. of the tongue | The GSE fibers are responsible for innervating the major portion of the tongue musculature | Lesions of the hypoglossal n. cause the tongue to deviate to the side of the lesion on protrusion |

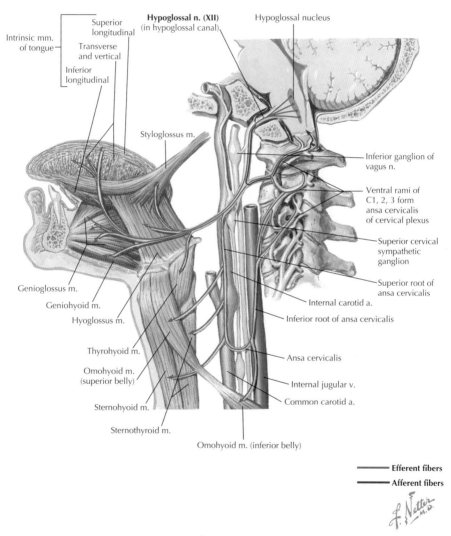

Figure 3-30

- The accessory nerve provides motor innervation to the sternocleidomastoid and trapezius muscles
- The accessory nerve courses close to the superficial cervical lymph nodes
  - This course makes it vulnerable to damage during biopsy or radical neck dissection in the posterior triangle
  - Damage to the accessory nerve also may result from a carotid endarterectomy
- In lesions located in the posterior triangle, the sternocleidomastoid muscle is unaffected, but the trapezius muscle is deinnervated
  - The shoulder droops, with mild winging of the scapula
  - Abduction of the arm also is affected when patient attempts to raise it above the horizontal plane

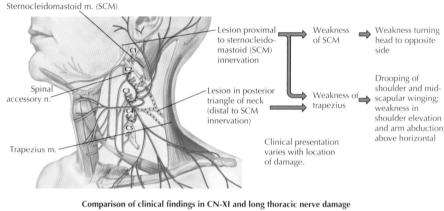

Sternocleidomastoid m. (SCM)

Spinal accessory n.

Trapezius m.

Lesion proximal to sternocleido-mastoid (SCM) innervation → Weakness of SCM → Weakness turning head to opposite side

Lesion in posterior triangle of neck (distal to SCM innervation) → Weakness of trapezius → Drooping of shoulder and mid-scapular winging; weakness in shoulder elevation and arm abduction above horizontal

Clinical presentation varies with location of damage.

**Comparison of clinical findings in CN-XI and long thoracic nerve damage**

**Spinal accessory nerve**

Upper trapezius atrophy

Spinal accessory nerve palsy

Drooping of scapula

Spinal accessory n. (CN-XI)

Trapezius m.

Scapula

Atrophy of the trapezius demonstrates loss of the contour of the neck and prominence of the rhomboids as well as drooping of the scapula.

*f. Netter M.D.*

with   JOHN A. CRAIG—AD

*Jauman* CMI   *K. marggn*

**Figure 3-31**

- The hypoglossal nerve provides motor innervation to a majority of the muscles of the tongue, including:
  - Genioglossus
  - Hyoglossus
  - Styloglossus
- Protrusion of the tongue is accomplished by the bilateral actions of the genioglossus muscles
- Paralysis of a genioglossus muscle causes the protruded tongue to deviate to the paralyzed side
- Paralysis of the hypoglossal nerve can be caused by:
  - Tumors
  - Neck trauma
  - Radiation therapy
- A similar paralysis can be caused by a stroke affecting the upper motor neurons on the side contralateral to the paralyzed muscles, owing to the crossing fibers of the upper motor neurons

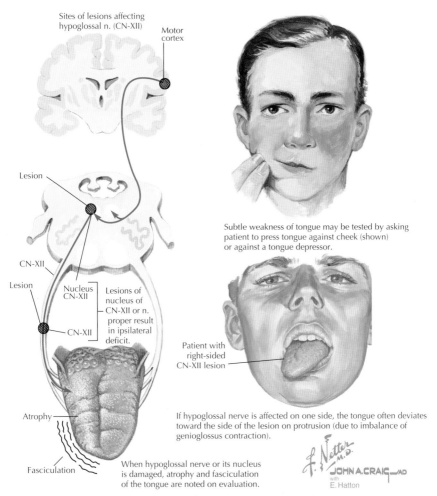

Sites of lesions affecting hypoglossal n. (CN-XII)

Motor cortex

Lesion

CN-XII

Lesion

Nucleus CN-XII

Lesions of nucleus of CN-XII or n. proper result in ipsilateral deficit.

CN-XII

Atrophy

Fasciculation

Subtle weakness of tongue may be tested by asking patient to press tongue against cheek (shown) or against a tongue depressor.

Patient with right-sided CN-XII lesion

If hypoglossal nerve is affected on one side, the tongue often deviates toward the side of the lesion on protrusion (due to imbalance of genioglossus contraction).

When hypoglossal nerve or its nucleus is damaged, atrophy and fasciculation of the tongue are noted on evaluation.

JOHN A. CRAIG—AD
with
E. Hatton

**Figure 3-32**

- The *neck* is the area between the base of the skull and inferior border of the mandible and the superior thoracic aperture
- The anterior portion of the neck contains the major visceral structures between the head and the thorax:
  - Pharynx
  - Larynx
  - Trachea
  - Esophagus
  - Thyroid and parathyroid glands
- For descriptive purposes, the neck is divided into 2 triangles:
  - Anterior triangle
  - Posterior triangle
- Skin is the most superficial structure covering the neck

FASCIA

- The neck is surrounded by 2 main layers of cervical fascia that can be further subdivided:
  - Superficial cervical fascia
  - Deep cervical fascia
    - Superficial layer of deep cervical fascia (also known as the investing layer)
    - Middle layer of deep cervical fascia (includes muscular and visceral parts such as the pretracheal)
    - Deep layer of deep cervical fascia (includes prevertebral and alar)
    - Carotid sheath (formed by other layers of deep cervical fascia)
- The contents of the superficial cervical fascia will vary depending upon location but include:
- Platysma (and cervical branch of facial nerve that innervate the muscle)
- Cutaneous nerves of the cervical plexus:
  - Lesser occipital
  - Great auricular
  - Transverse cervical (largest sensory contribution)
  - Supraclavicular
- Deep to the superficial cervical fascia is the investing (or superficial) layer of deep cervical fascia
- The superficial (or investing) layer of deep cervical fascia attaches posteriorly along the midline and passes anteriorly to surround the entire neck
- The superficial (or investing) layer of deep cervical fascia surrounds these muscles:
  - Trapezius
  - Sternocleidomastoid

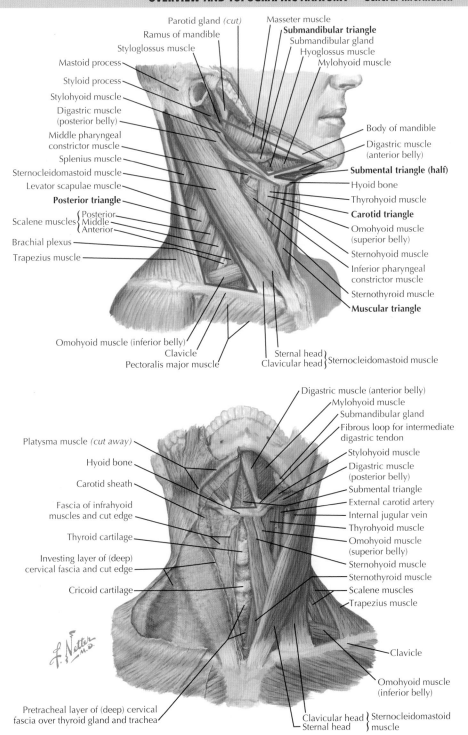

Parotid gland *(cut)*
Ramus of mandible
Styloglossus muscle
Mastoid process
Styloid process
Stylohyoid muscle
Digastric muscle (posterior belly)
Middle pharyngeal constrictor muscle
Splenius muscle
Sternocleidomastoid muscle
Levator scapulae muscle
**Posterior triangle**
Scalene muscles { Posterior, Middle, Anterior
Brachial plexus
Trapezius muscle

Masseter muscle
**Submandibular triangle**
Submandibular gland
Hyoglossus muscle
Mylohyoid muscle

Body of mandible
Digastric muscle (anterior belly)
**Submental triangle (half)**
Hyoid bone
Thyrohyoid muscle
**Carotid triangle**
Omohyoid muscle (superior belly)
Sternohyoid muscle
Inferior pharyngeal constrictor muscle
Sternothyroid muscle
**Muscular triangle**

Omohyoid muscle (inferior belly)
Clavicle
Pectoralis major muscle

Sternal head }
Clavicular head } Sternocleidomastoid muscle

Platysma muscle *(cut away)*
Hyoid bone
Carotid sheath
Fascia of infrahyoid muscles and cut edge
Thyroid cartilage
Investing layer of (deep) cervical fascia and cut edge
Cricoid cartilage

Digastric muscle (anterior belly)
Mylohyoid muscle
Submandibular gland
Fibrous loop for intermediate digastric tendon
Stylohyoid muscle
Digastric muscle (posterior belly)
Submental triangle
External carotid artery
Internal jugular vein
Thyrohyoid muscle
Omohyoid muscle (superior belly)
Sternohyoid muscle
Sternothyroid muscle
Scalene muscles
Trapezius muscle

Clavicle
Omohyoid muscle (inferior belly)

Pretracheal layer of (deep) cervical fascia over thyroid gland and trachea

Clavicular head } Sternocleidomastoid
Sternal head } muscle

**Figure 4-1**

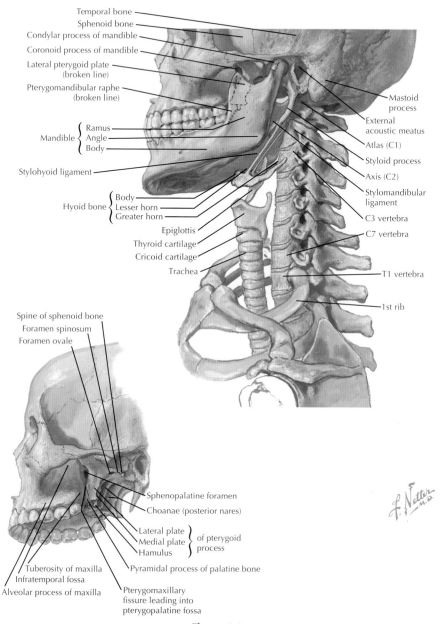

Temporal bone
Sphenoid bone
Condylar process of mandible
Coronoid process of mandible
Lateral pterygoid plate
(broken line)
Pterygomandibular raphe
(broken line)

Mandible { Ramus / Angle / Body

Stylohyoid ligament

Hyoid bone { Body / Lesser horn / Greater horn

Epiglottis
Thyroid cartilage
Cricoid cartilage
Trachea

Mastoid process
External acoustic meatus
Atlas (C1)
Styloid process
Axis (C2)
Stylomandibular ligament
C3 vertebra
C7 vertebra

T1 vertebra

1st rib

Spine of sphenoid bone
Foramen spinosum
Foramen ovale

Sphenopalatine foramen
Choanae (posterior nares)

Lateral plate }
Medial plate } of pterygoid
Hamulus } process

Pyramidal process of palatine bone

Tuberosity of maxilla
Infratemporal fossa
Alveolar process of maxilla

Pterygomaxillary
fissure leading into
pterygopalatine fossa

**Figure 4-2**

- Borders of the anterior triangle:
  - Anterior border of the sternocleidomastoid
  - Inferior border of the mandible (including a line from the angle of the mandible to the mastoid process)
  - Midline of the neck (continuous from the mandible to the suprasternal notch)
- Using the hyoid as a keystone, the omohyoid and digastric muscles subdivide the anterior triangle into:
  - Submental triangle
  - Submandibular triangle
  - Carotid triangle
  - Muscular triangle
- All of the triangles within the anterior triangle are paired except for the submental triangle, which spans the right and the left sides of the neck
- Hyoid bone divides the anterior triangle into 2 areas: suprahyoid and infrahyoid regions
- The *suprahyoid* region contains 4 muscles:
  - Mylohyoid
  - Digastric
  - Stylohyoid
  - Geniohyoid
- The *infrahyoid* region contains 4 muscles commonly called strap muscles:
  - Omohyoid
  - Sternohyoid
  - Sternothyroid
  - Thyrohyoid

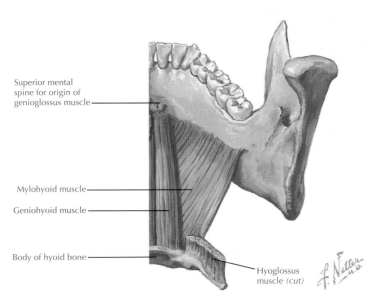

Superior mental spine for origin of genioglossus muscle

Mylohyoid muscle

Geniohyoid muscle

Body of hyoid bone

Hyoglossus muscle *(cut)*

**Figure 4-3**

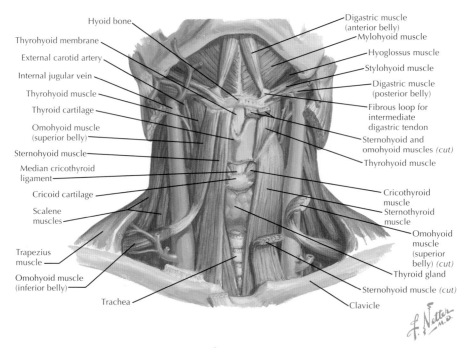

Hyoid bone

Thyrohyoid membrane

External carotid artery

Internal jugular vein

Thyrohyoid muscle

Thyroid cartilage

Omohyoid muscle
(superior belly)

Sternohyoid muscle

Median cricothyroid
ligament

Cricoid cartilage

Scalene
muscles

Trapezius
muscle

Omohyoid muscle
(inferior belly)

Trachea

Digastric muscle
(anterior belly)

Mylohyoid muscle

Hyoglossus muscle

Stylohyoid muscle

Digastric muscle
(posterior belly)

Fibrous loop for
intermediate
digastric tendon

Sternohyoid and
omohyoid muscles *(cut)*

Thyrohyoid muscle

Cricothyroid
muscle

Sternothyroid
muscle

Omohyoid
muscle
(superior
belly) *(cut)*

Thyroid gland

Sternohyoid muscle *(cut)*

Clavicle

**Figure 4-4**

- Borders of the submental triangle:
  - Body of hyoid
  - Anterior digastric on right
  - Anterior digastric on left
- Floor of the triangle is composed of the:
  - Mylohyoid
- Roof is made of the:
  - Skin
  - Superficial cervical fascia with platysma
  - Deep cervical fascia
- Submental triangle is unpaired

| MAJOR CONTENTS OF THE SUBMENTAL TRIANGLE | | | |
|---|---|---|---|
| **Artery** | **Vein** | **Nerve** | **Structures** |
| | Anterior jugular | | Submental lymph nodes |

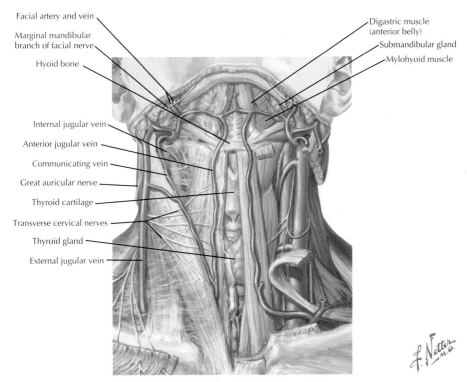

**Figure 4-5**

- Often called the digastric triangle
- Borders of the submandibular triangle:
  - Inferior border of the mandible (including a line from the angle of the mandible to the mastoid process)
  - Posterior digastric
  - Anterior digastric
- Floor of the triangle is composed of the:
  - Hyoglossus
  - Mylohyoid
  - Middle constrictor
- Roof is made of the:
  - Skin
  - Superficial cervical fascia with platysma
  - Deep cervical fascia
- Submandibular triangle is paired
- There are 3 clinically significant triangles found within the submandibular triangle:
  - Lesser's triangle
  - Pirogoff's triangle
  - Beclard's triangle
- All 3 triangles are small subdivision of the submandibular triangle, which aids in identifying the hypoglossal nerve (which lies superficial to the hyoglossus) and the lingual artery (which lies deep to the hyoglossus) which may be important for ligation during hemorrhage or surgery

## LESSER'S TRIANGLE

- Boundaries of Lesser's triangle:
  - Hypoglossal nerve
  - Anterior digastric
  - Posterior digastric

## PIROGOV'S TRIANGLE

- Boundaries of Pirogov's triangle:
  - Hypoglossal nerve
  - Intermediate tendon of the digastric
  - Mylohyoid (posterior border)

## BECLARD'S TRIANGLE

- Boundaries of Beclard's triangle:
  - Greater cornu of the hyoid
  - Posterior digastric
  - Hyoglossus (posterior border)

| MAJOR CONTENTS OF THE SUBMANDIBULAR TRIANGLE | | | |
|---|---|---|---|
| **Arteries** | **Veins** | **Nerves** | **Structures** |
| Facial | Facial | Mylohyoid | Submandibular gland |
| Submental | Submental | Hypoglossal | Submandibular lymph nodes |
| Lingual | Lingual | Lingual (hidden deep to deep portion of the submandibular gland) | Inferior portion of the parotid gland |
| | | Facial (branches of marginal mandibular and cervical) | |

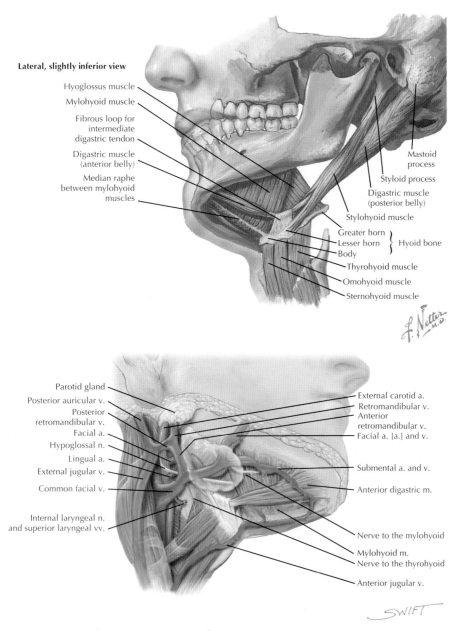

Lateral, slightly inferior view

Hyoglossus muscle
Mylohyoid muscle
Fibrous loop for intermediate digastric tendon
Digastric muscle (anterior belly)
Median raphe between mylohyoid muscles

Mastoid process
Styloid process
Digastric muscle (posterior belly)
Stylohyoid muscle
Greater horn ⎱
Lesser horn ⎰ Hyoid bone
Body ⎰
Thyrohyoid muscle
Omohyoid muscle
Sternohyoid muscle

Parotid gland
Posterior auricular v.
Posterior retromandibular v.
Facial a.
Hypoglossal n.
Lingual a.
External jugular v.
Common facial v.
Internal laryngeal n. and superior laryngeal vv.

External carotid a.
Retromandibular v.
Anterior retromandibular v.
Facial a. [a.] and v.
Submental a. and v.
Anterior digastric m.
Nerve to the mylohyoid
Mylohyoid m.
Nerve to the thyrohyoid
Anterior jugular v.

**Figure 4-6**

- Named because parts of all 3 carotid arteries are located within it
- Borders of the carotid triangle:
  - Anterior border of the sternocleidomastoid
  - Posterior digastric
  - Superior omohyoid
- Floor of the triangle is composed of the:
  - Hyoglossus
  - Thyrohyoid
  - Middle constrictor
  - Inferior constrictor
- Roof is made of the:
  - Skin
  - Superficial fascia with platysma
  - Deep cervical fascia
- Carotid triangle is paired

| MAJOR CONTENTS OF THE CAROTID TRIANGLE | | | |
|---|---|---|---|
| **Arteries** | **Veins** | **Nerves** | **Structures** |
| Common carotid (with carotid body)<br>• Internal carotid (with carotid sinus)<br>• External carotid<br>  • Superior thyroid (with superior laryngeal branch)<br>  • Lingual<br>  • Facial<br>  • Ascending pharyngeal<br>  • Occipital | Internal jugular<br>Common facial<br>Lingual<br>Superior thyroid<br>Middle thyroid | Vagus<br>• External laryngeal<br>• Internal laryngeal<br>Accessory (small portion)<br>Hypoglossal<br>Ansa cervicalis (superior limb)<br>Sympathetic trunk | Larynx (small portion)<br>Thyroid (small portion)<br>Lymph nodes |

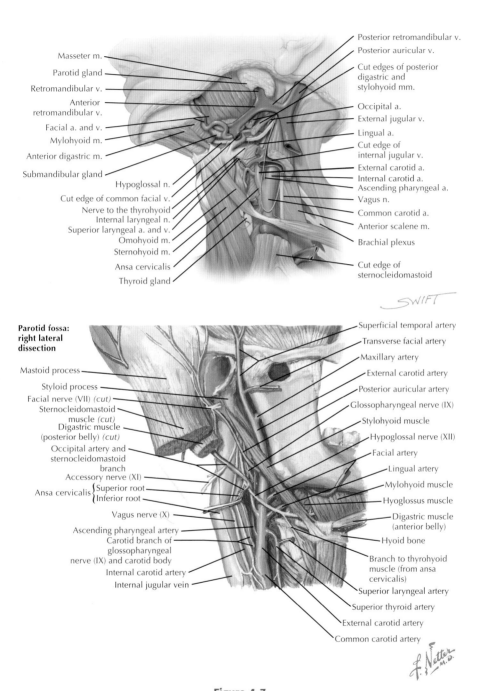

Masseter m.
Parotid gland
Retromandibular v.
Anterior retromandibular v.
Facial a. and v.
Mylohyoid m.
Anterior digastric m.
Submandibular gland
Hypoglossal n.
Cut edge of common facial v.
Nerve to the thyrohyoid
Internal laryngeal n.
Superior laryngeal a. and v.
Omohyoid m.
Sternohyoid m.
Ansa cervicalis
Thyroid gland

Posterior retromandibular v.
Posterior auricular v.
Cut edges of posterior digastric and stylohyoid mm.
Occipital a.
External jugular v.
Lingual a.
Cut edge of internal jugular v.
External carotid a.
Internal carotid a.
Ascending pharyngeal a.
Vagus n.
Common carotid a.
Anterior scalene m.
Brachial plexus
Cut edge of sternocleidomastoid

SWIFT

**Parotid fossa: right lateral dissection**

Mastoid process
Styloid process
Facial nerve (VII) *(cut)*
Sternocleidomastoid muscle *(cut)*
Digastric muscle (posterior belly) *(cut)*
Occipital artery and sternocleidomastoid branch
Accessory nerve (XI)
Ansa cervicalis { Superior root
Inferior root
Vagus nerve (X)
Ascending pharyngeal artery
Carotid branch of glossopharyngeal nerve (IX) and carotid body
Internal carotid artery
Internal jugular vein

Superficial temporal artery
Transverse facial artery
Maxillary artery
External carotid artery
Posterior auricular artery
Glossopharyngeal nerve (IX)
Stylohyoid muscle
Hypoglossal nerve (XII)
Facial artery
Lingual artery
Mylohyoid muscle
Hyoglossus muscle
Digastric muscle (anterior belly)
Hyoid bone
Branch to thyrohyoid muscle (from ansa cervicalis)
Superior laryngeal artery
Superior thyroid artery
External carotid artery
Common carotid artery

**Figure 4-7**

- Borders of the muscular triangle:
  - Anterior border of the sternocleidomastoid
  - Superior omohyoid
  - Midline
- Floor of the triangle is composed of the:
  - Sternohyoid
  - Sternothyroid
- Roof is made of the:
  - Skin
  - Superficial fascia with platysma
  - Deep cervical fascia
- Muscular triangle is paired

| MAJOR CONTENTS OF THE MUSCULAR TRIANGLE | | | |
|---|---|---|---|
| **Artery** | **Veins** | **Nerve** | **Structures** |
| Superior thyroid | Superior thyroid<br>Inferior thyroid<br>Anterior jugular | Ansa cervicalis | Strap muscles:<br>• Sternohyoid<br>• Sternothyroid<br>• Thyrohyoid<br>Thyroid gland<br>Parathyroid glands<br>Larynx<br>Trachea<br>Esophagus<br>Lymph nodes |

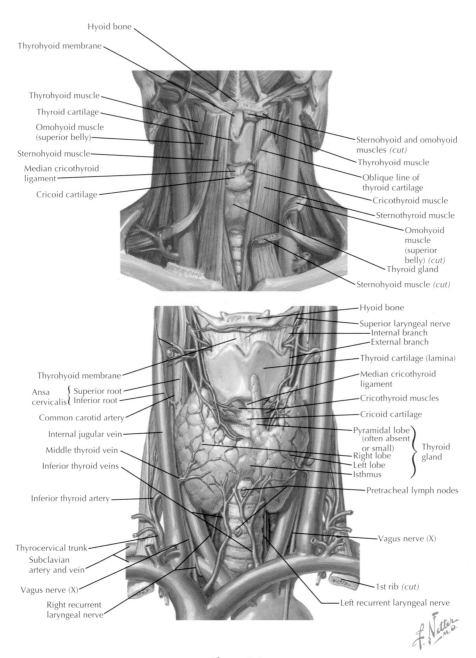

Hyoid bone

Thyrohyoid membrane

Thyrohyoid muscle

Thyroid cartilage

Omohyoid muscle
(superior belly)

Sternohyoid muscle

Median cricothyroid
ligament

Cricoid cartilage

Sternohyoid and omohyoid
muscles *(cut)*

Thyrohyoid muscle

Oblique line of
thyroid cartilage

Cricothyroid muscle

Sternothyroid muscle

Omohyoid
muscle
(superior
belly) *(cut)*

Thyroid gland

Sternohyoid muscle *(cut)*

Hyoid bone

Superior laryngeal nerve
Internal branch
External branch

Thyroid cartilage (lamina)

Median cricothyroid
ligament

Cricothyroid muscles

Cricoid cartilage

Thyrohyoid membrane

Ansa { Superior root
cervicalis { Inferior root

Common carotid artery

Internal jugular vein

Middle thyroid vein

Inferior thyroid veins

Inferior thyroid artery

Pyramidal lobe
(often absent
or small)         } Thyroid
Right lobe        } gland
Left lobe
Isthmus

Pretracheal lymph nodes

Vagus nerve (X)

Thyrocervical trunk
Subclavian
artery and vein

Vagus nerve (X)

Right recurrent
laryngeal nerve

1st rib *(cut)*

Left recurrent laryngeal nerve

**Figure 4-8**

- Borders of the posterior triangle:
  - Posterior border of the sternocleidomastoid
  - Middle third of the clavicle
  - Anterior border of the trapezius
- Located on the lateral side of the neck and spirals around the neck
- Is subdivided into 2 triangles by the omohyoid:
  - Omoclavicular (also called the supraclavicular triangle)
  - Occipital
- Roof of the posterior triangle includes:
  - Skin
  - Superficial fascia with platysma
  - Superficial (investing) layer of deep cervical fascia
- Floor of the posterior triangle includes:*
  - Semispinalis capitis (at apex)
  - Splenius capitis
  - Levator scapulae
  - Posterior scalene
  - Middle scalene
  - Anterior scalene
- Posterior triangle is paired

*These muscles are covered by the prevertebral layer of deep cervical fascia.

| MAJOR CONTENTS OF THE POSTERIOR TRIANGLE | | | |
|---|---|---|---|
| **Arteries** | **Veins** | **Nerves** | **Structures** |
| 3rd part of the subclavian<br>Occipital (occasionally)<br>Suprascapular<br>Transverse cervical<br>Dorsal scapular (usually) | External jugular (terminal part)<br>Occipital (occasionally)<br>Suprascapular<br>Transverse cervical | Cervical plexus<br>  (sensory branches):<br>• Lesser occipital<br>• Transverse cervical<br>• Great auricular<br>• Supraclavicular<br>Accessory<br>Rami and trunks of<br>  brachial plexus<br>• Dorsal scapular<br>• Long thoracic<br>• Suprascapular<br>Phrenic | Lymph nodes |

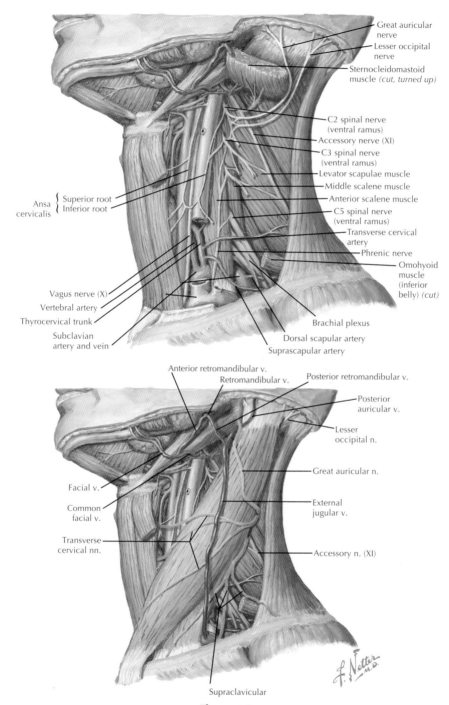

Great auricular
nerve

Lesser occipital
nerve

Sternocleidomastoid
muscle *(cut, turned up)*

C2 spinal nerve
(ventral ramus)

Accessory nerve (XI)

C3 spinal nerve
(ventral ramus)

Levator scapulae muscle

Middle scalene muscle

Anterior scalene muscle

C5 spinal nerve
(ventral ramus)

Transverse cervical
artery

Phrenic nerve

Omohyoid
muscle
(inferior
belly) *(cut)*

Ansa
cervicalis { Superior root
Inferior root

Vagus nerve (X)

Vertebral artery

Thyrocervical trunk

Subclavian
artery and vein

Brachial plexus

Dorsal scapular artery

Suprascapular artery

Anterior retromandibular v.

Retromandibular v.

Posterior retromandibular v.

Posterior
auricular v.

Lesser
occipital n.

Great auricular n.

Facial v.

Common
facial v.

Transverse
cervical nn.

External
jugular v.

Accessory n. (XI)

Supraclavicular

**Figure 4-9**

- Borders of the suboccipital triangle:
  - Obliquus capitis superior
  - Obliquus capitis inferior
  - Rectus capitis posterior major
- Roof of the suboccipital triangle includes:
  - Dense connective tissue
- Floor of the suboccipital triangle includes:
  - Posterior atlanto-occipital membrane
  - Posterior arch of the atlas
- Suboccipital triangle is paired

## VERTEBRAL ARTERIES

- These vessels enter the foramen transversarium of the 6th cervical vertebra, emerging above the 1st cervical vertebra to enter the suboccipital triangle
- They curve medially to lie in a groove on the posterior arch of the atlas
- Pass through the posterior atlanto-occipital membrane to enter the vertebral canal

| MAJOR CONTENTS OF THE SUBOCCIPITAL TRIANGLE | | | |
|---|---|---|---|
| **Artery** | **Vein** | **Nerves** | **Structures** |
| Vertebral | Vertebral (formed by tributaries of the internal vertebral venous plexus) Suboccipital plexus | Greater occipital Suboccipital | Muscles: • Rectus capitis posterior major • Rectus capitis posterior minor • Obliquus capitis superior • Obliquus capitis inferior |

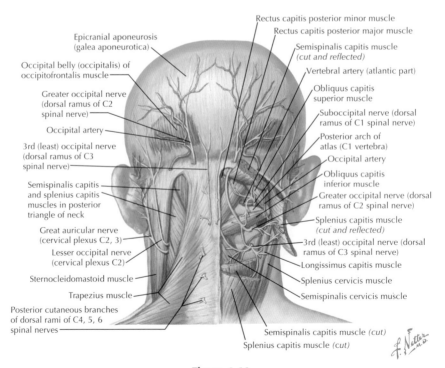

Figure 4-10

THYROID GLAND

- Highly vascular organ located on the anterior and lateral surfaces of the neck
- Formed by a right and a left lobe connected in the midline by an isthmus
- Lies roughly at a level between the 5th cervical and the 1st thoracic vertebrae
- The isthmus crosses at the 2nd and 3rd tracheal rings
- A pyramidal lobe often arises from the isthmus and extends superiorly
- Arterial supply arises from the superior and inferior thyroid arteries, with the major portion from the inferior thyroid artery
- A thyroidea ima vessel may supply the thyroid gland and arises from the brachiocephalic artery or as a direct branch from the aorta
- Venous drainage forms from a plexus on the surface of the thyroid gland that drains into the superior, middle, and inferior thyroid veins
- Microscopically, the thyroid is made of:
  - Thyroid follicular cells (which secrete thyroxine and triiodothyronine)
  - Parafollicular or C cells (which secrete calcitonin and develop from the 4th pharyngeal pouch)

PARATHYROID GLANDS

- Parathyroid glands normally are 4 small endocrine glands located on the posterior surface of the thyroid lobes
- Main role is to regulate calcium levels in the body
- The superior parathyroids are supplied by the superior thyroid artery and the inferior parathyroids are supplied by the inferior thyroid artery
- Microscopically, their cells are organized in cords
- There are 2 major cell types in the parathyroid gland:
  - Chief cells (which secrete parathyroid hormone)
  - Oxyphil cells
- Developed from the 3rd (inferior parathyroid) and 4th (superior parathyroid) pharyngeal pouches, which alter their final position through migration

LARYNX (refer to Chapter 16 on the Larynx for more information)

- Connection between the pharynx and the trachea
- Prevents foreign bodies from entering the airways
- Designed for the production of sound (phonation)
- Shorter in women and children
- Formed by 9 cartilages: 3 paired and 3 unpaired
- Located in the midline opposite the 3rd to 6th cervical vertebrae

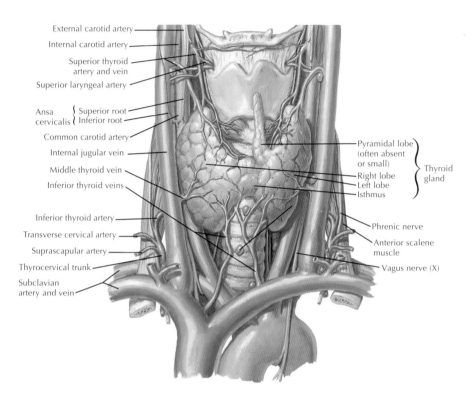

External carotid artery

Internal carotid artery

Superior thyroid
artery and vein

Superior laryngeal artery

Ansa { Superior root
cervicalis { Inferior root

Common carotid artery

Internal jugular vein

Middle thyroid vein

Inferior thyroid veins

Inferior thyroid artery

Transverse cervical artery

Suprascapular artery

Thyrocervical trunk

Subclavian
artery and vein

Pyramidal lobe
(often absent
or small)

Right lobe
Left lobe
Isthmus

} Thyroid
gland

Phrenic nerve

Anterior scalene
muscle

Vagus nerve (X)

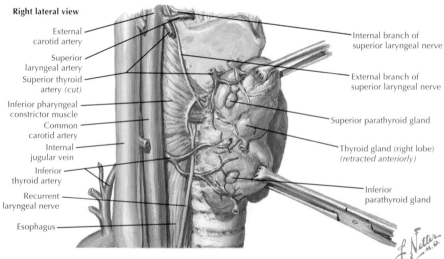

**Right lateral view**

External
carotid artery

Superior
laryngeal artery

Superior thyroid
artery *(cut)*

Inferior pharyngeal
constrictor muscle

Common
carotid artery

Internal
jugular vein

Inferior
thyroid artery

Recurrent
laryngeal nerve

Esophagus

Internal branch of
superior laryngeal nerve

External branch of
superior laryngeal nerve

Superior parathyroid gland

Thyroid gland (right lobe)
*(retracted anteriorly)*

Inferior
parathyroid gland

**Figure 4-11**

- Root of the neck connects the structures of the neck with the thoracic cavity
- The superior thoracic aperture is bounded by:
  - Manubrium
  - 1st rib and cartilage
  - 1st thoracic vertebra
- The apex of each lung extends into the root of the neck on the lateral side of the superior thoracic aperture

| MAJOR CONTENTS OF THE ROOT OF THE NECK | | | |
|---|---|---|---|
| **Arteries** | **Veins** | **Nerves** | **Structures** |
| Common carotid | Internal jugular | Vagus | Trachea |
| Subclavian | Subclavian | Recurrent laryngeal | Esophagus |
| Vertebral | Brachiocephalic | Phrenic | Thoracic duct |
| Thyrocervical trunk | Inferior thyroid | Sympathetic trunk | Right lymphatic duct |
| • Inferior thyroid | Vertebral | Brachial plexus | Lymph nodes |
| • Transverse cervical | | | |
| • Suprascapular | | | |
| • Ascending cervical | | | |

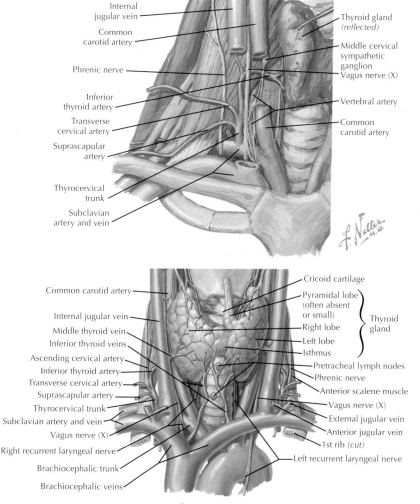

**Right anterior dissection**

Internal jugular vein

Common carotid artery

Phrenic nerve

Inferior thyroid artery

Transverse cervical artery

Suprascapular artery

Thyrocervical trunk

Subclavian artery and vein

Thyroid gland (reflected)

Middle cervical sympathetic ganglion

Vagus nerve (X)

Vertebral artery

Common carotid artery

Common carotid artery

Internal jugular vein

Middle thyroid vein

Inferior thyroid veins

Ascending cervical artery

Inferior thyroid artery

Transverse cervical artery

Suprascapular artery

Thyrocervical trunk

Subclavian artery and vein

Vagus nerve (X)

Right recurrent laryngeal nerve

Brachiocephalic trunk

Brachiocephalic veins

Cricoid cartilage

Pyramidal lobe (often absent or small)

Right lobe

Left lobe

Isthmus

} Thyroid gland

Pretracheal lymph nodes

Phrenic nerve

Anterior scalene muscle

Vagus nerve (X)

External jugular vein

Anterior jugular vein

1st rib (cut)

Left recurrent laryngeal nerve

**Figure 4-12**

## Major Borders of the Triangles

| Muscle | Origin | Insertion | Actions | Nerve Supply |
|---|---|---|---|---|
| Trapezius | External occipital protuberance<br>Superior nuchal line<br>Ligamentum nuchae<br>Spinous process of C7<br>Spinous processes of T1 to T12 | Spine of the scapula<br>Acromion<br>Lateral 1/3 of the clavicle | Elevate the scapula<br>Retract the scapula<br>Depress the scapula | Accessory n. also receives some branches from C3 and C4, thought to be proprioceptive |
| Sternocleidomastoid | Manubrium<br>Medial 1/3 of the clavicle | Mastoid process of the temporal bone<br>Superior nuchal line | Unilaterally:<br>• Face turns to contralateral side<br>• Head tilts to ipsilateral side<br>Bilaterally:<br>• Head is flexed | Accessory n. |

## Muscles That Subdivide the Triangles

| Muscle | Origin | Insertion | Actions | Nerve Supply |
|---|---|---|---|---|
| Digastric (posterior and anterior bellies connected by a tendon attached to the hyoid) | Mastoid process | Digastric fossa of the mandible | Elevates hyoid<br>Helps depress and retract the mandible | Facial n. (posterior belly)<br>Trigeminal n. (anterior belly) |
| Omohyoid (superior and inferior bellies connected by a tendon) | Superior border of the scapula | Body of the hyoid | Depresses the hyoid<br>Helps depress the larynx | Ansa cervicalis |

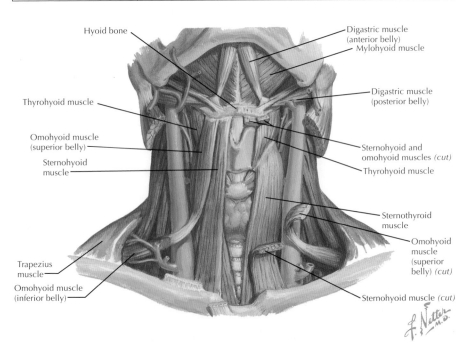

**Figure 4-13**

### Suprahyoid Muscles

| Muscle | Origin | Insertion | Actions | Nerve Supply |
|---|---|---|---|---|
| Stylohyoid | Styloid process | Body of the hyoid | Elevates the hyoid<br>Retracts the hyoid | Facial n. |
| Mylohyoid | Mylohyoid line of the mandible | Mylohyoid of opposite side at the raphe<br>Body of the hyoid | Elevates the hyoid<br>Elevates the floor of the oral cavity | Trigeminal n. (mandibular division) |
| Digastric (posterior and anterior bellies connected by a tendon attached to the hyoid) | Mastoid process | Digastric fossa of the mandible | Elevates hyoid<br>Helps depress and retract the mandible | Facial n. (posterior belly)<br>Trigeminal n. (anterior belly—mandibular division) |
| Geniohyoid | Inferior genial tubercle | Body of the hyoid | Helps move the hyoid and tongue anteriorly | C1 (ventral ramus, which follows the hypoglossal n.) |

### Infrahyoid Muscles

| Muscle | Origin | Insertion | Actions | Nerve Supply |
|---|---|---|---|---|
| Omohyoid (superior and inferior bellies connected by a tendon) | Superior border of the scapula | Body of the hyoid | Depresses the hyoid | Ansa cervicalis |
| Sternohyoid | Manubrium | Body of the hyoid | Depresses the hyoid | |
| Sternothyroid | Manubrium | Oblique line of the thyroid cartilage | Depresses the larynx | |
| Thyrohyoid | Oblique line of the thyroid cartilage | Greater cornu (horn) of the hyoid | Depresses the hyoid | C1 (ventral ramus, which follows the hypoglossal n.) |

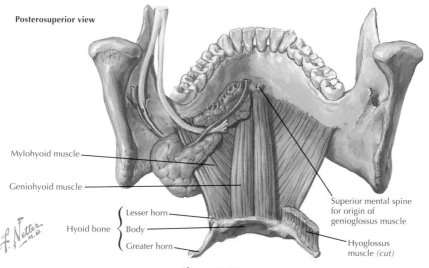

Posterosuperior view

Mylohyoid muscle

Geniohyoid muscle

Lesser horn

Hyoid bone — Body

Greater horn

Superior mental spine for origin of genioglossus muscle

Hyoglossus muscle *(cut)*

**Figure 4-14**

| Muscle | Origin | Insertion | Actions | Nerve Supply |
|---|---|---|---|---|
| Longus colli | | | Bilaterally:<br>• Flexion of neck<br>Unilaterally:<br>• Head rotates to ipsilateral side<br>• Head tilts to ipsilateral side | Ventral rami of C2 to C8 |
| *Superior oblique* | Transverse processes of C3 to C5 | Anterior arch of atlas | | |
| *Inferior oblique* | Vertebral bodies of T1 to T3 | Transverse process of C5 to C6 | | |
| *Vertical* | Vertebral bodies of C5 to C7 and T1 to T3 | Vertebral bodies of C2 to C4 | | |
| Longus capitis | Transverse processes of C3 to C6 | Basilar portion of the occipital bone | Bilaterally:<br>• Flexion of head<br>Unilaterally:<br>• Head rotates to ipsilateral side<br>• Head tilts to ipsilateral side | Ventral rami of C1 to C3 |
| Rectus capitis anterior | Lateral mass of the atlas<br><br>Transverse process of the atlas | | | Ventral rami of C1 and C2 |
| Rectus capitis lateralis | Transverse process of the atlas | Jugular portion of the occipital bone | Lateral flexion of the head | |
| Anterior scalene | Transverse processes (anterior tubercle) of C3 to C6 | Scalene tubercle on the 1st rib | Elevates 1st rib<br><br>Lateral flexion of the neck | Ventral rami of C4 to C6 |
| Middle scalene | Transverse processes (posterior tubercle) of C2 to C7 | 1st rib | Lateral flexion of the neck | Ventral rami of C5 to C8 |
| Posterior scalene | Transverse processes (posterior tubercle) of C5 to C7 | 2nd rib | | Ventral rami of C6 to C8 |

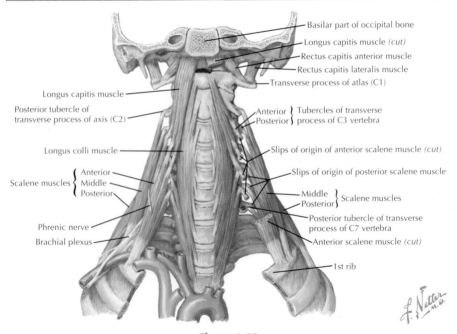

**Figure 4-15**

| Muscle | Origin | Insertion | Actions | Nerve Supply |
|--------|--------|-----------|---------|--------------|
| Obliquus capitis superior | Transverse process of the atlas | Occipital bone | Bilaterally:<br>• Extension of head<br>Unilaterally:<br>• Lateral flexion of head to ipsilateral side | Suboccipital n. (dorsal rami of C1) |
| Obliquus capitis inferior | Spinous process of the axis | Transverse process of the atlas | Rotates head to ipsilateral side | |
| Rectus capitis posterior major | | Inferior nuchal line (lateral portion) of the occipital bone | Bilaterally:<br>• Extension of head<br>Unilaterally:<br>• Head rotates to ipsilateral side | |
| Rectus capitis posterior minor | Posterior arch of the atlas | Inferior nuchal line (medial portion) of the occipital bone | Extends head | |

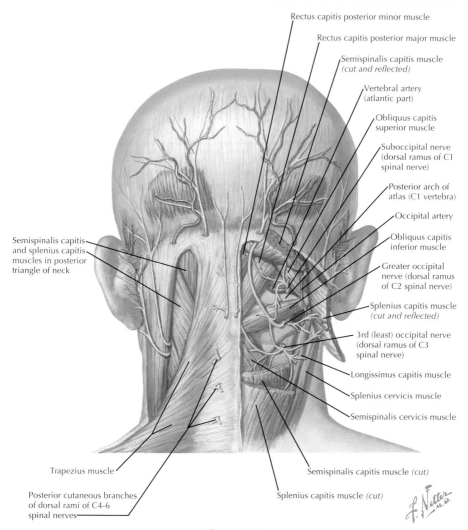

Figure 4-16

- The major arteries of the neck are the common carotid and the subclavian arteries

## SUBCLAVIAN

- Thyrocervical
- Costocervical
- Vertebral
- Dorsal scapular (usually)
- (Internal thoracic artery is located in the thorax)

## COMMON CAROTID

- Internal carotid
- External carotid
  - Superior thyroid
  - Lingual
  - Facial
  - Ascending pharyngeal
  - Occipital
- (Posterior auricular, maxillary, and superficial temporal arteries are located in the head)

| SUBCLAVIAN VASCULAR SUPPLY OF THE NECK | | |
|---|---|---|
| **Artery** | **Source** | **Comments** |
| Subclavian | Right subclavian a. is a branch of the brachiocephalic a.; left subclavian a. is a direct branch of the aorta | Both subclavian aa. travel lateral to the trachea into the root of the neck, passing between the anterior and middle scalene aa.<br>Divided into 3 parts based on its relationship to the anterior scalene m.:<br>• 1st part—extends from the beginning of the subclavian to the medial border of the anterior scalene, and all of the branches of the subclavian a. arise from the 1st part, except the left costocervical trunk, which often is a branch of the 2nd part<br>• 2nd part—located posterior to the anterior scalene<br>• 3rd part—located from the lateral margin of the anterior scalene to the lateral border of the 1st rib, where it becomes the axillary a. |
| *Thyrocervical* | A branch of the 1st part of the subclavian along the medial aspect of the anterior scalene m. | Immediately divides into 3 branches:<br>• Inferior thyroid—travels along the medial border of the anterior scalene posterior to the carotid sheath and anterior to the vertebral a. to the thyroid gland while accompanied by the recurrent laryngeal n.; it gives rise to the inferior laryngeal a. to the larynx and the ascending cervical a., which helps supply the muscles in the area and sends branches to the vertebral a.<br>• Suprascapular—travels inferior to and laterally across the anterior scalene m. and phrenic n. deep to the sternocleidomastoid m. and crosses the posterior triangle of the neck to reach the scapula, where it passes superior to the transverse lig. of the scapula<br>• Transverse cervical—travels across the posterior triangle of the neck to reach the anterior border of the trapezius m. |
| *Costocervical* | A branch of the 1st part of the right subclavian a. and the 2nd part of the left subclavian a. | Divides into 2 branches:<br>• Deep cervical—travels superiorly along the posterior part of the neck mainly to help supply the muscles<br>• Supreme intercostal—travels to supply the 1st and 2nd intercostal spaces |
| *Vertebral* | 1st part of the subclavian a. | Ascends to enter the foramen transversarium of C6<br>Passes around the atlas and then through the foramen magnum to enter the skull, where it unites with the vertebral a. from the other side to form the basilar a. along the ventral surface of the pons |
| *Dorsal scapular* | 2nd or 3rd part of the subclavian a. | Arises from the subclavian a. in about 70% to 75% of people and the transverse cervical a. in the other 25% to 30%<br>When arising from the subclavian a., it passes posteriorly between the trunks of the brachial plexus to travel across the posterior triangle of the neck to reach the anterior border of the trapezius m. |

**Right anterior dissection**

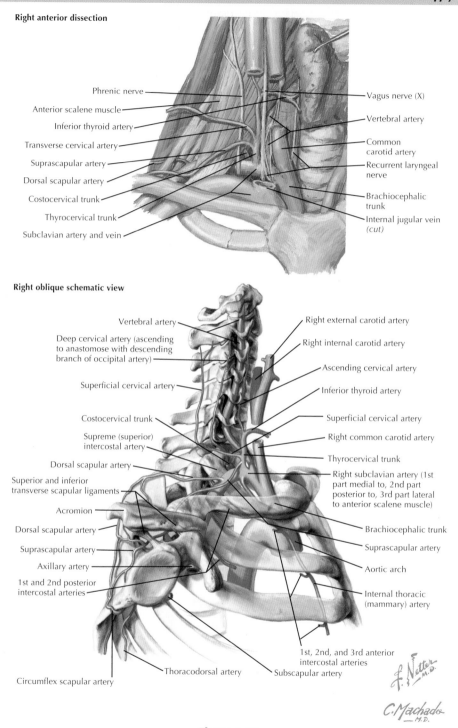

Phrenic nerve

Anterior scalene muscle

Inferior thyroid artery

Transverse cervical artery

Suprascapular artery

Dorsal scapular artery

Costocervical trunk

Thyrocervical trunk

Subclavian artery and vein

Vagus nerve (X)

Vertebral artery

Common carotid artery

Recurrent laryngeal nerve

Brachiocephalic trunk

Internal jugular vein (cut)

**Right oblique schematic view**

Vertebral artery

Deep cervical artery (ascending to anastomose with descending branch of occipital artery)

Superficial cervical artery

Costocervical trunk

Supreme (superior) intercostal artery

Dorsal scapular artery

Superior and inferior transverse scapular ligaments

Acromion

Dorsal scapular artery

Suprascapular artery

Axillary artery

1st and 2nd posterior intercostal arteries

Circumflex scapular artery

Thoracodorsal artery

Right external carotid artery

Right internal carotid artery

Ascending cervical artery

Inferior thyroid artery

Superficial cervical artery

Right common carotid artery

Thyrocervical trunk

Right subclavian artery (1st part medial to, 2nd part posterior to, 3rd part lateral to anterior scalene muscle)

Brachiocephalic trunk

Suprascapular artery

Aortic arch

Internal thoracic (mammary) artery

1st, 2nd, and 3rd anterior intercostal arteries

Subscapular artery

**Figure 4-17**

THE NECK **131**

| CAROTID VASCULAR SUPPLY OF THE NECK | | |
|---|---|---|
| **Artery** | **Source** | **Comments** |
| Common carotid | Right common carotid a. is a branch of the brachiocephalic a.; left common carotid a. is a direct branch of the aorta | Both common carotids ascend posterior to the sternoclavicular joint into the neck and bifurcate at the superior border of the thyroid cartilage at C3 into the: <br>• External carotid a. <br>• Internal carotid a. <br>There are no branches of the common carotid a. in the neck <br>*Carotid body*: <br>A chemoreceptor located along the common carotid a. <br>Usually receives its sensory innervation from the carotid branch of the glossopharyngeal n. |
| *Internal carotid* | The 2 branches of the common carotid a.; arise at the superior border of the thyroid cartilage at C3 | There are no branches of the internal carotid a. in the neck <br>Passes superiorly in the neck within the carotid sheath along with the internal jugular v. and the vagus n. anterior to the transverse processes of the upper cervical vertebrae <br>*Carotid sinus*: <br>A baroreceptor located as a dilation at the beginning of the internal carotid a. <br>Usually receives its sensory innervation from the carotid branch of the glossopharyngeal n. |
| *External carotid* | | Gives rise to a majority of the branches to the neck <br>Located external to the carotid sheath and travels anteriorly and superiorly in the neck posterior to the mandible and deep to the posterior belly of the digastric and stylohyoid mm. to enter the parotid gland |
| • *Superior thyroid* | The 1st branch of the external carotid a.; arises in the carotid triangle | Passes inferiorly along the inferior constrictor m. on its path to the thyroid gland <br>The superior laryngeal a. arises from the superior thyroid a. and passes through the thyrohyoid membrane to supply the larynx |
| • *Lingual* | External carotid a.; arises within the carotid triangle | Passes superiorly and medially toward the greater cornu of the hyoid bone in an oblique fashion and makes a loop by passing anteriorly and inferiorly while traveling superficial to the middle constrictor m. <br>While forming a loop, the artery is crossed superficially by the hypoglossal n. <br>The lingual a. passes deep to the posterior belly of the digastric and stylohyoid mm. as it travels anteriorly <br>At this region, it gives rise to a hyoid branch that travels on the superior surface of the hyoid bone supplying the muscles in the area <br>Passes deep to the hyoglossus m. and travels anteriorly between the hyoglossus and genioglossus mm. to supply the tongue |

*Continued on next page*

| | SUBCLAVIAN VASCULAR SUPPLY OF THE NECK *Continued* | |
|---|---|---|
| **Artery** | **Source** | **Comments** |
| • *Facial* | External carotid a. in the carotid triangle of the neck | Passes superiorly immediately deep to the posterior belly of the digastric and stylohyoid mm. |
| | | Passes along the submandibular gland giving rise to the submental a., which helps supply the gland |
| | | Passes superiorly over the body of the mandible at the masseter m. in a tortuous pattern to supply the face |
| • *Ascending pharyngeal* | Posterior portion of the external carotid a. near the bifurcation of the common carotid a. | The smallest branch of the external carotid |
| | | Ascends superiorly between the lateral side of the pharynx and the internal carotid a. |
| | | Has a series of branches: |
| | | 3 to 4 pharyngeal branches supply the superior and middle constrictor mm. |
| | | The most superior branch passes through the gap superior to the superior constrictor m. |
| | | Gives rise to an inferior tympanic branch, which supplies the middle ear cavity |
| | | Gives rise to a posterior meningeal branch, which supplies the bones of the posterior cranial fossa and dura mater |
| • *Occipital* | External carotid a. in the carotid triangle of the neck | Branches along the inferior margin of the posterior belly of the digastric and stylohyoid mm. |
| | | The hypoglossal n. wraps around the occipital a. from the posterior part of the vessel, traveling anteriorly |
| | | Passes posteriorly along the mastoid process, making a groove on the bone |
| | | Pierces the fascia that connects the attachment of the trapezius with the sternocleidomastoid m. |
| | | Ascends in the connective tissue layer of the scalp, dividing into many branches |
| | | Anastomoses with the posterior auricular and superficial temporal aa. |
| | | The terminal part of the artery is accompanied by the greater occipital n. |

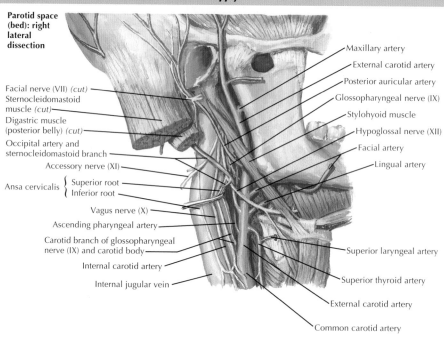

**Parotid space (bed): right lateral dissection**

Maxillary artery

External carotid artery

Posterior auricular artery

Glossopharyngeal nerve (IX)

Stylohyoid muscle

Hypoglossal nerve (XII)

Facial artery

Lingual artery

Facial nerve (VII) *(cut)*

Sternocleidomastoid muscle *(cut)*

Digastric muscle (posterior belly) *(cut)*

Occipital artery and sternocleidomastoid branch

Accessory nerve (XI)

Ansa cervicalis { Superior root / Inferior root }

Vagus nerve (X)

Ascending pharyngeal artery

Carotid branch of glossopharyngeal nerve (IX) and carotid body

Internal carotid artery

Internal jugular vein

Superior laryngeal artery

Superior thyroid artery

External carotid artery

Common carotid artery

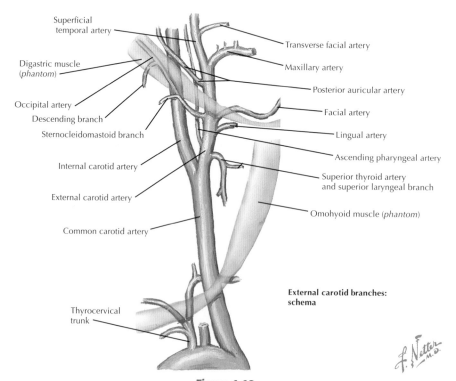

Superficial temporal artery

Transverse facial artery

Maxillary artery

Posterior auricular artery

Digastric muscle *(phantom)*

Occipital artery

Descending branch

Sternocleidomastoid branch

Facial artery

Lingual artery

Ascending pharyngeal artery

Internal carotid artery

External carotid artery

Superior thyroid artery and superior laryngeal branch

Omohyoid muscle *(phantom)*

Common carotid artery

**External carotid branches: schema**

Thyrocervical trunk

**Figure 4-18**

- Highly variable, with inconsistent drainage

## MAJOR VEINS OF THE NECK

- Internal jugular
  - Occipital
  - Common facial
    - Facial
  - Lingual
  - Pharyngeal
  - Superior thyroid
  - Middle thyroid
- Subclavian
  - Vertebral
  - External Jugular
    - Transverse cervical
    - Suprascapular
    - Anterior jugular
- Brachiocephalic
  - Inferior thyroid

| JUGULAR VASCULAR SUPPLY OF THE NECK | |
|---|---|
| **Vein** | **Comments** |
| Internal jugular | Continuous with the sigmoid sinus within the cranial cavity |
| | Begins at the base of the skull at a dilation called the superior bulb |
| | Lies posterior to the internal carotid a. and the glossopharyngeal, vagus, and spinal accessory nn. as it initially descends |
| | Travels lateral to the internal carotid a. within the carotid sheath with the vagus n. posterior to the vessels |
| | Unites with the subclavian v. to form the brachiocephalic v. at the root of the neck |
| | Receives a series of branches |
| *Occipital* | Begins on the posterior portion of the scalp at the vertex |
| | Passes from superficial to deep by passing through the attachment of the sternocleidomastoid m. |
| | Has a mastoid emissary v. that connects it to the transverse sinus |
| | The vein's termination is variable, but it usually passes inferiorly to join the internal jugular v. |
| *Common facial* | In the submandibular triangle, the facial v. joins the anterior branch of the retromandibular to form the common facial v. |
| | Common facial v. drains into the internal jugular v. |
| • *Facial* | Has no valves to allow blood to backflow |
| | Begins as the angular v. |
| | Passes inferiorly along the side of the nose, receiving the lateral nasal v. |
| | Continues in a posterior and inferior path across the angle of the mouth to the cheek, receiving the superior and inferior labial vv. |
| | While passing toward the mandible, the deep facial v. connects the facial v. to the pterygoid plexus |
| | In the submandibular triangle, the facial v. joins the anterior branch of the retromandibular to form the common facial v. |
| *Lingual* | Passes with the lingual a., deep to the hyoglossus m., and ends in the internal jugular v. |
| | The vena comitans nervi hypoglossi, or accompanying v. of the hypoglossal n., begins at the apex of the tongue and either joins the lingual v. or accompanies the hypoglossal n. and enters the common facial v., draining into the internal jugular v. |

*Continued on next page*

| JUGULAR VASCULAR SUPPLY OF THE NECK *Continued* | |
|---|---|
| **Vein** | **Comments** |
| *Pharyngeal* | Pharyngeal vv. pass from the pharyngeal plexus of vv. along the posterior portion of the pharynx<br>Drain into the internal jugular v. |
| *Superior thyroid* | Forms a venous plexus on the thyroid gland with the middle and inferior thyroid vv. before draining into the internal jugular v. |
| *Middle thyroid* | Forms a venous plexus on the thyroid gland with the superior and inferior thyroid vv. before draining into the internal jugular v. |
| External jugular | Formed by the combination of the posterior branch of the retromandibular and posterior auricular vv. in the parotid gland<br>Lies deep to the platysma m. but superficial to the sternocleidomastoid m. as it descends vertically<br>Passes into the posterior triangle of the neck, where it drains into the subclavian v. immediately lateral to the anterior scalene m. |
| *Transverse cervical* | Passes from the anterior border of the trapezius m. through the posterior triangle to drain into the external jugular v. |
| *Suprascapular* | Arises from the scapula above the transverse scapular lig. to pass through the posterior triangle of the neck to drain into the external jugular v. |
| *Anterior jugular* | Arises by the joining of a series of superficial veins in the submental region<br>Descends anterior to the sternocleidomastoid m. and passes deep to the muscle before draining into the external jugular or the subclavian |
| Brachiocephalic | The right and left brachiocephalic vv. are formed posterior to the right and left sternoclavicular joints by the merging of the internal jugular v. and subclavian v. from their respective sides<br>Both brachiocephalic vv. merge to form the superior vena cava |
| *Inferior thyroid* | Forms a venous plexus on the thyroid gland with the superior and middle thyroid vv.<br>Typically, right and left inferior thyroid vv. form and drain into the right and left brachiocephalic vv. |
| Subclavian | The continuation of the axillary v.<br>Located along the lateral border of the 1st rib until it unites with the internal jugular v.<br>Passes anterior to the anterior scalene m. |
| *Vertebral* | Begins as a plexus in the suboccipital triangle and descends through the foramen transversarium of all of the cervical vertebrae before draining into the subclavian v. or, more commonly, the brachiocephalic v. |

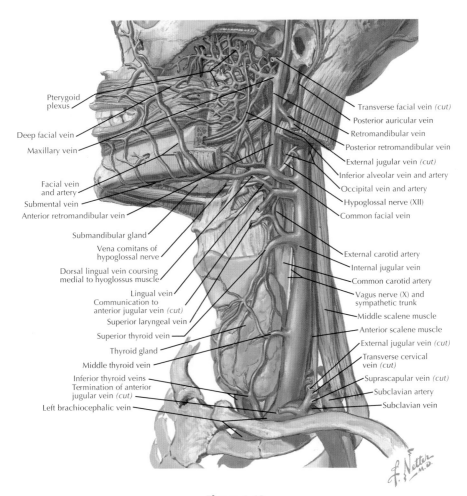

Pterygoid plexus

Deep facial vein

Maxillary vein

Facial vein and artery

Submental vein

Anterior retromandibular vein

Submandibular gland

Vena comitans of hypoglossal nerve

Dorsal lingual vein coursing medial to hyoglossus muscle

Lingual vein

Communication to anterior jugular vein *(cut)*

Superior laryngeal vein

Superior thyroid vein

Thyroid gland

Middle thyroid vein

Inferior thyroid veins

Termination of anterior jugular vein *(cut)*

Left brachiocephalic vein

Transverse facial vein *(cut)*

Posterior auricular vein

Retromandibular vein

Posterior retromandibular vein

External jugular vein *(cut)*

Inferior alveolar vein and artery

Occipital vein and artery

Hypoglossal nerve (XII)

Common facial vein

External carotid artery

Internal jugular vein

Common carotid artery

Vagus nerve (X) and sympathetic trunk

Middle scalene muscle

Anterior scalene muscle

External jugular vein *(cut)*

Transverse cervical vein *(cut)*

Suprascapular vein *(cut)*

Subclavian artery

Subclavian vein

**Figure 4-19**

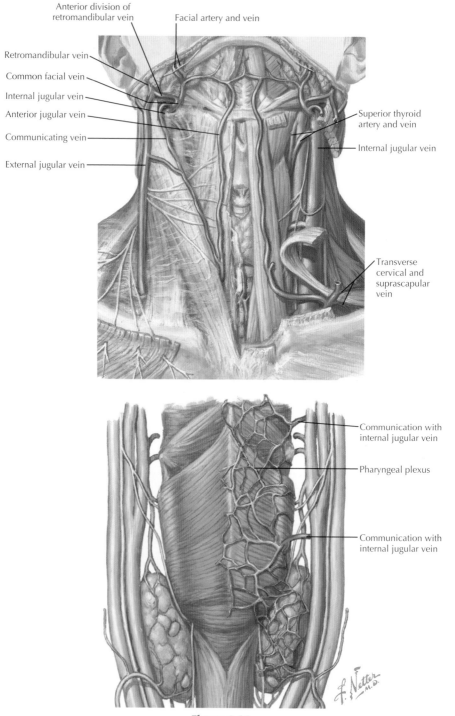

Anterior division of retromandibular vein

Facial artery and vein

Retromandibular vein

Common facial vein

Internal jugular vein

Anterior jugular vein

Communicating vein

External jugular vein

Superior thyroid artery and vein

Internal jugular vein

Transverse cervical and suprascapular vein

Communication with internal jugular vein

Pharyngeal plexus

Communication with internal jugular vein

**Figure 4-20**

- The nerve supply to the neck is extensive; it is made up of:
  - Cranial nerves
    - Glossopharyngeal
    - Vagus
    - Accessory
    - Hypoglossal
  - Cervical plexus
  - Brachial plexus
    - Dorsal scapular
    - Long thoracic
    - Suprascapular
  - Phrenic
  - Other cervical ventral rami

## Cranial Nerves of the Neck

| GLOSSOPHARYNGEAL NERVE |
|---|
| • Also known as cranial nerve IX |
| • Branches from the medulla oblongata and passes through the jugular foramen with the vagus and spinal accessory nn. |
| • Immediately after passing through the jugular foramen, it gives off the tympanic branch |
| • As the glossopharyngeal passes through the foramen, it passes between the internal carotid a. and internal jugular v. in an inferior direction |
| • Gives rise to the carotid branch that passes between the internal and external carotid aa. to the carotid body and carotid sinus |
| • The main glossopharyngeal n. continues to pass inferiorly, giving rise to the pharyngeal branch, which is the sensory nerve to the pharyngeal plexus that perforates the muscles of the pharynx and supplies the mucous membranes (mainly oropharynx region) |
| • Continues to pass inferiorly; travels posterior to the stylopharyngeus m. and innervates it |
| • Passes anteriorly with the stylopharyngeus and travels between the superior and middle constrictor mm. to be located by the palatine tonsils |
| • Small lingual branches arise from it and distribute general somatic afferent (GSA) fibers to the mucous membrane of the posterior 1/3 of the tongue, in addition to the fauces, and special visceral afferent (SVA) fibers to the taste buds |

| VAGUS NERVE |
|---|
| • Also known as cranial nerve X |
| • Branches from the medulla oblongata and passes through the jugular foramen with the glossopharyngeal and spinal accessory nn. |
| • As the vagus n. passes through the foramen, it passes between the internal carotid a. and internal jugular v. |
| • A series of nerves branch from the vagus n. as it passes from the base of the skull through the neck: auricular, pharyngeal, superior laryngeal, recurrent laryngeal, and cardiac vagal branches |

| Auricular Branch |
|---|
| • Arises from the superior ganglion, travels posterior to the internal jugular v., and passes along the temporal bone to enter the mastoid canaliculus and give branches that innervate the skin of the back of the auricle and the posterior portion of the external acoustic meatus |

| Pharyngeal Branch |
|---|
| • Arises from the upper part of the inferior ganglion of the vagus n. and serves as the motor component to the pharyngeal plexus |

| Superior Laryngeal n. |
|---|
| • Travels inferiorly posterior to the internal carotid and on the side of the pharynx, and divides into the: |
|   • Internal laryngeal n.–passes inferiorly to the larynx through the thyrohyoid membrane along with the superior laryngeal vessels to distribute the GSA fibers to the base of the tongue at the epiglottic region, and to the mucous membranes of the larynx as far inferiorly as the false vocal folds; and SVA fibers to the taste buds in the area |
|   • External laryngeal n.–travels inferiorly along the inferior constrictor to supply the cricothyroid muscle and the inferior portion of the inferior constrictor |

*Continued on next page*

| Recurrent Laryngeal n. |
|---|
| • Arises from the vagus n. differently, depending on the side of the body |
| • The right recurrent laryngeal n. loops under the right subclavian, whereas the left recurrent laryngeal n. loops under the ligamentum arteriosum posterior to the aorta |
| • Ascends on the lateral side of the trachea until reaching the pharynx where it passes deep to the inferior constrictor m. to reach the larynx, innervating the mucous membranes below the false vocal folds and all of the intrinsic muscles of the larynx except the cricothyroid |

| Cardiac Vagal Branches |
|---|
| • Descend to form the parasympathetic portion of the cardiac plexus |

| **ACCESSORY NERVE** |
|---|
| • Also known as cranial nerve XI |
| • Classically described as being formed from 2 parts: cranial and spinal |

| Cranial Part |
|---|
| • Begins in the nucleus ambiguus from the medulla as 4 to 5 branches just inferior to the roots of the vagus n. and passes laterally to the jugular foramen, where it merges with the fibers of the spinal part of the accessory n. |
| • While united for a short distance, it also is connected by 1 or 2 branches with the inferior ganglion of the vagus n. |
| • Exits through the jugular foramen, separates from the spinal part, and continues over the surface of the inferior ganglion of the vagus n. to be distributed mainly to the pharyngeal branches of the vagus to form the motor portion of the pharyngeal plexus, which innervates the muscles in the pharynx, soft palate, and 1 tongue muscle |

| Spinal Part |
|---|
| • Begins in the upper cervical levels of the spinal cord and after separating from the cranial part provides innervation to the sternocleidomastoid m. and passes obliquely through the posterior triangle of the neck to innervate the trapezius m. |

| **HYPOGLOSSAL NERVE** |
|---|
| • Also known as cranial nerve XII |
| • Arises as a series of rootlets from the medulla oblongata and passes through the hypoglossal canal |
| • Travels inferiorly, located between the internal carotid a. and the internal jugular v. |
| • Passes anteriorly as it wraps around the occipital a. inferior to the posterior belly of the digastric m. |
| • Passes superficial to the external carotid a. and the loop of the lingual a. in its anterior path |
| • Passes deep to the posterior belly of the digastric and stylohyoid mm. and lies superficial to the hyoglossus m. with the accompanying v. of the hypoglossal n. |
| • Passes deep to the mylohyoid m. and continues anterior in the genioglossus m. |
| • Gives rise to muscular branches that supply all the intrinsic tongue muscles and the hyoglossus, genioglossus, and styloglossus mm. |

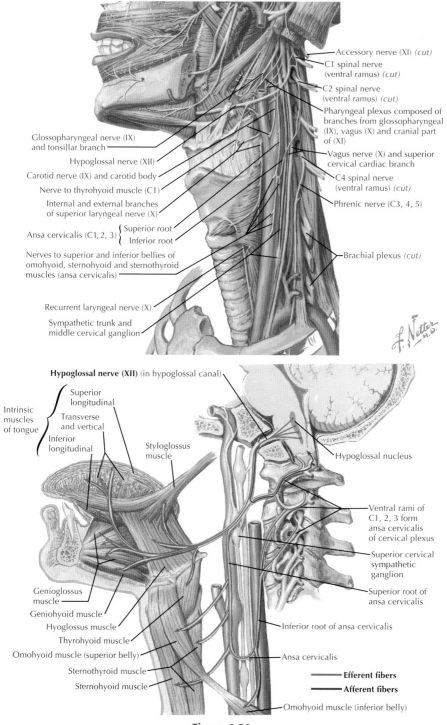

Accessory nerve (XI) *(cut)*

C1 spinal nerve (ventral ramus) *(cut)*

C2 spinal nerve (ventral ramus) *(cut)*

Pharyngeal plexus composed of branches from glossopharyngeal (IX), vagus (X) and cranial part of (XI)

Vagus nerve (X) and superior cervical cardiac branch

C4 spinal nerve (ventral ramus) *(cut)*

Phrenic nerve (C3, 4, 5)

Brachial plexus *(cut)*

Glossopharyngeal nerve (IX) and tonsillar branch

Hypoglossal nerve (XII)

Carotid nerve (IX) and carotid body

Nerve to thyrohyoid muscle (C1)

Internal and external branches of superior laryngeal nerve (X)

Ansa cervicalis (C1, 2, 3) { Superior root / Inferior root

Nerves to superior and inferior bellies of omohyoid, sternohyoid and sternothyroid muscles (ansa cervicalis)

Recurrent laryngeal nerve (X)

Sympathetic trunk and middle cervical ganglion

**Hypoglossal nerve (XII)** (in hypoglossal canal)

Intrinsic muscles of tongue { Superior longitudinal / Transverse and vertical / Inferior longitudinal

Styloglossus muscle

Hypoglossal nucleus

Ventral rami of C1, 2, 3 form ansa cervicalis of cervical plexus

Superior cervical sympathetic ganglion

Superior root of ansa cervicalis

Genioglossus muscle

Geniohyoid muscle

Hyoglossus muscle

Thyrohyoid muscle

Omohyoid muscle (superior belly)

Sternothyroid muscle

Sternohyoid muscle

Inferior root of ansa cervicalis

Ansa cervicalis

Efferent fibers

Afferent fibers

Omohyoid muscle (inferior belly)

**Figure 4-21**

- Skin of the neck receives sensory innervation from both dorsal and ventral rami
- Dorsal ramus of C1 lacks sensory fibers and does not contribute to the sensory distribution to the neck
- Dorsal rami of C6 to C8 lack sensory fibers and do not contribute to the sensory distribution to the neck
- Ventral rami provide most of the sensory innervation to the neck through the sensory branches of the cervical plexus

## CERVICAL PLEXUS

- Formed by C1 to C4 ventral rami
- Originates deep to the sternocleidomastoid
- Sensory branches pass along midpoint of the posterior border of the muscle to travel to their destinations

| VENTRAL RAMI | | |
|---|---|---|
| **Nerve** | **Source** | **Comments** |
| Lesser occipital | Cervical plexus by contributions from the ventral ramus of C2 | Passes posterior to the midpoint of the sternocleidomastoid m. <br> Ascends posterior to the sternocleidomastoid along the posterior portion of the head <br> Continues on the head posterior to the auricle supplying the skin in the region |
| Great auricular | Cervical plexus formed by contributions of ventral rami C2 and C3 | Passes posterior to the midpoint of the sternocleidomastoid m. <br> Ascends along the sternocleidomastoid, dividing into anterior and posterior branches: <br> • Anterior branch innervates the skin of the face over the parotid gland <br> • Posterior branch innervates the skin over the mastoid process, the posterior portion of the auricle, and the concha and lobule |
| Transverse cervical | | Passes posterior to the midpoint of the sternocleidomastoid m. <br> Crosses anteriorly along the sternocleidomastoid, dividing into ascending and descending branches <br> Ascending and descending branches pass through the platysma m. to supply the skin of the neck from the region between the mandible and the manubrium |
| Supraclavicular | Cervical plexus formed by contributions of ventral rami C3 and C4 | Passes posterior to the midpoint of the sternocleidomastoid m. <br> Travels inferiorly in an oblique direction through the posterior triangle of the neck <br> *Divides into 3 major branches:* <br> • Medial supraclavicular—supplies the skin up to the midline <br> • Middle supraclavicular—supplies the skin over the pectoralis major and deltoid m. region <br> • Lateral supraclavicular—supplies the skin along the deltoid and anterior trapezius mm. |
| DORSAL RAMI | | |
| Greater occipital | Dorsal ramus of C2 | Ascends after emerging from the suboccipital triangle obliquely between the inferior oblique and semispinalis capitis mm. <br> Passes through the trapezius m. and ascends to innervate the skin along the posterior part of the scalp to the vertex |
| 3rd occipital | Branch of the dorsal ramus of C3 deep to the trapezius m. | Passes through the trapezius m. and ascends along in the skin of the inferior portion of the posterior surface of the head near the midline |
| Dorsal ramus of C4 | Dorsal ramus of C4 deep to the trapezius m. | Passes through the trapezius m. and ascends along in the skin of the inferior portion of the posterior surface of the head near the midline |
| Dorsal ramus of C5 | Dorsal ramus of C5 deep to the trapezius m. | Passes through the trapezius m. and ascends along in the skin of the inferior portion of the posterior surface of the head near the midline |

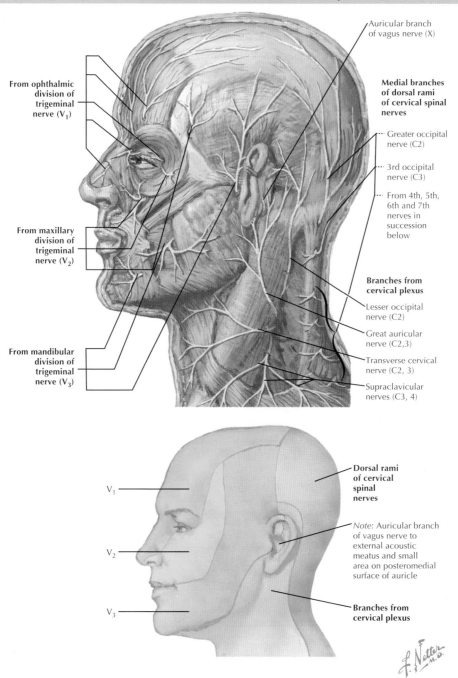

From ophthalmic
division of
trigeminal
nerve (V₁)

From maxillary
division of
trigeminal
nerve (V₂)

From mandibular
division of
trigeminal
nerve (V₃)

Auricular branch
of vagus nerve (X)

**Medial branches
of dorsal rami
of cervical spinal
nerves**

Greater occipital
nerve (C2)

3rd occipital
nerve (C3)

From 4th, 5th,
6th and 7th
nerves in
succession
below

**Branches from
cervical plexus**

Lesser occipital
nerve (C2)

Great auricular
nerve (C2,3)

Transverse cervical
nerve (C2, 3)

Supraclavicular
nerves (C3, 4)

V₁

V₂

V₃

**Dorsal rami
of cervical
spinal
nerves**

*Note*: Auricular branch
of vagus nerve to
external acoustic
meatus and small
area on posteromedial
surface of auricle

**Branches from
cervical plexus**

**Figure 4-22**

- Arises from the ventral rami of C1 to C4
- Divided into 2 parts:
  - Ansa cervicalis (motor component)
  - Cutaneous branches (sensory component):
    - Lesser occipital
    - Transverse cervical
    - Great auricular
    - Supraclavicular

| ANSA CERVICALIS | |
|---|---|
| **Source** | **Comments** |
| Ventral rami of C1 to C3 | The motor component of the cervical plexus<br>Innervates the:<br>• Omohyoid<br>• Sternohyoid<br>• Sternothyroid<br>**Divisions:**<br>Superior root (descendens hypoglossi)<br>    Arises from the ventral ramus of C1, which passes anteriorly and joins the hypoglossal n., and the fibers travel together without mixing<br>    As the hypoglossal n. passes anteriorly toward the tongue, some of the fibers of C1 branch inferiorly to form the superior root of the ansa cervicalis<br>    Superior root joins the inferior root along the lateral border of the carotid sheath<br>    Some of the fibers from C1 continue to follow the hypoglossal n. to innervate the geniohyoid and thyrohyoid mm.<br>Inferior root (descendens cervicalis)<br>    Arises from the ventral rami of C2 and C3<br>These branches unite to form the inferior root that unites with the superior root along the lateral border of the carotid sheath |

| CUTANEOUS BRANCHES | | |
|---|---|---|
| **Nerve** | **Source** | **Comments** |
| Lesser occipital | Cervical plexus by contributions from the ventral ramus of C2 | Passes posterior to the midpoint of the sternocleidomastoid m.<br>Ascends posterior to the sternocleidomastoid along the posterior portion of the head<br>Continues on the head posterior to the auricle supplying the skin in the region |
| Great auricular | Cervical plexus formed by contributions of ventral rami C2 and C3 | Passes posterior to the midpoint of the sternocleidomastoid m.<br>Ascends along the sternocleidomastoid, dividing into anterior and posterior branches:<br>• Anterior branch innervates the skin of the face over the parotid gland<br>• Posterior branch innervates the skin over the mastoid process, the posterior portion of the auricle, and the concha and lobule |
| Transverse cervical | | Passes posterior to the midpoint of the sternocleidomastoid m.<br>Crosses anteriorly along the sternocleidomastoid dividing into ascending and descending branches<br>Ascending and descending branches pass through the platysma to supply the skin of the neck from the region between the mandible and the manubrium |
| Supraclavicular | Cervical plexus formed by contributions of ventral rami C3 and C4 | Passes posterior to the midpoint of the sternocleidomastoid m.<br>Travels inferiorly in an oblique direction through the posterior triangle of the neck<br>*Divides into 3 major branches:*<br>• Medial supraclavicular—supplies the skin up to the midline<br>• Middle supraclavicular—supplies the skin over the pectoralis major and deltoid m. region<br>• Lateral supraclavicular—supplies the skin along the deltoid and anterior trapezius mm. |

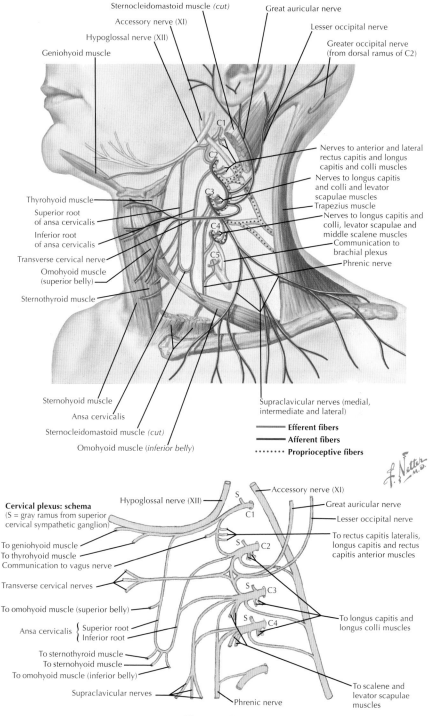

Sternocleidomastoid muscle *(cut)*
Accessory nerve (XI)
Hypoglossal nerve (XII)
Geniohyoid muscle
Great auricular nerve
Lesser occipital nerve
Greater occipital nerve
(from dorsal ramus of C2)

C1
C2
C3
C4
C5

Nerves to anterior and lateral
rectus capitis and longus
capitis and colli muscles
Nerves to longus capitis
and colli and levator
scapulae muscles
Trapezius muscle
Nerves to longus capitis and
colli, levator scapulae and
middle scalene muscles
Communication to
brachial plexus
Phrenic nerve

Thyrohyoid muscle
Superior root
of ansa cervicalis
Inferior root
of ansa cervicalis
Transverse cervical nerve
Omohyoid muscle
(superior belly)
Sternothyroid muscle

Sternohyoid muscle
Ansa cervicalis
Sternocleidomastoid muscle *(cut)*
Omohyoid muscle *(inferior belly)*

Supraclavicular nerves (medial,
intermediate and lateral)

── **Efferent fibers**
── **Afferent fibers**
······ **Proprioceptive fibers**

Cervical plexus: schema
(S = gray ramus from superior
cervical sympathetic ganglion)

Hypoglossal nerve (XII)
S
C1
Accessory nerve (XI)
Great auricular nerve
Lesser occipital nerve

To geniohyoid muscle
To thyrohyoid muscle
Communication to vagus nerve
S
C2

To rectus capitis lateralis,
longus capitis and rectus
capitis anterior muscles

Transverse cervical nerves
S
C3

To omohyoid muscle (superior belly)
Ansa cervicalis { Superior root
Inferior root
S
C4

To longus capitis and
longus colli muscles

To sternothyroid muscle
To sternohyoid muscle
To omohyoid muscle (inferior belly)
Supraclavicular nerves
Phrenic nerve

To scalene and
levator scapulae
muscles

**Figure 4-23**

| Nerve | Source | Comments |
|-------|--------|----------|
| Phrenic | Arises from the ventral rami of C3 to C5 | Passes inferiorly along the anterior surface of the anterior scalene m.<br><br>Eventually passes through the thorax to innervate the diaphragm |
| Brachial plexus | Ventral rami of C5 to C8 and T1 form the brachial plexus, which provides motor and sensory function to the upper limb | These rami pass between the anterior and middle scalene mm.<br><br>Ventral rami of C5 and C6 unite to form the upper trunk<br><br>Ventral ramus of C7 continues as the middle trunk<br><br>Ventral ramus of C8 and T1 form the inferior trunk<br><br>These trunks continue to form the divisions of the brachial plexus that enter the axilla<br><br>3 branches of the brachial plexus are contained in the posterior triangle of the neck:<br><br>• Dorsal scapular—arises from C5 and passes through the middle scalene before passing obliquely to the levator scapulae, which it innervates (along with the rhomboid major and minor mm.)<br><br>• Long thoracic—arises from the ventral rami C5 to C7 to pass through the middle scalene before passing inferiorly to the serratus anterior, which it innervates<br><br>• Suprascapular—arises from the upper trunk to pass through the posterior triangle of the neck to reach the supraspinatus and infraspinatus mm. by passing below the transverse scapular lig. |

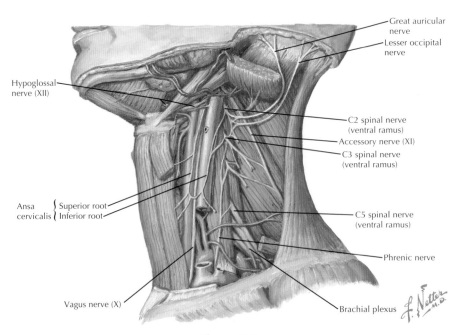

**Figure 4-24**

- Sympathetic trunk extends into the neck from the thorax
- In the neck, the sympathetic trunk typically has 3 ganglia:
  - Superior cervical ganglion—located at the base of the skull
  - Middle cervical ganglion—located at C6
  - Inferior cervical ganglion—located immediately posterior to the vertebral artery near the vessel's origin
- Often the inferior cervical ganglion unites with the 1st thoracic ganglion to create the stellate ganglion
- Sympathetics for the head and neck arise in the intermediolateral horn column of the spinal cord from T1 to T4
- These preganglionic fibers ascend through the sympathetic trunk to reach the cervical ganglia and synapse with the postganglionic neurons
- Postganglionic neurons follow either of 2 paths:
  - May travel to the spinal nerves via the gray ramus
  - May follow the arterial supply to the effector organs of the head

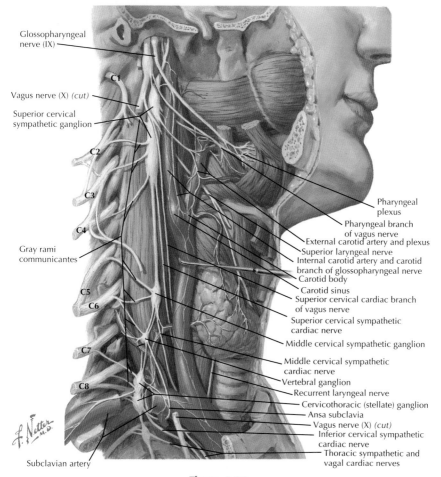

**Figure 4-25**

- Torticollis, also known as "wryneck," is a disorder in which the muscles of the neck are flexed, extended, or twisted in an abnormal position
- The sternocleidomastoid is the most commonly affected muscle
- The neck typically twists to 1 side, leading to abnormal movements and postures of the head
- In congenital muscular torticollis, the bent neck is caused by a tight sternocleidomastoid on 1 side of the body
- Early treatment is important in preventing permanent deformities
- Certain drugs, such as neuroleptic agents, can cause *dystonia*, a condition in which involuntary muscle contraction occurs in the neck, back, and trunk

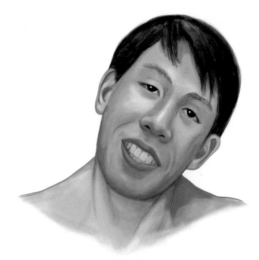

Young man with muscular torticollis. Head tilted to left with chin turned slightly to right because of contracture of left sternocleidomastoid muscle.

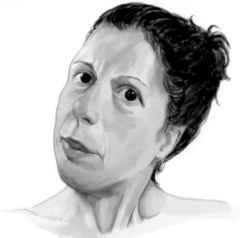

Untreated torticollis in middle-aged woman. Thick, fibrotic, tendon-like bands have replaced sternocleidomastoid muscle, making head appear tethered to clavicle. 2 heads of left sternocleidomastoid muscle are prominent.

**Figure 4-26**

### Nonmuscular Causes of Torticollis

**Atlantoaxial rotatory subluxation and fixation** (after Fielding and Hawkins)

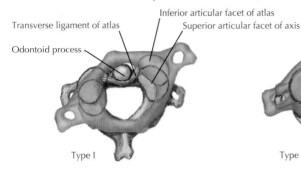

Transverse ligament of atlas

Inferior articular facet of atlas
Superior articular facet of axis

Odontoid process

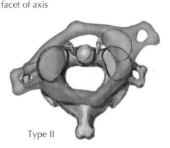

**Type I**

Rotatory subluxation of atlas about dens but transverse ligament intact. No anterior displacement

**Type II**

1 articular facet subluxated, other acts as pivot; transverse ligament defective. Anterior displacement of 3–5 mm

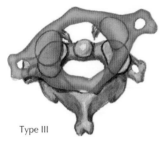

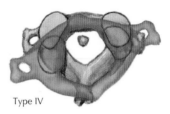

**Type III**

Both articular facets subluxated, transverse ligament defective. Anterior displacement of >5 mm

**Type IV**

Posterior rotatory subluxation (rare). Os odontoideum or absent or defective dens

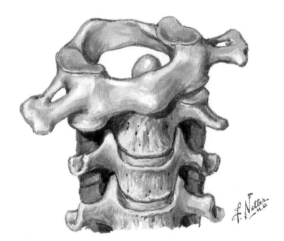

Type I rotatory subluxation

**Figure 4-27**

- Condition in which the thyroid gland does not produce enough thyroid hormones
- The pituitary gland regulates the thyroid's normal production of the hormones thyroxine and triiodothyronine
- The lack of hormones leads to an overall slowing of mental and physical activities
- Congenital hypothyroidism is known as cretinism

### CAUSES

- Hashimoto's thyroiditis—immune system of the body attacks the gland
- Irradiation of the gland
- Surgical removal of the gland
- Congenital defects

### RISK FACTORS

- Obesity
- Age older than 50 years
- Female gender

### CLINICAL MANIFESTATIONS

- Fatigue
- Weakness
- Slow pulse
- Edema of face
- Cold sensations
- Dry and coarse skin
- Coarse voice

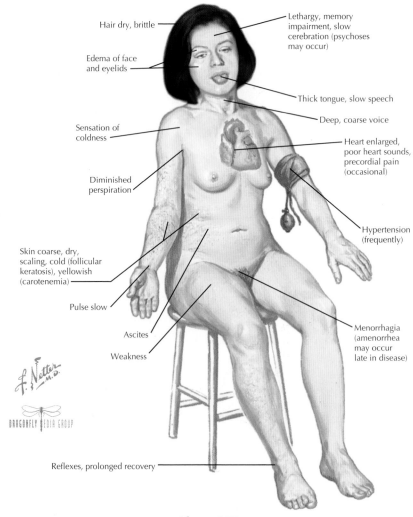

Hair dry, brittle

Edema of face and eyelids

Lethargy, memory impairment, slow cerebration (psychoses may occur)

Thick tongue, slow speech

Deep, coarse voice

Sensation of coldness

Heart enlarged, poor heart sounds, precordial pain (occasional)

Diminished perspiration

Hypertension (frequently)

Skin coarse, dry, scaling, cold (follicular keratosis), yellowish (carotenemia)

Pulse slow

Ascites

Weakness

Menorrhagia (amenorrhea may occur late in disease)

Reflexes, prolonged recovery

**Figure 4-28**

- Characterized by hypermetabolism and elevated levels of thyroid hormones
- Can lead to thyrotoxicosis, a toxic condition caused by excess thyroid hormones regardless of the cause

## CAUSES

- Graves' disease—most common cause (in greater than 80% of all cases of hyperthyroidism), in which the body produces antibodies that stimulate the thyroid to synthesize excess thyroid hormones
- Benign growths of the thyroid or pituitary gland
- Thyroiditis

- Ingestion of excess thyroid hormones or iodine
- Gonadal tumors

## CLINICAL MANIFESTATIONS

- Loss of weight
- Restlessness
- Nervousness
- Increased appetite
- Fatigue
- Goiter

## TREATMENT

- Radioactive iodine—but too much can lead to hypothyroidism
- Surgery
- Antithyroid agents

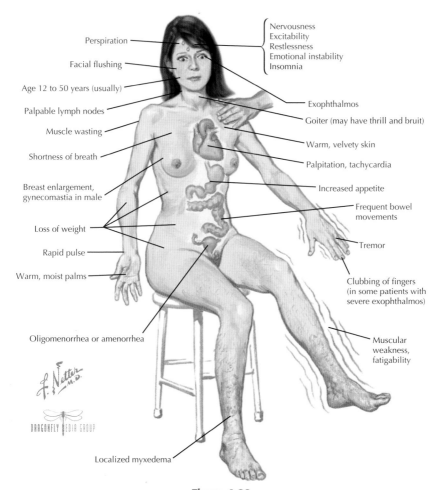

Nervousness
Excitability
Restlessness
Emotional instability
Insomnia

Perspiration

Facial flushing

Age 12 to 50 years (usually)

Palpable lymph nodes

Muscle wasting

Shortness of breath

Breast enlargement, gynecomastia in male

Loss of weight

Rapid pulse

Warm, moist palms

Oligomenorrhea or amenorrhea

Localized myxedema

Exophthalmos

Goiter (may have thrill and bruit)

Warm, velvety skin

Palpitation, tachycardia

Increased appetite

Frequent bowel movements

Tremor

Clubbing of fingers (in some patients with severe exophthalmos)

Muscular weakness, fatigability

**Figure 4-29**

# SCALP AND MUSCLES OF FACIAL EXPRESSION

SCALP

- The area bordered by the forehead, superior part of the cranium, and occipital area immediately superior to the superior nuchal line
- The lateral portion of the scalp blends with the temporal area because it extends inferiorly to the zygomatic arch
- Anatomy of the scalp is important because of frequent trauma in this region

FACE

- The area bordered within the hairline, anterior border of the auricles, and the chin
- Major contents: eyes, nose, mouth, muscles of facial expression, muscles of mastication, parotid gland, trigeminal nerve, and facial nerve
- There is no deep fascia along the face
- The superficial fascia of the face has varying amounts of adipose tissue
- The superficial muscular aponeurotic system (SMAS) is deep to the superficial fascia and provides a surgical plane for surgery of the face
- The skin, superficial fascia, and SMAS form an anatomic structure similar to the scalp proper
- The skin is attached to the underlying bone by retaining ligaments, which are in constant locations on the face
- The release of the retaining ligaments is important during facial surgeries to achieve a desired aesthetic outcome

BONES

- Bones of the facial skeleton:
  - Frontal bone
  - Zygomatic bone (zygoma)
  - Maxilla
  - Palatine bone
  - Nasal bone
  - Mandible
- Besides the nasal bone, the most commonly fractured bone of the facial skeleton is the zygomatic bone

MUSCLES OF FACIAL EXPRESSION

- The muscles of facial expression also are called mimetic muscles
- Innervated by the facial nerve
- Derivatives of the 2nd pharyngeal arch
- Originate from either bone or fascia and insert on the skin
- The SMAS provides an anatomic plane for the muscles of facial expression and is maneuvered in a rhytidectomy (facelift)

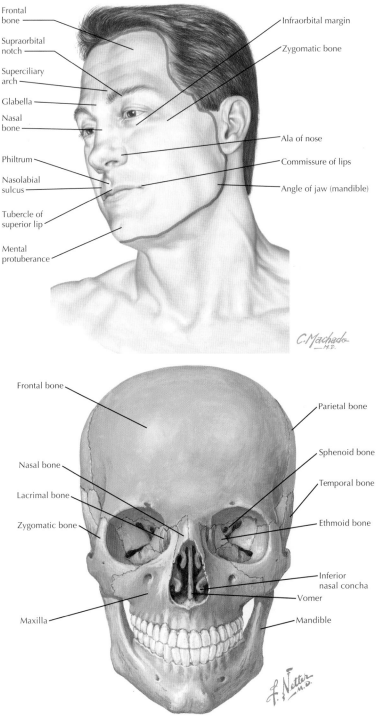

Frontal bone

Supraorbital notch

Superciliary arch

Glabella

Nasal bone

Philtrum

Nasolabial sulcus

Tubercle of superior lip

Mental protuberance

Infraorbital margin

Zygomatic bone

Ala of nose

Commissure of lips

Angle of jaw (mandible)

Frontal bone

Nasal bone

Lacrimal bone

Zygomatic bone

Maxilla

Parietal bone

Sphenoid bone

Temporal bone

Ethmoid bone

Inferior nasal concha

Vomer

Mandible

**Figure 5-1**

SCALP AND MUSCLES OF FACIAL EXPRESSION **155**

| Layer | Description |
|---|---|
| Skin | Thickest layer of the scalp<br>Contains the hair follicles |
| Connective tissue | Heavily vascularized<br>Arteries, veins, and nerves of the scalp are located here<br>Emissary veins connect this layer to the dural venous sinuses, providing channel for infections to spread<br>Head wounds that pierce the skin and connective tissue layers bleed profusely<br>Continuous with superficial fascia of the posterior part of the neck |
| Aponeurosis | Also called galea aponeurotica<br>Continuous with the occipitofrontalis m.: anteriorly with the frontalis, posteriorly with the occipitalis<br>Blends laterally with the temporal fascia<br>Its surgical manipulation is important in cosmetic surgery<br>Head wounds that pierce the skin, connective tissue, and aponeurosis layers bleed and gape open from the pull of the 2 bellies of the occipitofrontalis<br>Skin, connective tissue, and aponeurosis layers are adherent and often called "scalp proper" |
| Loose areolar connective tissue | Thin and mobile<br>Helps form a subaponeurotic layer that extends from the eyebrows to the superior nuchal line and external occipital protuberance<br>Allows substances such as bacteria and blood to pass freely<br>Separates with scalp avulsion |
| Pericranium | Covers the outer surface of the cranium |

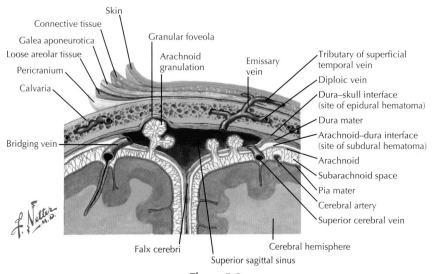

**Figure 5-2**

- Highly vascularized; the vessels anastomose freely on the scalp
- Arteries are derived from the external and the internal carotid arteries
- The neurovascular supply arises from the anterior, lateral, and posterior scalp regions

| ARTERIAL SUPPLY | | |
|---|---|---|
| **Artery** | **Source** | **Course** |
| Supratrochlear | Ophthalmic a. from the internal carotid a. | Exits the orbit at the medial angle accompanied by supratrochlear n.<br>Ascends up to the scalp at the frontal notch<br>Anastomoses with the contralateral supraorbital and supratrochlear aa. |
| Supraorbital | | Branches from the ophthalmic a. as the artery passes the optic n.<br>Passes medially to the levator palpebrae superioris and superior rectus mm. to join the supraorbital n.<br>Passes through the supraorbital foramen (notch) and ascends superiorly along the scalp<br>Anastomoses with the supratrochlear and superficial temporal aa. |
| Superficial temporal | External carotid a. | Begins posterior to the neck of the mandible and travels superiorly as a continuation of the external carotid a.<br>Joined by the auriculotemporal n.<br>Anastomoses with a majority of other branches supplying the scalp |
| Posterior auricular | | Arises within the parotid gland<br>Passes superiorly between the mastoid process and the cartilage of the ear<br>Anastomoses with the superficial temporal and occipital aa. |
| Occipital | | Branches along the inferior margin of the posterior belly of the digastric and stylohyoid mm.<br>Hypoglossal n. wraps around it from the posterior part of the vessel, traveling anteriorly<br>Passes posteriorly along the mastoid process, making a groove on the bone<br>Pierces the fascia that connects the attachment of the trapezius with the sternocleidomastoid m.<br>Ascends in the connective tissue layer of the scalp, dividing into many branches<br>The terminal part is accompanied by the greater occipital n.<br>Anastomoses with the posterior auricular and superficial temporal aa. |
| VENOUS DRAINAGE | | |
| **Vein** | **Course** | |
| Supratrochlear | Begins on the forehead, where it communicates with the superficial temporal v.<br>Passes inferiorly along the forehead parallel with the vein of the opposite side<br>At the medial angle of the orbit, it joins the supraorbital and the angular v. | |
| Supraorbital | Begins on the forehead, where it communicates with the superficial temporal v.<br>Passes inferiorly superficial to the frontalis m. and joins the supratrochlear v. at the medial angle of the orbit and the angular v. | |
| Superficial temporal | Descends posterior to the zygomatic root of the temporal bone alongside the auriculotemporal n. to enter the substance of the parotid gland<br>Unites with the maxillary v. to form the retromandibular v. | |
| Posterior auricular | Begins on the side of the scalp, posterior to the auricle<br>Passes inferiorly and joins the posterior division of the retromandibular v. to form the external jugular v. | |
| Occipital | Begins on the posterior portion of the scalp at the vertex<br>Passes from superficial to deep by passing through the attachment of the sternocleidomastoid m. to the skull<br>Has a mastoid emissary v. that connects it to the transverse sinus<br>The vein's termination is variable, but it usually passes inferiorly to join the internal jugular v. | |

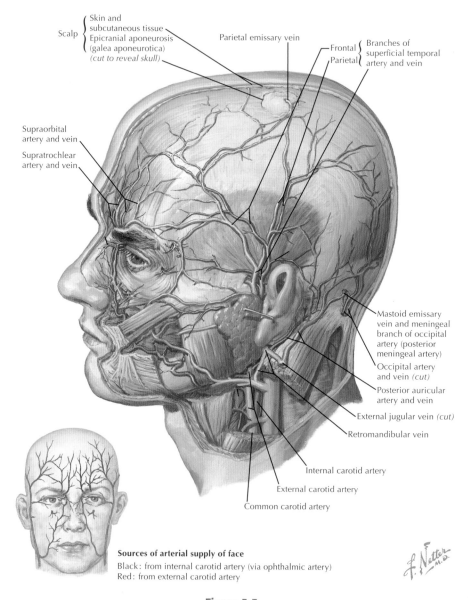

Scalp
{ Skin and
subcutaneous tissue
Epicranial aponeurosis
(galea aponeurotica)
*(cut to reveal skull)*

Parietal emissary vein

Frontal
Parietal { Branches of
superficial temporal
artery and vein

Supraorbital
artery and vein

Supratrochlear
artery and vein

Mastoid emissary
vein and meningeal
branch of occipital
artery (posterior
meningeal artery)

Occipital artery
and vein *(cut)*

Posterior auricular
artery and vein

External jugular vein *(cut)*

Retromandibular vein

Internal carotid artery

External carotid artery

Common carotid artery

**Sources of arterial supply of face**
Black: from internal carotid artery (via ophthalmic artery)
Red: from external carotid artery

**Figure 5-3**

- Sensory supply is derived from all 3 divisions of the trigeminal nerve, branches of the cervical plexus, and upper cervical dorsal rami
- These nerves travel in the scalp's connective tissue layer

| SENSORY NERVES OF THE SCALP | | |
|---|---|---|
| **Nerve** | **Source** | **Course** |
| Supratrochlear | Ophthalmic division of the trigeminal n. | The frontal nerve passes anteriorly in the orbit after branching from the ophthalmic division of the trigeminal<br>The frontal nerve divides into supratrochlear and supraorbital nerves<br>The supratrochlear continues to pass anteriorly toward the trochlea once the supratrochlear a. joins it within the orbit<br>In the trochlear region, it exits the orbit at the frontal notch<br>Ascends along the scalp, at first deep to the musculature in the region, before piercing them to reach the cutaneous innervation along the scalp |
| Supraorbital | | 1 of the 2 terminal branches of the frontal n. in the orbit<br>Passes between the levator palpebrae superioris m. and periosteum of the orbit<br>Continues anteriorly to the supraorbital foramen (notch)<br>At the level of the supraorbital margin, it sends nerve supply to the frontal sinus, skin, and conjunctiva of the upper eyelid<br>Continues to ascend superiorly along the scalp<br>Divides into medial and lateral branches, which travel up to the vertex of the scalp |
| Zygomaticotemporal | Maxillary division of the trigeminal n. | Arises from the zygomatic n. in the pterygopalatine fossa, and passes through the inferior orbital fissure to enter the lateral wall of the orbit and branches into the zygomaticotemporal and zygomaticofacial branches<br>Passes on the lateral wall of the orbit in a groove in the zygomatic bone, then through a foramen in the zygomatic bone to enter the temporal fossa region<br>Within the temporal fossa, it passes superiorly between the bone and the temporalis m. to pierce the temporal fascia superior to the zygomatic arch<br>Passes along the skin of the side of the scalp |
| Auriculotemporal | Posterior division of the mandibular division of the trigeminal n. | Normally arises as 2 roots, between which the middle meningeal a. passes<br>Runs posteriorly just inferior to the lateral pterygoid and continues to the medial aspect of the neck of the mandible<br>While passing posterior to the mandible, it provides sensory innervation to the temporomandibular joint<br>Turns superiorly with the superficial temporal vessels between the auricle and the condyle of the mandible deep to the parotid gland<br>On exiting the parotid gland, ascends over the zygomatic arch and divides into branches along the scalp |
| Lesser occipital | Arises from the cervical plexus from the ventral ramus of C2 | Wraps around and travels superiorly along the posterior border of the sternocleidomastoid<br>At the skull, it passes through the investing layer of deep cervical fascia and continues superiorly posterior to the auricle to supply the skin in the area |
| Greater occipital | Dorsal ramus of C2 | Ascends between the obliquus capitis inferior and semispinalis capitis mm. in the suboccipital triangle<br>Passes through the semispinalis capitis and trapezius mm. near their bony attachments<br>Ascends on the back of the head with the occipital a. to supply the skin as far anterior as the vertex |
| 3rd occipital | Dorsal ramus of C3 | Arises deep to the trapezius m., passes through it, and ascends in the skin of the inferior portion of the posterior surface of the head near the midline |

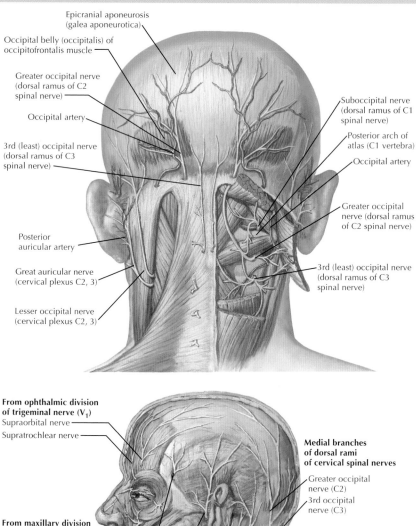

Epicranial aponeurosis
(galea aponeurotica)

Occipital belly (occipitalis) of
occipitofrontalis muscle

Greater occipital nerve
(dorsal ramus of C2
spinal nerve)

Occipital artery

3rd (least) occipital nerve
(dorsal ramus of C3
spinal nerve)

Suboccipital nerve
(dorsal ramus of C1
spinal nerve)

Posterior arch of
atlas (C1 vertebra)

Occipital artery

Greater occipital
nerve (dorsal ramus
of C2 spinal nerve)

Posterior
auricular artery

Great auricular nerve
(cervical plexus C2, 3)

Lesser occipital nerve
(cervical plexus C2, 3)

3rd (least) occipital nerve
(dorsal ramus of C3
spinal nerve)

**From ophthalmic division
of trigeminal nerve (V$_1$)**
Supraorbital nerve
Supratrochlear nerve

**Medial branches
of dorsal rami
of cervical spinal nerves**

Greater occipital
nerve (C2)
3rd occipital
nerve (C3)

**From maxillary division
of trigeminal nerve (V$_2$)**

Zygomaticotemporal nerve

**Branches from
cervical plexus**
Lesser occipital
nerve (C2)

**From mandibular division
of trigeminal nerve (V$_3$)**

Auriculotemporal nerve

**Figure 5-4**

- Innervated by the facial nerve
- Derivatives of the 2nd pharyngeal arch
- Insert into the skin to provide movement
- Most muscles of facial expression are localized around the facial orifices
- There is no deep fascia along the face

**Muscle Attachments
of the Face: Anterior View**

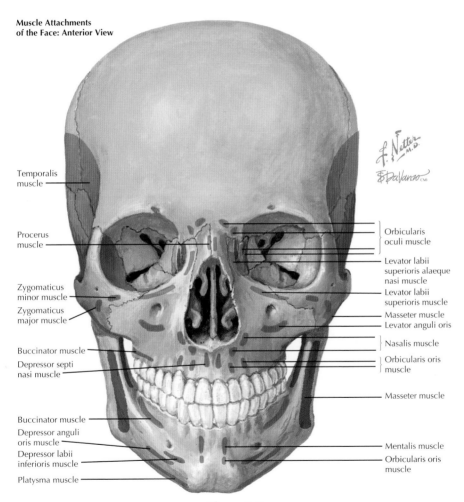

Temporalis muscle

Procerus muscle

Zygomaticus minor muscle

Zygomaticus major muscle

Buccinator muscle

Depressor septi nasi muscle

Buccinator muscle

Depressor anguli oris muscle

Depressor labii inferioris muscle

Platysma muscle

Orbicularis oculi muscle

Levator labii superioris alaeque nasi muscle

Levator labii superioris muscle

Masseter muscle

Levator anguli oris

Nasalis muscle

Orbicularis oris muscle

Masseter muscle

Mentalis muscle

Orbicularis oris muscle

**Figure 5-5**

**Muscle Attachments of the Face:**
**Lateral View and Inferior View**

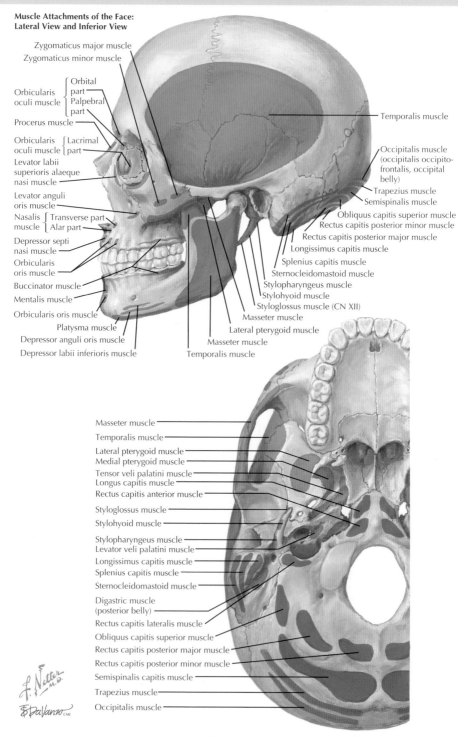

Zygomaticus major muscle
Zygomaticus minor muscle

Orbicularis
oculi muscle {
Orbital part
Palpebral part

Procerus muscle

Orbicularis
oculi muscle { Lacrimal part

Levator labii
superioris alaeque
nasi muscle

Levator anguli
oris muscle

Nasalis { Transverse part
muscle { Alar part

Depressor septi
nasi muscle

Orbicularis
oris muscle

Buccinator muscle

Mentalis muscle

Orbicularis oris muscle

Platysma muscle

Depressor anguli oris muscle

Depressor labii inferioris muscle

Temporalis muscle

Occipitalis muscle
(occipitalis occipito-
frontalis, occipital
belly)

Trapezius muscle
Semispinalis muscle

Obliquus capitis superior muscle
Rectus capitis posterior minor muscle
Rectus capitis posterior major muscle
Longissimus capitis muscle

Splenius capitis muscle
Sternocleidomastoid muscle
Stylopharyngeus muscle
Stylohyoid muscle
Styloglossus muscle (CN XII)
Masseter muscle
Lateral pterygoid muscle
Masseter muscle

Masseter muscle
Temporalis muscle
Lateral pterygoid muscle
Medial pterygoid muscle
Tensor veli palatini muscle
Longus capitis muscle
Rectus capitis anterior muscle

Styloglossus muscle
Stylohyoid muscle

Stylopharyngeus muscle
Levator veli palatini muscle
Longissimus capitis muscle
Splenius capitis muscle

Sternocleidomastoid muscle

Digastric muscle
(posterior belly)

Rectus capitis lateralis muscle

Obliquus capitis superior muscle

Rectus capitis posterior major muscle

Rectus capitis posterior minor muscle

Semispinalis capitis muscle

Trapezius muscle

Occipitalis muscle

**Figure 5-6**

| Muscle | Origin | Insertion | Actions | Nerve | Comments |
|--------|--------|-----------|---------|-------|----------|
| Orbicularis oris | *Bone*: anterior midline of the maxilla and mandible<br>*Muscular*: angle of the mouth where fibers blend with levator anguli oris, depressor anguli oris, zygomaticus major mm., and risorius mm. | Skin along the mouth | Closes lips<br>Protrusion of lips<br>Pursing of lips | Facial (buccal and mandibular branches) | Sphincter of the mouth<br>Muscle fibers encircle the mouth |
| Depressor anguli oris | Mandible along area near the external oblique line | Angle of the mouth<br>Some fibers blend and provide origin for the orbicularis oris m.<br>Fibers overlap those of the depressor labii inferioris m. | Depresses the corners of the mouth in an inferior and lateral direction | Facial (buccal and mandibular branches) | Antagonizes levator anguli oris m. |
| Levator anguli oris | Canine fossa of the maxilla (inferior to the infraorbital foramen) | Angle of the mouth<br>Some fibers blend and provide origin for the orbicularis oris m. | Elevates the angle of the mouth (e.g., in smiling)<br>Makes nasolabial furrow more pronounced | Facial (zygomatic and buccal branches) | In an infraorbital injection, the needle lies between the levator anguli oris and levator labii superioris mm. |
| Zygomaticus major | Zygomatic bone (anterior to the zygomaticotemporal suture) | | Moves the angle of the mouth superiorly and laterally (e.g., with broad smile and laughing) | | Dimples typically are caused by deformities in this muscle (e.g., muscle is bifid)<br>Also called the "laughing muscle" owing to its action |
| Zygomaticus minor | Zygomatic bone (anterior to the zygomaticus major) | Lateral upper lip (just medial to Zygomaticus major attachment) | Helps elevate the upper lip | | Inserts between the levator labii superioris and zygomaticus major mm. |

*Continued on next page*

| Muscle | Origin | Insertion | Actions | Nerve | Comments |
|---|---|---|---|---|---|
| Levator labii superioris | Maxilla (superior to the infraorbital foramen along the inferior margin of the orbit) | Lateral upper lip<br>Some fibers blend and provide origin for the orbicularis oris m. | Elevates the upper lip | Facial (zygomatic and buccal branches) | In an infraorbital injection, the needle lies between the levator anguli oris and levator labii superioris mm. |
| Levator labii superioris alaeque nasi | Maxilla (near the bridge of the nose) | Alar cartilage of the nose<br>Lateral upper lip (blending with orbicularis oris and levator labii superioris mm.) | Elevates the upper lip<br>Dilates the nostril | | Also called the angular part of the levator labii superioris m. |
| Risorius | Fascia overlying the parotid gland | Angle of the mouth | Moves the angle of the mouth laterally (e.g., with grinning, smiling, laughing) | Facial (buccal branch) | Commonly called the "grinning muscle" |
| Depressor labii inferioris | Mandible (inferior to the mental foramen) | Lower lip<br>Fibers blend and provide origin for the orbicularis oris m. | Depresses the lower lip (e.g., in "pouting") | Facial (mandibular branch) | Fibers of the depressor anguli oris m. overlap the fibers of the depressor labii inferioris m. |
| Mentalis | Incisive fossa of the mandible | Skin of the chin | Elevates lower lip<br>Protrudes lower lip (e.g., while drinking) | | Used in "pouting" |
| Buccinator | Pterygomandibular raphe<br>Alveolar margins of the maxilla and mandible | Some fibers blend and provide origin for the orbicularis oris<br>Some fibers blend into the upper and lower lips | Aids in mastication, keeping the bolus between cheek and teeth<br>Helps forcibly expel air<br>Helps create a sucking action | Facial (buccal branch) | Creates the framework of the cheek |

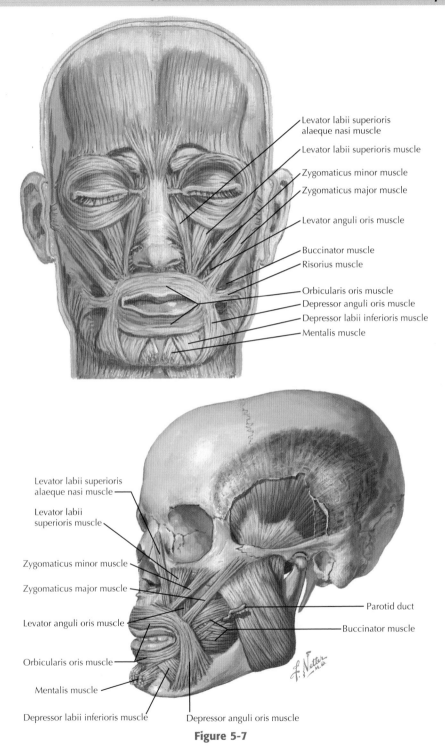

**Figure 5-7**

## NASAL GROUP

| Muscle | Parts | Origin | Insertion | Actions | Nerve | Comment |
|--------|-------|--------|-----------|---------|-------|---------|
| Nasalis | Compressor naris (Transverse part) | Maxilla | Compressor naris m. of opposite side | Compresses the nostril | Facial n.: buccal branch | Antagonist to the dilator naris |
| | Dilator naris (Alar part) | | Nasal cartilage | Dilates the nostril | | Allows flaring of the nostrils |
| Depressor septi | | | Nasal septum | Draws nasal septum and tip of nose anteriorly | | Variable and occasionally absent |
| Procerus | | Nasal bone (lower portion) Lateral nasal cartilage | Skin of the forehead between the eyes | Brings skin together producing transverse wrinkles on the bridge of the nose (e.g., in frowning) | Facial n.: temporal and zygomatic branches | Partially excised in some facelift procedures (rhytidectomy) Also common area for Botox injections |

## ORBITAL GROUP

| Muscle | Parts | Origin | Insertion | Actions | Nerve | Comment |
|--------|-------|--------|-----------|---------|-------|---------|
| Orbicularis oculi | Orbital | Frontal process of maxilla Nasal portion of frontal bone Medial palpebral ligament | Around the orbit | Voluntary closure of the eye (as in squinting) | Facial n.: temporal and zygomatic branches | Fat that accumulates around the eye from aging may be removed surgically (blepharoplasty) Because the orbicularis oculi m. moves the skin around the eye, its attachment is extremely important |
| | Lacrimal | Lacrimal bone | Lacrimal fascia around the lacrimal canaliculi | Pulls lacrimal papilla and eyelids medially, which aids the flow of tears | | |
| | Palpebral | Medial palpebral ligament | Lateral palpebral raphe | Closure of eyelids gently (as in sleeping and blinking) | | |
| Corrugator supercilii | | Frontal bone (medial end of superciliary arch) | Middle of the eyebrow | Draws the eyebrows medially and inferiorly (as in squinting) | Facial n.: temporal branch | Fibers lie deep to the orbicularis oculi m. |

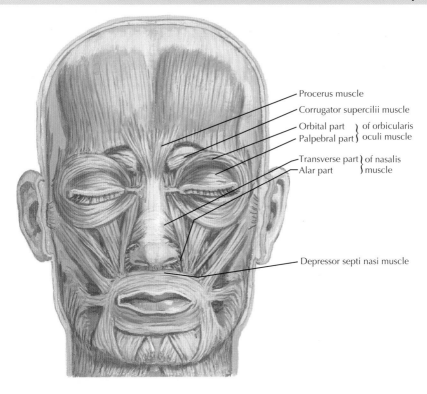

Procerus muscle

Corrugator supercilii muscle

Orbital part } of orbicularis
Palpebral part } oculi muscle

Transverse part } of nasalis
Alar part } muscle

Depressor septi nasi muscle

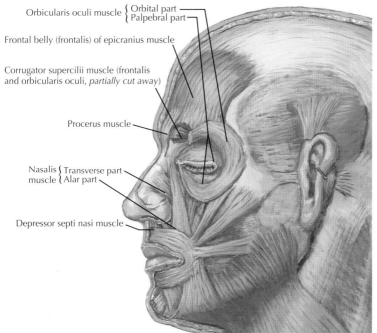

Orbicularis oculi muscle { Orbital part
                           Palpebral part

Frontal belly (frontalis) of epicranius muscle

Corrugator supercilii muscle (frontalis
and orbicularis oculi, *partially cut away*)

Procerus muscle

Nasalis { Transverse part
muscle { Alar part

Depressor septi nasi muscle

**Figure 5-8**

## AURICULAR GROUP

| Muscle | Parts | Origin | Insertion | Actions | Nerve | Comment |
|--------|-------|--------|-----------|---------|-------|---------|
| Auricular | Anterior | Galea aponeurosis | Helix | Draws auricle anteriorly | Facial n.: temporal branch | These muscles usually provide little movement and tend to not always be voluntary |
| | Superior | | Superior part of the auricle | Draws auricle superiorly | | |
| | Posterior | Mastoid process | Posterior part of the auricle | Draws auricle posteriorly | Facial n.: posterior auricular branch | |

## SCALP GROUP (OCCIPITOFRONTALIS)

| Muscle | Origin | Insertion | Actions | Nerve | Comment |
|--------|--------|-----------|---------|-------|---------|
| Frontalis | Skin and superficial fascia along eyebrows and adjacent facial muscles (corrugator supercilii, orbicularis oculi, and procerus) | Galea aponeurosis | Elevates eyebrows Wrinkles forehead | Facial n.: temporal branch | Has no bony attachment Surgical management important in cosmetic surgery |
| Occipitalis | Superior nuchal line Mastoid process | | Wrinkles the back of the head | Facial n: posterior auricular branch | |

## NECK GROUP

| Muscle | Origin | Insertion | Actions | Nerve | Comment |
|--------|--------|-----------|---------|-------|---------|
| Platysma | Fascia of upper part of the pectoralis major m. and deltoid | Inferior border of the mandible Some fibers blend with the skin of the neck and lower face | Tenses the skin of the neck (i.e. - causing the skin of the neck to wrinkle) Depresses the skin of the lower face | Facial n.: cervical branch | The external jugular lies deep to the platysma m. |

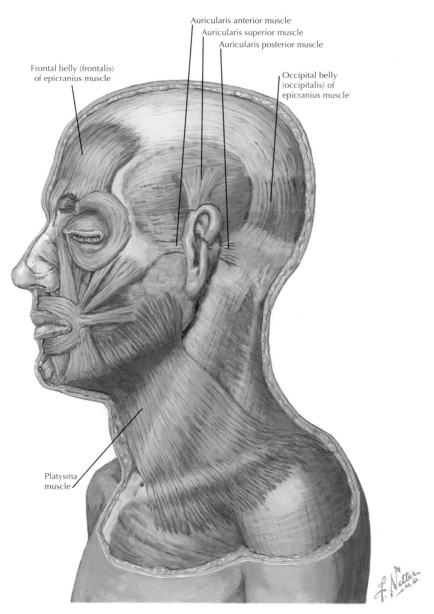

Auricularis anterior muscle
Auricularis superior muscle
Auricularis posterior muscle

Frontal belly (frontalis) of epicranius muscle

Occipital belly (occipitalis) of epicranius muscle

Platysma muscle

**Figure 5-9**

- Most of the arterial supply to the face arises from the superficial temporal artery and facial branches of the external carotid artery
- The maxillary branch of the external carotid supplies most areas that the superficial temporal and facial branches do not supply
- The internal carotid artery supplies the anterior portion of the forehead and dorsal surface of the nose via ophthalmic artery branches
- The arteries of the face anastomose freely

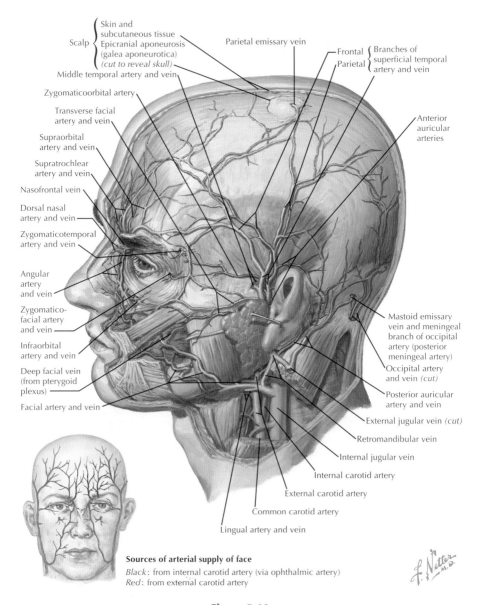

**Sources of arterial supply of face**

*Black*: from internal carotid artery (via ophthalmic artery)
*Red*: from external carotid artery

**Figure 5-10**

| EXTERNAL CAROTID ARTERY AND ITS BRANCHES IN THE FACE | | |
|---|---|---|
| **Artery** | **Source** | **Course** |
| Facial | External carotid a. | Arises in the carotid triangle of the neck |
| | | Passes superiorly immediately deep to the posterior belly of the digastric m. and the stylohyoid mm. |
| | | Passes along the submandibular gland, giving rise to the submental a. that helps supply the gland |
| | | Passes superiorly over the body of the mandible at the masseter m. |
| | | Continues anterosuperiorly across the cheek to the angle of the mouth, giving rise to the *superior and inferior labial* aa. |
| | | Passes superiorly along the side of the nose, giving rise to the *lateral nasal* a. |
| | | Continues on the side of the nose as the *angular* a. to terminate along the medial aspect of the eye |
| | | Tortuous |
| *Superior labial* | Facial a. | Supplies the upper lip |
| | | Gives rise to the septal branch that travels to the nasal septum |
| *Inferior labial* | | Supplies the lower lip |
| *Lateral nasal* | | Supplies the ala and nose |
| *Angular* | | The facial a.'s terminal branch |
| | | Passes superiorly to terminate at the medial angle of the orbit |
| Superficial temporal | External carotid a. | 1 of the 2 terminal branches of the external carotid |
| | | Arises posterior to the neck of the mandible and travels superiorly as a continuation of the external carotid a. |
| | | Joined by the auriculotemporal n. |
| *Transverse facial* | Superficial temporal a. | Passes transversely before it exits the parotid gland |
| | | Passes immediately superior to the parotid duct across the masseter m. and face |
| Maxillary | External carotid a. | 1 of the 2 terminal branches of the external carotid a. |
| | | Gives rise to a series of branches; only 3 provide blood supply to the face: the *infraorbital*, *buccal*, and *mental* |
| *Infraorbital* | Maxillary a. | The continuation of the 3rd part of the maxillary a. |
| | | Accompanied by the infraorbital n. and v. |
| | | Passes forward in the infraorbital groove and infraorbital canal and exits the infraorbital foramen |
| | | On exiting the infraorbital foramen, it lies between the levator labii superioris and levator anguli oris mm. and follows the branching pattern of the nerve: |
| | | Inferior palpebral (supplies the lower eyelid) |
| | | Nasal (supplies the lateral side of the nose) |
| | | Superior labial (supplies the upper lip) |
| *Buccal* | | A branch of the 2nd part of the maxillary |
| | | A small artery that runs obliquely in an anterior direction between the medial pterygoid m. and the insertion of the temporalis m. until it reaches the outer surface of the buccinator m. to supply it and the face |
| *Mental* | | A terminal branch of the inferior alveolar a., which arises from the 1st part of the maxillary a. |
| | | Emerges from the mental foramen to supply the chin region |

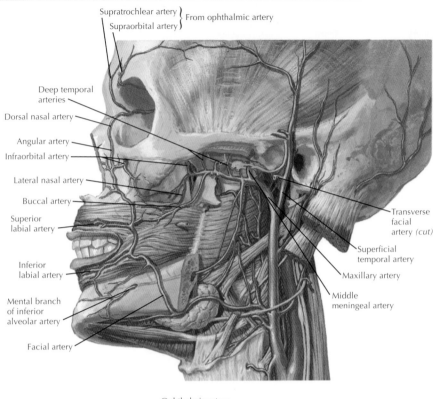

Supratrochlear artery ⎱
Supraorbital artery ⎰ From ophthalmic artery

Deep temporal arteries

Dorsal nasal artery

Angular artery

Infraorbital artery

Lateral nasal artery

Buccal artery

Superior labial artery

Inferior labial artery

Mental branch of inferior alveolar artery

Facial artery

Transverse facial artery *(cut)*

Superficial temporal artery

Maxillary artery

Middle meningeal artery

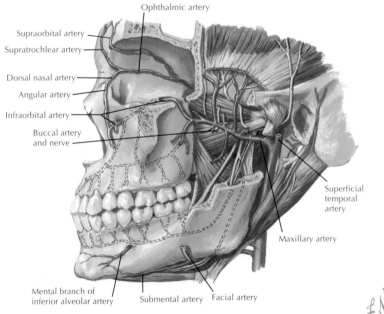

Ophthalmic artery

Supraorbital artery

Supratrochlear artery

Dorsal nasal artery

Angular artery

Infraorbital artery

Buccal artery and nerve

Superficial temporal artery

Maxillary artery

Mental branch of inferior alveolar artery

Submental artery

Facial artery

**Figure 5-11**

| OPHTHALMIC ARTERY AND ITS BRANCHES | |
|---|---|
| **Artery** | **Course** |
| Ophthalmic | A branch of the internal carotid |
| | Enters the orbit through the optic foramen immediately inferior and lateral to the optic n. |
| | Crosses the optic n. to reach the medial part of the orbit |
| | Within the orbit, besides the orbital branches, it gives rise to 5 major branches that supply the face (either directly or indirectly): |
| | • Supratrochlear |
| | • Supraorbital |
| | • Lacrimal |
| | • Anterior ethmoid (from which the external nasal arises) |
| | • Dorsal nasal |
| Supratrochlear | Exits the orbit at the medial angle accompanied by supratrochlear n. |
| | Ascends on the scalp, anastomosing with the supraorbital and supratrochlear aa. from the opposite side |
| Supraorbital | Arises as the ophthalmic a. passes the optic n. |
| | Passes on the medial side of the levator palpebrae superioris and superior rectus mm. to join the supraorbital n. |
| | Passes through the supraorbital foramen (notch) and ascends superiorly along the scalp |
| | Anastomoses with the supratrochlear and superficial temporal aa. |
| Lacrimal | Arises near the optic foramen |
| | 1 of the largest branches of the ophthalmic a. |
| | Follows the lacrimal n. along the superior border of the lateral rectus m. of the eye to reach and supply the lacrimal gland |
| | Gives rise to a series of terminal branches that pass to the eyelids and conjunctivae |
| | Gives rise to a zygomatic branch that divides into the zygomaticotemporal and zygomaticofacial aa., to supply those facial regions |
| External nasal | A terminal branch of the anterior ethmoid a. |
| | Supplies the area along the external nose at the junction of the nasal bone and the lateral nasal cartilage |
| Dorsal nasal | 1 of the terminal branches of the ophthalmic a. |
| | Exits the orbit along the superomedial border along with the infratrochlear n. |
| | Supplies the area along the bridge of the nose |

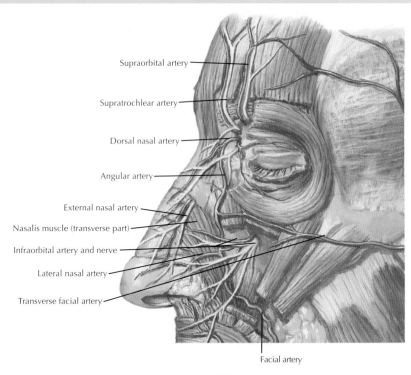

Supraorbital artery

Supratrochlear artery

Dorsal nasal artery

Angular artery

External nasal artery

Nasalis muscle (transverse part)

Infraorbital artery and nerve

Lateral nasal artery

Transverse facial artery

Facial artery

**Anterior view**

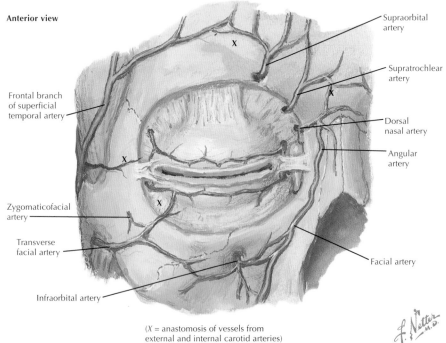

Frontal branch
of superficial
temporal artery

Zygomaticofacial
artery

Transverse
facial artery

Infraorbital artery

Supraorbital
artery

Supratrochlear
artery

Dorsal
nasal artery

Angular
artery

Facial artery

(*X* = anastomosis of vessels from
external and internal carotid arteries)

**Figure 5-12**

- Facial veins have similar distribution pattern as the arteries
- Highly variable
- 4 major veins connect the superficial veins of the nose, cheeks, and upper lip to the deeper vessels (pterygoid plexus and cavernous sinus), creating the "danger triangle of the face"—it provides a pathway for infections to spread to the cavernous sinus (cavernous sinus thrombosis)

| SUPERFICIAL VEINS | |
|---|---|
| **Vein** | **Course** |
| Facial | Begins as the angular v. |
| | Passes inferiorly along the side of the nose, receiving the lateral nasal v. |
| | Continues posteroinferiorly across the angle of the mouth to the cheek, receiving the superior and inferior labial vv. |
| | While passing toward the mandible, the deep facial v. connects it to the pterygoid plexus |
| | In the submandibular triangle, it joins the anterior branch of the retromandibular to form the common facial v. |
| | Has no valves that can allow blood to backflow |
| Superior labial | Drains the upper lip and joins the facial v. |
| Inferior labial | Drains the lower lip and joins the facial v. |
| Lateral nasal | Drains the ala and nose and joins the facial v. |
| Angular | Forms from the confluence of the supraorbital and supratrochlear vv. along the medial part of the eye |
| | Travels along the lateral aspect of the nose to become the facial v. |
| Supraorbital | Begins on the forehead, where it communicates with the superficial temporal |
| | Passes inferiorly superficial to the frontalis m. and joins the supratrochlear v. at the medial angle of the orbit to form the angular v. |
| Supratrochlear | Begins on the forehead, where it communicates with the superficial temporal vv. |
| | Passes inferiorly along the forehead parallel with the vein of the opposite side |
| | At the medial angle of the orbit, it joins the supraorbital v. to form the angular v. |
| Superficial temporal | Descends posterior to the zygomatic root of the temporal bone alongside the auriculotemporal n. to enter the substance of the parotid gland |
| | Unites with the maxillary v. to form the retromandibular v. |
| Transverse facial | Travels posteriorly to enter the parotid gland and join the superficial temporal v. |
| Buccal | Drains the cheek and joins the pterygoid plexus |
| Mental | Drains the chin and joins the pterygoid plexus |

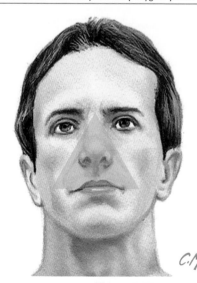

**Figure 5-13**

| COMMUNICATING VEINS | |
|---|---|
| **Vein** | **Course** |
| Superior ophthalmic | Receives blood from the roof of the orbit and the scalp<br>Travels posteriorly to communicate with the pterygoid plexus and cavernous sinus |
| Inferior ophthalmic | Receives blood from the floor of the orbit<br>Travels posteriorly with the infraorbital v., which passes through the inferior orbital fissure to communicate with the pterygoid plexus and the cavernous sinus |
| Infraorbital | Receives blood from the midface via the lower eyelid, lateral aspect of the nose, and the upper lip<br>Eventually communicates with the pterygoid plexus |
| Deep facial | Connects the facial v. with the pterygoid plexus |
| **DEEP VEINS** | |
| **Vein** | **Course** |
| Cavernous sinus | A reticulated venous structure on the lateral body of the sphenoid bone<br>Drains posteriorly into the superior and inferior petrosal sinuses<br>Receives blood from the superior and inferior ophthalmic vv.<br>The oculomotor and trochlear nn. and ophthalmic and maxillary divisions of the trigeminal n. lie along the lateral wall of the sinus<br>Abducens n. and internal carotid artery lie in the sinus |
| Pterygoid plexus | An extensive network of veins that parallels the 2nd and 3rd parts of the maxillary a.<br>Receives branches that correspond to the maxillary a.'s branches<br>Tributaries of the pterygoid plexus eventually converge to form a short maxillary v.<br>Communicates with the cavernous sinus, pharyngeal venous plexus, facial v. via the deep facial v., and ophthalmic vv. |

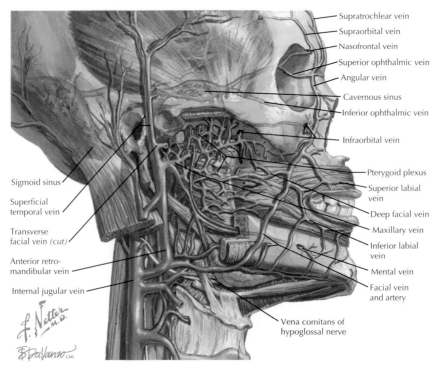

Supratrochlear vein
Supraorbital vein
Nasofrontal vein
Superior ophthalmic vein
Angular vein
Cavernous sinus
Inferior ophthalmic vein
Infraorbital vein
Pterygoid plexus
Superior labial vein
Deep facial vein
Maxillary vein
Inferior labial vein
Mental vein
Facial vein and artery

Sigmoid sinus
Superficial temporal vein
Transverse facial vein *(cut)*
Anterior retro-mandibular vein
Internal jugular vein

Vena comitans of hypoglossal nerve

**Figure 5-14**

- Many motor and sensory nerves supply the face
- All motor nerves are from the facial nerve and supply the muscles of facial expression
- Sensory nerves of the face are derived mainly from the 3 divisions of the trigeminal nerve ($V_1$, $V_2$, $V_3$)
- Some sensory branches are from the cervical plexus

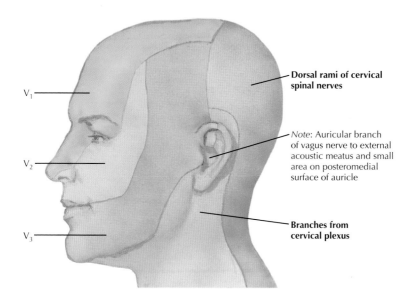

$V_1$

$V_2$

$V_3$

**Dorsal rami of cervical spinal nerves**

*Note*: Auricular branch of vagus nerve to external acoustic meatus and small area on posteromedial surface of auricle

**Branches from cervical plexus**

Facial nerve (VII)

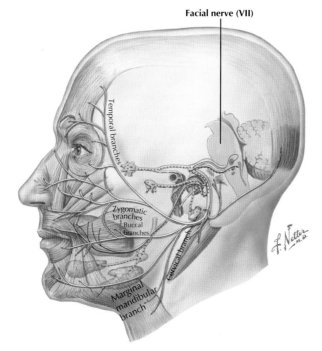

Temporal branches

Zygomatic branches

Buccal branches

Cervical branch

Marginal mandibular branch

**Figure 5-15**

| TRIGEMINAL NERVE: OPHTHALMIC DIVISION | | |
|---|---|---|
| **Nerve** | **Source** | **Course** |
| Ophthalmic division | Trigeminal n. in the middle cranial fossa | Passes anteriorly on the lateral wall of the cavernous sinus immediately inferior to the oculomotor and trochlear nn., but superior to the maxillary division of the trigeminal n. |
| | | Immediately before entering the orbit, through the superior orbital fissure, it divides into 3 major branches: *lacrimal, frontal,* and *nasociliary* |
| *Supratrochlear* | From the ophthalmic division; the 2 terminal branches of the frontal n. in the orbit | 1 of the 2 terminal branches of the frontal n. in the orbit |
| | | Once the supratrochlear a. joins it within the orbit, it continues to pass anteriorly toward the trochlear n. |
| | | In the trochlear region, it exits the orbit at the frontal notch |
| | | Ascends along the scalp, at first deep to the musculature in the region, before piercing these muscles to reach the cutaneous innervation along the scalp |
| *Supraorbital* | | 1 of the 2 terminal branches of the frontal n. in the orbit |
| | | Passes between the levator palpebrae superioris m. and periosteum of the orbit |
| | | Continues anteriorly to the supraorbital foramen (notch) |
| | | At the level of the supraorbital margin, it sends nerve supply to the frontal sinus, skin, and conjunctiva of the upper eyelid |
| | | Continues to ascend superiorly along the scalp |
| | | Divides into medial and lateral branches, which travel up to the vertex of the scalp |
| *Lacrimal* | The smallest branch of the ophthalmic division | Smallest of the major branches of the ophthalmic division of the trigeminal n. |
| | | Passes anteriorly to enter the orbit through the superior orbital fissure |
| | | In the orbit it travels superolaterally on the superior border of the lateral rectus with the lacrimal a. |
| | | Before reaching the lacrimal gland, it communicates with the zygomatic branch of the maxillary division of the trigeminal n. to receive autonomic nervous fibers |
| | | Enters the lacrimal gland and supplies it and the conjunctiva before piercing the orbital septum to supply the skin of the upper eyelid |
| *Infratrochlear* | 1 of the terminal branches of the nasociliary | Passes anteriorly on the superior border of the medial rectus m. |
| | | Passes inferior to the trochlea toward the medial angle of the eye |
| | | Supplies the skin of the eyelids and bridge of the nose, the conjunctivae, and all of the lacrimal structures |
| *External nasal* | Arises from the anterior ethmoid n. (from the nasociliary n.) | Terminal branch of the anterior ethmoid n. |
| | | Exits between the lateral nasal cartilage and the inferior border of the nasal bone |
| | | Supplies the skin of the ala and apex of the nose around the nares |

| TRIGEMINAL NERVE: MAXILLARY DIVISION | | |
|---|---|---|
| **Nerve** | **Source** | **Course** |
| Maxillary division | Trigeminal n. in the middle cranial fossa | Travels along the lateral wall of the cavernous sinus |
| | | Before exiting the middle cranial fossa, it gives off a meningeal branch that innervates the dura mater |
| | | Passes from the middle cranial fossa into the pterygopalatine fossa via the foramen rotundum |
| | | Within the pterygopalatine fossa, it gives rise to 4 branches: *posterior superior alveolar n., zygomatic n., ganglionic branches*, and *infraorbital n.* |
| *Zygomaticotemporal* | Zygomatic branch of the maxillary division | Arises from the zygomatic n. in the pterygopalatine fossa, which passes through the inferior orbital fissure to enter the orbit, dividing into the zygomaticotemporal and zygomaticofacial |
| | | Passes on the lateral wall of the orbit in a groove in the zygomatic bone, then through a foramen in the zygomatic fossa to enter the temporal fossa region |
| | | Within the temporal fossa, it passes superiorly between the bone and the temporalis m. to pierce the temporal fascia superior to the zygomatic arch |
| | | Continues along the skin of the side of the scalp |
| *Zygomaticofacial* | Zygomatic branch of the maxillary division | Passes on the lateral wall of the orbit before emerging on the face through the zygomaticofacial foramen in the zygomatic bone |
| | | Supplies the skin on the prominence of the cheek |
| *Infraorbital* | The continuation of the maxillary division of the trigeminal n. | Passes through the inferior orbital fissure to enter the orbit, then anteriorly through the infraorbital groove, infraorbital canal, and exits onto the face via the infraorbital foramen |
| | | Within the infraorbital canal, it gives rise to the anterior superior alveolar and middle superior alveolar nn. |
| | | It exits onto the face and divides into 3 terminal branches: |
| | | • Inferior palpebral (supplies the skin of the lower eyelid) |
| | | • Nasal (supplies the ala of the nose) |
| | | • Superior labial (supplies the skin of the upper lip) |

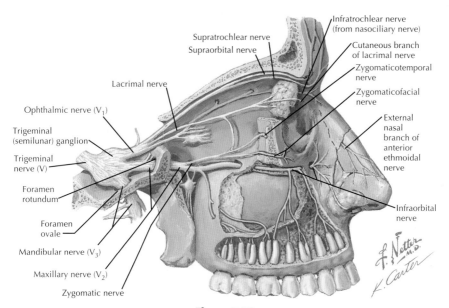

Figure 5-16

| TRIGEMINAL NERVE: MANDIBULAR DIVISION | | |
|---|---|---|
| **Nerve** | **Source** | **Course** |
| Mandibular division | Trigeminal n. in the middle cranial fossa | The largest of the trigeminal n.'s 3 divisions<br><br>Created by a large sensory and a small motor root that unite just after passing through the foramen ovale to enter the infratemporal fossa<br><br>Immediately gives rise to a meningeal branch and a medial pterygoid branch before dividing into anterior and posterior divisions:<br>• Anterior division—smaller and mainly motor, with 1 sensory branch (buccal n.)<br>• Posterior division—larger and mainly sensory, with 1 motor branch (mylohyoid n.) |
| *Auriculotemporal* | Posterior division of mandibular division of the trigeminal n. | Normally arises by 2 roots, between which the middle meningeal a. passes<br><br>Runs posteriorly just inferior to the lateral pterygoid and continues to the medial aspect of the neck of the mandible<br><br>While passing posterior to the mandible, it provides sensory innervation to the temporomandibular joint<br><br>Turns superiorly with the superficial temporal vessels between the auricle and the condyle of the mandible deep to the parotid gland<br><br>On exiting the substance of the parotid gland, it ascends over the zygomatic arch and divides into superficial temporal branches |
| *Buccal* | Anterior division of the mandibular division of the trigeminal n. | Passes anterior between the 2 heads of the lateral pterygoid m.<br><br>Descends inferiorly along the lower part of the temporalis to emerge deep to the anterior border of the masseter m.<br><br>Supplies the skin over the buccinator m. before passing through it to supply the mucous membrane lining its inner surface and the gingiva along the mandibular molars |
| *Mental* | 1 of the 2 terminal branches of the inferior alveolar n. | Emerges through the mental foramen of the mandible in the region of the 2nd mandibular premolar<br><br>Supplies the skin of the lower lip, chin, and facial gingiva as far posteriorly as the 2nd mandibular premolar |

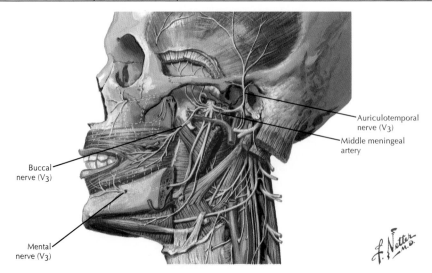

Auriculotemporal nerve (V3)

Middle meningeal artery

Buccal nerve (V3)

Mental nerve (V3)

**Figure 5-17**

| CERVICAL PLEXUS | | |
|---|---|---|
| **Nerve** | **Source** | **Course** |
| Great auricular | Arises from the cervical plexus formed by contributions of C2 and C3 ventral rami | Passes posterior to the midpoint of the sternocleidomastoid m. |
| | | Ascends along the sternocleidomastoid dividing into anterior and posterior branches |
| | | Anterior branch continues along the superficial aspect of the parotid gland's inferior part |
| | | Innervates the superficial and inferior portions of the parotid gland |
| Transverse cervical | | Passes posterior to the midpoint of the sternocleidomastoid m. |
| | | Crosses the sternocleidomastoid to pass anteriorly toward the neck |
| | | Perforates the investing layer of deep cervical fascia, dividing deep to the platysma m. into ascending and descending branches |
| | | Innervates the skin to the anterolateral region of the neck and lower face around the mandible |

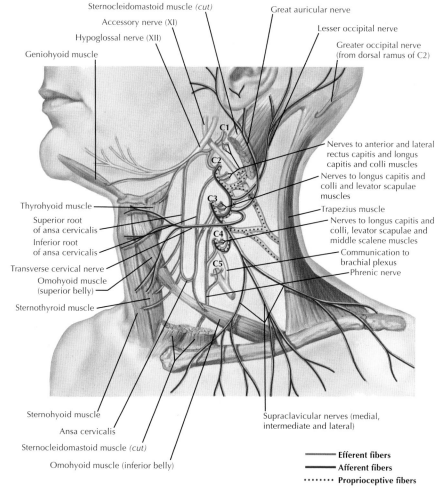

Sternocleidomastoid muscle *(cut)*
Accessory nerve (XI)
Hypoglossal nerve (XII)
Geniohyoid muscle
Great auricular nerve
Lesser occipital nerve
Greater occipital nerve (from dorsal ramus of C2)
C1
C2
C3
C4
C5
Nerves to anterior and lateral rectus capitis and longus capitis and colli muscles
Nerves to longus capitis and colli and levator scapulae muscles
Trapezius muscle
Nerves to longus capitis and colli, levator scapulae and middle scalene muscles
Communication to brachial plexus
Phrenic nerve
Thyrohyoid muscle
Superior root of ansa cervicalis
Inferior root of ansa cervicalis
Transverse cervical nerve
Omohyoid muscle (superior belly)
Sternothyroid muscle
Sternohyoid muscle
Ansa cervicalis
Sternocleidomastoid muscle *(cut)*
Omohyoid muscle (inferior belly)
Supraclavicular nerves (medial, intermediate and lateral)

——— Efferent fibers
——— Afferent fibers
······· Proprioceptive fibers

**Figure 5-18**

SCALP AND MUSCLES OF FACIAL EXPRESSION    **181**

| Nerve | Course |
|---|---|
| Facial | Exits the stylomastoid foramen and gives rise to the posterior auricular n. |
| | Enters the parotid fossa by passing between the stylohyoid m. and posterior belly of the digastric m. |
| | Small muscular branches innervate the stylohyoid m., the posterior belly of the digastric m., and the auricularis mm. |
| | Once in the fossa, it splits the parotid gland into a superficial lobe and a deep lobe that are connected by an isthmus |
| | Within the gland, it divides into temporofacial and cervicofacial trunks |
| | The trunks form a loop anterior to the gland superficial to the parotid duct and give rise to 5 major branches before emerging from the gland: *temporal, zygomatic, buccal, mandibular,* and *cervical* |
| *Temporal* | Exits the superior portion of the parotid gland from the temporofacial trunk |
| | Crosses the zygomatic arch along the temporal fossa to innervate the forehead |
| *Zygomatic* | The zygomatic branches from the temporofacial trunk pass across the zygomatic bone to the lateral angle of the orbit |
| | Innervates muscles in the region |
| *Buccal* | Branches arise from both the temporofacial and the cervicofacial trunks |
| | Innervates muscles of the cheek |
| *Marginal mandibular* | Branches arise from the cervicofacial trunk and pass anteriorly |
| | Innervates muscles of the lower lip and chin |
| *Cervical* | Branches arise from the cervicofacial trunk and pass anteriorly and inferiorly to innervate the platysma m. |

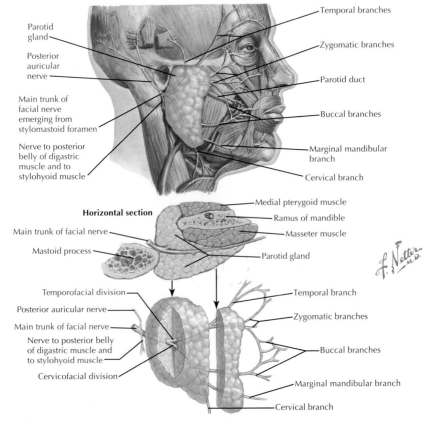

**Figure 5-19**

- Also called tic douloureux
- Usually affects the maxillary ($V_2$) or mandibular ($V_3$) division of the trigeminal nerve; rarely affects the ophthalmic division ($V_1$)
- Bilateral involvement suggests other factors such as multiple sclerosis
- More common in the 5th and 6th decades of life
- Cause is unknown—theories involve nerve irritation from abnormal vascularity or tumor compression, or a nerve injury

CLINICAL MANIFESTATIONS

- Periods of intense (lasting 1 to 2 minutes), paroxysmal pain along 1 of the divisions of the trigeminal nerve
- Usually unilateral
- Pain normally is initiated by a particular sensory stimulus, such as light touch (putting on makeup, washing the face, shaving, a light breeze), mastication, or brushing teeth

TREATMENT

- Commonly, trigeminal neuralgia is treated pharmacologically with anticonvulsants, such as carbamazepine (Tegretol)
- If drug therapy is unsuccessful, neurosurgery may be required, such as percutaneous radiofrequency rhizotomy of the nerve, glycerol injection of the trigeminal ganglion, or nerve decompression
- Alternative and complementary medicine treatments have included acupuncture and meditation

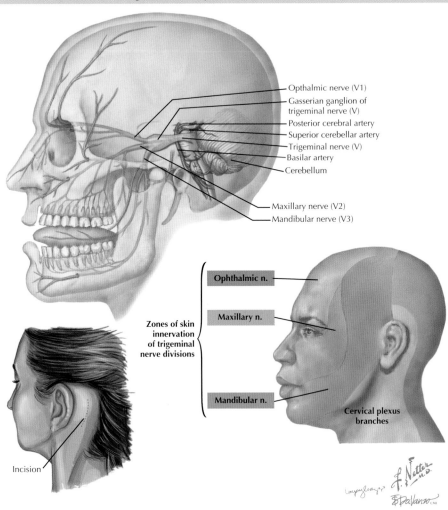

Opthalmic nerve (V1)
Gasserian ganglion of trigeminal nerve (V)
Posterior cerebral artery
Superior cerebellar artery
Trigeminal nerve (V)
Basilar artery
Cerebellum

Maxillary nerve (V2)
Mandibular nerve (V3)

Zones of skin innervation of trigeminal nerve divisions

Ophthalmic n.

Maxillary n.

Mandibular n.

Cervical plexus branches

Incision

**Microvascular decompression**

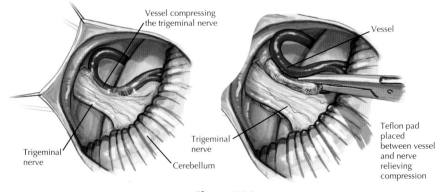

Vessel compressing the trigeminal nerve

Vessel

Trigeminal nerve

Trigeminal nerve

Trigeminal nerve

Cerebellum

Teflon pad placed between vessel and nerve relieving compression

**Figure 5-20**

- Pathologic condition involving the cavernous sinus that is often caused by a thrombosis, tumor, aneurysm, fistula, or trauma
- When caused by a thrombosis, the syndrome usually occurs as a sepsis from the central portion of the face or paranasal sinuses from their connection to the cavernous sinus
- Before the advent of antibiotics, death was the usual outcome from the sepsis
- It affects the contents of the cavernous sinus, including:
  - Internal carotid artery with sympathetics
  - Cranial nerve III
  - Cranial nerve IV
  - Cranial nerve $V_1$
  - Cranial nerve $V_2$
  - Cranial nerve VI
- Common clinical manifestations include:
  - Ophthalmoplegia with diminished pupillary light reflexes
  - Venous congestion leading to periorbital edema
  - Exophthalmos

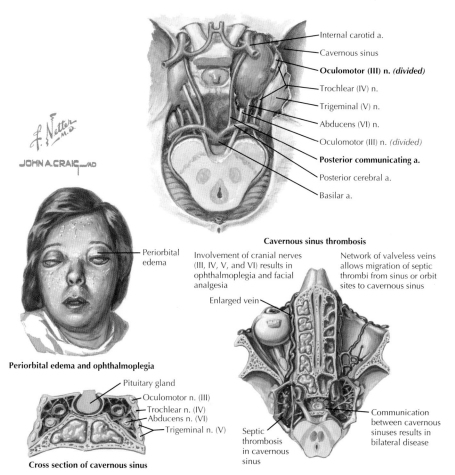

F. Netter M.D.

JOHN A.CRAIG—AD

Internal carotid a.

Cavernous sinus

**Oculomotor (III) n.** *(divided)*

Trochlear (IV) n.

Trigeminal (V) n.

Abducens (VI) n.

Oculomotor (III) n. *(divided)*

**Posterior communicating a.**

Posterior cerebral a.

Basilar a.

**Cavernous sinus thrombosis**

Periorbital edema

Involvement of cranial nerves (III, IV, V, and VI) results in ophthalmoplegia and facial analgesia

Network of valveless veins allows migration of septic thrombi from sinus or orbit sites to cavernous sinus

Enlarged vein

**Periorbital edema and ophthalmoplegia**

Pituitary gland

Oculomotor n. (III)

Trochlear n. (IV)

Abducens n. (VI)

Trigeminal n. (V)

Septic thrombosis in cavernous sinus

Communication between cavernous sinuses results in bilateral disease

**Cross section of cavernous sinus**

**Figure 5-21**

SCALP AND MUSCLES OF FACIAL EXPRESSION **185**

# PAROTID FOSSA AND GLAND

- The largest of all the major salivary glands, which weighs approximately 25 g
- Responsible for 20% to 25% of saliva formed by salivary glands
- Entirely serous in secretion
- Pyramidal in shape, with up to 5 processes (or extensions)
- The gland's capsule is extremely tough and derived from the deep cervical fascia (although evidence supports that the superficial portion is continuous with the platysma fascia, and it is classified as part of the superficial muscular aponeurotic system [SMAS])

### Anatomic Landmarks

- Approximately 75% or more of the parotid gland overlies the masseter muscle; the rest is retromandibular
- Facial nerve enters the parotid fossa by passing between the stylohyoid muscle and the posterior belly of the digastric muscle, which splits the gland into a "superficial lobe" and a "deep lobe" that are connected by an isthmus
- Deep lobe lies adjacent to the lateral pharyngeal space—thus tumors of the deep lobe are observed as swellings in the oropharynx
- Transverse facial artery parallels the parotid duct slightly superior to the duct
- Buccal and zygomatic branches of the facial nerve form an anastomosing loop superficial to the parotid duct

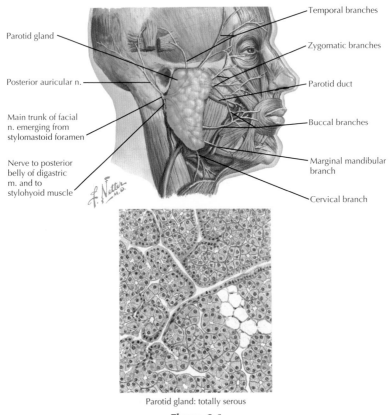

Parotid gland: totally serous

**Figure 6-1**

| Borders | Structures |
|---|---|
| Anterior | Masseter m.<br>Ramus of mandible |
| Anteromedial | Medial pterygoid m.<br>Stylomandibular fascia |
| Medial | Styloid process superomedially<br>Transverse process of the atlas inferomedially |
| Posteromedial | Stylohyoid m.<br>Posterior belly of the digastric m. |
| Posterior | Mastoid process of the temporal bone<br>Sternocleidomastoid m. |
| Lateral | Investing layer of deep cervical fascia helping form the capsule |
| Superior | External acoustic meatus<br>Condylar head of the mandible articulating in the glenoid fossa |
| Inferior | Angular tract of Eisler between the angle of the mandible and the sternocleidomastoid m. |

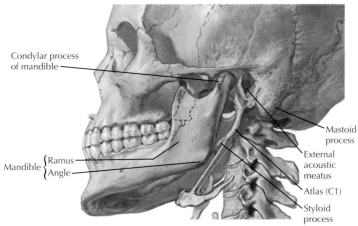

Condylar process
of mandible

Mastoid
process

External
acoustic
meatus

Mandible { Ramus
{ Angle

Atlas (C1)

Styloid
process

**Horizontal section below
lingula of mandible (superior
view) demonstrating bed
of parotid gland**

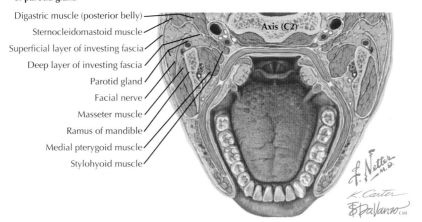

Digastric muscle (posterior belly)

Sternocleidomastoid muscle

Superficial layer of investing fascia

Deep layer of investing fascia

Parotid gland

Facial nerve

Masseter muscle

Ramus of mandible

Medial pterygoid muscle

Stylohyoid muscle

Axis (C2)

**Figure 6-2**

| Structure | Features |
|---|---|
| Parotid gland | The largest of all of the major salivary glands, entirely serous in secretion |
| | Pyramidal in shape, with up to 5 processes (or extensions) |
| | The gland's capsule is from the deep cervical fascia |
| | About 75% or more of the parotid gland overlies the masseter m.; the rest is retromandibular |
| Facial nerve | Facial n. exits the stylomastoid foramen and gives rise to the posterior auricular n. |
| | Enters the parotid fossa by passing between the stylohyoid m. and the posterior belly of the digastric m. |
| | Small muscular branches innervate the stylohyoid m., the posterior belly of the digastric m., and the auricularis mm. |
| | Once in the fossa, it splits the parotid gland into a superficial lobe and a deep lobe that are connected by an isthmus |
| | Parotid gland's deep lobe lies adjacent to the lateral pharyngeal space |
| | Within the gland, the facial n. divides into temporofacial and cervicofacial trunks |
| | The trunks form a loop anterior to the gland superficial to the parotid duct and give rise to 5 major branches before emerging from the gland: |
| | • Temporal |
| | • Zygomatic |
| | • Buccal |
| | • Marginal mandibular |
| | • Cervical |
| | Although it passes through the parotid gland, the facial n. does not provide any innervation to it |
| | Buccal and zygomatic branches of the facial n. form an anastomosing loop superficial to the parotid duct |
| Parotid duct | Also known as Stensen's duct |
| | The duct typically is 5 cm in length |
| | Forms within the deep lobe and passes from the anterior border of the gland across the masseter superficially, through the buccinator into the oral cavity opposite the 2nd maxillary molar |
| | Accessory parotid tissue often follows the parotid duct |
| External carotid artery | The external carotid a. travels through the parotid gland and gives off branches within the gland: |
| | • Posterior auricular a. |
| | • Maxillary a. |
| | • Superficial temporal a. |
| | • Transverse facial a. |
| Retromandibular vein | The retromandibular vein is located superficial to the external carotid artery within the parotid gland |
| | The retromandibular vein is formed by the union of: |
| | • Superficial temporal v. (a small transverse facial v. drains into this vein) |
| | • Maxillary v. |
| | Typically, the retromandibular v. exits the inferior portion of the parotid gland and divides into: |
| | • Anterior division of the retromandibular (which joins the facial v. to form the common facial v.) |
| | • Posterior division of the retromandibular (which joins the posterior auricular v. to form the external jugular v.) |

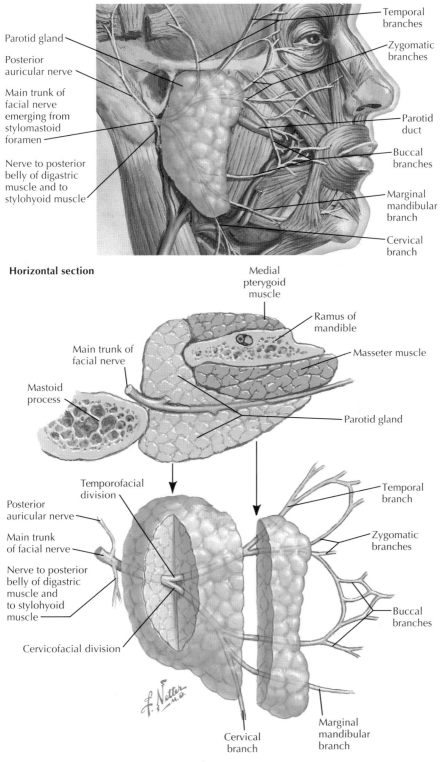

Temporal branches

Zygomatic branches

Parotid gland

Posterior auricular nerve

Main trunk of facial nerve emerging from stylomastoid foramen

Nerve to posterior belly of digastric muscle and to stylohyoid muscle

Parotid duct

Buccal branches

Marginal mandibular branch

Cervical branch

**Horizontal section**

Medial pterygoid muscle

Ramus of mandible

Main trunk of facial nerve

Masseter muscle

Mastoid process

Parotid gland

Temporofacial division

Temporal branch

Posterior auricular nerve

Zygomatic branches

Main trunk of facial nerve

Nerve to posterior belly of digastric muscle and to stylohyoid muscle

Cervicofacial division

Buccal branches

Marginal mandibular branch

Cervical branch

**Figure 6-3**

| ARTERIAL SUPPLY | | |
|---|---|---|
| **Artery** | **Source** | **Course** |
| External carotid | The bifurcation of the common carotid a. (most commonly located at vertebral level C3) | Ascends superiorly posterior to the mandible and deep to the posterior belly of the digastric m. and the stylohyoid m. to enter the parotid gland |
| | | Within the parotid gland, it gives branches to the gland and the posterior auricular a. |
| | | Then branches into the superficial temporal and maxillary aa. within the gland |
| | | The transverse facial a. arises from the superficial temporal a. within the gland |
| *Posterior auricular* | External carotid a. within the parotid gland | Passes superiorly between the mastoid process and cartilage of the ear |
| *Maxillary* | The 2 terminal branches of the external carotid a. within the parotid gland | Begins posterior to the neck of the mandible and travels anteromedially between the sphenomandibular lig. and the ramus of the mandible |
| | | On exiting the parotid gland, passes either superficial or deep to the lateral pterygoid muscle |
| *Superficial temporal* | | Begins posterior to the neck of the mandible and travels superiorly as a continuation of the external carotid |
| | | Joined by the auriculotemporal n. |
| • *Transverse facial* | Superficial temporal a. before it exits the parotid gland | Passes transversely to exit the gland |
| | | Passes immediately superior to the parotid duct across the masseter m. and face |

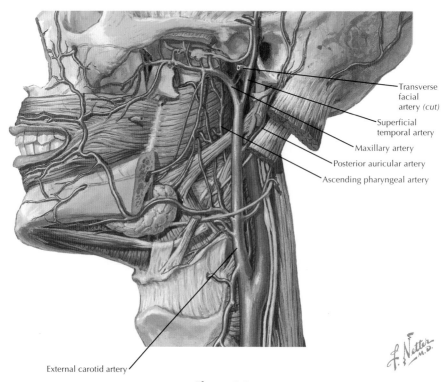

Figure 6-4

| VENOUS DRAINAGE | |
|---|---|
| **Vein** | **Course** |
| Superficial temporal | Descends posterior to the zygomatic root of the temporal bone alongside the auriculotemporal n. to enter the parotid gland |
| | Unites with the maxillary v. to form the retromandibular v. |
| *Transverse facial* | Travels posteriorly to enter the parotid gland and join the superficial temporal v. |
| Maxillary | A short, sometimes paired vein, formed by the convergence of the tributaries of the pterygoid plexus |
| | Enters the parotid gland traveling posteriorly between the sphenomandibular lig. and the neck of the mandible |
| | Unites with the superficial temporal v. to form the retromandibular v. |
| Retromandibular | Arises from the joining of the superficial temporal and maxillary vv. within the parotid gland |
| | Descends superficial to the external carotid a. in the gland, where it branches into: |
| | • Anterior division of the retromandibular (which joins the facial v. to form the common facial v.) |
| | • Posterior division of the retromandibular (which joins the posterior auricular to form the external jugular v.) |
| *Anterior division of the retromandibular* | 1 of the terminal divisions of the retromandibular vein |
| | Typically branches once the retromandibular vein has exited the parotid gland inferiorly |
| | Joins the facial v to form the common facial v., which drains into the internal jugular v. |
| *Posterior division of the retromandibular* | 1 of the terminal divisions of the retromandibular vein |
| | Typically branches once the retromandibular vein has exited the parotid gland inferiorly |
| | Joins the posterior auricular v. (which arises as a plexus of veins created by the occipital and superficial temporal vv.) to form the external jugular v., which drains into subclavian v. |

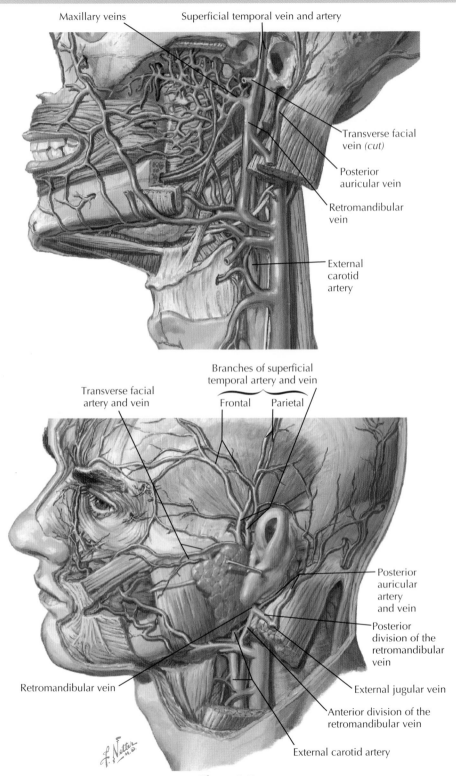

Maxillary veins

Superficial temporal vein and artery

Transverse facial vein *(cut)*

Posterior auricular vein

Retromandibular vein

External carotid artery

Branches of superficial temporal artery and vein

Transverse facial artery and vein

Frontal　Parietal

Posterior auricular artery and vein

Posterior division of the retromandibular vein

Retromandibular vein

External jugular vein

Anterior division of the retromandibular vein

External carotid artery

**Figure 6-5**

| SENSORY NERVES OF THE PAROTID | | |
|---|---|---|
| **Nerve** | **Source** | **Course** |
| Auriculotemporal | Mandibular division of the trigeminal n. | Often arises as 2 roots surrounding the middle meningeal a. that unite |
| | | Passes inferior to the lateral pterygoid toward the neck of the mandible |
| | | Passes posterior to the neck of the mandible to ascend with the superficial temporal a. |
| | | Provides sensory fibers to the parotid gland |
| Great auricular | The cervical plexus formed by contributions of C2 and C3 ventral rami | After passing posterior to the midpoint of the sternocleidomastoid, it ascends along the sternocleidomastoid m., dividing into anterior and posterior branches |
| | | The anterior branch continues along the superficial aspect of the inferior part of the parotid gland |
| | | Helps supply parotid capsule |

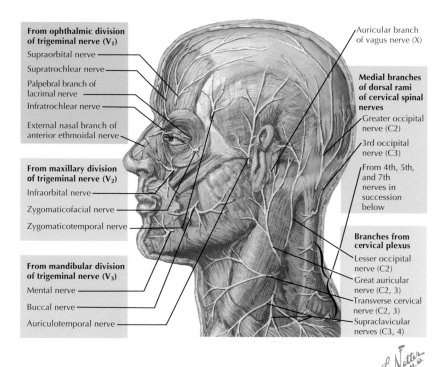

**From ophthalmic division of trigeminal nerve (V₁)**
Supraorbital nerve
Supratrochlear nerve
Palpebral branch of lacrimal nerve
Infratrochlear nerve
External nasal branch of anterior ethmoidal nerve

**From maxillary division of trigeminal nerve (V₂)**
Infraorbital nerve
Zygomaticofacial nerve
Zygomaticotemporal nerve

**From mandibular division of trigeminal nerve (V₃)**
Mental nerve
Buccal nerve
Auriculotemporal nerve

Auricular branch of vagus nerve (X)

**Medial branches of dorsal rami of cervical spinal nerves**
Greater occipital nerve (C2)
3rd occipital nerve (C3)
From 4th, 5th, and 7th nerves in succession below

**Branches from cervical plexus**
Lesser occipital nerve (C2)
Great auricular nerve (C2, 3)
Transverse cervical nerve (C2, 3)
Supraclavicular nerves (C3, 4)

**Figure 6-6**

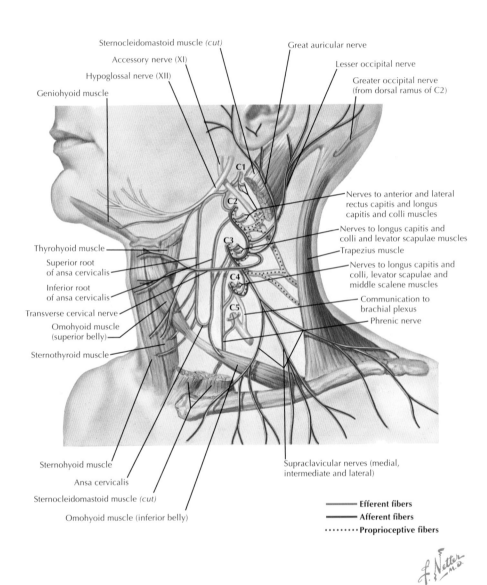

Sternocleidomastoid muscle *(cut)*

Accessory nerve (XI)

Hypoglossal nerve (XII)

Geniohyoid muscle

Great auricular nerve

Lesser occipital nerve

Greater occipital nerve
(from dorsal ramus of C2)

C1

C2

C3

C4

C5

Nerves to anterior and lateral
rectus capitis and longus
capitis and colli muscles

Nerves to longus capitis and
colli and levator scapulae muscles

Trapezius muscle

Nerves to longus capitis and
colli, levator scapulae and
middle scalene muscles

Communication to
brachial plexus

Phrenic nerve

Thyrohyoid muscle

Superior root
of ansa cervicalis

Inferior root
of ansa cervicalis

Transverse cervical nerve

Omohyoid muscle
(superior belly)

Sternothyroid muscle

Sternohyoid muscle

Ansa cervicalis

Sternocleidomastoid muscle *(cut)*

Omohyoid muscle (inferior belly)

Supraclavicular nerves (medial,
intermediate and lateral)

———— Efferent fibers
———— Afferent fibers
········ Proprioceptive fibers

**Figure 6-7**

| ANATOMIC PATHWAY FOR PARASYMPATHETICS OF THE PAROTID GLAND | | | |
|---|---|---|---|
| **Type of Neuron** | **Name of Cell Body** | **Characteristics of Cell Body** | **Course of the Neuron** |
| Preganglionic neuron | Inferior salivatory nucleus | A collection of nerve cell bodies located in the medulla | Preganglionic parasympathetic fibers arise from the inferior salivatory nucleus in the medulla<br><br>These fibers travel through the glossopharyngeal n. (IX) and exit the jugular foramen<br><br>Gives rise to the tympanic branch of IX, which reenters the skull via the tympanic canaliculus<br><br>Tympanic branch of IX forms the tympanic plexus along the promontory of the ear<br><br>The plexus re-forms as the lesser petrosal n., typically exiting the foramen ovale to enter the infratemporal fossa<br><br>Lesser petrosal n. joins the otic ganglion |
| Postganglionic neuron | Otic ganglion | A collection of nerve cell bodies located inferior to the foramen ovale medial to the mandibular division of the trigeminal n. | Postganglionic parasympathetic fibers arise in the otic ganglion<br><br>These fibers travel to the auriculotemporal branch of the trigeminal n.<br><br>Auriculotemporal n. travels to the parotid gland<br><br>Postganglionic parasympathetic fibers innervate the parotid gland |

| ANATOMIC PATHWAY FOR SYMPATHETICS OF THE PAROTID GLAND | | | |
|---|---|---|---|
| **Type of Neuron** | **Name of Cell Body** | **Characteristics of Cell Body** | **Course of the Neuron** |
| Preganglionic neuron | Intermediolateral horn nucleus | Collection of nerve cell bodies located in the lateral horn nucleus of the spinal cord between spinal segments T1 and T3 (and possibly T4) | Arise from the intermediolateral horn nuclei from T1 and T3(4)<br><br>Travel through the ventral root of the spinal cord to the spinal nerve<br><br>Enter the sympathetic chain via white rami communicantes<br><br>Once in the sympathetic chain, the preganglionic fibers for the eye will ascend and synapse with postganglionic fibers in the superior cervical ganglion |
| Postganglionic neuron | Superior cervical ganglion | Collection of nerve cell bodies located in the superior cervical ganglion, which is located at the base of the skull | Arise in the superior cervical ganglion<br><br>Postganglionic fibers will follow the external carotid a.<br><br>Branches from the external carotid follow the arteries that supply the parotid gland |

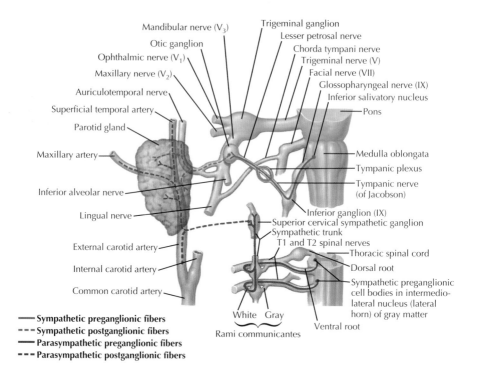

Mandibular nerve (V₃)
Otic ganglion
Ophthalmic nerve (V₁)
Maxillary nerve (V₂)
Auriculotemporal nerve
Superficial temporal artery
Parotid gland
Maxillary artery
Inferior alveolar nerve
Lingual nerve
External carotid artery
Internal carotid artery
Common carotid artery

Trigeminal ganglion
Lesser petrosal nerve
Chorda tympani nerve
Trigeminal nerve (V)
Facial nerve (VII)
Glossopharyngeal nerve (IX)
Inferior salivatory nucleus
Pons
Medulla oblongata
Tympanic plexus
Tympanic nerve (of Jacobson)
Inferior ganglion (IX)
Superior cervical sympathetic ganglion
Sympathetic trunk
T1 and T2 spinal nerves
Thoracic spinal cord
Dorsal root
Sympathetic preganglionic cell bodies in intermediolateral nucleus (lateral horn) of gray matter
Ventral root

White   Gray
Rami communicantes

—— Sympathetic preganglionic fibers
--- Sympathetic postganglionic fibers
—— Parasympathetic preganglionic fibers
--- Parasympathetic postganglionic fibers

**Lateral view**

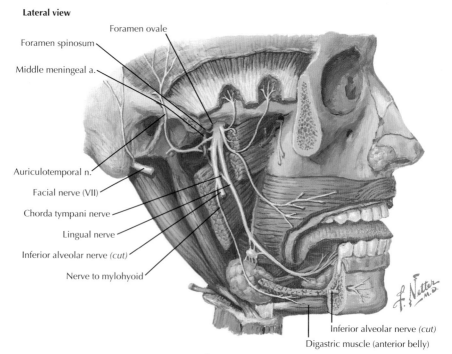

Foramen ovale
Foramen spinosum
Middle meningeal a.
Auriculotemporal n.
Facial nerve (VII)
Chorda tympani nerve
Lingual nerve
Inferior alveolar nerve *(cut)*
Nerve to mylohyoid
Inferior alveolar nerve *(cut)*
Digastric muscle (anterior belly)

**Figure 6-8**

- Unilateral facial paralysis from facial nerve (cranial nerve VII) damage

CAUSES

- Approximately 80% of cases have unclear etiology
- Evidence suggests herpes simplex virus (HSV-1) infection as a cause
  - *Proposed mechanism*: When the virus becomes active at the facial nerve, if the inflammation is in the bony facial canal, limited room for expansion results in nerve compression
- Bacterial infections also have been implicated
  - In some cases of otitis media, bacteria may enter the facial canal, and any resulting inflammatory response could compress the facial nerve
- Temporary Bell's palsy can result from dental procedures if inferior alveolar nerve block anesthetic is improperly administered in the parotid fossa; signs and symptoms disappear when the anesthetic effects wear off

PROGNOSIS

- Mild cases produce a facial nerve neurapraxia; the prognosis for complete recovery is very good, usually within 2 to 3 weeks
- In more moderate cases, an axonotmesis may occur, producing wallerian degeneration; full recovery may take 2 to 3 months
- In a small percentage of cases, function is never completely recovered

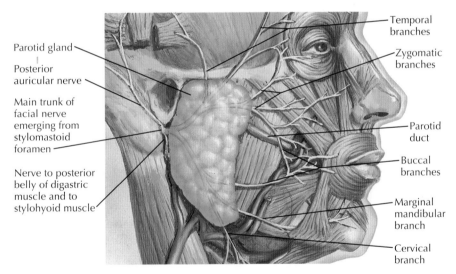

**Horizontal section**

**Course and distribution of facial (VII) nerve**

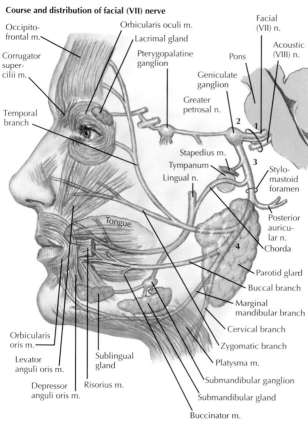

Occipito-frontal m.
Orbicularis oculi m.
Lacrimal gland
Corrugator super-cilii m.
Pterygopalatine ganglion
Facial (VII) n.
Acoustic (VIII) n.
Pons
Geniculate ganglion
Greater petrosal n.
Temporal branch
Stapedius m.
Tympanum
Lingual n.
Stylo-mastoid foramen
Tongue
Posterior auricu-lar n.
Chorda
Parotid gland
Buccal branch
Marginal mandibular branch
Cervical branch
Zygomatic branch
Platysma m.
Submandibular ganglion
Submandibular gland
Buccinator m.
Orbicularis oris m.
Levator anguli oris m.
Sublingual gland
Depressor anguli oris m.
Risorius m.

**Sites of lesions and their manifestations**

1. Intracranial and/or internal auditory meatus. All symptoms of 2, 3, and 4, plus deafness due to involvement of 8th cranial nerve.

2. Geniculate ganglion. All symptoms of 3 and 4, plus pain behind ear. Herpes of tympanum and of external auditory meatus may occur.

3. Facial canal. All symptoms of 4, plus loss of taste in anterior tongue and decreased salivation on affected side due to chorda tympani involvement. Hyperacusia due to effect on nerve branch to stapedius muscle.

4. Below stylomastoid foramen (parotid gland tumor, trauma) Facial paralysis (mouth draws to opposite side; on affected side, patient unable to close eye or wrinkle forehead; food collects between teeth and cheek due to paralysis of buccinator muscle).

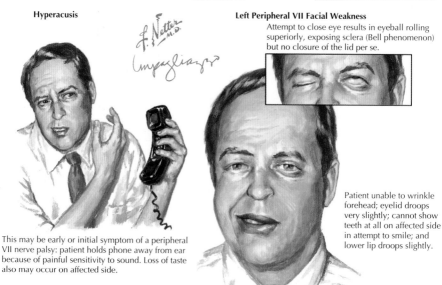

**Hyperacusis**

This may be early or initial symptom of a peripheral VII nerve palsy: patient holds phone away from ear because of painful sensitivity to sound. Loss of taste also may occur on affected side.

**Left Peripheral VII Facial Weakness**

Attempt to close eye results in eyeball rolling superiorly, exposing sclera (Bell phenomenon) but no closure of the lid per se.

Patient unable to wrinkle forehead; eyelid droops very slightly; cannot show teeth at all on affected side in attempt to smile; and lower lip droops slightly.

**Figure 6-9**

- Caused by regeneration of the auriculotemporal autonomic fibers in an abnormal fashion, innervating the sweat glands near the parotid gland after a parotidectomy
- Symptoms include sweating and redness in the distribution of the auriculotemporal nerve during eating
- Diagnosis is via Minor's starch iodine test—creates a dark spot over the gustatory sweating area
- Treatments include tympanic neurectomy (severing the parasympathetic component) and the topical anticholinergic glycopyrrolate (Robinul)

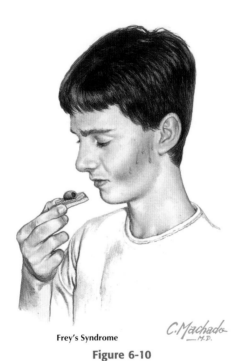

**Frey's Syndrome**

C. Machado
_M.D.

**Figure 6-10**

- 80% of parotid tumors are benign
- The most common benign tumor is a pleomorphic adenoma, which, if present for many years, can convert to a highly malignant carcinoma
- When pleomorphic adenomas extend through the capsule, they must be removed to reduce recurrence
- Because of the proximity, these tumors can extend into the lateral pharyngeal space
- Removal of the tumor with its surrounding capsule and tissue is important to obtain a low recurrence rate
  - Histologically, pleomorphic adenomas have extensions through the tumor capsule into adjacent tissue, so simple enucleation would allow recurrence from tumor cells left behind

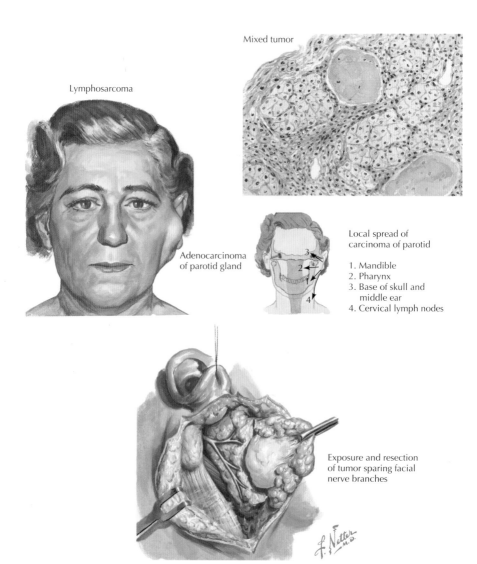

Mixed tumor

Lymphosarcoma

Adenocarcinoma of parotid gland

Local spread of carcinoma of parotid

1. Mandible
2. Pharynx
3. Base of skull and middle ear
4. Cervical lymph nodes

Exposure and resection of tumor sparing facial nerve branches

**Figure 6-11**

- An inflammation of the parotid glands that typically is caused by a bacterial or viral infection
- Can also be caused by other diseases, such as Sjögren's syndrome, tuberculosis, and human immunodeficiency virus (HIV) infection
- Pain on mandibular movement is the result of the compression of the deep lobe of the gland by the mandibular ramus

## BACTERIAL PAROTITIS

- Less common since the introduction of antibiotics, proper hydration, and better oral hygiene
- Mortality rate in the early 19th century was as high as 70% to 80%
- Most cases now seen in patients on anticholinergic medication, especially the elderly, because it inhibits the salivary flow, which makes it easier for the bacteria to be transported in retrograde fashion along the parotid duct into the gland, where they may settle to cause an infection

## VIRAL PAROTITIS

- Known as mumps
- Causative virus is a paramyxovirus that infects different body parts, notably the parotid glands
- Usually is spread through saliva, coughing, and sneezing
- Parotid glands typically swell and become very painful
- With the introduction of mumps vaccination in the 1970s, now rare in most developed nations

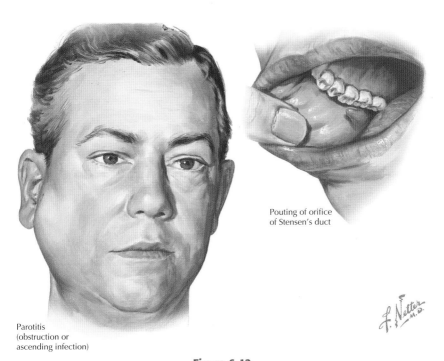

Pouting of orifice of Stensen's duct

Parotitis (obstruction or ascending infection)

**Figure 6-12**

- *Xerostomia*: "dry mouth"
- Dry mouth is a symptom that increases the affected person's susceptibility to dental caries
- Can be caused by any medication that reduces salivary outflow, commonly many antihistamines, antidepressants, chemotherapy agents, antihypertensives, and analgesics, as well as by therapeutic irradiation
- Occurs in disease processes such as depression, stress, endocrine disorders, Sjögren's syndrome, and improper nutrition
- Can lead to the formation of sialoliths, calculi that form in the duct or gland, although they are more commonly associated with infections of the submandibular gland than of the parotid gland and duct

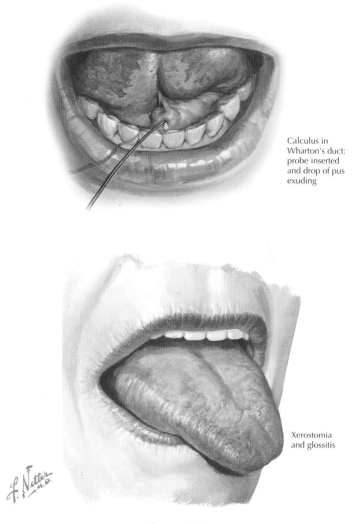

Calculus in Wharton's duct: probe inserted and drop of pus exuding

Xerostomia and glossitis

**Figure 6-13**

- *Parotid fistula*: a communication between the skin and the parotid gland or duct that may lead to the formation of a sialocele, a cyst filled with a collection of mucoid saliva in the tissues surrounding the gland

## CAUSES

- Both parotid fistulas and sialoceles often occur as the result of trauma during surgery
- May also be caused by:
  - Section or injury of the duct or 1 of its branches during operation for cancer of the cheek or face
  - Removal of parotid tumors, especially those of the accessory lobe
  - Primary or secondary malignant tumors that ulcerate the skin
  - Incision and drainage for acute bacterial parotitis
  - Ulceration and infection associated with large salivary calculi
  - Fistula may develop after a mastoid or fenestration operation
  - Congenital
  - Infection (actinomycosis, tuberculosis, syphilis, cancrum oris)

## TREATMENT

- Fistulas that lead directly into the oral cavity need no treatment
- Fistulas on the skin may or may not need surgical intervention
- Anticholinergics are useful agents to diminish the salivation during treatment
- Sialoceles often resolve with aspiration or compression and normally do not require drain placement
- Injury to the parotid gland or duct should be repaired to prevent formation of fistulas and sialoceles

## COMMON REPAIRS

- Repair of the duct using a stent
- Ligation of the duct
- Creating a fistula from the duct into the oral cavity

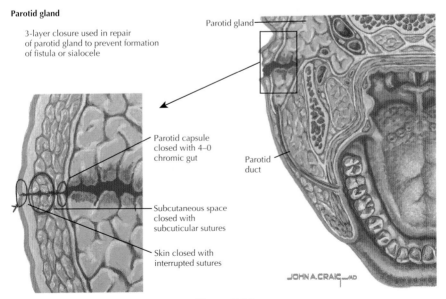

**Parotid gland**

3-layer closure used in repair of parotid gland to prevent formation of fistula or sialocele

Parotid gland

Parotid capsule closed with 4–0 chromic gut

Parotid duct

Subcutaneous space closed with subcuticular sutures

Skin closed with interrupted sutures

JOHN A. CRAIG—AD

**Figure 6-14**

# TEMPORAL AND INFRATEMPORAL FOSSAE

- The entire temporal area consists of 2 fossae divided by the zygomatic arch

## TEMPORAL FOSSA

- Related to the temple of the head
- Communicates with the infratemporal fossa beneath the zygomatic arch

## INFRATEMPORAL FOSSA

- An irregularly shaped fossa inferior and medial to the zygomatic arch
- Communicates with the pterygopalatine fossa at the pterygomaxillary fissure

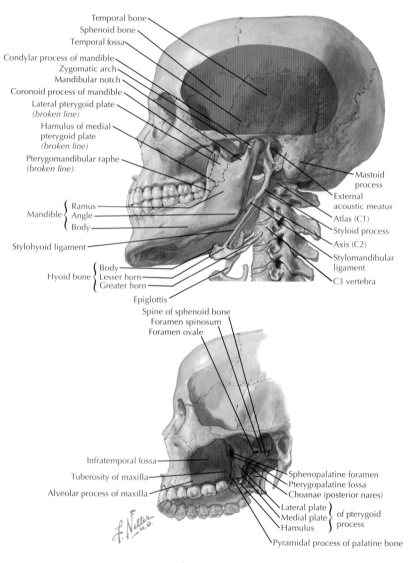

**Figure 7-1**

| Border | Structures |
|--------|-----------|
| Superior | Superior temporal line<br>Inferior temporal line |
| Inferior | Zygomatic arch (laterally)<br>Infratemporal crest of greater wing of sphenoid (medially) |
| Anterior | Frontal process of the zygoma<br>Zygomatic process of the frontal bone |
| Posterior | Supramastoid crest<br>Posterior portion of superior temporal line (which arches inferiorly to the supramastoid crest) |
| Medial | Frontal<br>Greater wing of the sphenoid<br>Squamous part of the temporal<br>Parietal |
| Lateral | Temporal fascia |

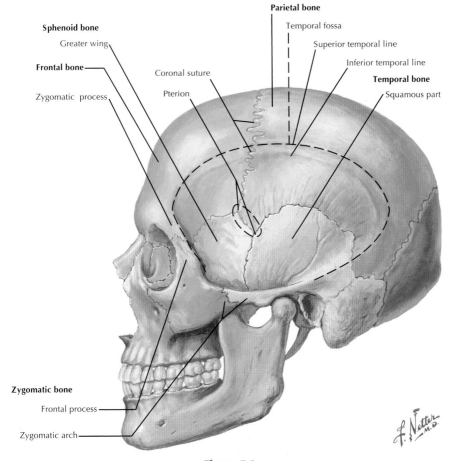

**Figure 7-2**

| ARTERIAL SUPPLY | | |
|---|---|---|
| **Artery** | **Source** | **Course** |
| Superficial temporal | A terminal branch of the external carotid a. that arises within the parotid gland | Within the substance of the parotid gland, it gives off a transverse facial a.<br><br>Emerges from the superior part of the parotid gland immediately posterior to the temporomandibular joint and anterior to the external auditory meatus<br><br>Passes superficial to the root of the zygomatic arch just anterior to the auriculotemporal n. and the auricle<br><br>Immediately superior to the root of the zygomatic arch, it gives rise to the middle temporal a. that pierces deep into the temporalis fascia and muscle<br><br>As it continues to pass superiorly, it divides into anterior and posterior branches |
| *Middle temporal* | Superficial temporal a. after it passes superior to the root of the zygomatic arch | Passes deep into the temporalis fascia and temporalis m., where it anastomoses with the anterior and posterior deep temporal vessels |
| Anterior and posterior deep temporal | Branches of the 2nd part of the maxillary a. | Pass between the skull and the temporalis m.<br><br>Supply the temporalis throughout their course<br><br>While ascending, they anastomose with the middle temporal a. |

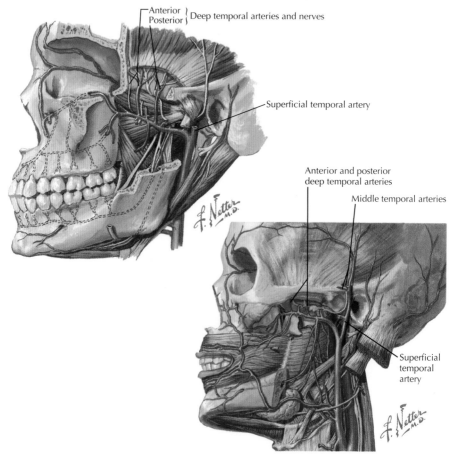

Anterior ⎫ Deep temporal arteries and nerves
Posterior ⎭

Superficial temporal artery

Anterior and posterior deep temporal arteries

Middle temporal arteries

Superficial temporal artery

**Figure 7-3**

| VENOUS DRAINAGE | |
| --- | --- |
| **Vein** | **Course** |
| Superficial temporal | Begins at the vertex and lateral aspect of the skull |
| | Forms a venous plexus along the scalp by communicating with the supraorbital, posterior auricular, occipital vv. and corresponding veins from the opposite side |
| | Forms an anterior and a posterior branch of the superficial temporal v. that pass inferiorly immediately anterior to the artery |
| | A middle temporal v. joins the superficial temporal before the vessel passes inferior to the root of the zygomatic arch |
| | Enters the parotid gland, where it receives the transverse facial v. |
| | Joins the maxillary v. to form the retromandibular v. |
| Middle temporal | Arises deep within the temporalis m. and fascia |
| | Within the temporalis m. and fascia, it anastomoses with the anterior and posterior deep temporal vessels |
| | Joins the superficial temporal a. immediately before it passes inferior to the root of the zygomatic arch |
| Anterior and posterior deep temporal | Drain into the pterygoid plexus of veins |
| | Also communicate with the middle temporal v. |

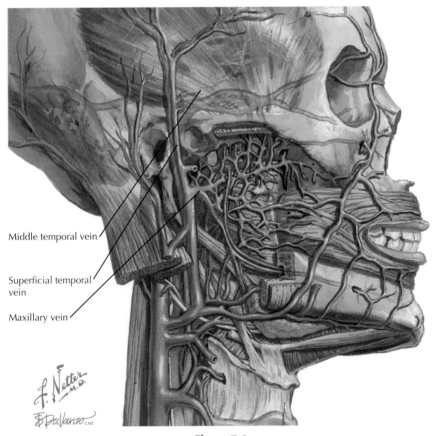

Middle temporal vein

Superficial temporal vein

Maxillary vein

**Figure 7-4**

| Nerve | Source | Course |
|-------|--------|--------|
| Mandibular division of the trigeminal | The largest of the 3 divisions of the trigeminal n. <br><br> Created by a large sensory and small motor root that unite just after passing through the foramen ovale to enter the infratemporal fossa | Immediately gives rise to a meningeal branch and medial pterygoid branch before it divides into anterior and posterior divisions <br><br> The anterior division is smaller and mainly motor, with 1 sensory branch (buccal n.) <br><br> The posterior division is larger and mainly sensory, with 1 motor branch (mylohyoid n.) |
| *Anterior and posterior deep temporal* | Arise from the anterior division of the mandibular division of the trigeminal n. | Pass superior to the lateral pterygoid m. between the skull and the temporalis m. while passing deep to the muscle to innervate it |
| *Auriculotemporal* | Arises from the posterior division of the mandibular division of the trigeminal n. | Normally arises from 2 roots, between which the middle meningeal a. passes <br><br> Runs posteriorly just inferior to the lateral pterygoid and continues to the medial side of the neck of the mandible <br><br> While passing posterior to the mandible, it provides sensory innervation to the temporomandibular joint <br><br> Turns superiorly with the superficial temporal vessels between the auricle and the condyle of the mandible deep to the parotid gland <br><br> On exiting the substance of the parotid gland, it ascends over the zygomatic arch and divides into superficial temporal branches |
| Temporal branches of the facial | Motor branches that arise in the substance of the parotid gland | Cross the zygomatic arch to the temporal region <br><br> Supply the muscles in the area, including the frontalis, anterior auricular, superior auricular, orbicularis oculi, procerus, and corrugator supercilii mm. |

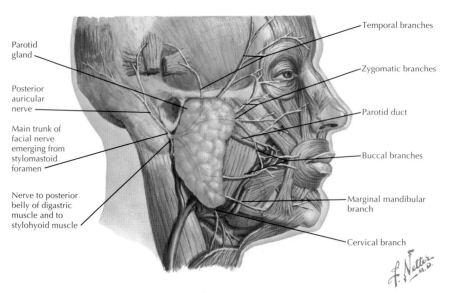

Parotid gland

Posterior auricular nerve

Main trunk of facial nerve emerging from stylomastoid foramen

Nerve to posterior belly of digastric muscle and to stylohyoid muscle

Temporal branches

Zygomatic branches

Parotid duct

Buccal branches

Marginal mandibular branch

Cervical branch

**Figure 7-5**

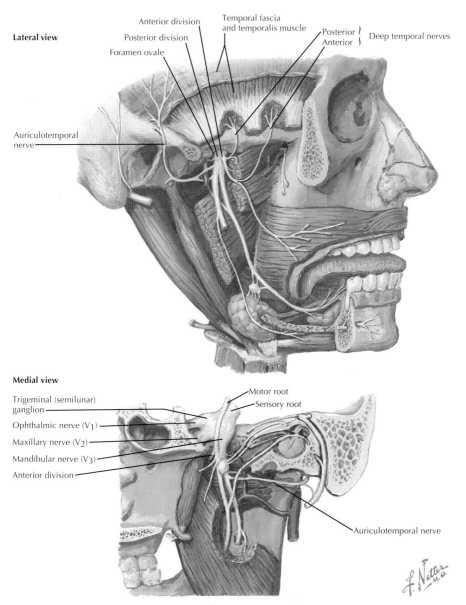

**Lateral view**

Anterior division

Posterior division

Foramen ovale

Temporal fascia
and temporalis muscle

Posterior
Anterior } Deep temporal nerves

Auriculotemporal
nerve

**Medial view**

Trigeminal (semilunar)
ganglion

Ophthalmic nerve (V₁)

Maxillary nerve (V₂)

Mandibular nerve (V₃)

Anterior division

Motor root

Sensory root

Auriculotemporal nerve

**Figure 7-6**

| Border | Structure(s) |
|--------|-------------|
| Superior | Infratemporal surface of the greater wing of the sphenoid (with the foramen ovale and foramen spinosum)<br>Infratemporal surface of the temporal bone |
| Inferior | No anatomic floor—the boundary of the fossa ends where the medial pterygoid attaches to the mandible |
| Lateral | Ramus of the mandible (medial surface) |
| Medial | Lateral pterygoid plate of the sphenoid (lateral surface)<br>Pyramidal process of the palatine bone |
| Anterior | Posterior portion of the maxilla |
| Posterior | Styloid process<br>Condylar process of the mandible |

MUSCLES
- Temporalis
- Lateral pterygoid
- Medial pterygoid

ARTERIES
- Maxillary and its branches

VEINS
- Pterygoid plexus of veins and tributaries

NERVES
- Mandibular division of the trigeminal n. and branches
- Posterior superior alveolar (branch of maxillary division of trigeminal)
- Chorda tympani (branch of the facial n.)
- Otic ganglion
- Lesser petrosal

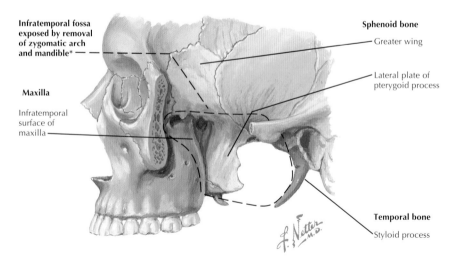

Infratemporal fossa exposed by removal of zygomatic arch and mandible*

Sphenoid bone
Greater wing

Lateral plate of pterygoid process

Maxilla

Infratemporal surface of maxilla

Temporal bone
Styloid process

*Superficially, mastoid process forms posterior boundary

**Figure 7-7**

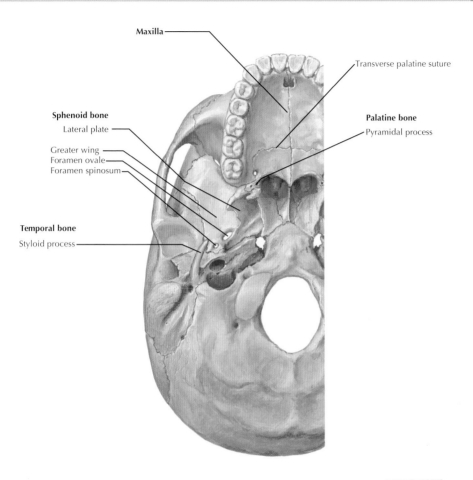

Maxilla

Transverse palatine suture

**Sphenoid bone**
Lateral plate

**Palatine bone**
Pyramidal process

Greater wing
Foramen ovale
Foramen spinosum

**Temporal bone**
Styloid process

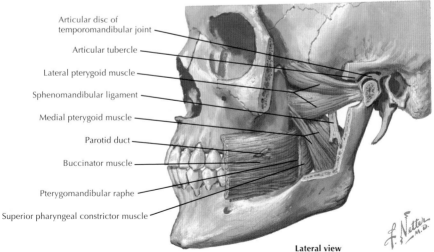

Articular disc of
temporomandibular joint

Articular tubercle

Lateral pterygoid muscle

Sphenomandibular ligament

Medial pterygoid muscle

Parotid duct

Buccinator muscle

Pterygomandibular raphe

Superior pharyngeal constrictor muscle

**Lateral view**

**Figure 7-8**

| MAXILLARY ARTERY |
|---|
| • The larger of the 2 terminal branches of the external carotid a. (superficial temporal a.) |
| • Arises posterior to the condylar neck of the mandible within the parotid gland |
| • Exits the parotid gland and passes anteriorly between the ramus of the mandible and the sphenomandibular lig. within the infratemporal fossa |
| • Takes a course that is either superficial or deep to the lateral pterygoid until reaching the pterygopalatine fossa via the pterygomaxillary fissure |
| • Supplies the deep structures of the face and may be divided into 3 parts as it passes medially through the infratemporal fossa: |
| • 1st part—mandibular part |
| • 2nd part—pterygoid part |
| • 3rd part—pterygopalatine part |

Maxillary Artery: 1st Part (Mandibular Part)

| Artery | Course |
|---|---|
| 1st part (mandibular part) | Passes between the ramus of the mandible and the sphenomandibular lig.<br>Lies parallel to and inferior to the auriculotemporal n.<br>Crosses the inferior alveolar n. and passes on the inferior border of the lateral pterygoid<br>Gives rise to 5 branches: *anterior tympanic, deep auricular, middle meningeal, accessory meningeal,* and the *inferior alveolar* |
| Deep auricular | Given off in the same area as the anterior tympanic<br>Lies in the parotid gland, posterior to the temporomandibular joint, where it gives branches to supply the temporomandibular joint and continues along the osseous and cartilaginous portions of the auditory tube, supplying them as well as a small part of the tympanic membrane |
| Anterior tympanic | Given off in the same area as for the the deep auricular a.<br>Passes superiorly immediately posterior to the temporomandibular joint, where it gives branches to supply the temporomandibular joint<br>Enters the tympanic cavity through the petrotympanic fissure and aids in supplying the tympanic membrane, along with branches of the posterior auricular a., artery of the pterygoid canal, deep auricular a., and caroticotympanic branch from the internal carotid a. |
| Middle meningeal | Passes superiorly between the sphenomandibular lig. and the lateral pterygoid between the 2 roots of the auriculotemporal n. to the foramen spinosum of the sphenoid bone<br>In the middle cranial fossa, passes anteriorly in a groove on the greater wing of the sphenoid, dividing into an anterior and a posterior branch |
| Accessory meningeal | Arises from the maxillary or middle meningeal a.<br>Enters the skull through the foramen ovale to supply the trigeminal ganglion and dura mater |
| Inferior alveolar | Descends inferiorly following the inferior alveolar n. to enter the mandibular foramen |

Maxillary Artery: 2nd Part (Pterygoid Part)

| Artery | Course |
|---|---|
| 2nd part (pterygoid part) | Passes obliquely and anterosuperiorly between the ramus of the mandible and insertion of the temporalis m.<br>Then passes on the superficial surface of the lateral pterygoid to travel between the muscle's 2 heads<br>Has 5 branches: *anterior* and *posterior deep temporal, masseteric, pterygoid,* and *buccal* |
| Anterior and posterior deep temporal | Pass between the skull and the temporalis m.<br>Supply the temporalis throughout their course<br>While ascending, these arteries anastomose with the middle temporal a. from the superficial temporal a. |
| Masseteric | Small; passes laterally through the mandibular notch to supply the deep surface of the masseter m. |
| Pterygoid | An irregular number of arteries supplying the pterygoid mm. |
| Buccal | A small artery that runs obliquely in an anterior direction between the medial pterygoid m. and the insertion of the temporalis m. until it reaches the outer surface of the buccinator m. to supply it, anastomosing with the facial and infraorbital branches |

| MAXILLARY ARTERY | |
| --- | --- |
| Maxillary Artery: 3rd Part (Pterygopalatine Part) | |
| **Artery** | **Course** |
| 3rd part (pterygopalatine part) | Passes from the infratemporal fossa into the pterygopalatine fossa via the pterygomaxillary fissure |
| | Before passing through the pterygomaxillary fissure, it gives off the posterior superior alveolar a. (the only artery off the 3rd part of the maxillary a. that does not normally branch off within the pterygopalatine fossa) |
| *Posterior superior alveolar* | Arises in the infratemporal fossa |
| | Descends on the maxillary tuberosity to enter the posterior surface of the maxilla to supply the molars and premolars, lining of the maxillary sinus, and the gums |

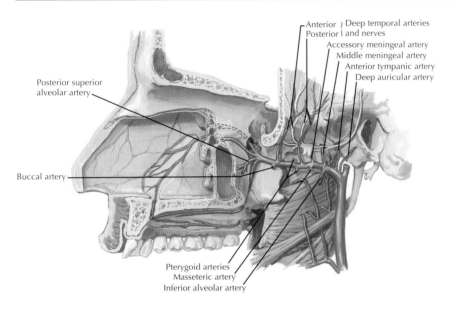

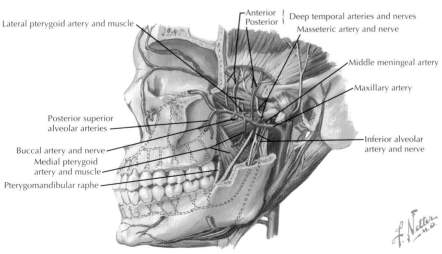

Figure 7-9

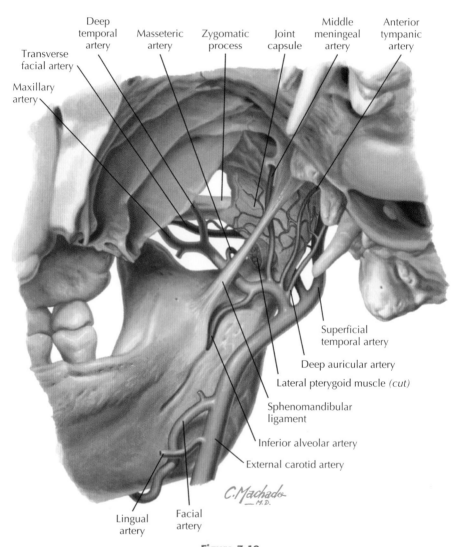

Transverse facial artery

Maxillary artery

Deep temporal artery

Masseteric artery

Zygomatic process

Joint capsule

Middle meningeal artery

Anterior tympanic artery

Superficial temporal artery

Deep auricular artery

Lateral pterygoid muscle *(cut)*

Sphenomandibular ligament

Inferior alveolar artery

External carotid artery

Lingual artery

Facial artery

C. Machado
_M.D.

**Figure 7-10**

| VENOUS DRAINAGE | |
|---|---|
| **Vein** | **Course** |
| Pterygoid plexus | An extensive network of veins that parallel the 2nd and 3rd parts of the maxillary a.<br>Receives branches that correspond with the same branches of the maxillary a.<br>The tributaries of the pterygoid plexus eventually converge to form a short maxillary v.<br>Communicates with the cavernous sinus, pharyngeal venous plexus, facial v. via the deep facial v., and ophthalmic vv. |
| Deep facial | Connects the facial v. with the pterygoid plexus |
| Maxillary | A short, sometimes paired vein, formed by the convergence of the tributaries of the pterygoid plexus<br>Enters the parotid gland traveling posteriorly between the sphenomandibular lig. and the neck of the mandible<br>Unites with the superficial temporal v. to form the retromandibular v. |

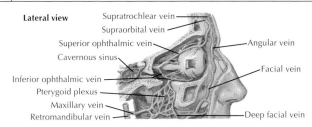

Lateral view

Supratrochlear vein — Supraorbital vein — Superior ophthalmic vein — Cavernous sinus — Inferior ophthalmic vein — Pterygoid plexus — Maxillary vein — Retromandibular vein — Angular vein — Facial vein — Deep facial vein

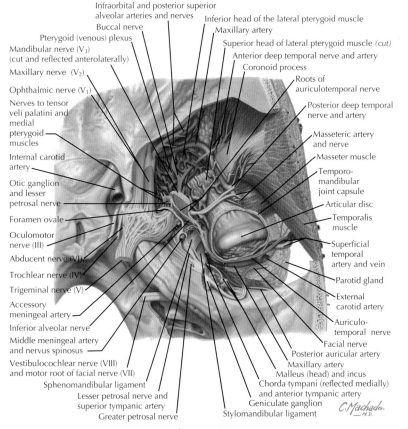

Infraorbital and posterior superior alveolar arteries and nerves — Buccal nerve — Pterygoid (venous) plexus — Mandibular nerve (V₃) (cut and reflected anterolaterally) — Maxillary nerve (V₂) — Ophthalmic nerve (V₁) — Nerves to tensor veli palatini and medial pterygoid muscles — Internal carotid artery — Otic ganglion and lesser petrosal nerve — Foramen ovale — Oculomotor nerve (III) — Abducent nerve (VI) — Trochlear nerve (IV) — Trigeminal nerve (V) — Accessory meningeal artery — Inferior alveolar nerve — Middle meningeal artery and nervus spinosus — Vestibulocochlear nerve (VIII) and motor root of facial nerve (VII) — Sphenomandibular ligament — Lesser petrosal nerve and superior tympanic artery — Greater petrosal nerve — Inferior head of the lateral pterygoid muscle — Maxillary artery — Superior head of lateral pterygoid muscle (cut) — Anterior deep temporal nerve and artery — Coronoid process — Roots of auriculotemporal nerve — Posterior deep temporal nerve and artery — Masseteric artery and nerve — Masseter muscle — Temporomandibular joint capsule — Articular disc — Temporalis muscle — Superficial temporal artery and vein — Parotid gland — External carotid artery — Auriculotemporal nerve — Facial nerve — Posterior auricular artery — Maxillary artery — Malleus (head) and incus — Chorda tympani (reflected medially) and anterior tympanic artery — Geniculate ganglion — Stylomandibular ligament

C. Machado, M.D.

**Figure 7-11**

| MANDIBULAR DIVISION |
|---|

- Mandibular division (V₃) is the largest of the 3 divisions of the trigeminal n.
- Has motor *and* sensory functions
- Created by a large sensory and a small motor root that unite just after passing through the foramen ovale to enter the infratemporal fossa
- Immediately gives rise to a meningeal branch and a medial pterygoid branch before dividing into anterior and posterior divisions

| Branches From the Undivided Trunk | |
|---|---|
| **Branch** | **Course** |
| Meningeal (nervus spinosum) | After passing through the foramen ovale, the undivided trigeminal trunk is located between the tensor veli palatini and the lateral pterygoid |
| | The undivided trunk then gives rise to a lateral branch called the meningeal nerve |
| | The branch travels through the foramen spinosum to enter the middle cranial fossa and innervate the dura mater |
| Medial pterygoid | After passing through the foramen ovale, the undivided trigeminal trunk is located between the tensor veli palatini and the lateral pterygoid |
| | The undivided trunk then gives rise to a medial branch to the medial pterygoid |
| | This branch continues to supply the tensor veli palatini and the tensor tympani |

*Anterior Division*

- Smaller; mainly motor with 1 sensory branch (buccal):
  - Masseteric
  - Anterior and posterior deep temporal
  - Medial pterygoid
  - Lateral pterygoid
  - Buccal

*Posterior Division*

- Larger, mainly sensory with 1 motor branch (mylohyoid n.):
  - Auriculotemporal
  - Lingual
  - Inferior alveolar
  - Mylohyoid n.

| Anterior Division of the Mandibular Division | |
|---|---|
| **Branch** | **Course** |
| Masseteric | Passes laterally superior to the lateral pterygoid |
| | Lies anterior to the temporomandibular joint and posterior to the tendon of the temporalis m. |
| | Crosses the mandibular notch with the masseteric a. to innervate the masseter m. |
| | Also provides a small branch to the temporomandibular joint |
| Anterior and posterior deep temporal | Pass superior to the lateral pterygoid m. between the skull and the temporalis m. while passing deep to the muscle to innervate it |
| | Provides a small branch to the temporomandibular joint |
| Lateral pterygoid | Passes into the deep surface of the muscle |
| | Often arises from the buccal n. |
| Buccal | Passes anteriorly between the 2 heads of the lateral pterygoid m. |
| | Descends inferiorly along the lower part of the temporalis m. to appear from deep to the anterior border of the masseter m. |
| | Supplies the skin over the buccinator m. before passing through it to supply the mucous membrane lining its inner surface and the gingiva along the mandibular molars |

| MANDIBULAR DIVISION | |
|---|---|
| Posterior Division of the Mandibular Division | |
| **Branch** | **Course** |
| Auriculotemporal | Normally arises from 2 roots, between which the middle meningeal a. passes |
| | Runs posteriorly just inferior to the lateral pterygoid and continues to the medial aspect of the neck of the mandible |
| | While passing posterior to the mandible, it provides sensory innervation to the temporomandibular joint |
| | Then it turns superiorly with the superficial temporal vessels between the auricle and condyle of the mandible deep to the parotid gland |
| | On exiting the parotid gland, it ascends over the zygomatic arch and divides into superficial temporal branches |
| Lingual | Lies inferior to the lateral pterygoid and medial and anterior to the inferior alveolar n. |
| | The chorda tympani n. also joins the posterior part |
| | The lingual n. passes between the medial pterygoid and the ramus of the mandible to pass obliquely to enter the oral cavity bounded by the superior pharyngeal constrictor m., medial pterygoid m., and the mandible |
| | Supplies the mucous membrane of the anterior 2/3 of the tongue and gingiva on the lingual aspect of the mandibular teeth |
| Inferior alveolar | The largest branch of the mandibular division |
| | Descends following the inferior alveolar a. inferior to the lateral pterygoid and, finally, between the sphenomandibular lig. and the ramus of the mandible until it enters the mandibular foramen |
| | Innervates all mandibular teeth and the gingiva from the premolars anteriorly to the midline via the mental branch |
| Mylohyoid | Branches from the inferior alveolar n. immediately before it enters the mandibular foramen |
| | Descends in a groove on the deep side of the ramus of the mandible until it reaches the superficial surface of the mylohyoid m. |
| | Supplies the mylohyoid m. and the anterior belly of the digastric m. |
| **MAXILLARY NERVE** | |
| **Branch** | **Course** |
| Posterior superior alveolar | Passes through the pterygomaxillary fissure to enter the infratemporal fossa |
| | In the infratemporal fossa, it passes on the posterior surface of the maxilla along the region of the maxillary tuberosity |
| | Gives rise to a gingival branch that innervates the buccal gingiva alongside the maxillary molars |
| | Enters the posterior surface of the maxilla and supplies the maxillary sinus and the maxillary molars, with the possible exception of the mesiobuccal root of the 1st maxillary molar |

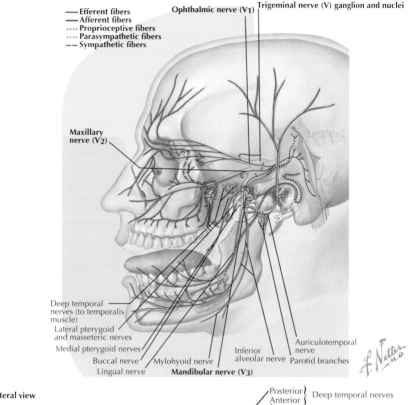

— Efferent fibers
— Afferent fibers
···· Proprioceptive fibers
···· Parasympathetic fibers
– – Sympathetic fibers

Ophthalmic nerve (V₁)   Trigeminal nerve (V) ganglion and nuclei

Maxillary nerve (V₂)

Deep temporal nerves (to temporalis muscle)
Lateral pterygoid and masseteric nerves
Medial pterygoid nerves
Buccal nerve   Mylohyoid nerve
Lingual nerve   **Mandibular nerve (V₃)**
Inferior alveolar nerve
Auriculotemporal nerve   Parotid branches

Lateral view

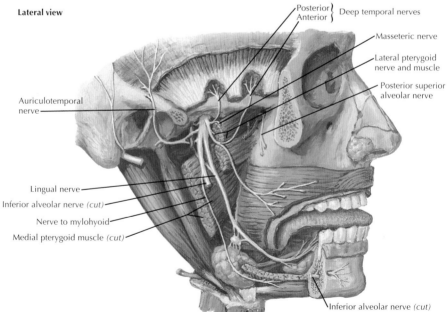

Posterior }
Anterior  }   Deep temporal nerves

Masseteric nerve

Lateral pterygoid nerve and muscle

Posterior superior alveolar nerve

Auriculotemporal nerve

Lingual nerve
Inferior alveolar nerve *(cut)*
Nerve to mylohyoid
Medial pterygoid muscle *(cut)*

Inferior alveolar nerve *(cut)*

**Figure 7-12**

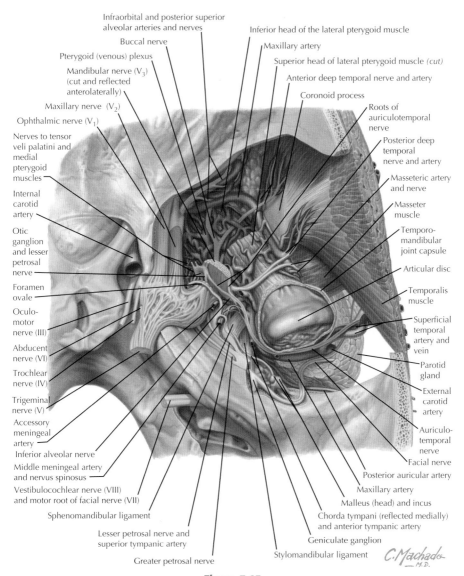

Infraorbital and posterior superior alveolar arteries and nerves

Buccal nerve

Pterygoid (venous) plexus

Mandibular nerve ($V_3$) (cut and reflected anterolaterally)

Maxillary nerve ($V_2$)

Ophthalmic nerve ($V_1$)

Nerves to tensor veli palatini and medial pterygoid muscles

Internal carotid artery

Otic ganglion and lesser petrosal nerve

Foramen ovale

Oculomotor nerve (III)

Abducent nerve (VI)

Trochlear nerve (IV)

Trigeminal nerve (V)

Accessory meningeal artery

Inferior alveolar nerve

Middle meningeal artery and nervus spinosus

Vestibulocochlear nerve (VIII) and motor root of facial nerve (VII)

Sphenomandibular ligament

Lesser petrosal nerve and superior tympanic artery

Greater petrosal nerve

Inferior head of the lateral pterygoid muscle

Maxillary artery

Superior head of lateral pterygoid muscle *(cut)*

Anterior deep temporal nerve and artery

Coronoid process

Roots of auriculotemporal nerve

Posterior deep temporal nerve and artery

Masseteric artery and nerve

Masseter muscle

Temporomandibular joint capsule

Articular disc

Temporalis muscle

Superficial temporal artery and vein

Parotid gland

External carotid artery

Auriculotemporal nerve

Facial nerve

Posterior auricular artery

Maxillary artery

Malleus (head) and incus

Chorda tympani (reflected medially) and anterior tympanic artery

Geniculate ganglion

Stylomandibular ligament

C. Machado
—M.D.

**Figure 7-13**

| CHORDA TYMPANI, LESSER PETROSAL NERVE, AND OTIC GANGLION | | |
|---|---|---|
| **Nerve** | **Source** | **Course** |
| Chorda tympani | Branch from the facial n. in the tympanic cavity | Carries the preganglionic parasympathetic fibers to the submandibular ganglion and taste fibers to the anterior 2/3 of the tongue |
| | | Passes anteriorly to enter the tympanic cavity and lies along the tympanic membrane and malleus until exiting the petrotympanic fissure |
| | | Once it exits the petrotympanic fissure, it joins the posterior border of the lingual n. in the infratemporal fossa |
| | | The lingual n. is distributed to the anterior 2/3 of the tongue, and the SVA* fibers from the chorda tympani travel to the taste buds in this region |
| Lesser petrosal | Tympanic plexus along the promontory of the ear re-forms as the lesser petrosal n. | Forms in the middle ear cavity |
| | | Carries the preganglionic parasympathetic (from the tympanic branch of glossopharyngeal n. [IX]) and postganglionic sympathetic (from the caroticotympanic branch of the internal carotid a. plexus) that are traveling to the parotid gland |
| | | The nerve passes along the groove for the lesser petrosal n. on the petrous portion of the temporal bone toward the foramen ovale |
| | | Normally enters the infratemporal fossa by passing through the foramen ovale |
| | | Joins the otic ganglion |
| **Nerve Cell Body** | **Characteristics of Cell Body** | **Course** |
| Otic ganglion | A collection of nerve cell bodies located in the infratemporal fossa | Postganglionic parasympathetic fibers arise in the otic ganglion and travel to the auriculotemporal branch of the trigeminal n. |
| | This very small stellate-shaped ganglion is inferior to the foramen ovale and medial to the mandibular division of the trigeminal n. | Auriculotemporal n. travels to the parotid gland |
| | | These postganglionic parasympathetic fibers innervate the: |
| | | • Parotid gland—secretion of saliva |

*SVA, special visceral afferent. See Chapter 3 for a discussion of the SVA and other functional columns.

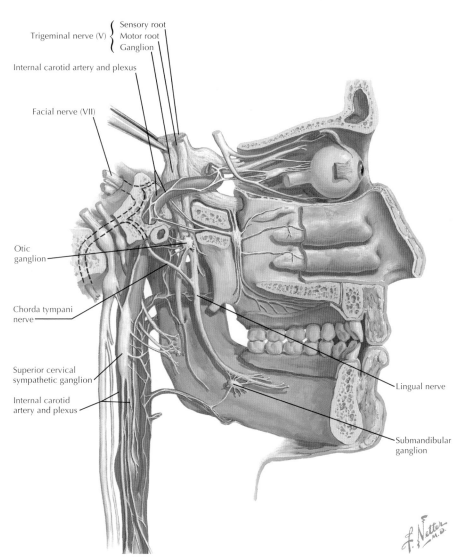

Trigeminal nerve (V) { Sensory root
Motor root
Ganglion

Internal carotid artery and plexus

Facial nerve (VII)

Otic ganglion

Chorda tympani nerve

Superior cervical sympathetic ganglion

Internal carotid artery and plexus

Lingual nerve

Submandibular ganglion

**Figure 7-14**

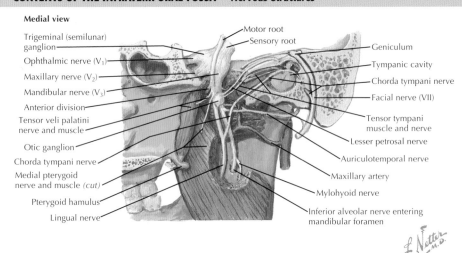

**Medial view**

Trigeminal (semilunar) ganglion
Ophthalmic nerve (V₁)
Maxillary nerve (V₂)
Mandibular nerve (V₃)
Anterior division
Tensor veli palatini nerve and muscle
Otic ganglion
Chorda tympani nerve
Medial pterygoid nerve and muscle *(cut)*
Pterygoid hamulus
Lingual nerve

Motor root
Sensory root
Geniculum
Tympanic cavity
Chorda tympani nerve
Facial nerve (VII)
Tensor tympani muscle and nerve
Lesser petrosal nerve
Auriculotemporal nerve
Maxillary artery
Mylohyoid nerve
Inferior alveolar nerve entering mandibular foramen

**Figure 7-15**

| ANATOMIC PATHWAY FOR PARASYMPATHETICS OF THE PAROTID GLAND | | | |
| --- | --- | --- | --- |
| **Type of Neuron** | **Name of Cell Body** | **Characteristics of Cell Body** | **Course of the Neuron** |
| Preganglionic neuron | Inferior salivatory nucleus | A collection of nerve cell bodies located in the medulla | Preganglionic parasympathetic fibers arise from the inferior salivatory nucleus in the medulla |
| | | | Travel through the glossopharyngeal n. (IX) and exit the jugular foramen |
| | | | The glossopharyngeal n. gives rise to the tympanic branch of IX, which reenters the skull via the tympanic canaliculus |
| | | | Tympanic branch of IX forms the tympanic plexus along the promontory of the ear |
| | | | The plexus re-forms as the lesser petrosal n., which typically exits the foramen ovale to enter the infratemporal fossa |
| | | | Lesser petrosal n. joins the otic ganglion |
| Postganglionic neuron | Otic ganglion | A collection of nerve cell bodies | Postganglionic parasympathetic fibers arise in the otic ganglion |
| | | This very small stellate-shaped ganglion is located inferior to the foramen ovale, medial to the mandibular division of the trigeminal n. | These fibers travel to the auriculotemporal branch of the trigeminal n. |
| | | | Auriculotemporal n. travels to the parotid gland |
| | | | These postganglionic parasympathetic fibers innervate the: |
| | | | • Parotid gland—secretion of saliva |

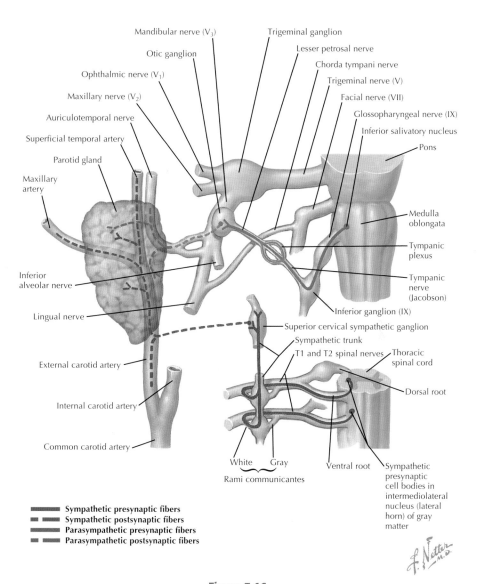

Figure 7-16

Mandibular nerve (V₃)
Otic ganglion
Ophthalmic nerve (V₁)
Maxillary nerve (V₂)
Auriculotemporal nerve
Superficial temporal artery
Parotid gland
Maxillary artery
Inferior alveolar nerve
Lingual nerve
External carotid artery
Internal carotid artery
Common carotid artery

Trigeminal ganglion
Lesser petrosal nerve
Chorda tympani nerve
Trigeminal nerve (V)
Facial nerve (VII)
Glossopharyngeal nerve (IX)
Inferior salivatory nucleus
Pons
Medulla oblongata
Tympanic plexus
Tympanic nerve (Jacobson)
Inferior ganglion (IX)
Superior cervical sympathetic ganglion
Sympathetic trunk
T1 and T2 spinal nerves
Thoracic spinal cord
Dorsal root
Ventral root
Sympathetic presynaptic cell bodies in intermediolateral nucleus (lateral horn) of gray matter

White   Gray
Rami communicantes

Sympathetic presynaptic fibers
Sympathetic postsynaptic fibers
Parasympathetic presynaptic fibers
Parasympathetic postsynaptic fibers

# MUSCLES OF MASTICATION

- *Mastication* is the process of chewing food in preparation for deglutition (swallowing) and digestion
- All muscles of mastication originate on the skull and insert on the mandible
- All muscles of mastication are innervated by the mandibular division of the trigeminal nerve
- All muscles of mastication are derivatives of the 1st pharyngeal arch
- Movements of the mandible are classified as:
  - Elevation
  - Depression
  - Protrusion
  - Retrusion
  - Side-to-side (lateral) excursion

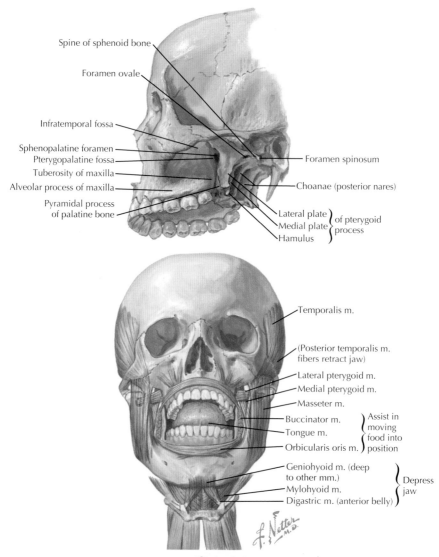

Spine of sphenoid bone

Foramen ovale

Infratemporal fossa

Sphenopalatine foramen
Pterygopalatine fossa
Tuberosity of maxilla
Alveolar process of maxilla

Pyramidal process
of palatine bone

Foramen spinosum

Choanae (posterior nares)

Lateral plate
Medial plate } of pterygoid process
Hamulus

Temporalis m.

(Posterior temporalis m. fibers retract jaw)

Lateral pterygoid m.
Medial pterygoid m.
Masseter m.

Buccinator m.
Tongue m.
Orbicularis oris m. } Assist in moving food into position

Geniohyoid m. (deep to other mm.)
Mylohyoid m.
Digastric m. (anterior belly) } Depress jaw

**Figure 8-1**

| MASSETER | | | | | |
|---|---|---|---|---|---|
| Parts | Origin | Insertion | Main Actions | Nerve Supply | Comments |
| Superficial head (larger part) | Inferior border of the anterior 2/3 of the zygomatic arch<br><br>Maxillary process of the zygomatic bone | Angle of mandible<br><br>Inferior and lateral parts of the mandibular ramus | Elevates mandible<br><br>Protrudes mandible (superficial head)<br><br>Aids in lateral excursion of the mandible | Masseteric branch from the anterior division of the mandibular division of the trigeminal n. | Superficial head's fibers run posteroinferiorly<br><br>The parotid duct, transverse facial a., and branches of the facial n. pass superficial to the masseter m. |
| Deep head (smaller part) | Medial border of the zygomatic arch<br><br>Inferior border of the posterior 1/3 of the zygomatic arch | Superior and lateral mandibular ramus<br><br>Coronoid process | | | Some evidence suggests the presence of middle fibers, which corresponds to part of the traditionally described deep head of the masseter |

| TEMPORALIS | | | | | |
|---|---|---|---|---|---|
| | Entire temporal fossa: along the inferior temporal line including the temporal fascia | Coronoid process: along the apex, anterior and posterior borders, medial surface extending inferiorly on the anterior border of the mandibular ramus (temporal crest) to the 3rd molar tooth | Elevates mandible<br><br>Retrudes mandible (posterior fibers)<br><br>Aids in lateral excursion of the mandible | Anterior and posterior deep temporal branches from the anterior division of the mandibular division of the trigeminal n. (Anterior deep temporal may branch from the buccal n., and the posterior deep temporal may branch from the masseteric n.) | The main postural muscle—maintains the mandible in rest position |

| MEDIAL PTERYGOID | | | | | |
|---|---|---|---|---|---|
| Deep head | Medial surface of lateral pterygoid plate | Medial surface of ramus and angle of the mandible (pterygoid tubercles) | Elevates mandible<br><br>Protrudes mandible<br><br>Lateral excursion of the mandible (side-to-side movements) (Acting unilaterally, it causes the mandible to deviate to the contralateral side, rotating around axis created by contralateral condyle, which is important in grinding on ipsilateral side) | Medial pterygoid branch from the mandibular division of the trigeminal n. (main trunk before it divides into anterior and posterior divisions) | The deepest muscle of mastication<br><br>Forms the pterygomasseteric sling with the masseter<br><br>If anesthetic is injected into the medial pterygoid m. during an inferior alveolar nerve block, trismus will result |
| Superficial head | Maxillary tuberosity<br><br>Pyramidal process of the palatine | | | | |

| LATERAL PTERYGOID | | | | | |
|---|---|---|---|---|---|
| Upper head | Infratemporal crest of the greater wing of the sphenoid | Anterior and medial portions of the articular disc<br><br>Capsule of the temporomandibular joint<br><br>Pterygoid fovea (upper portion) | Protrudes mandible<br><br>Depresses mandible (as result of protrusion)<br><br>Lateral excursion of the mandible (side-to-side movements) (Acting unilaterally, it causes the mandible to deviate to the contralateral side, rotating around axis created by contralateral condyle, which is important in grinding on ipsilateral side) | Lateral pterygoid branches (for each head) from the anterior division of the mandibular division of the trigeminal n., which exits the foramen ovale, lying medial to the lateral pterygoid (often this innervation is observed to be a branch from the buccal branch of the trigeminal n.) | Maxillary a. runs either superficial or deep to it<br><br>Surrounded by the pterygoid venous plexus<br><br>Buccal branch of the trigeminal n. passes between the 2 heads |
| Lower head | Lateral surface of the lateral pterygoid plate | Pterygoid fovea on the neck of the condyle of the mandible | | | |

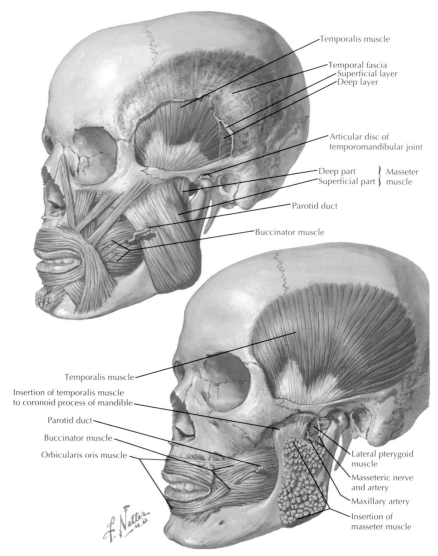

Temporalis muscle

Temporal fascia
Superficial layer
Deep layer

Articular disc of
temporomandibular joint

Deep part $\}$ Masseter
Superficial part $\}$ muscle

Parotid duct

Buccinator muscle

Temporalis muscle

Insertion of temporalis muscle
to coronoid process of mandible

Parotid duct

Buccinator muscle

Orbicularis oris muscle

Lateral pterygoid
muscle

Masseteric nerve
and artery

Maxillary artery

Insertion of
masseter muscle

**Figure 8-2**

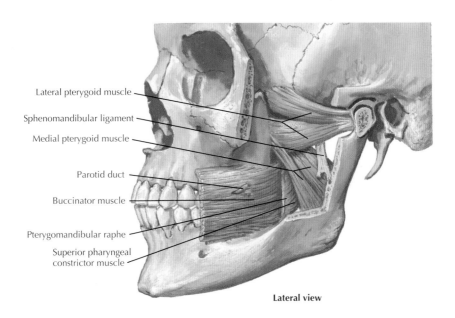

Lateral pterygoid muscle

Sphenomandibular ligament

Medial pterygoid muscle

Parotid duct

Buccinator muscle

Pterygomandibular raphe

Superior pharyngeal
constrictor muscle

**Lateral view**

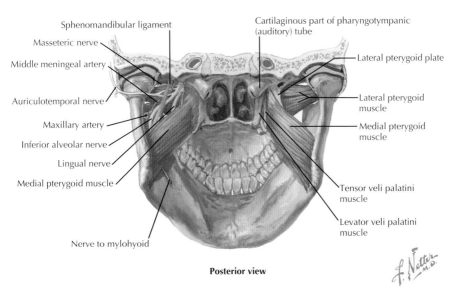

Sphenomandibular ligament

Masseteric nerve

Middle meningeal artery

Auriculotemporal nerve

Maxillary artery

Inferior alveolar nerve

Lingual nerve

Medial pterygoid muscle

Nerve to mylohyoid

Cartilaginous part of pharyngotympanic
(auditory) tube

Lateral pterygoid plate

Lateral pterygoid
muscle

Medial pterygoid
muscle

Tensor veli palatini
muscle

Levator veli palatini
muscle

**Posterior view**

**Figure 8-3**

| Artery | Source | Course |
|---|---|---|
| Maxillary | Larger of the 2 terminal branches of the external carotid a. (superficial temporal a. is the other terminal branch) | Arises posterior to the condylar neck of the mandible within the parotid gland<br><br>Exits the parotid gland and passes anteriorly between the condylar neck of the mandible and the sphenomandibular ligament within the infratemporal fossa<br><br>Takes a course that is either superficial or deep to the lateral pterygoid until reaching the pterygopalatine fossa via the pterygomaxillary fissure<br><br>Supplies the deep structures of the face and is divided into 3 parts as it passes medially through the infratemporal fossa:<br>• 1st part: mandibular<br>• 2nd part: pterygoid<br>• 3rd part: pterygopalatine<br>1st and 3rd parts do not supply the muscles of mastication<br>2nd part also feeds the buccinator m., which is not a muscle of mastication |
| 2nd part: (pterygoid part) | External carotid a. | Passes obliquely in an anterior and superior direction between the ramus of the mandible and insertion of the temporalis m.<br><br>Courses on the superficial surface of the lateral pterygoid m. to travel between the 2 heads of the muscle<br><br>Provides the muscular branches to the muscles of mastication and the buccinator m.<br><br>Gives rise to 5 branches: *anterior* and *posterior deep temporal, masseteric, pterygoid branches,* and *buccal* |
| *Anterior and posterior deep temporal* | Pterygoid (2nd part of the maxillary a.) | Pass between the skull and the temporalis m.<br>Supply the temporalis throughout their course<br>While ascending, they anastomose with the middle temporal a. from the superficial temporal a. |
| *Masseteric* | | Typically arises between the condylar neck of the mandible and the sphenomandibular lig.<br>Passes laterally through the mandibular notch with the nerve<br>Supplies the deep surface of the masseter |
| *Pterygoid* | | An irregular number of branches supply the medial and lateral pterygoids |
| *Buccal* | | A small artery that runs obliquely in an anterior direction between the medial pterygoid and the insertion of the temporalis m. until it reaches the outer surface of the buccinator, which it supplies<br><br>Occasionally a small lingual branch is observed, which accompanies the lingual nerve into the oral cavity |
| Middle temporal | Superficial temporal a. after it passes superior to the root of the zygomatic arch | Passes deep into the temporalis fascia and temporalis m.<br>Anastomoses with the anterior and posterior deep temporal vessels |
| Transverse facial | Superficial temporal a. before it exits the parotid gland | Passes transversely to exit the gland<br>Passes immediately superior to the parotid duct across the masseter m. and face, providing vascular supply along the way |

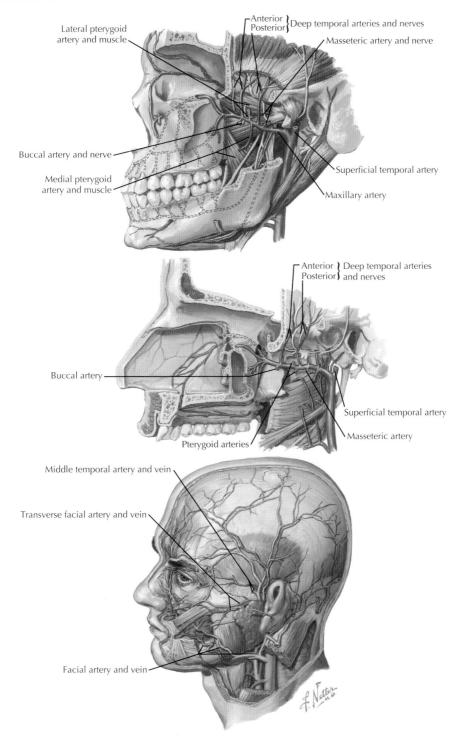

Lateral pterygoid artery and muscle

Anterior
Posterior } Deep temporal arteries and nerves

Masseteric artery and nerve

Buccal artery and nerve

Superficial temporal artery

Medial pterygoid artery and muscle

Maxillary artery

Anterior
Posterior } Deep temporal arteries and nerves

Buccal artery

Superficial temporal artery

Masseteric artery

Pterygoid arteries

Middle temporal artery and vein

Transverse facial artery and vein

Facial artery and vein

**Figure 8-4**

| Vein | Course |
|------|--------|
| Pterygoid plexus | An extensive network of veins that parallel the 2nd and 3rd parts of the maxillary a.<br>Receives branches that correspond with the same branches of the maxillary a.<br>Tributaries of the pterygoid plexus eventually converge to form a short maxillary v.<br>Communicates with the cavernous sinus, pharyngeal venous plexus, facial v. via the deep facial v., and ophthalmic vv. |
| Maxillary | Formed by the convergence of the pterygoid plexus of veins<br>Is a short vein that parallels the 1st part of the maxillary a.<br>Passes posteriorly between the condylar neck and the sphenomandibular ligament into the parotid gland<br>In the parotid gland, it joins the superficial temporal v. to form the retromandibular v. |
| Middle temporal | Arises from deep within the temporalis m. and fascia, where it anastomoses with the anterior and posterior deep temporal vessels<br>Joins the superficial temporal v. immediately before it passes inferior to the root of the zygomatic arch |
| Transverse facial | Travels posteriorly to enter the parotid gland and join the superficial temporal v. |
| Anterior and posterior deep temporal | Join the pterygoid plexus of veins<br>Also communicate with the middle temporal v. |
| Masseteric | Join the pterygoid plexus of veins |
| Pterygoid | |
| Buccal | |

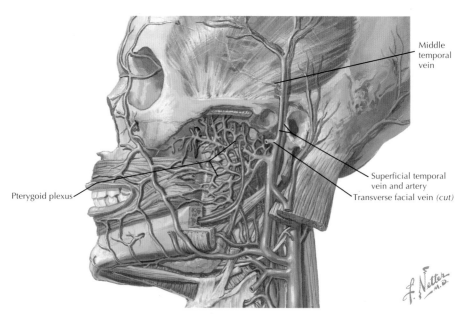

Pterygoid plexus

Middle temporal vein

Superficial temporal vein and artery
Transverse facial vein *(cut)*

**Figure 8-5**

## MANDIBULAR DIVISION OF THE TRIGEMINAL

- Largest of the 3 divisions of the trigeminal n.
- Created by a large sensory and a small motor root that unite just after passing through the foramen ovale to enter the infratemporal fossa
- Upon passing through the foramen ovale, the mandibular division of the trigeminal is located between the lateral pterygoid m. (lateral to the nerve) and the tensor veli palatine m. (medial to the nerve)
- Immediately gives rise to 2 branches:
  - meningeal (sensory to the dura mater)
  - medial pterygoid (which provides branches to the):
    - tensor veli palatini
    - tensor tympani
- The mandibular division divides into anterior and posterior divisions
  - Anterior division (smaller)—mainly motor with 1 sensory branch (buccal n.)
  - Posterior division (larger)—mainly sensory with 1 motor branch (mylohyoid n.)
- The anterior division provides motor innervation to most of the muscles of mastication

## MOTOR BRANCH FROM THE UNDIVIDED TRUNK

| Branch | Course |
|---|---|
| Medial pterygoid | Passes through the otic ganglion to provide motor and proprioceptive innervation to the medial pterygoid m. |
| | Passes anteriorly and inferiorly to enter the medial pterygoid |
| | This branch continues to supply the tensor veli palatini and the tensor tympani |

## ANTERIOR DIVISION OF THE MANDIBULAR DIVISION

| Branch | Course |
|---|---|
| Anterior and posterior deep temporal | Arises from the anterior part of the mandibular division of the trigeminal n. |
| | The anterior deep temporal n. sometimes arises from the buccal n. |
| | Pass superior to the lateral pterygoid m. between the skull and the temporalis m. while passing deep to the temporalis to innervate it |
| | Innervates the temporalis |
| | Posterior deep temporal n. also provides slight innervation to the temporomandibular joint |
| Masseteric | Arises from the anterior part of the mandibular division of the trigeminal n., but occasionally arises from a common branch with the posterior deep temporal n. |
| | Runs superior to the lateral pterygoid m. and continues on the lateral aspect of the muscle as it approaches the mandible |
| | Lies anterior to the temporomandibular joint and posterior to the tendon of the temporalis m. |
| | Passes though the masseteric notch with the masseteric vessels |
| | Enters the masseter m.'s deep surface to innervate it |
| | Also provides innervation to the temporomandibular joint |
| Lateral pterygoid | Arises from the anterior part of the mandibular division of the trigeminal n., but sometimes arises as a branch from the buccal n. |
| | These branches, 1 for each muscular head, enter the deep surface of the lateral pterygoid m. to innervate it |
| | Occasionally receives innervation from a branch from the buccal n. |

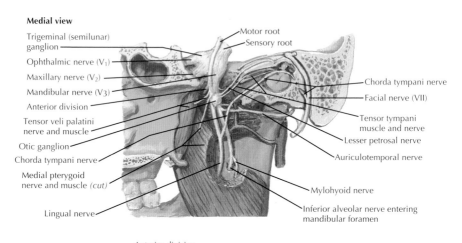

**Medial view**

Trigeminal (semilunar) ganglion

Ophthalmic nerve (V₁)

Maxillary nerve (V₂)

Mandibular nerve (V₃)

Anterior division

Tensor veli palatini nerve and muscle

Otic ganglion

Chorda tympani nerve

Medial pterygoid nerve and muscle *(cut)*

Lingual nerve

Motor root

Sensory root

Chorda tympani nerve

Facial nerve (VII)

Tensor tympani muscle and nerve

Lesser petrosal nerve

Auriculotemporal nerve

Mylohyoid nerve

Inferior alveolar nerve entering mandibular foramen

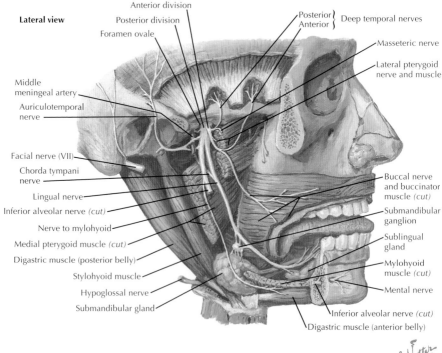

**Lateral view**

Anterior division

Posterior division

Foramen ovale

Posterior } Anterior } Deep temporal nerves

Masseteric nerve

Lateral pterygoid nerve and muscle

Middle meningeal artery

Auriculotemporal nerve

Facial nerve (VII)

Chorda tympani nerve

Lingual nerve

Inferior alveolar nerve *(cut)*

Nerve to mylohyoid

Medial pterygoid muscle *(cut)*

Digastric muscle (posterior belly)

Stylohyoid muscle

Hypoglossal nerve

Submandibular gland

Buccal nerve and buccinator muscle *(cut)*

Submandibular ganglion

Sublingual gland

Mylohyoid muscle *(cut)*

Mental nerve

Inferior alveolar nerve *(cut)*

Digastric muscle (anterior belly)

**Figure 8-6**

- Mastication prepares food by chewing for deglutition and digestion
- It is the 1st step in the breakdown of food by:
  - Making smaller pieces from larger pieces (thus increasing the surface area for digestive breakdown)
  - Helping soften and lubricate the food with saliva

## BONES INVOLVED

- Base of the skull and the mandible
- They articulate at the temporomandibular joint (between the squamous portion of the temporal bone [skull] and the condyle of the mandible)

## MUSCLES INVOLVED

- 4 muscles of mastication:
  - Masseter
  - Temporalis
  - Medial pterygoid
  - Lateral pterygoid
- All muscles of mastication are innervated by the mandibular division of the trigeminal nerve (nerve of the 1st pharyngeal arch)
- Mastication involves using the 4 muscles in different combinations to move the mandible in 1 of 3 planes in an antagonistic fashion:
  - Elevation/depression
  - Protrusion/retrusion
  - Side-to-side excursion
- Although the buccinator is not a muscle of mastication, it aids in keeping the bolus of food against the teeth to help in mastication

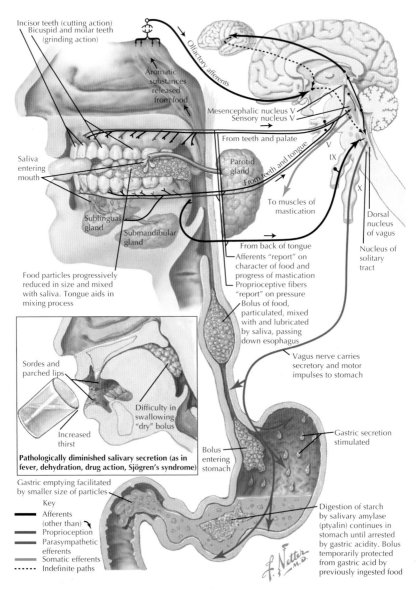

Incisor teeth (cutting action)
Bicuspid and molar teeth (grinding action)

Olfactory afferents

Aromatic substances released from food

Mesencephalic nucleus V
Sensory nucleus V

From teeth and palate

Saliva entering mouth

Parotid gland

From teeth and tongue

V
IX

To muscles of mastication

Dorsal nucleus of vagus

Sublingual gland

Submandibular gland

From back of tongue
Afferents "report" on character of food and progress of mastication
Proprioceptive fibers "report" on pressure
Bolus of food, particulated, mixed with and lubricated by saliva, passing down esophagus

Nucleus of solitary tract

X

Food particles progressively reduced in size and mixed with saliva. Tongue aids in mixing process

Vagus nerve carries secretory and motor impulses to stomach

Sordes and parched lips

Difficulty in swallowing "dry" bolus

Increased thirst

Gastric secretion stimulated

Bolus entering stomach

**Pathologically diminished salivary secretion (as in fever, dehydration, drug action, Sjögren's syndrome)**

Gastric emptying facilitated by smaller size of particles

Key
Afferents (other than)
Proprioception
Parasympathetic efferents
Somatic efferents
Indefinite paths

Digestion of starch by salivary amylase (ptyalin) continues in stomach until arrested by gastric acidity. Bolus temporarily protected from gastric acid by previously ingested food

**Figure 8-7**

# TEMPOROMANDIBULAR JOINT

- The *temporomandibular joint* (TMJ) is the articulation between the squamous portion of the temporal bone and the condyle of the mandible
- It is a ginglymoarthrodial joint because it has both a hinge and a gliding action

## STRUCTURAL COMPONENTS

- The TMJ comprises 2 types of synovial joints—*hinge* and *sliding*—and consists of the following:
  - Squamous portion of the temporal bone
  - Articular disc (contained within the TMJ)
  - Condyle of the mandible
  - Ligaments (also serve as boundaries)

## TMJ DYSFUNCTION

- Affects 33% of the population and may be severe
- Causes include arthritis, trauma, infection, bruxism, and disc displacement
- More common in females

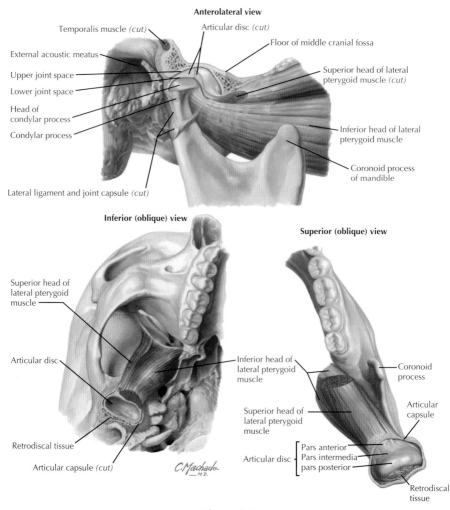

**Anterolateral view**

Temporalis muscle *(cut)*
Articular disc *(cut)*
Floor of middle cranial fossa
External acoustic meatus
Upper joint space
Lower joint space
Superior head of lateral pterygoid muscle *(cut)*
Head of condylar process
Condylar process
Inferior head of lateral pterygoid muscle
Coronoid process of mandible
Lateral ligament and joint capsule *(cut)*

**Inferior (oblique) view**

**Superior (oblique) view**

Superior head of lateral pterygoid muscle
Articular disc
Inferior head of lateral pterygoid muscle
Coronoid process
Superior head of lateral pterygoid muscle
Articular capsule
Retrodiscal tissue
Articular capsule *(cut)*
Articular disc { Pars anterior / Pars intermedia / pars posterior
Retrodiscal tissue

C.Machado—M.D.

**Figure 9-1**

| OSSEOUS STRUCTURES |
|---|

| Squamous Portion of the Temporal Bone |
|---|

- The TMJ articulation is located on the squamous portion of the temporal bone
- Has an avascular articular surface composed primarily of fibrous connective tissue and some fibrocartilage instead of hyaline cartilage
- The main load-bearing areas are on the lateral aspect of the squamous portion, condyle, and articular disc
- The dense fibrous connective tissue is thickest in the load-bearing areas
- Relations of the squamous portion of the temporal bone:
  - Anterior—articular eminence
  - Intermediate—glenoid fossa
  - Posterior—tympanic plate tapering to the postglenoid tubercle

| Structure | Comments |
|---|---|
| Articular eminence | The strong bony prominence on the base of the zygomatic process |
| Articular tubercle | The lateral part of the articular eminence is referred to as the articular tubercle and provides attachment for the capsule and lateral temporomandibular ligament |
| Glenoid fossa | The depression into which the condyle is located<br>Superior to this thin plate of bone is the middle cranial fossa<br>The anterior boundary of the glenoid fossa is the articular eminence<br>The posterior boundary of the glenoid fossa is the tympanic plate<br>The glenoid fossa can be divided into 2 parts by the squamotympanic fissure (lateral) and the petrotympanic fissure (medial):<br>• Anterior articular area—squamosal part of the temporal bone (this is where the articulation occurs)<br>• Posterior nonarticular area—tympanic portion (parotid gland may extend into this area) |
| Tympanic plate | The vertical plate located anterior to the external auditory meatus |
| Postglenoid tubercle | An inferior extension of the squamous portion of the temporal bone<br>Makes the posterior aspect of the glenoid fossa<br>Provides attachment for the capsule and retrodiscal pad |

| Mandibular Condyles |
|---|

- Articulate with the articular disc
- Ovoid in shape:
  - Mediolateral—20 mm
  - Anteroposterior—10 mm
- Articular surface is avascular fibrous connective tissue instead of hyaline cartilage
- The main load-bearing areas are on the lateral aspect

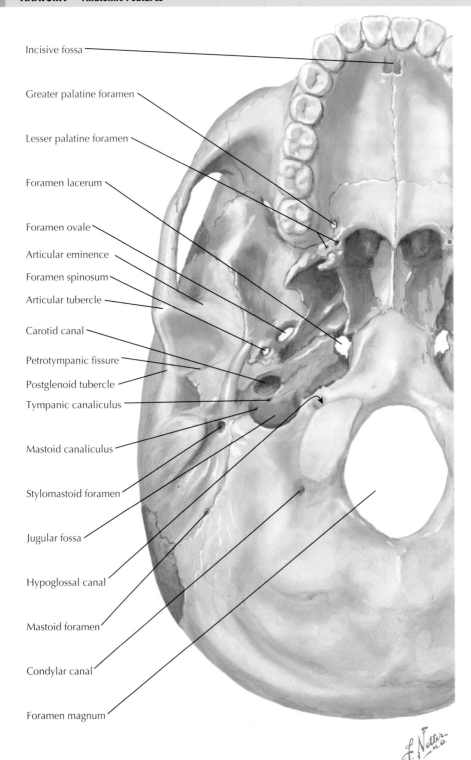

Incisive fossa

Greater palatine foramen

Lesser palatine foramen

Foramen lacerum

Foramen ovale

Articular eminence

Foramen spinosum

Articular tubercle

Carotid canal

Petrotympanic fissure

Postglenoid tubercle

Tympanic canaliculus

Mastoid canaliculus

Stylomastoid foramen

Jugular fossa

Hypoglossal canal

Mastoid foramen

Condylar canal

Foramen magnum

**Figure 9-2**

| **ARTICULAR DISC** |
|---|
| • Composed of dense fibrous connective tissue<br>• Located between the squamous portion of the temporal bone and the condyle<br>• Is avascular and aneural in its central part but is vascular and innervated in the peripheral areas, where load-bearing is minimal<br>• The main load-bearing areas are located on the lateral aspect; this is an area of potential perforation<br>• Merges around its periphery, attaching to the capsule<br>• Divided into 3 bands:<br>  • Anterior—this thick band lies just anterior to the condyle with the mouth closed<br>  • Intermediate—this band, the thinnest part, is located along the articular eminence with the mouth closed<br>  • Posterior—this thick band is located superior to the disc with the mouth closed<br>• Additional attachments:<br>  • Medial/lateral—strong medial and lateral collateral ligaments anchor the disc to the condyle<br>  • Anterior—the disc is attached to the capsule and the superior head of the lateral pterygoid, but not the condyle, allowing the disc to rotate over the condyle in an anteroposterior direction<br>  • Posterior—the disc is contiguous with the bilaminar zone that blends with the capsule |

| **BILAMINAR ZONE (Posterior Attachment Complex)** |
|---|
| • A bilaminar structure located posterior to the articular disc<br>• Highly distortable, especially on opening the mouth<br>• Composed of:<br>  • Superior lamina (stratum)—contains elastic fibers and anchors the superior aspect of the posterior portion of the disc to the capsule and bone at the postglenoid tubercle and tympanic plate<br>  • Retrodiscal pad—the highly vascular and neural portion of the TMJ, made of collagen, elastic fibers, fat, nerves, and blood vessels (a large venous plexus fills with blood when the condyle moves anteriorly)<br>  • Inferior lamina (stratum)—contains mainly collagen fibers and anchors the inferior aspect of the posterior portion of the disc to the condyle |

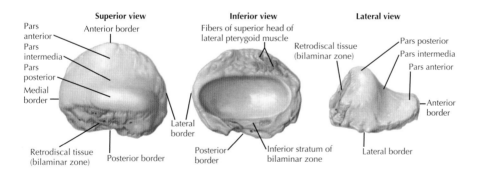

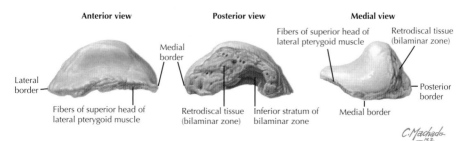

**Figure 9-3**

## TMJ COMPARTMENTS

- The articular disc divides the TMJ into superior and inferior compartments
- The internal surface of both compartments contains specialized endothelial cells that form a synovial lining that produces synovial fluid, making the TMJ a synovial joint
- Synovial fluid acts as:
  - A lubricant
  - A medium for providing the metabolic requirements to the articular surfaces of the TMJ

| | |
|---|---|
| Superior compartment | Between the squamous portion of the temporal bone and the articular disc<br>Volume = 1.2 mL<br>Provides for the translational movement of the TMJ |
| Inferior compartment | Between the articular disc and the condyle<br>Volume = 0.9 mL<br>Provides for the rotational movement of the TMJ |

## CAPSULE AND LIGAMENTS

### Capsule

- Completely encloses the articular surface of the temporal bone and the condyle
- Composed of fibrous connective tissue
- Toughened along the medial and lateral aspects by ligaments
- Lined by a highly vascular synovial membrane
- Has various sensory receptors including nociceptors
- Attachments:
  - Superior—along the rim of the temporal articular surfaces
  - Inferior—along the condylar neck
  - Medial—blends along the medial collateral ligament
  - Lateral—blends along the lateral collateral ligament
  - Anterior—blends with the superior head of the lateral pterygoid m.
  - Posterior—along the retrodiscal pad

### Ligaments

| | |
|---|---|
| Collateral ligaments | • Composed of 2 ligaments:<br>   *Medial collateral ligament*—connects the medial aspect of the articular disc to the medial pole of the condyle<br>   *Lateral collateral ligament*—connects the lateral aspect of the articular disc to the lateral pole of the condyle<br>• Frequently called the discal ligaments<br>• Composed of collagenous connective tissue; thus, they are not designed to stretch |
| Temporomandibular (lateral) ligament | The thickened ligament on the lateral aspect of the capsule<br>Prevents posterior displacement of the condyle<br>Composed of 2 separate bands:<br>   *Outer oblique part*—largest portion; attached to the articular tubercle; travels posteroinferiorly to attach immediately inferior to the condyle; this limits the opening of the mandible<br>   *Inner horizontal part*—smaller band attached to the articular tubercle running horizontally to attach to the lateral part of the condyle and disc; this limits posterior movement of the articular disc and the condyle |
| Stylomandibular ligament | Composed of a thickening of deep cervical fascia<br>Extends from the styloid process to the posterior margin of the angle and the ramus of the mandible<br>Helps limit anterior protrusion of the mandible |
| Sphenomandibular ligament | Remnant of Meckel's cartilage<br>Extends from the spine of the sphenoid to the lingula of the mandible<br>Some authors suggest it may help act as a pivot on the mandible by maintaining the same amount of tension during both opening and closing of the mouth<br>Some authors suggest it may help limit anterior protrusion of the mandible<br>Is the ligament most frequently damaged in an inferior alveolar nerve block |

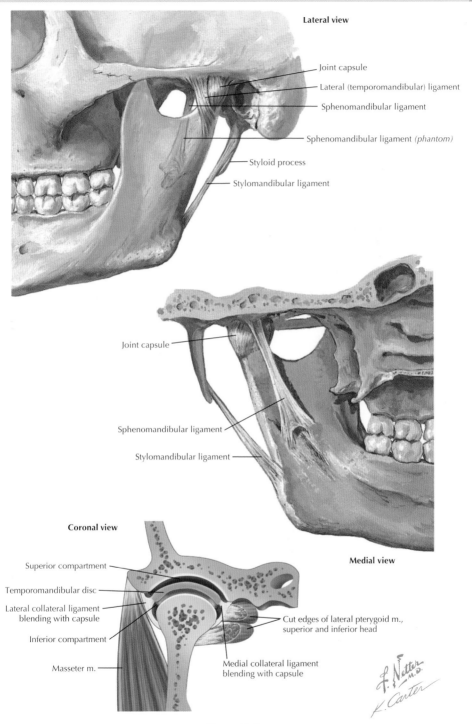

Lateral view

Joint capsule

Lateral (temporomandibular) ligament

Sphenomandibular ligament

Sphenomandibular ligament *(phantom)*

Styloid process

Stylomandibular ligament

Joint capsule

Sphenomandibular ligament

Stylomandibular ligament

Medial view

Coronal view

Superior compartment

Temporomandibular disc

Lateral collateral ligament blending with capsule

Inferior compartment

Masseter m.

Cut edges of lateral pterygoid m., superior and inferior head

Medial collateral ligament blending with capsule

**Figure 9-4**

| Artery | Source | Course |
|--------|--------|--------|
| Superficial temporal | Terminal branch of the external carotid a. | Begins in the parotid gland and initially is located posterior to the mandible, where it provides small branches to the TMJ |
| Deep auricular | Maxillary a. | Arising in the same area as that of the anterior tympanic a.<br><br>Lies in the parotid gland, posterior to the TMJ, where it gives branches to the TMJ |
| Anterior tympanic | | Arising in the same area as that of the deep auricular a.<br><br>Passes superiorly behind the TMJ to enter the tympanic cavity through the petrotympanic fissure, where it gives branches to the TMJ |

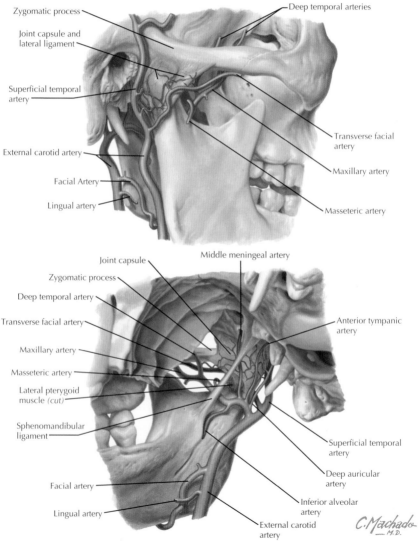

**Figure 9-5**

| Vein | Course |
|------|--------|
| Superficial temporal | Receives some branches from the TMJ<br>Then joins the maxillary v. to form the retromandibular v. |
| Maxillary | Receives some branches from the TMJ<br>Joins the superficial temporal v. to form the retromandibular v. |

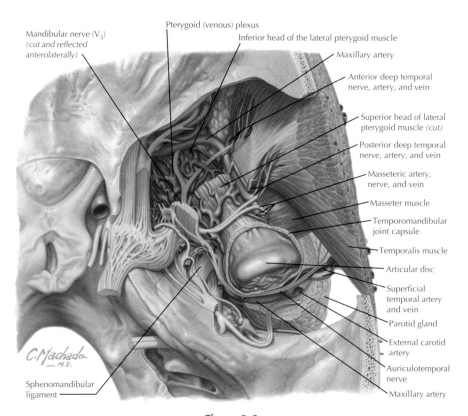

Mandibular nerve (V₃)
*(cut and reflected anterolaterally)*

Pterygoid (venous) plexus

Inferior head of the lateral pterygoid muscle

Maxillary artery

Anterior deep temporal nerve, artery, and vein

Superior head of lateral pterygoid muscle *(cut)*

Posterior deep temporal nerve, artery, and vein

Masseteric artery, nerve, and vein

Masseter muscle

Temporomandibular joint capsule

Temporalis muscle

Articular disc

Superficial temporal artery and vein

Parotid gland

External carotid artery

Auriculotemporal nerve

Maxillary artery

Sphenomandibular ligament

**Figure 9-6**

| Nerve | Source | Comment |
|---|---|---|
| Auriculotemporal | Posterior division of the mandibular division of the trigeminal n. | From the posterior division of the mandibular division of the trigeminal n. |
| | | Splits around the middle meningeal a. and passes between the sphenomandibular ligament and the condylar neck |
| | | Supplies sensory branches all along the capsule |
| | | Sensory but carries autonomic function to the parotid gland |
| Masseteric | Anterior division of the mandibular division of the trigeminal n. | Lies anterior to the TMJ and provides branches to the joint before passing over the masseteric notch to reach the masseter m. |
| | | Sensory branches aid the auriculotemporal n. |
| Posterior deep temporal | | Lies anterior to the TMJ and provides branches to the joint before innervating the temporalis m. |
| | | Sensory branches aid the auriculotemporal n. in supplying the anterior part of the TMJ |
| | | Mainly motor, but carries additional sensory function to the TMJ |

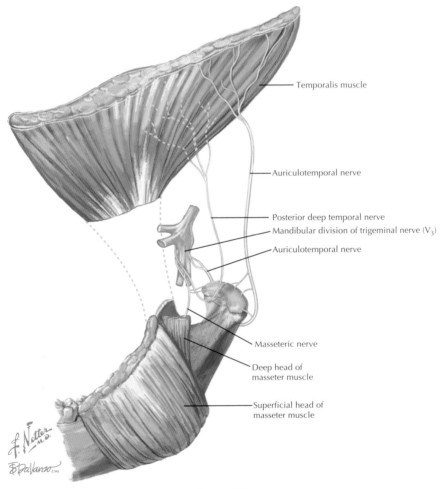

Temporalis muscle

Auriculotemporal nerve

Posterior deep temporal nerve
Mandibular division of trigeminal nerve (V₃)
Auriculotemporal nerve

Masseteric nerve

Deep head of masseter muscle

Superficial head of masseter muscle

**Figure 9-7**

- Up to 33% of adults have a TMJ-related problem
- Perforations of the articular disc typically occur in the later stages of TMJ dysfunction
- Women have a higher prevalence of disc perforations than men
- Many factors may contribute to changes in the disc:
  - Bruxism
  - Trauma
  - Lateral pterygoid muscle abnormal activity
  - Overloading
- Most disc perforations occur in the lateral or posterior portions of the disc and vary in size
- Crepitus and clicking sounds on opening the mouth are common clinical manifestations
- Anterior disc displacement also is common

**Anterosuperior view of condylar process and articular discs**

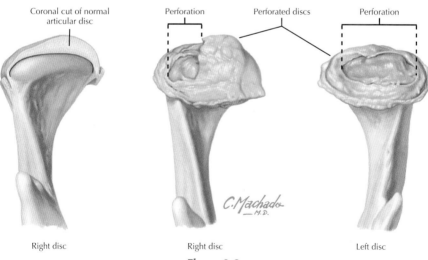

Coronal cut of normal articular disc    Perforation    Perforated discs    Perforation

Right disc      Right disc      Left disc

**Figure 9-8**

- *Mandibular dislocation* (or subluxation of the TMJ) occurs when the condyle moves anterior to the articular eminence
  - With dislocation, the mouth appears "wide open"
  - Because the condyle is displaced anterior to the articular eminence, a depression can be palpated posterior to the condyle
- Spontaneous dislocations can occur from a variety of actions ranging from a simple yawn to an extended dental treatment
- Because the mandible is dislocated, the patient has a great deal of difficulty verbalizing his or her predicament
- Relocation involves repositioning the condyle posterior to the articular eminence

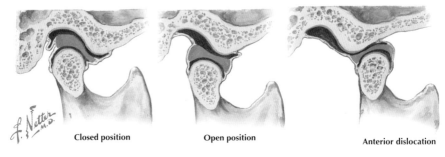

Closed position      Open position      Anterior dislocation

**Figure 9-9**

- Opening the mandible involves a complex series of movements
- Initial movement is *rotational,* which occurs in the lower TMJ compartment:
  - Lateral pterygoid (inferior head) initiates the opening of the jaw (the superior head of the lateral pterygoid is described as being active during elevation of the mandible in a "power stroke")
  - As the mandible is depressed, the medial and collateral ligaments tightly attach the condyle to the articular disc, thereby allowing for only rotational movement
  - Once the TMJ becomes taut, no further rotation of the condyle can occur
  - Normally, rotational movement continues until the upper and the lower teeth are about 20 mm away from each other
- For additional/further opening of the mandible, *translational* movement must occur:
  - A translational movement occurs in the upper TMJ compartment and provides for most of the mandible's ability to open
  - In this movement, the articular disc and the condyle complex slide inferiorly on the articular eminences, allowing for maximum depression of the mandible

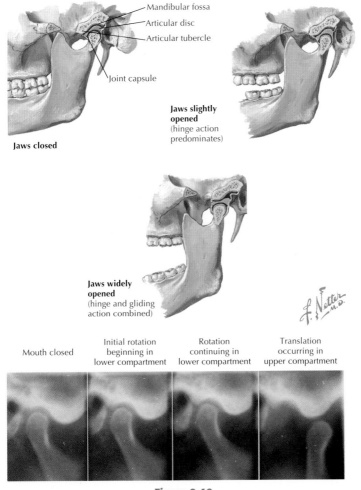

Mandibular fossa
Articular disc
Articular tubercle
Joint capsule

**Jaws closed**

**Jaws slightly opened** (hinge action predominates)

**Jaws widely opened** (hinge and gliding action combined)

| Mouth closed | Initial rotation beginning in lower compartment | Rotation continuing in lower compartment | Translation occurring in upper compartment |

**Figure 9-10**

**Opening the mouth**

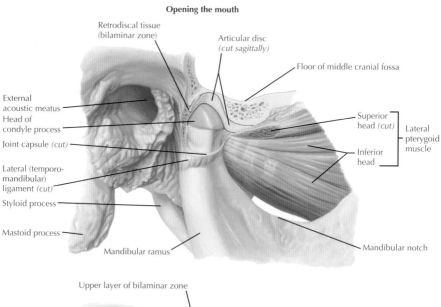

Retrodiscal tissue (bilaminar zone)

Articular disc *(cut sagittally)*

Floor of middle cranial fossa

External acoustic meatus

Head of condyle process

Joint capsule *(cut)*

Lateral (temporomandibular) ligament *(cut)*

Styloid process

Mastoid process

Mandibular ramus

Superior head *(cut)*

Inferior head

Lateral pterygoid muscle

Mandibular notch

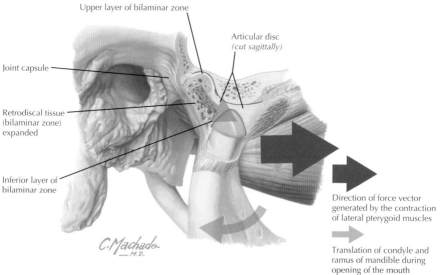

Upper layer of bilaminar zone

Articular disc *(cut sagittally)*

Joint capsule

Retrodiscal tissue (bilaminar zone) expanded

Inferior layer of bilaminar zone

*C.Machado* —M.D.

Direction of force vector generated by the contraction of lateral pterygoid muscles

Translation of condyle and ramus of mandible during opening of the mouth

**Figure 9-11**

## ARTHRITIS

- *Arthritis* is the most common cause of pathologic changes in the TMJ
- When rheumatoid arthritis occurs, usually both TMJs are affected, and other joints tend to be affected before the TMJ
- Radiologic images in the *initial* disease stages show decreased joint space without osseous changes
- Radiologic images in the *late* disease stages show decreased joint space with osseous changes, possibly including ankylosis
- In osteoarthritis, causes include normal wear, trauma, and bruxism, and clinical manifestations may range from mild to severe

## ANKLYOSIS

- *Ankylosis* is an obliteration of the TMJ space with abnormal osseous morphologic features, which often occurs as a result of trauma or infection
- Classified as either *true* (intracapsular) or *false* (extracapsular, usually associated with an abnormally large coronoid process or zygomatic arch) ankylosis
- Treatment varies in accordance with the cause but may include a prosthetic replacement or condylectomy

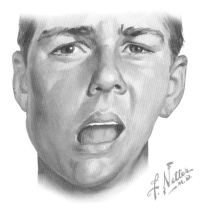

Unilateral ankylosis

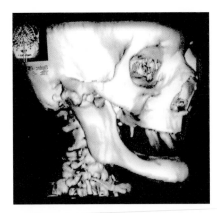

Ankylosis

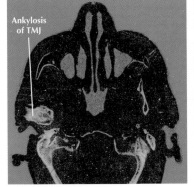

Ankylosis of TMJ

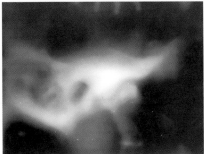

Osteoarthritis

**Figure 9-12**

# PTERYGOPALATINE FOSSA

- The *pterygopalatine fossa* is a pyramid-shaped fossa on the lateral aspect of the skull between the maxilla's infratemporal surface and the pterygoid process of the sphenoid
- Is located inferior to the apex of the orbit
- Is located between the infratemporal fossa and the nasal cavity
- Is a major pathway for the spread of infections and tumors from the head and neck into the skull base
- Allows the infratemporal fossa, middle cranial fossa, nasopharynx, nasal cavity, orbit, and oral cavity to communicate
- Contains major nerves and vessels:
  - Maxillary division of the trigeminal nerve and branches
  - Pterygopalatine (sphenopalatine, Meckel's) ganglion
  - 3rd part of the maxillary artery and branches (with corresponding veins)
- Clinically, the pterygopalatine fossa is often described as being divided into:
  - Anterior (Vascular) Compartment–location of 3rd part of maxillary a. and its branches
  - Posterior (Neural) Compartment–location of maxillary division of the trigeminal n., pterygopalatine ganglion, and n. of the pterygoid canal
- 7 openings (foramina/fissures/canals) allow passage of nerves and vessels

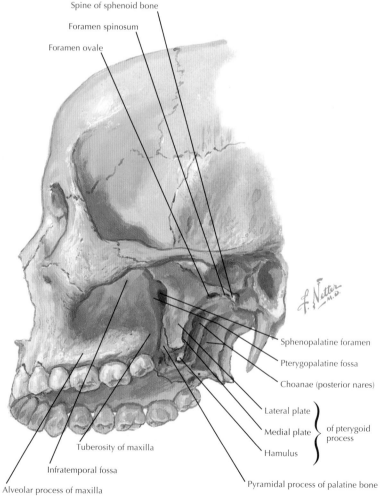

Spine of sphenoid bone

Foramen spinosum

Foramen ovale

Sphenopalatine foramen

Pterygopalatine fossa

Choanae (posterior nares)

Lateral plate

Medial plate } of pterygoid process

Hamulus

Tuberosity of maxilla

Infratemporal fossa

Alveolar process of maxilla

Pyramidal process of palatine bone

**Figure 10-1**

| Border | Structure(s) | Opening(s) |
|---|---|---|
| Anterior | Infratemporal surface of the posterior maxilla | |
| Posterior | Pterygoid process of the sphenoid | Foramen rotundum<br>Pterygoid (vidian) canal<br>Palatovaginal (pharyngeal) canal |
| Medial | Perpendicular plate of the palatine | Sphenopalatine foramen |
| Lateral | Pterygomaxillary fissure | Pterygomaxillary fissure |
| Superior | Inferior surface of the sphenoid and the orbital plate of the palatine bone | Inferior orbital fissure |
| Inferior | Pyramidal process of the palatine | Greater palatine canal |

## Openings

| Opening | Location | Communicates With | Transmitted Structures |
|---|---|---|---|
| Pterygomaxillary fissure | Lateral part of the pterygopalatine fossa | Infratemporal fossa | Posterior superior alveolar n. from the pterygopalatine fossa into the infratemporal fossa<br>3rd part of the maxillary a. from the infratemporal fossa into the pterygopalatine fossa<br>A variable network of veins, such as the sphenopalatine, into the pterygoid plexus of vv. |
| Sphenopalatine foramen | Medial wall of the pterygopalatine fossa<br>Often located posterior to the middle nasal concha | Nasal cavity | Nasopalatine n.<br>Posterior superior nasal n. (medial and lateral branches)<br>Sphenopalatine a. and v. |
| Inferior orbital fissure | Superior part of the pterygopalatine fossa<br>Continues posteriorly with the superior part of the pterygomaxillary fissure | Orbit | Infraorbital n. from the maxillary division of the trigeminal n.<br>Zygomatic n. from the maxillary division of the trigeminal<br>Infraorbital a. and v.<br>Orbital branches from the maxillary division of the trigeminal<br>Inferior ophthalmic v. that connects with the pterygoid plexus of veins |
| Greater palatine canal | Inferior part of the pterygopalatine fossa<br>Eventually terminates into the greater and lesser palatine foramina | Oral cavity | Greater palatine n. and vessels (through the greater palatine foramen) onto the hard palate<br>Lesser palatine n. and vessels (through the lesser palatine foramen) onto the soft palate |
| Foramen rotundum | Posterolateral part of the pterygopalatine fossa | Middle cranial fossa | Maxillary division of the trigeminal n. |
| Pterygoid (vidian) canal | Posterior part of the pterygopalatine fossa<br>Between the pterygopalatine fossa and the foramen lacerum<br>Inferior and medial to the foramen rotundum | Middle cranial fossa | Nerve of the pterygoid canal (vidian n.)<br>Artery (and vein) of the pterygoid canal |
| Palatovaginal (pharyngeal) canal | Posteromedial part of the pterygopalatine fossa<br>Medial to the pterygoid canal | Nasopharynx | Pharyngeal n.<br>Pharyngeal a. and v. |

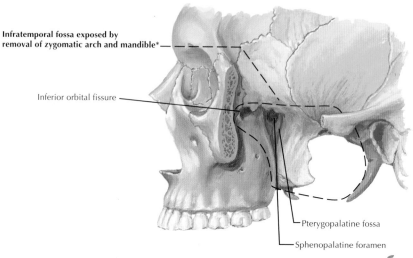

Infratemporal fossa exposed by
removal of zygomatic arch and mandible*

Inferior orbital fissure

Pterygopalatine fossa

Sphenopalatine foramen

*Superficially, mastoid process forms posterior boundary

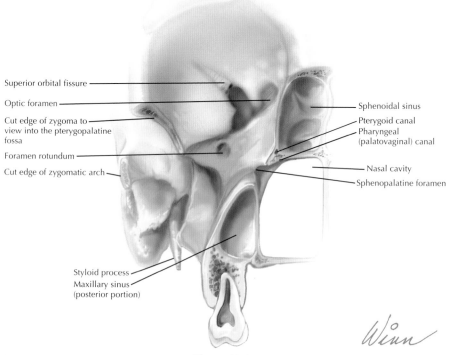

Superior orbital fissure

Optic foramen

Cut edge of zygoma to
view into the pterygopalatine
fossa

Foramen rotundum

Cut edge of zygomatic arch

Sphenoidal sinus

Pterygoid canal

Pharyngeal
(palatovaginal) canal

Nasal cavity

Sphenopalatine foramen

Styloid process
Maxillary sinus
(posterior portion)

**Figure 10-2**

**Posterior – Red border**

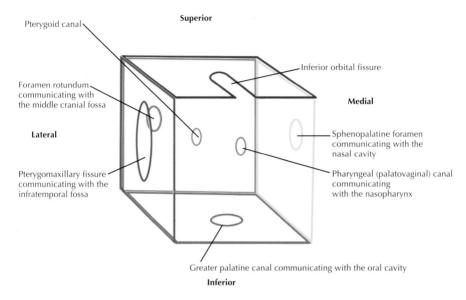

**Superior**

Pterygoid canal

Inferior orbital fissure

Foramen rotundum
communicating with
the middle cranial fossa

**Medial**

**Lateral**

Sphenopalatine foramen
communicating with the
nasal cavity

Pterygomaxillary fissure
communicating with the
infratemporal fossa

Pharyngeal (palatovaginal) canal
communicating
with the nasopharynx

Greater palatine canal communicating with the oral cavity

**Inferior**

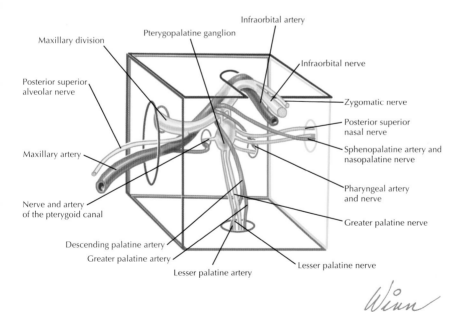

Infraorbital artery

Pterygopalatine ganglion

Maxillary division

Infraorbital nerve

Posterior superior
alveolar nerve

Zygomatic nerve

Posterior superior
nasal nerve

Maxillary artery

Sphenopalatine artery and
nasopalatine nerve

Nerve and artery
of the pterygoid canal

Pharyngeal artery
and nerve

Greater palatine nerve

Descending palatine artery

Greater palatine artery

Lesser palatine nerve

Lesser palatine artery

**Figure 10-3**

| ARTERIAL SUPPLY | | |
|---|---|---|
| **Artery** | **Source** | **Course** |
| Maxillary (3rd part) | External carotid a. | Passes from the infratemporal fossa into the pterygopalatine fossa via the pterygomaxillary fissure<br><br>Prior to passing through the pterygomaxillary fissure, it gives off the posterior superior alveolar a. (the only artery from the 3rd part of the maxillary a. that does not normally branch off within the pterygopalatine fossa) |
| *Infraorbital* | The continuation of the 3rd part of the maxillary a. | Accompanied by the infraorbital n. and v.<br><br>The artery passes forward in the infraorbital groove, infraorbital canal, and exits the infraorbital foramen<br><br>In the infraorbital canal, it gives rise to various orbital branches that aid in supplying the lacrimal gland and extraocular muscles<br><br>In the infraorbital canal, it also gives rise to the anterior and middle (if present) superior alveolar aa. that supply the maxillary teeth from the central incisors to the premolars (where they anastomose with the posterior superior alveolar a.) and the mucous membrane of the maxillary sinus<br><br>On exiting the infraorbital foramen, the artery is located between the levator labii superioris and levator anguli oris mm. and follows the branching pattern of the nerve:<br>• Inferior palpebral branch (supplies the lower eyelid)<br>• Nasal branch (supplies the lateral side of the nose)<br>• Superior labial branch (supplies the upper lip) |
| *Descending palatine* | 3rd part of the maxillary a. | Descends into the greater palatine canal<br><br>Within the canal, the artery splits into the greater and lesser palatine aa.<br><br>Greater palatine a. exits the greater palatine foramen and passes anteriorly toward the incisive foramen and supplies the hard palate gingiva, mucosa, and palatal glands and anastomoses with the terminal branch of the sphenopalatine a. that exits the incisive foramen<br><br>Lesser palatine a. supplies the soft palate and palatine tonsil |
| *Artery of the pterygoid canal* | | Passes posteriorly into the pterygoid canal, accompanying the nerve of the pterygoid canal (vidian n.)<br><br>Helps supply the auditory tube and sphenoid sinus |
| *Pharyngeal* | | Passes posteromedially into the palatovaginal canal<br><br>Helps supply the auditory tube and nasopharynx |
| *Sphenopalatine* | | Passes medially into the sphenopalatine foramen to enter the nasal cavity<br><br>It then gives rise to the posterior lateral nasal branches and posterior septal branches, which supply the nasal concha, mucous membranes, and nasal septum<br><br>The sphenopalatine a. continues along the nasal septum to enter the hard palate via the incisive canal |

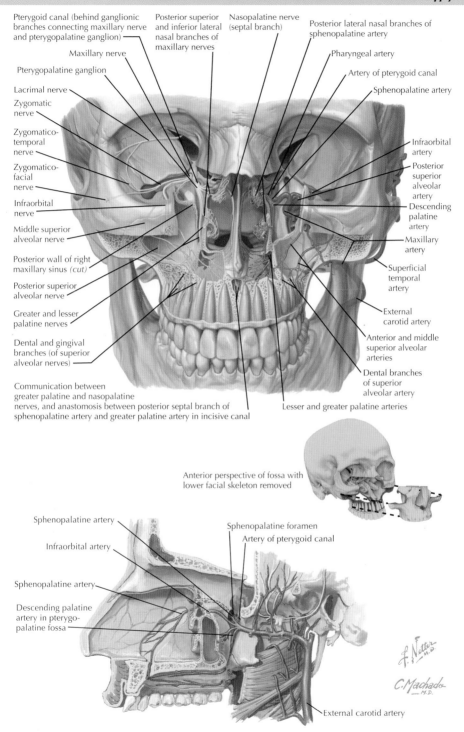

Pterygoid canal (behind ganglionic branches connecting maxillary nerve and pterygopalatine ganglion)

Maxillary nerve

Pterygopalatine ganglion

Lacrimal nerve

Zygomatic nerve

Zygomatico-temporal nerve

Zygomatico-facial nerve

Infraorbital nerve

Middle superior alveolar nerve

Posterior wall of right maxillary sinus *(cut)*

Posterior superior alveolar nerve

Greater and lesser palatine nerves

Dental and gingival branches (of superior alveolar nerves)

Communication between greater palatine and nasopalatine nerves, and anastomosis between posterior septal branch of sphenopalatine artery and greater palatine artery in incisive canal

Posterior superior and inferior lateral nasal branches of maxillary nerves

Nasopalatine nerve (septal branch)

Posterior lateral nasal branches of sphenopalatine artery

Pharyngeal artery

Artery of pterygoid canal

Sphenopalatine artery

Infraorbital artery

Posterior superior alveolar artery

Descending palatine artery

Maxillary artery

Superficial temporal artery

External carotid artery

Anterior and middle superior alveolar arteries

Dental branches of superior alveolar artery

Lesser and greater palatine arteries

Anterior perspective of fossa with lower facial skeleton removed

Sphenopalatine artery

Infraorbital artery

Sphenopalatine artery

Descending palatine artery in pterygo-palatine fossa

Sphenopalatine foramen

Artery of pterygoid canal

External carotid artery

**Figure 10-4**

| VENOUS DRAINAGE | | |
|---|---|---|
| **Vein** | **Course** | |
| Posterior superior alveolar | Receives blood from the posterior teeth and soft tissue | Eventually communicate with the pterygoid plexus of veins |
| Pharyngeal | Receives blood from the nasopharynx | |
| Descending palatine | Receives blood from the hard and soft palate | |
| Infraorbital | Receives blood from the midface via the lower eyelid, lateral side of the nose, and the upper lip | |
| Sphenopalatine | Receives blood from the nasal cavity and the nasal septum | |
| Vein of the pterygoid canal | Receives blood from the foramen lacerum region and the sphenoid sinus | |
| Inferior ophthalmic | Receives blood from the floor of the orbit<br><br>Branches into 2 parts<br><br>The 1st branch travels posteriorly with the infraorbital v. that passes through the inferior orbital fissure to communicate with the pterygoid plexus and the cavernous sinus<br><br>The main branch travels posteriorly to communicate with the superior ophthalmic vein in the superior orbital fissure or travels posteriorly in the fissure to join the cavernous sinus | |
| Pterygoid plexus | An extensive network of veins that parallels the 2nd and 3rd parts of the maxillary a.<br><br>The tributaries of the pterygoid plexus eventually converge to form a short maxillary v. | |

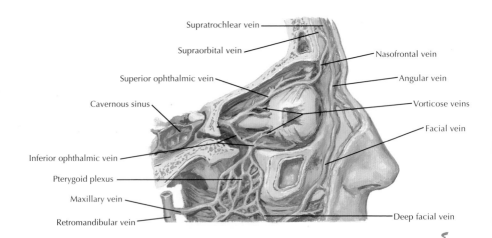

Figure 10-5

| MAXILLARY NERVE | | |
|---|---|---|
| **Nerve** | **Source** | **Course** |
| Maxillary division of the trigeminal n. | Trigeminal n. | Sensory in function<br><br>Travels along the lateral wall of the cavernous sinus<br><br>Before exiting the middle cranial fossa, it gives off a meningeal branch that innervates the dura mater<br><br>Passes from the middle cranial fossa into the pterygopalatine fossa via the foramen rotundum<br><br>Within the pterygopalatine fossa, gives rise to 4 branches:<br>• Posterior superior alveolar n.<br>• Zygomatic n.<br>• Ganglionic branches<br>• Infraorbital n. |
| Posterior superior alveolar | Maxillary division of the trigeminal n. in pterygopalatine fossa | Passes through the pterygomaxillary fissure to enter the infratemporal fossa<br><br>In the infratemporal fossa, it passes on the posterior surface of the maxilla along the region of the maxillary tuberosity<br><br>Gives rise to a gingival branch that innervates the buccal gingiva and adjacent mucosa alongside the maxillary molars<br><br>Enters the posterior surface of the maxilla and supplies the maxillary sinus and the maxillary molars, with the possible exception of the mesiobuccal root of the 1st maxillary molar |
| Zygomatic | | Passes through the inferior orbital fissure to enter the orbit<br><br>Passes on the lateral wall of the orbit and branches into the zygomaticotemporal and zygomaticofacial branches<br><br>A communicating branch from it joins the lacrimal n. from the ophthalmic division of the trigeminal to carry autonomics to the lacrimal gland |
| Ganglionic branches | | Usually 1 or 2 ganglionic branches that connect the maxillary division of the trigeminal to the pterygopalatine ganglion<br><br>Contain sensory fibers that pass through the pterygopalatine ganglion (without synapsing) to be distributed with the nerves that arise from the pterygopalatine ganglion<br><br>Also contain postganglionic autonomic fibers to the lacrimal gland that pass through the pterygopalatine ganglion (parasympathetic fibers form a synapse here, between the preganglionic fibers from the vidian n. and the postganglionic fibers) |
| Infraorbital | Considered the continuation of the maxillary division of the trigeminal n. | Passes through the inferior orbital fissure to enter the orbit<br><br>Passes anteriorly through the infraorbital groove, infraorbital canal, and exits onto the face via the infraorbital foramen<br><br>Within the infraorbital canal, it gives rise to:<br>• Anterior superior alveolar (supplies the maxillary sinus; maxillary central incisor, lateral incisor, and canine; gingiva and mucosa alongside the same teeth)<br>• A small branch of the anterior superior alveolar (supplies the nasal cavity)<br>• Middle superior alveolar (present about 30% of the time; supplies the maxillary sinus, maxillary premolars and often the mesiobuccal root of the 1st maxillary molar, and gingiva and mucosa alongside the same teeth) |

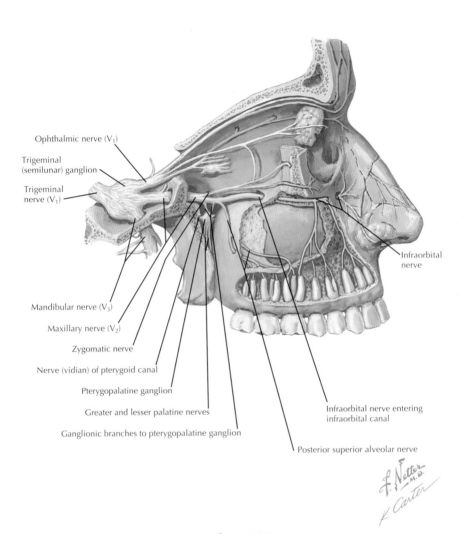

Ophthalmic nerve (V₁)

Trigeminal (semilunar) ganglion

Trigeminal nerve (V₁)

Mandibular nerve (V₃)

Maxillary nerve (V₂)

Zygomatic nerve

Nerve (vidian) of pterygoid canal

Pterygopalatine ganglion

Greater and lesser palatine nerves

Ganglionic branches to pterygopalatine ganglion

Infraorbital nerve

Infraorbital nerve entering infraorbital canal

Posterior superior alveolar nerve

**Figure 10-6**

| BRANCHES OF THE MAXILLARY DIVISION OF THE TRIGEMINAL NERVE ASSOCIATED WITH THE PTERYGOPALATINE GANGLION | | |
|---|---|---|

- A parasympathetic ganglion named because it is a collection of cell bodies in the peripheral nervous system (postganglionic cell bodies)
- The ganglionic branches are of the maxillary division of the trigeminal n. that pass through the pterygopalatine ganglion
- The vidian n. connects to the pterygopalatine ganglion
- 3 sets of nerve fibers travel through the pterygopalatine ganglion:
  - General sensory fibers from the trigeminal n. (without synapsing)
  - Postganglionic sympathetic fibers (carried to the pterygopalatine ganglion via the vidian n, without synapsing)
  - Preganglionic parasympathetic fibers (carried to the pterygopalatine ganglion via the vidian n. and formed by synapsing in the pterygopalatine ganglion with the postganglionic parasympathetic fibers)
- All branches arising from the pterygopalatine ganglion carry these 3 sets of fibers to the areas where they terminate
- These nerves of the maxillary division travel through the pterygopalatine ganglion:
  - Nasopalatine n.
  - Posterior superior nasal n.
  - Greater palatine n.
  - Lesser palatine n.
  - Pharyngeal n.
  - Orbital branches

| Branch(es) | Source | Course |
|---|---|---|
| Vidian (nerve of the pterygoid canal) | Formed by the greater and deep petrosal nn. | An autonomic nerve: <br>• Greater petrosal n. carries the preganglionic parasympathetic fibers<br>• Deep petrosal n. carries the postganglionic sympathetic fibers<br>Communicates with the pterygopalatine ganglion, which allows the autonomics to be distributed along any nerve connected to the ganglion |
| Nasopalatine | A nerve of the maxillary division of the trigeminal n., which branches off the pterygopalatine ganglion in the pterygopalatine fossa | Passes through the sphenopalatine foramen to enter the nasal cavity<br>Passes along the superior portion of the nasal cavity to the nasal septum; then travels anteroinferiorly to the incisive canal<br>Exits the incisive foramen on the hard palate and supplies the palatal gingiva and mucosa from the region of the central incisors to the canines |
| Posterior superior nasal | | Passes through the sphenopalatine foramen to enter the nasal cavity, where it divides into 2 nerves:<br>• Lateral posterior superior (supplies the lateral wall of the nasal cavity)<br>• Medial posterior superior nasal (supplies the posterosuperior portion of the nasal septum) |
| Greater palatine | | Passes through the greater palatine canal to enter the hard palate via the greater palatine foramen<br>Supplies the palatal gingiva and mucosa from the area in the premolar region to the posterior border of the hard palate to the midline |
| Lesser palatine | | Passes through the greater palatine canal to enter and supply the soft palate via the lesser palatine foramen |
| Pharyngeal | | Passes through the palatovaginal (pharyngeal) canal to enter and supply the nasopharynx |
| Orbital | Several branches arising from the maxillary division of the trigeminal n., which branch off of the pterygopalatine ganglion in the pterygopalatine fossa | Pass through the inferior orbital fissure to enter the orbit (supplying orbital periosteum) and some fibers continue through the posterior ethmoid foramen supplying the sphenoid and posterior ethmoid sinuses |

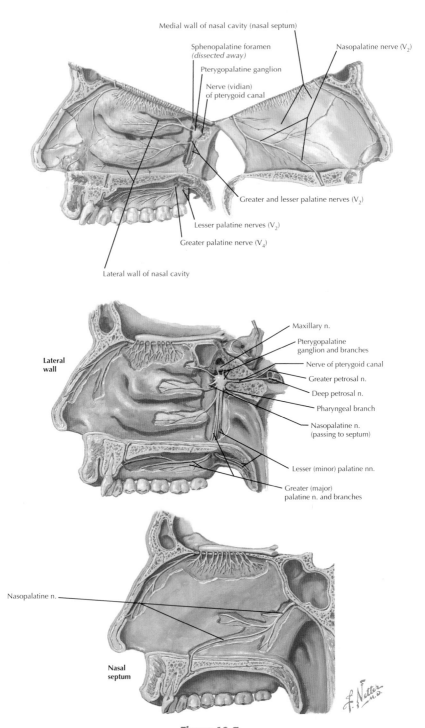

Medial wall of nasal cavity (nasal septum)

Sphenopalatine foramen
*(dissected away)*

Pterygopalatine ganglion

Nerve (vidian)
of pterygoid canal

Nasopalatine nerve (V₂)

Greater and lesser palatine nerves (V₂)

Lesser palatine nerves (V₂)

Greater palatine nerve (V₄)

Lateral wall of nasal cavity

Lateral
wall

Maxillary n.

Pterygopalatine
ganglion and branches

Nerve of pterygoid canal

Greater petrosal n.

Deep petrosal n.

Pharyngeal branch

Nasopalatine n.
(passing to septum)

Lesser (minor) palatine nn.

Greater (major)
palatine n. and branches

Nasopalatine n.

Nasal
septum

**Figure 10-7**

| AUTONOMICS TRAVERSING THE PTERYGOPALATINE FOSSA | | | |
|---|---|---|---|
| Type of Neuron | Name of Cell Body | Characteristics of Cell Body | Course of the Neuron |
| Anatomic Pathway for Parasympathetics Associated With the Maxillary Division of the Trigeminal Nerve | | | |
| Preganglionic neuron | Superior salivatory nucleus | A collection of nerve cell bodies located in the pons<br>Travel through the nervus intermedius of the facial n. into the internal acoustic meatus<br>In the facial canal, the facial n. gives rise to 2 parasympathetic branches:<br>• Greater petrosal n.<br>• Chorda tympani n. | **Greater Petrosal Nerve**<br>Greater petrosal n. exits along the hiatus for the greater petrosal n. toward the foramen lacerum, where it joins the deep petrosal n. (sympathetics) to form the nerve of the pterygoid canal (vidian n.)<br>Vidian n. passes through the pterygoid canal and enters the pterygopalatine fossa, where it joins with the pterygopalatine ganglion |
| Postganglionic neuron | Pterygopalatine ganglion | Pterygopalatine ganglion is a collection of nerve cell bodies located in the pterygopalatine fossa<br>Postganglionic parasympathetic fibers that arise in the pterygopalatine ganglion are distributed to the ophthalmic and maxillary divisions of the trigeminal n. to the:<br>• Lacrimal gland<br>• Nasal glands (in respiratory epithelium)<br>• Paranasal sinus glands (in respiratory epithelium)<br>• Palatine glands<br>• Pharyngeal glands | **Ophthalmic Division Distribution**<br>Postganglionic fibers travel along the zygomatic branch of the maxillary division for a short distance to enter the orbit<br>A short communicating branch joins the lacrimal n. of the ophthalmic division of the trigeminal n.<br>These fibers innervate the lacrimal gland to cause the secretion of tears<br>**Maxillary Division Distribution**<br>Postganglionic fibers travel along the maxillary division of the trigeminal n. to be distributed along its branches that are located in the nasal cavity, paranasal sinuses, oral cavity, and pharynx (e.g., nasopalatine, greater palatine)<br>These fibers innervate:<br>• Nasal glands<br>• Paranasal glands<br>• Palatine glands<br>• Pharyngeal glands |

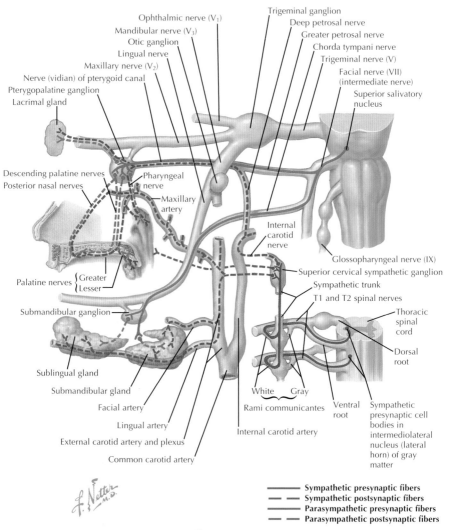

Ophthalmic nerve (V₁)
Mandibular nerve (V₃)
Otic ganglion
Lingual nerve
Maxillary nerve (V₂)
Nerve (vidian) of pterygoid canal
Pterygopalatine ganglion
Lacrimal gland

Trigeminal ganglion
Deep petrosal nerve
Greater petrosal nerve
Chorda tympani nerve
Trigeminal nerve (V)
Facial nerve (VII)
(intermediate nerve)
Superior salivatory
nucleus

Descending palatine nerves
Posterior nasal nerves
Pharyngeal
nerve
Maxillary
artery

Internal
carotid
nerve

Glossopharyngeal nerve (IX)
Superior cervical sympathetic ganglion
Sympathetic trunk
T1 and T2 spinal nerves

Palatine nerves { Greater
Lesser

Submandibular ganglion

Thoracic
spinal
cord

Dorsal
root

Sublingual gland
Submandibular gland
Facial artery
Lingual artery
External carotid artery and plexus
Common carotid artery

White     Gray
Rami communicantes

Ventral
root

Internal carotid artery

Sympathetic
presynaptic cell
bodies in
intermediolateral
nucleus (lateral
horn) of gray
matter

——————— Sympathetic presynaptic fibers
— — — Sympathetic postsynaptic fibers
——————— Parasympathetic presynaptic fibers
— — — Parasympathetic postsynaptic fibers

**Figure 10-8**

| AUTONOMICS TRAVERSING THE PTERYGOPALATINE FOSSA | | | |
|---|---|---|---|
| **Type of Neuron** | **Name of Cell Body** | **Characteristics of Cell Body** | **Course of the Neuron** |
| Anatomic Pathway for Sympathetics Associated With the Maxillary Division of the Trigeminal Nerve | | | |
| Preganglionic neuron | Intermediolateral horn nucleus | Collection of nerve cell bodies located in the lateral horn nucleus of the spinal cord between spinal segments T1 and T3 (and possibly T4) | Arise from the intermediolateral horn nuclei from T1 to T3 (or T4)<br><br>Travel through the ventral root of the spinal cord to the spinal n.<br><br>Enter the sympathetic chain via a white ramus communicans<br><br>Once in the sympathetic chain, the preganglionic fibers for the eye will ascend and synapse with postganglionic fibers in the superior cervical ganglion |
| Postganglionic neuron | Superior cervical ganglion | Collection of nerve cell bodies located in the superior cervical ganglion, which is located at the base of the skull<br><br>Postganglionic sympathetic fibers follow the internal carotid or external carotid a. to pass near their respective effector organs:<br>• Nasal cavity<br>• Paranasal sinuses<br>• Palate<br>• Lacrimal gland | **Nasal Cavity, Paranasal Sinuses, and Palate**<br>• Postganglionic sympathetic fibers follow both the *internal* and *external* carotid aa.<br>• Postganglionic fibers that will follow the internal carotid a. will form the internal carotid n., which travels along the internal carotid a., forming the internal carotid plexus<br>• Postganglionic sympathetic fibers from the internal carotid plexus branch in the region of the foramen lacerum to form the deep petrosal n.<br>• The deep petrosal n. joins the greater petrosal n. (parasympathetics) to form the nerve of the pterygoid canal (vidian n.)<br>• Postganglionic sympathetic fibers travel along the branches of the maxillary division of the trigeminal n. associated with the pterygopalatine ganglion to be distributed along its branches in the nasal cavity, paranasal sinuses, and palate<br>• Postganglionic sympathetic fibers that will follow the external carotid travel to the external carotid a. and branch and follow the maxillary a.<br>• These fibers travel along the branches of the maxillary a. to be distributed along the nasal cavity, paranasal sinuses, and palate<br>**Lacrimal Gland**<br>• Postganglionic sympathetic fibers follow the internal carotid a.<br>• Postganglionic fibers that will follow the internal carotid a. will form the internal carotid n., which travels along the internal carotid a., forming the internal carotid plexus<br>• Postganglionic sympathetic fibers from the internal carotid plexus branch off in the region of the foramen lacerum to form the deep petrosal n.<br>• The deep petrosal n. joins the greater petrosal n. (parasympathetics) to form the nerve of the pterygoid canal (vidian n.)<br>• Postganglionic fibers travel along the zygomatic branch of the maxillary division for a short distance to enter the orbit<br>• A short communicating branch joins the lacrimal n. of the ophthalmic division of the trigeminal n.<br>• These fibers are distributed to the lacrimal gland |

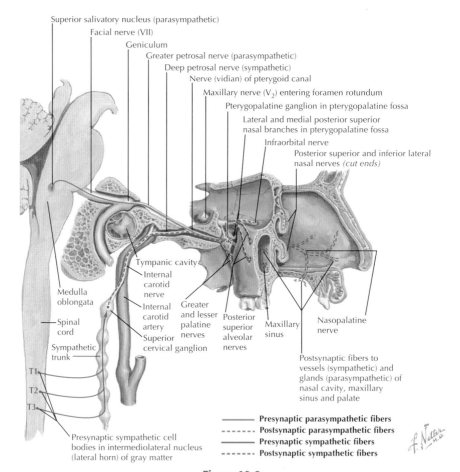

Superior salivatory nucleus (parasympathetic)
Facial nerve (VII)
Geniculum
Greater petrosal nerve (parasympathetic)
Deep petrosal nerve (sympathetic)
Nerve (vidian) of pterygoid canal
Maxillary nerve (V₂) entering foramen rotundum
Pterygopalatine ganglion in pterygopalatine fossa
Lateral and medial posterior superior nasal branches in pterygopalatine fossa
Infraorbital nerve
Posterior superior and inferior lateral nasal nerves (cut ends)

Tympanic cavity
Internal carotid nerve
Medulla oblongata
Internal carotid artery
Greater and lesser palatine nerves
Posterior superior alveolar nerves
Spinal cord
Superior cervical ganglion
Maxillary sinus
Nasopalatine nerve
Sympathetic trunk

T1
T2
T3

Presynaptic sympathetic cell bodies in intermediolateral nucleus (lateral horn) of gray matter

Postsynaptic fibers to vessels (sympathetic) and glands (parasympathetic) of nasal cavity, maxillary sinus and palate

———— Presynaptic parasympathetic fibers
- - - - Postsynaptic parasympathetic fibers
———— Presynaptic sympathetic fibers
- - - - Postsynaptic sympathetic fibers

**Figure 10-9**

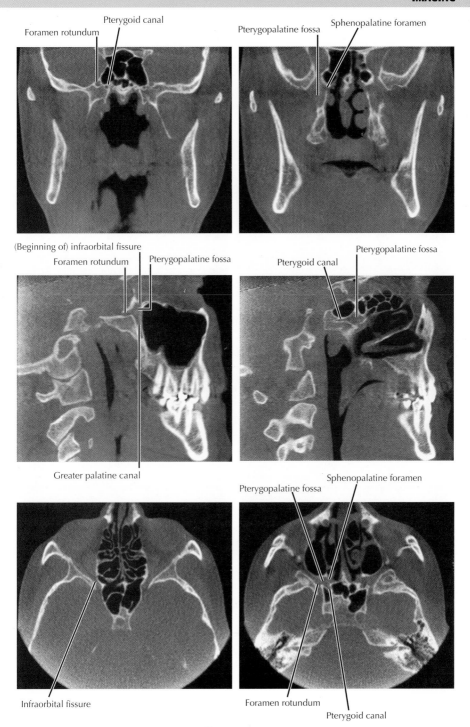

Foramen rotundum

Pterygoid canal

Pterygopalatine fossa

Sphenopalatine foramen

(Beginning of) infraorbital fissure

Foramen rotundum

Pterygopalatine fossa

Pterygoid canal

Pterygopalatine fossa

Greater palatine canal

Infraorbital fissure

Pterygopalatine fossa

Sphenopalatine foramen

Foramen rotundum

Pterygoid canal

**Figure 10-10**

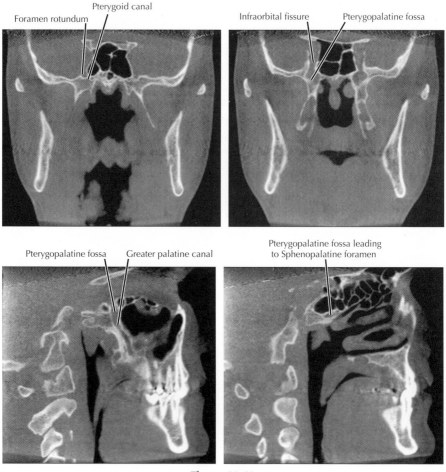

**Figure 10-11**

### NOSE

- The prominent anatomic structure located inferior and medial to the eyes
- Helps in breathing and olfaction

### NASAL CAVITY

- The complex chamber located posterior to the vestibule and atrium of the nose

### RESPIRATORY EPITHELIUM

- Pseudostratified columnar epithelium with cilia
- Highly vascular and easily congested
- When this tissue is irritated, its blood vessels reflexively dilate and the glands secrete, normally leading to sneezing

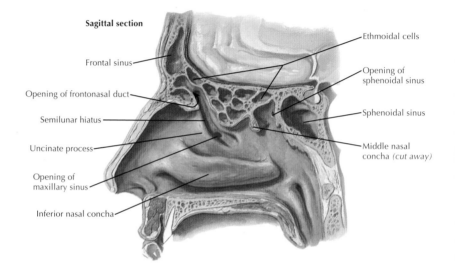

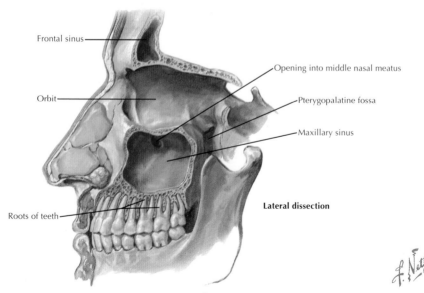

**Figure 11-1**

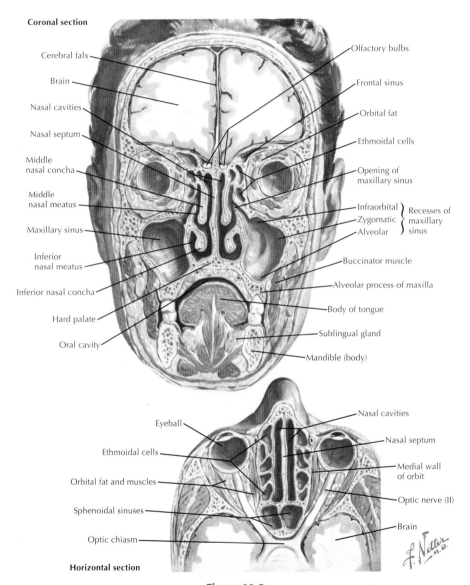

Coronal section

Cerebral falx

Brain

Nasal cavities

Nasal septum

Middle nasal concha

Middle nasal meatus

Maxillary sinus

Inferior nasal meatus

Inferior nasal concha

Hard palate

Oral cavity

Olfactory bulbs

Frontal sinus

Orbital fat

Ethmoidal cells

Opening of maxillary sinus

Infraorbital ⎫
Zygomatic ⎬ Recesses of maxillary sinus
Alveolar ⎭

Buccinator muscle

Alveolar process of maxilla

Body of tongue

Sublingual gland

Mandible (body)

Eyeball

Ethmoidal cells

Orbital fat and muscles

Sphenoidal sinuses

Optic chiasm

Horizontal section

Nasal cavities

Nasal septum

Medial wall of orbit

Optic nerve (II)

Brain

Figure 11-2

- The nose is pyramidal in form
- Fractures of the nasal bones are common—these are the most frequently broken bones in the face
- The opening in the skull is the piriform aperture and is bounded by 2 bones:
  - Nasal
  - Maxilla
- 3 pairs of *bones* form the root of the nose:
  - Frontal (nasal process)
  - Maxilla (frontal process)
  - Nasal
- Because the root of the nose is made of bone, it is fixed
- 3 different major *cartilages* form the dorsum and apex of the nose:
  - Septal
  - Lateral nasal (upper nasal)
  - Major alar (lower nasal)
- Minor cartilages that complete the nose are the:
  - Lesser alar (3 to 4 cartilages)
  - Vomeronasal
- Because the dorsum and apex are cartilaginous, the nose is quite mobile
- The cavity of the nose opposite the alar cartilage is called the vestibule and is lined by many coarse hairs called vibrissae
- The skin over the nose is keratinized stratified squamous epithelium
- The cavity posterior to the vestibule is the atrium
- At the apex are found the 2 nostrils, or anterior nares, which are separated by the septum connecting the apex to the philtrum of the upper lip
- Fibrous tissue helps connect the cartilages together and posteriorly to the maxilla
- The primary lymphatic drainage of the nose is into the submandibular lymph nodes

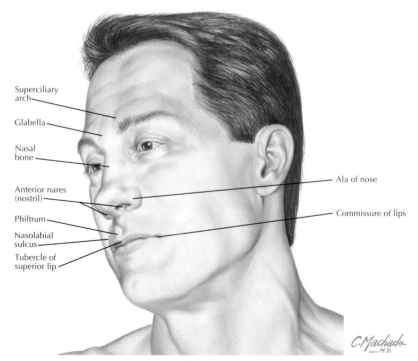

Superciliary arch

Glabella

Nasal bone

Anterior nares (nostril)

Philtrum

Nasolabial sulcus

Tubercle of superior lip

Ala of nose

Commissure of lips

C. Machado —M.D.

**Figure 11-3**

Anterolateral view

Frontal bone
Nasal bones
Frontal process of maxilla
Lateral process of
septal nasal cartilages
Septal cartilage
Minor alar cartilage
Accessory nasal cartilage
Major alar cartilage { Lateral crus
Medial crus
Septal nasal cartilage
Anterior nasal spine of maxilla
Alar fibrofatty tissue
Infraorbital foramen

Inferior view
Major alar cartilage
Lateral crus — Medial crus
Alar fibrofatty tissue
Septal nasal cartilage
Anterior nasal spine of maxilla
Intermaxillary suture

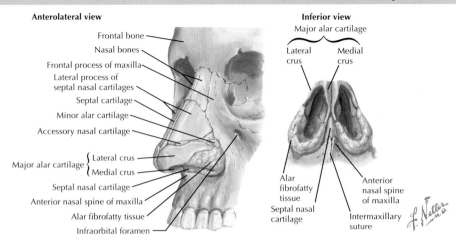

Figure 11-4

## Vascular Supply of the Nose

- The blood supply to the nose arises from 3 major *arteries:*
  - Ophthalmic
  - Maxillary
  - Facial
- These vessels are derived from the external and internal carotid arteries
- These arteries anastomose along the nose
- Many nosebleeds are due to trauma to the septal branch of the superior labial artery from the facial artery

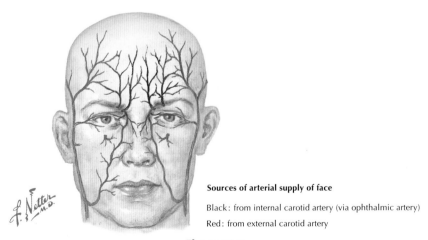

Sources of arterial supply of face

Black: from internal carotid artery (via ophthalmic artery)

Red: from external carotid artery

Figure 11-5

| ARTERIAL SUPPLY | | |
|---|---|---|
| **Artery** | **Source** | **Course** |
| Ophthalmic | Internal carotid a. | Enters the orbit through the optic foramen immediately inferior and lateral to the optic n.<br>Crosses the optic n. to reach the medial part of the orbit<br>While in the orbit, besides other branches including the orbital vessels, it gives rise to 2 major branches that supply the nose:<br>• Dorsal nasal<br>• External nasal from the anterior ethmoidal a. |
| *Dorsal nasal* | Ophthalmic a. | 1 of 2 terminal branches of the ophthalmic a.<br>Exits the orbit along the superomedial border along with the infratrochlear n.<br>Supplies the area along the bridge of the nose |
| *External nasal* | Anterior ethmoid a. | A terminal branch of the anterior ethmoid a.<br>Supplies the area along the external nose at the junction between the nasal bone and the lateral nasal cartilage |
| Maxillary | External carotid a. | Gives rise to a series of branches; only 1 provides blood supply to the nose: nasal branch of the infraorbital a. |
| *Nasal branch of the infraorbital* | Maxillary a. | Infraorbital is the continuation of the maxillary a.<br>Arises with the inferior palpebral branch and the superior labial branch<br>Supplies the lateral aspect of the nose |
| Facial | External carotid a. | Passes superiorly immediately deep to the posterior belly of the digastric m. and the stylohyoid m.<br>Passes along the submandibular gland, giving rise to the submental a., which helps supply the gland<br>Passes superiorly over the body of the mandible at the masseter, giving rise to the:<br>• Premasseteric a.<br>Continues anterosuperiorly across the cheek to the angle of the mouth, giving rise to the:<br>• Superior labial a.<br>• Inferior labial a.<br>Passes superiorly along the side of the nose, giving rise to the:<br>• Lateral nasal a.<br>Following the last branch, it continues on the side of the nose as the angular a. that terminates along the medial side of the eye<br>Tortuous |
| *(Nasal) septal* | Superior labial a. | Supplies the septum |
| *Alar* | Superior labial a. | Supplies the ala of the nose |
| *Lateral nasal* | Facial a. | Supplies the ala and dorsal surface of nose |

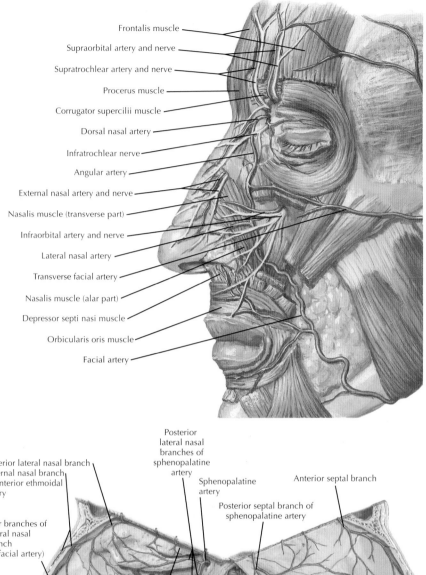

Frontalis muscle

Supraorbital artery and nerve

Supratrochlear artery and nerve

Procerus muscle

Corrugator supercilii muscle

Dorsal nasal artery

Infratrochlear nerve

Angular artery

External nasal artery and nerve

Nasalis muscle (transverse part)

Infraorbital artery and nerve

Lateral nasal artery

Transverse facial artery

Nasalis muscle (alar part)

Depressor septi nasi muscle

Orbicularis oris muscle

Facial artery

Anterior lateral nasal branch
External nasal branch
of anterior ethmoidal
artery

Posterior
lateral nasal
branches of
sphenopalatine
artery

Sphenopalatine
artery

Anterior septal branch

Posterior septal branch of
sphenopalatine artery

Alar branches of
lateral nasal
branch
(of facial artery)

Maxillary
artery

External carotid
artery

Nasal septal branch
of superior labial
branch (of facial
artery)

Lateral wall of nasal cavity

Greater palatine foramen and artery

Lesser palatine foramen and artery

**Figure 11-6**

| VENOUS DRAINAGE | |
|---|---|
| **Vein** | **Course** |
| Facial | Begins as the angular v.<br>Passes inferiorly along the side of the nose, receiving the lateral nasal v.<br>Continues in a posteroinferior path across the angle of the mouth to the cheek, receiving the superior and inferior labial vv.<br>While passing toward the mandible, the deep facial v. connects the facial vein to the pterygoid plexus<br>In the submandibular triangle, the facial v. joins the anterior branch of the retromandibular to form the common facial v.<br>Has no valves that can allow blood to backflow |
| Angular | From the confluence of the supraorbital and supratrochlear vv. along the medial part of the eye<br>Travels along the lateral side of the nose to become the facial v. |
| Superior ophthalmic | Receives blood from the roof of the orbit and the scalp<br>Anastomoses with the angular v.<br>Travels posteriorly to communicate with the pterygoid plexus |
| Inferior ophthalmic | Receives blood from the floor of the orbit<br>Anastomoses with the angular v.<br>Travels posteriorly with the infraorbital v. that passes through the inferior orbital fissure to communicate with the pterygoid plexus |

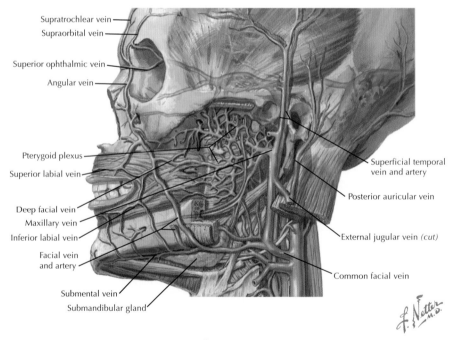

**Figure 11-7**

- The sensory supply to the nose arises from branches of the ophthalmic and maxillary divisions of the trigeminal nerve

| OPHTHALMIC DIVISION OF THE TRIGEMINAL |
|---|
| Arises from the trigeminal in the middle cranial fossa |
| Passes anterior on the lateral wall of the cavernous sinus immediately inferior to the oculomotor and trochlear nn., but superior to the maxillary division of the trigeminal n. |
| Immediately prior to entering the orbit, through the superior orbital fissure, the ophthalmic division divides into 3 major branches: |
| • Lacrimal |
| • Frontal |
| • Nasociliary |
| The nasociliary branch terminates as the: |
| • Anterior ethmoid n. |
| • Infratrochlear n. |

| Nerve | Source | Course |
|---|---|---|
| *External nasal* | Anterior ethmoid n. | Exits between the lateral nasal cartilage and the inferior border of the nasal bone |
| | | Supplies the skin of the ala and apex of the nose around the nares |
| *Internal nasal* | | Supplies the skin on the internal surface of the vestibule as the: |
| | | • Medial internal nasal n. |
| | | • Lateral internal nasal n. |
| *Infratrochlear* | Nasociliary n. | Passes anteriorly on the superior border of the medial rectus m. |
| | | Passes inferior to the trochlea toward the medial angle of the eye |
| | | Supplies the skin of the bridge of the nose |
| | | Also supplies the eyelids, the conjunctiva, and all lacrimal structures |

| MAXILLARY DIVISION OF THE TRIGEMINAL |
|---|
| Travels along the lateral wall of the cavernous sinus |
| Passes from the middle cranial fossa into the pterygopalatine fossa via the foramen rotundum *4 branches:* |
| • Infraorbital—this is the continuation of the maxillary division |
| • Posterior superior alveolar |
| • Zygomatic |
| • Ganglionic |

| *Infraorbital* | Continuation of maxillary division of the trigeminal n. | Passes through the inferior orbital fissure to enter the orbit |
|---|---|---|
| | | Passes anteriorly through the infraorbital groove and infraorbital canal and exits onto the face via the infraorbital foramen |
| | | Once it exits onto the face, it divides into *3 terminal branches:* |
| | | • Nasal (supplies the ala of the nose) |
| | | • Inferior palpebral (supplies the skin of the lower eyelid) |
| | | • Superior labial (supplies the skin of the upper lip) |
| *Nasal branch of the infraorbital* | Infraorbital n. | Supplies the ala of the nose |

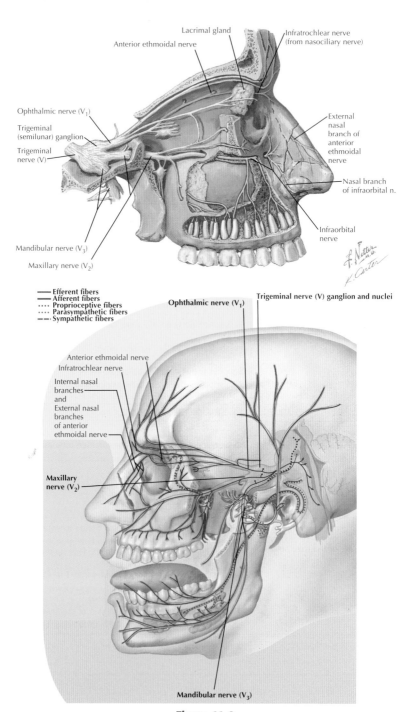

Lacrimal gland

Infratrochlear nerve
(from nasociliary nerve)

Anterior ethmoidal nerve

Ophthalmic nerve (V₁)

Trigeminal
(semilunar) ganglion

Trigeminal
nerve (V)

External
nasal
branch of
anterior
ethmoidal
nerve

Nasal branch
of infraorbital n.

Mandibular nerve (V₃)

Maxillary nerve (V₂)

Infraorbital
nerve

—— Efferent fibers
—— Afferent fibers
···· Proprioceptive fibers
···· Parasympathetic fibers
—·— Sympathetic fibers

Ophthalmic nerve (V₁)

Trigeminal nerve (V) ganglion and nuclei

Anterior ethmoidal nerve

Infratrochlear nerve

Internal nasal
branches
and
External nasal
branches
of anterior
ethmoidal nerve

**Maxillary
nerve (V₂)**

Mandibular nerve (V₃)

**Figure 11-8**

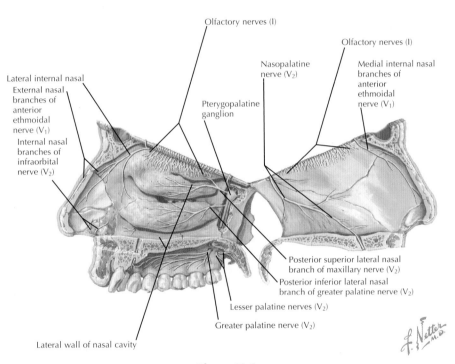

Olfactory nerves (I)

Olfactory nerves (I)

Nasopalatine nerve (V₂)

Medial internal nasal branches of anterior ethmoidal nerve (V₁)

Lateral internal nasal

External nasal branches of anterior ethmoidal nerve (V₁)

Pterygopalatine ganglion

Internal nasal branches of infraorbital nerve (V₂)

Posterior superior lateral nasal branch of maxillary nerve (V₂)

Posterior inferior lateral nasal branch of greater palatine nerve (V₂)

Lesser palatine nerves (V₂)

Greater palatine nerve (V₂)

Lateral wall of nasal cavity

**Figure 11-9**

- Lined by pseudostratified columnar epithelium with cilia
- Inferior portion is larger than superior portion
- Olfactory epithelium is located at the superior part of the nasal cavity around the cribriform plate

## PIRIFORM APERTURE

- Anterior opening bounded by the nasal bones and maxilla

## NASAL SEPTUM

- Frequently deviates to 1 side, giving rise to unequal chambers

## LATERAL WALLS

- Composed of large venous plexuses that have the appearance of erectile tissue
- 3 large elevations, known as conchae, protrude from the lateral wall
- All of the paranasal sinuses and the nasolacrimal duct drain into the lateral walls of the nasal cavity
- The sphenopalatine foramen, located in the posterior portion of the lateral walls, connects the nasal cavity to the pterygopalatine fossa

## CHOANAE

- Also known as the posterior nasal apertures, these openings connect the nasal cavity to the nasopharynx

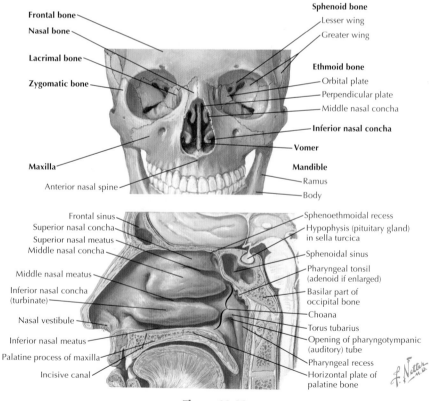

**Figure 11-10**

| BOUNDARIES | |
|---|---|
| **Border** | **Structure(s)** |
| Superior | Nasal, frontal, cribriform plate of the ethmoid, body of the sphenoid |
| Inferior | Palatine process of the maxilla, horizontal plate of the palatine |
| Anterior | External nose |
| Posterior | Choanae (posterior nasal aperture) |
| Medial | Ethmoid (perpendicular plate), vomer, septal cartilage |
| Lateral | Maxilla, ethmoid, palatine, sphenoid (medial pterygoid plate), and inferior nasal concha, lacrimal |
| **RELATIONS** | |
| **Border** | **Structure(s)** |
| Superior | Frontal sinus, sphenoid sinus, anterior cranial fossa with frontal lobe of the brain |
| Inferior | Palate, oral cavity |
| Medial | Other half of nasal cavity |
| Lateral | Maxillary sinus, ethmoid sinuses, orbit, and pterygopalatine fossa |

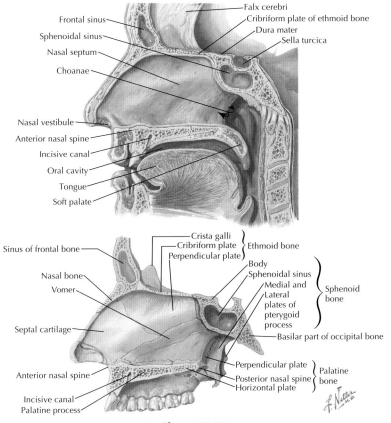

**Figure 11-11**

NOSE AND NASAL CAVITY **287**

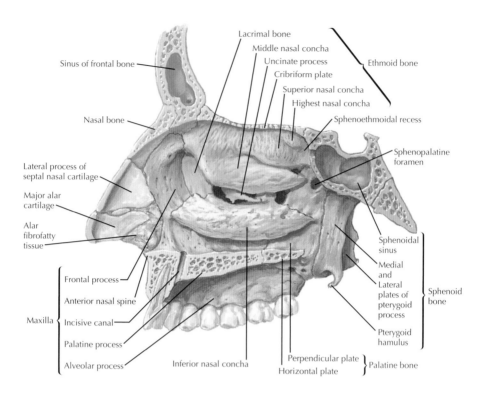

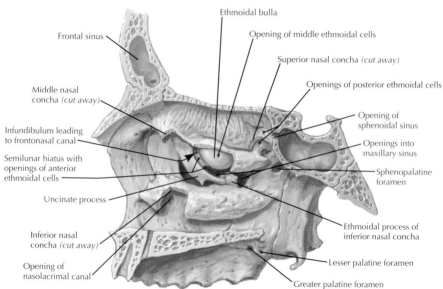

**Figure 11-12**

| Concha | Regions Drained | Location | Structures Drained |
|---|---|---|---|
| Superior | Sphenoethmoidal recess | Superior to the superior meatus | Sphenoidal sinus |
| | Superior meatus | Inferior to the superior meatus | Posterior ethmoid sinus |
| Middle | Middle meatus | Inferior to the middle meatus | Anterior ethmoidal sinus<br>Middle ethmoidal sinus<br>Maxillary sinus<br>Frontal sinus |
| Inferior | Inferior meatus | Inferior to the inferior meatus | Nasolacrimal duct |

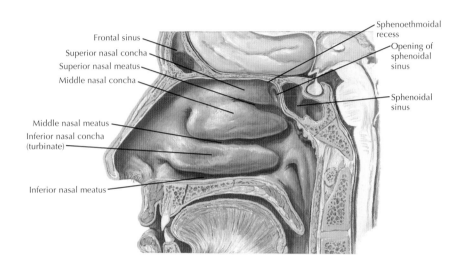

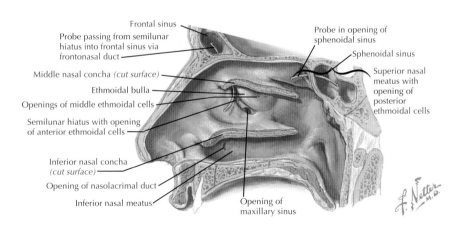

**Figure 11-13**

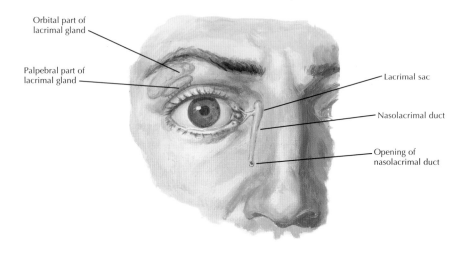

Orbital part of
lacrimal gland

Palpebral part of
lacrimal gland

Lacrimal sac

Nasolacrimal duct

Opening of
nasolacrimal duct

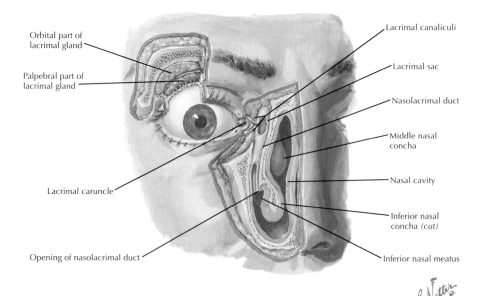

Orbital part of
lacrimal gland

Palpebral part of
lacrimal gland

Lacrimal caruncle

Opening of nasolacrimal duct

Lacrimal canaliculi

Lacrimal sac

Nasolacrimal duct

Middle nasal
concha

Nasal cavity

Inferior nasal
concha *(cut)*

Inferior nasal meatus

**Figure 11-14**

- The blood supply to the nasal cavity arises from *3 major arteries*:
  - Ophthalmic
  - Maxillary
  - Facial
- These 3 vessels are derived from the external and internal carotid arteries and generally follow the paths of the nerves
- Kiesselbach's plexus is the anastomosis along the nasal septum formed by:
  - Anterior ethmoid a.
  - Sphenopalatine a.
  - Greater palatine a.
  - Septal branch from the superior labial a.
- The *veins* generally correspond to the arteries

| ARTERIAL SUPPLY | | |
|---|---|---|
| **Artery** | **Source** | **Course** |
| Ophthalmic | Internal carotid a. | Enters the orbit through the optic foramen immediately inferior and lateral to the optic n. |
| | | Crosses the optic n. to reach the medial part of the orbit |
| | | While in the orbit, besides the orbital branches, it gives rise to 2 major branches that supply the nasal cavity: |
| | | • Anterior ethmoid |
| | | • Posterior ethmoid |
| *Anterior ethmoid* | Ophthalmic a. | Travels with the nasociliary n. through the anterior ethmoidal foramen |
| | | Enters the anterior cranial fossa, where it gives rise to a meningeal branch |
| | | Continues its path to give rise to nasal branches that descend into the nasal cavity: |
| | | • Lateral branch |
| | | • Septal branch |
| | | Supplies branches to the lateral wall and septum of the nose before giving rise to the external nasal a., which supplies the external nose |
| *Posterior ethmoid* | Ophthalmic a. | Travels through the posterior ethmoidal foramen |
| | | Enters the anterior cranial fossa, where it gives rise to a meningeal branch |
| | | Continues its path to give rise to nasal branches that descend into the nasal cavity through the cribriform plate: |
| | | • Lateral branch |
| | | • Septal branch |
| | | Supplies part of the lateral wall near the superior nasal concha and the posterosuperior portion of the nasal septum |
| Maxillary | External carotid a. | Gives rise to a series of branches; 2 provide blood supply to the nasal cavity: |
| | | • Sphenopalatine |
| | | • Greater palatine |
| *Sphenopalatine* | 3rd part of the maxillary a. | After passing through the sphenopalatine foramen, enters the nasal cavity, where it gives rise to the posterior nasal branches: |
| | | • The posterior *lateral* nasal branch supplies the nasal concha, mucous membranes, and lateral wall |
| | | • The posterior septal branch continues along the nasal septum to enter the hard palate via the incisive canal |

*Continued on next page*

| ARTERIAL SUPPLY *Continued* | | |
|---|---|---|
| **Artery** | **Source** | **Course** |
| *Greater palatine* | Descending palatine from the maxillary a. | Travels in the palatine canal, where it splits into the lesser palatine a. (supplies the soft palate and palatine tonsil), and greater palatine a., which exits the greater palatine foramen and passes anteriorly toward the incisive foramen (supplies the hard palate gingiva, mucosa, and palatal glands) and anastomoses with the terminal branch of the sphenopalatine a. that exits the incisive foramen<br><br>Also provides branches that supply the area of the inferior meatus |
| Facial | External carotid a. | Tortuous<br><br>Passes superiorly immediately deep to the posterior belly of the digastric and the stylohyoid mm.<br><br>Passes along the submandibular gland, giving rise to the submental a. that helps supply the gland<br><br>Passes superiorly over the body of the mandible at the masseter m.<br><br>Continues anterosuperiorly across the cheek to the angle of the mouth, giving rise to the superior and inferior labial aa.<br><br>Passes superiorly along the side of the nose, giving rise to the lateral nasal a.<br><br>Continues on the side of the nose as the angular a. that terminates along the medial aspect of the eye |
| *Superior labial* | Facial | Supplies the upper lip<br><br>Gives rise to the septal branch that travels to the nasal septum<br><br>The major blood supply to the anterior part of the nasal septum |

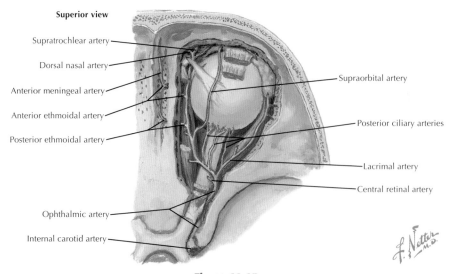

Superior view

Supratrochlear artery

Dorsal nasal artery

Anterior meningeal artery

Anterior ethmoidal artery

Posterior ethmoidal artery

Supraorbital artery

Posterior ciliary arteries

Lacrimal artery

Central retinal artery

Ophthalmic artery

Internal carotid artery

**Figure 11-15**

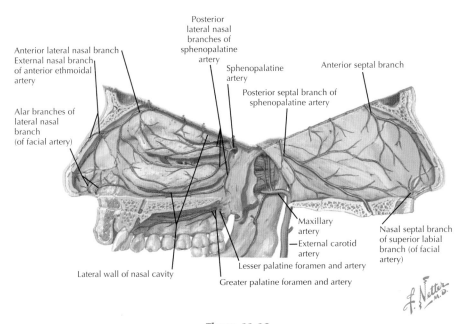

Posterior lateral nasal branches of sphenopalatine artery

Anterior lateral nasal branch
External nasal branch of anterior ethmoidal artery

Sphenopalatine artery

Anterior septal branch

Posterior septal branch of sphenopalatine artery

Alar branches of lateral nasal branch (of facial artery)

Maxillary artery

External carotid artery

Nasal septal branch of superior labial branch (of facial artery)

Lateral wall of nasal cavity

Lesser palatine foramen and artery

Greater palatine foramen and artery

**Figure 11-16**

| VENOUS DRAINAGE | |
|---|---|
| **Vein** | **Course** |
| • A well-developed cavernous plexus lies deep to the mucous membrane <br> • The plexus drains into the following series of veins: | |
| Emissary | Vein from the cavernous plexus in the nasal cavity passes through the foramen cecum to drain into the superior sagittal sinus |
| Sphenopalatine | Blood from the venous plexus along the posterior portion of the nasal cavity drains to the sphenopalatine v. <br><br> Travels through the sphenopalatine foramen to enter the pterygoid plexus |
| Anterior ethmoid | Blood from the venous plexus in the anterior portion of the nasal cavity drains into the anterior ethmoid, which terminates in the ophthalmic v. and/or facial v. |
| Posterior ethmoid | Blood from the venous plexus in the posterior portion of the nasal cavity drains into posterior ethmoid, which terminates in the ophthalmic v. and/or facial v. |
| Septal branch of the superior labial | Blood from the anterior portion drains into the septal branch of the superior labial, which drains into the facial v. |

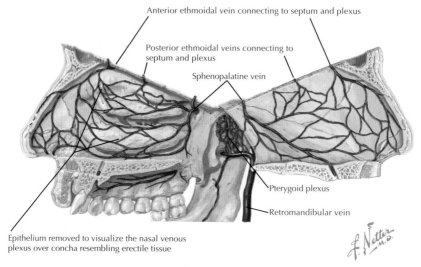

Anterior ethmoidal vein connecting to septum and plexus

Posterior ethmoidal veins connecting to septum and plexus

Sphenopalatine vein

Pterygoid plexus

Retromandibular vein

Epithelium removed to visualize the nasal venous plexus over concha resembling erectile tissue

**Figure 11-17**

- 2 major types of sensory innervation to the nasal cavity:
  - Olfaction (special visceral afferent) via the olfactory nerve
  - General sensation (general somatic afferent) via ophthalmic and maxillary divisions of the trigeminal nerve

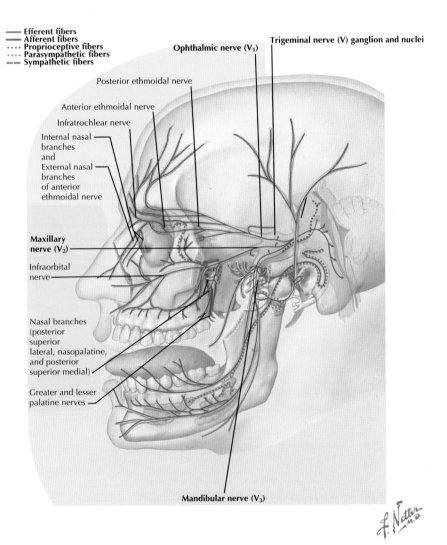

**Figure 11-18**

| Olfaction |
| --- |
| • The olfactory epithelium is found in the roof of the nasal cavity including the adjacent superior portions of the lateral wall of the nasal cavity and the nasal septum<br>• Roughly 20 to 25 small olfactory n. fibers, which collectively form the olfactory nerves per side, travel superiorly through the cribriform plate into the anterior cranial fossa to join the olfactory bulb |

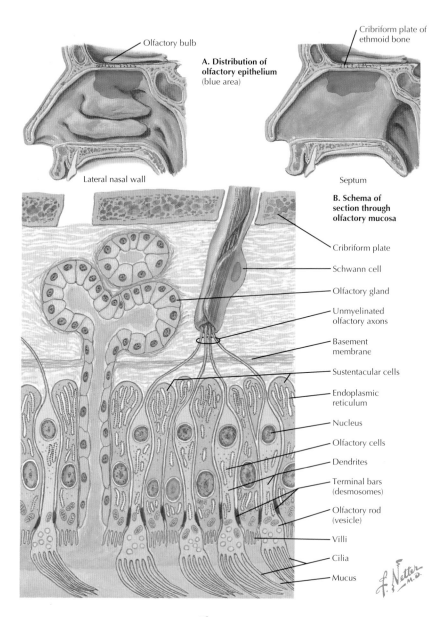

Olfactory bulb

Cribriform plate of ethmoid bone

**A. Distribution of olfactory epithelium** (blue area)

Lateral nasal wall

Septum

**B. Schema of section through olfactory mucosa**

Cribriform plate

Schwann cell

Olfactory gland

Unmyelinated olfactory axons

Basement membrane

Sustentacular cells

Endoplasmic reticulum

Nucleus

Olfactory cells

Dendrites

Terminal bars (desmosomes)

Olfactory rod (vesicle)

Villi

Cilia

Mucus

**Figure 11-19**

| | | |
|---|---|---|
| **OPHTHALMIC DIVISION OF THE TRIGEMINAL** | | |

Sensory

Arises from the main nerve in the middle cranial fossa

Passes anterior on the lateral wall of the cavernous sinus immediately inferior to the oculomotor and trochlear nn., but superior to the maxillary division of the trigeminal n.

Immediately before entering the orbit, through the superior orbital fissure, it divides into 3 major branches:

- Lacrimal
- Frontal
- Nasociliary

The nasociliary branch terminates as the:

- Anterior ethmoid n.
- Infratrochlear n.

| Nerve | Source | Course |
|---|---|---|
| *Anterior ethmoid* | Nasociliary n. | Enters the anterior ethmoid foramen and travels through the canal to enter the anterior cranial fossa |
| | | While descending toward the nasal cavity, it provides innervation to the anterior parts of the middle and inferior conchae, as well as the region anterior to the nasal concha |
| | | Specifically, it supplies the skin on the internal surface of the nasal cavity as the: |
| | | • Medial internal nasal n. |
| | | • Lateral internal nasal n. |

| | | |
|---|---|---|
| **MAXILLARY DIVISION OF THE TRIGEMINAL** | | |

Sensory

Travels along the lateral wall of the cavernous sinus

Passes from the middle cranial fossa into the pterygopalatine fossa via the foramen rotundum

Within the pterygopalatine fossa, it gives rise to 4 branches:

- Infraorbital—this is the continuation of the maxillary
- Posterior superior alveolar
- Zygomatic
- Ganglionic

| Infraorbital | Continuation of maxillary division of the trigeminal n. | Passes through the inferior orbital fissure to enter the orbit |
|---|---|---|
| | | Passes anteriorly through the infraorbital groove and infraorbital canal and exits onto the face via the infraorbital foramen |
| | | While in the infraorbital canal, it gives rise to the: |
| | | • Anterior superior alveolar n. |
| | | The anterior superior alveolar n. has a small branch that supplies the nasal cavity in the region of the inferior meatus and inferior corresponding portion of the nasal septum (in addition to supplying the maxillary sinus; the maxillary central incisor, lateral incisor, and canine teeth; and the gingiva and mucosa alongside these teeth) |
| *Nasopalatine* | Pterygopalatine ganglion | Passes through the sphenopalatine foramen to enter the nasal cavity |
| | | Passes along the superior portion of the nasal cavity to the nasal septum, where it travels anteroinferiorly to the incisive canal supplying the septum |

*Continued on next page*

| MAXILLARY DIVISION OF THE TRIGEMINAL *Continued* | | |
|---|---|---|
| *Posterior inferior lateral nasal* | Greater palatine | The greater palatine n. branches from the pterygopalatine ganglion in the pterygopalatine fossa<br><br>It descends through the greater palatine canal to enter the hard palate via the greater palatine foramen<br><br>While descending in the palatine canal, it gives rise to a:<br>• Posterior inferior lateral nasal branch<br><br>Supplies the posterior part of the lateral wall of the nasal cavity in the region of the middle meatus |
| *Posterior superior nasal* | Pterygopalatine ganglion | Passes through the sphenopalatine foramen to enter the nasal cavity and branches into 2 nerves:<br>• Posterior superior medial nasal<br>• Posterior superior lateral nasal |
| *Posterior superior lateral nasal* | Posterior superior nasal n. from the pterygopalatine ganglion | Supplies the posterosuperior portion of the lateral wall of the nasal cavity in the region of the superior and middle concha |
| *Posterior superior medial nasal* | | Supplies the posterior portion of the nasal septum |

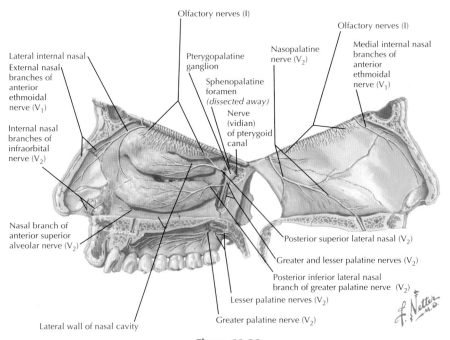

Figure 11-20

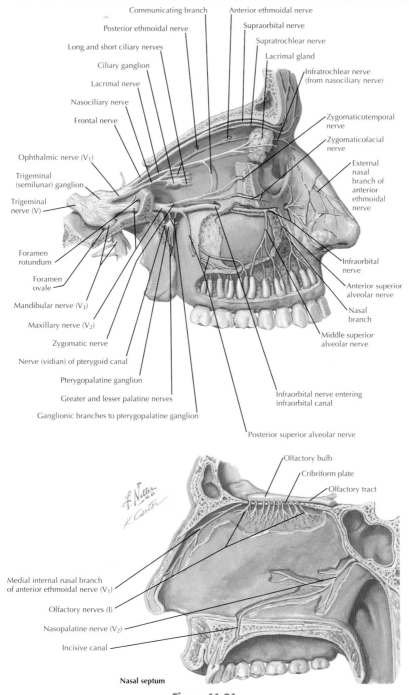

Communicating branch
Posterior ethmoidal nerve
Long and short ciliary nerves
Ciliary ganglion
Lacrimal nerve
Nasociliary nerve
Frontal nerve
Ophthalmic nerve (V₁)
Trigeminal (semilunar) ganglion
Trigeminal nerve (V)
Foramen rotundum
Foramen ovale
Mandibular nerve (V₃)
Maxillary nerve (V₂)
Zygomatic nerve
Nerve (vidian) of pterygoid canal
Pterygopalatine ganglion
Greater and lesser palatine nerves
Ganglionic branches to pterygopalatine ganglion

Anterior ethmoidal nerve
Supraorbital nerve
Supratrochlear nerve
Lacrimal gland
Infratrochlear nerve (from nasociliary nerve)
Zygomaticotemporal nerve
Zygomaticofacial nerve
External nasal branch of anterior ethmoidal nerve
Infraorbital nerve
Anterior superior alveolar nerve
Nasal branch
Middle superior alveolar nerve
Infraorbital nerve entering infraorbital canal
Posterior superior alveolar nerve

Olfactory bulb
Cribriform plate
Olfactory tract

Medial internal nasal branch of anterior ethmoidal nerve (V₁)
Olfactory nerves (I)
Nasopalatine nerve (V₂)
Incisive canal

Nasal septum

**Figure 11-21**

NOSE AND NASAL CAVITY **299**

- Autonomic fibers are distributed through the sensory branches of the maxillary division of the trigeminal nerve via the pterygopalatine ganglion (parasympathetics) and the superior cervical ganglion (sympathetics)
- Autonomics travel to the glands and blood vessels of the nasal cavity

| AUTONOMIC INNERVATION | | | |
|---|---|---|---|
| Anatomic Pathway for Parasympathetics of the Nasal Cavity | | | |
| **Type of Neuron** | **Name of Cell Body** | **Characteristics of Cell Body** | **Course of the Neuron** |
| Preganglionic neuron | Superior salivatory nucleus | A collection of nerve cell bodies located in the pons<br><br>Travel through the nervus intermedius of the facial nerve into the internal acoustic meatus<br><br>In the *facial canal*, the facial nerve gives rise to 2 parasympathetic branches:<br>• Greater petrosal n.<br>• Chorda tympani n. | **Greater Petrosal Nerve**<br>Greater petrosal n. exits the hiatus for the greater petrosal n. toward the foramen lacerum, where it joins the deep petrosal n. (sympathetics) to form the nerve of the pterygoid canal (vidian n.)<br>Vidian n. passes through the pterygoid canal and enters the pterygopalatine fossa, where it joins with the pterygopalatine ganglion |
| Postganglionic neuron | Pterygopalatine ganglion | Pterygopalatine ganglion is a collection of nerve cell bodies located in the pterygopalatine fossa<br><br>Postganglionic parasympathetic fibers that arise in the pterygopalatine ganglion are distributed to the ophthalmic and maxillary divisions of the trigeminal n. to the:<br>• Lacrimal gland<br>• Nasal glands<br>• Palatine glands<br>• Pharyngeal glands<br>• Paranasal sinus glands | **Maxillary Division Distribution**<br>Postganglionic fibers travel along the maxillary division of the trigeminal n. to be distributed along its branches that are located in the nasal cavity, oral cavity, and pharynx (e.g., nasopalatine, greater palatine)<br>These fibers innervate:<br>• Nasal glands<br>• Palatine glands<br>• Pharyngeal glands<br>• Paranasal sinus glands |
| Anatomic Pathway for Sympathetics of the Nasal Cavity | | | |
| **Type of Neuron** | **Name of Cell Body** | **Characteristics of Cell Body** | **Course of the Neuron** |
| Preganglionic neuron | Intermediolateral horn nucleus | Collection of nerve cell bodies located in the lateral horn nucleus of the spinal cord between spinal segments T1 and T3 (and possibly T4) | Arise from the intermediolateral horn nuclei from T1 to T3 (4)<br><br>Travel through the ventral root of the spinal cord to the spinal nerve<br><br>Enter the sympathetic chain via a white ramus communicans<br><br>Once in the sympathetic chain, the preganglionic fibers for the eye ascend and synapse with postganglionic fibers in the superior cervical ganglion |

*Continued on next page*

| | | **AUTONOMIC INNERVATION** *Continued* | |
|---|---|---|---|
| | | Anatomic Pathway for Sympathetics of the Nasal Cavity | |
| **Type of Neuron** | **Name of Cell Body** | **Characteristics of Cell Body** | **Course of the Neuron** |
| Postganglionic neuron | Superior cervical ganglion | Collection of nerve cell bodies located in the superior cervical ganglion, which is located at the base of the skull<br><br>Postganglionic sympathetic fibers follow the internal carotid or external carotid a. to pass near their respective effector organs (e.g., nasal cavity) | **Nasal Cavity, Paranasal Sinuses, and Palate**<br>• Postganglionic sympathetic fibers follow both the *internal* and *external carotid* aa.<br>• Postganglionic fibers will form the internal carotid nerve, which travels along the internal carotid a. forming the internal carotid plexus<br>• Postganglionic sympathetic fibers from the internal carotid plexus branch in the region of the foramen lacerum to form the deep petrosal n.<br>• The deep petrosal n. joins the greater petrosal n. (parasympathetics) to form the nerve of the pterygoid canal (vidian n.)<br>• Postganglionic sympathetic fibers travel along the branches of the maxillary division of the trigeminal n. associated with the pterygopalatine ganglion to be distributed along its branches in the nasal cavity, paranasal sinuses, and palate<br>• Postganglionic sympathetic fibers from the external carotid branch and follow the maxillary a.<br>• These fibers travel along the branches of the maxillary a. to be distributed along the nasal cavity, paranasal sinuses, and palate |

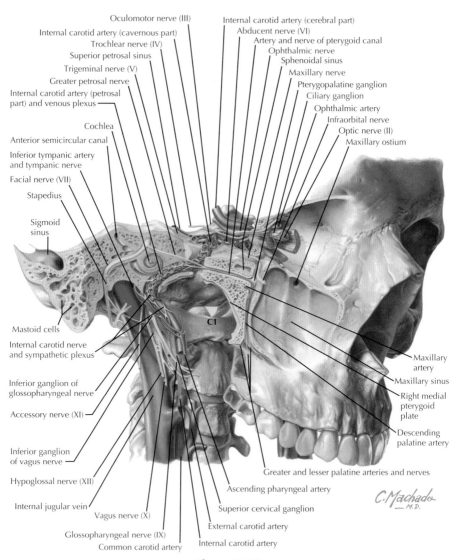

Oculomotor nerve (III)
Internal carotid artery (cavernous part)
Trochlear nerve (IV)
Superior petrosal sinus
Trigeminal nerve (V)
Greater petrosal nerve
Internal carotid artery (petrosal part) and venous plexus
Cochlea
Anterior semicircular canal
Inferior tympanic artery and tympanic nerve
Facial nerve (VII)
Stapedius
Sigmoid sinus

Internal carotid artery (cerebral part)
Abducent nerve (VI)
Artery and nerve of pterygoid canal
Ophthalmic nerve
Sphenoidal sinus
Maxillary nerve
Pterygopalatine ganglion
Ciliary ganglion
Ophthalmic artery
Infraorbital nerve
Optic nerve (II)
Maxillary ostium

Mastoid cells
Internal carotid nerve and sympathetic plexus

Inferior ganglion of glossopharyngeal nerve
Accessory nerve (XI)

Inferior ganglion of vagus nerve
Hypoglossal nerve (XII)

Internal jugular vein
Vagus nerve (X)
Glossopharyngeal nerve (IX)
Common carotid artery

C1

Maxillary artery
Maxillary sinus
Right medial pterygoid plate
Descending palatine artery

Greater and lesser palatine arteries and nerves
Ascending pharyngeal artery
Superior cervical ganglion
External carotid artery
Internal carotid artery

*C.Machado*
_M.D._

**Figure 11-22**

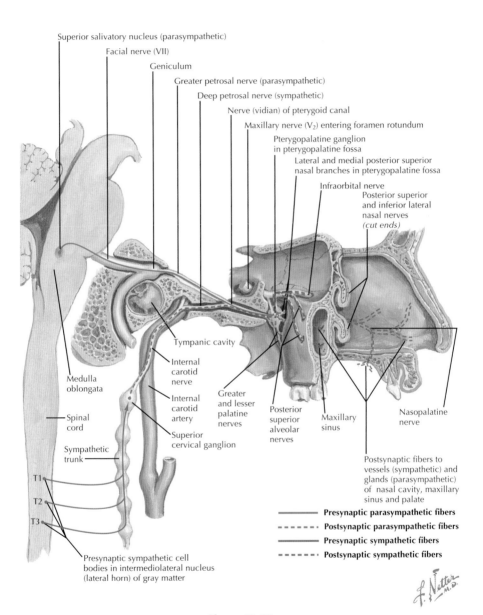

Superior salivatory nucleus (parasympathetic)

Facial nerve (VII)

Geniculum

Greater petrosal nerve (parasympathetic)

Deep petrosal nerve (sympathetic)

Nerve (vidian) of pterygoid canal

Maxillary nerve (V₂) entering foramen rotundum

Pterygopalatine ganglion
in pterygopalatine fossa

Lateral and medial posterior superior
nasal branches in pterygopalatine fossa

Infraorbital nerve

Posterior superior
and inferior lateral
nasal nerves
*(cut ends)*

Tympanic cavity

Medulla
oblongata

Spinal
cord

Sympathetic
trunk

Internal
carotid
nerve

Internal
carotid
artery

Superior
cervical ganglion

Greater
and lesser
palatine
nerves

Posterior
superior
alveolar
nerves

Maxillary
sinus

Nasopalatine
nerve

Postsynaptic fibers to
vessels (sympathetic) and
glands (parasympathetic)
of nasal cavity, maxillary
sinus and palate

T1

T2

T3

Presynaptic sympathetic cell
bodies in intermediolateral nucleus
(lateral horn) of gray matter

Presynaptic parasympathetic fibers

Postsynaptic parasympathetic fibers

Presynaptic sympathetic fibers

Postsynaptic sympathetic fibers

**Figure 11-23**

- *Epistaxis,* or nosebleed, is a hemorrhage from the nasal cavity or nose
- Classified by bleeding location:
  - Anterior
  - Posterior

## CAUSES

- May be localized or systemic:
  - Trauma (blows to the face, fractures, nose picking)
  - Sinus infections
  - Rhinitis
  - Arid environment
  - Hypertension
  - Hematologic disorders
  - Neoplasms

## ANTERIOR EPISTAXIS

- The most common form (in about 90% of cases)
- Usually found along the nasal septum and results from bleeding along Kiesselbach's plexus
- Many nosebleeds are due to trauma to the septal branch of the superior labial artery from the facial artery
- Typically managed with local pressure
- May be controlled by means of cautery with a silver nitrate stick or with use of anterior nasal packing if bleeding is persistent
- With anterior epistaxis, another treatment, although somewhat drastic, is septal dermoplasty
  - The thin septal mucosa is replaced by a thicker graft of skin
  - Often used to treat nosebleeds caused by hereditary hemorrhagic telangiectasia or septal perforations

## POSTERIOR EPISTAXIS

- Usually found along the posterior part of the nasal cavity
- More difficult to treat; use of posterior nasal packing or a balloon catheter usually is successful
- Severe posterior epistaxis may require ligation of the maxillary artery

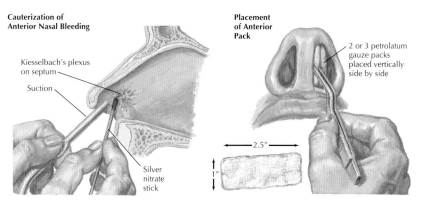

Cauterization of Anterior Nasal Bleeding

Kiesselbach's plexus on septum

Suction

Silver nitrate stick

Placement of Anterior Pack

2 or 3 petrolatum gauze packs placed vertically side by side

2.5"

1"

Septal Dermoplasty for Recurrent Severe Anterior Epistaxis

A. Incision

B. Flap elevated exposing telangiectasia on septal mucosa

C. Septal mucosa excised in area of telangiectasia; perichondrium preserved

D. Split-thickness skin graft applied

E. Flap sutured; intranasal pack (finger cot) then applied over Silastic sheet

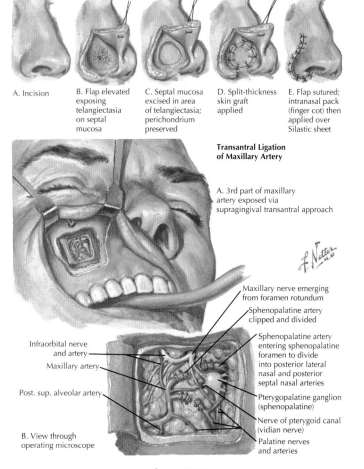

Transantral Ligation of Maxillary Artery

A. 3rd part of maxillary artery exposed via supragingival transantral approach

Maxillary nerve emerging from foramen rotundum

Sphenopalatine artery clipped and divided

Sphenopalatine artery entering sphenopalatine foramen to divide into posterior lateral nasal and posterior septal nasal arteries

Pterygopalatine ganglion (sphenopalatine)

Nerve of pterygoid canal (vidian nerve)

Palatine nerves and arteries

Infraorbital nerve and artery

Maxillary artery

Post. sup. alveolar artery

B. View through operating microscope

**Figure 11-24**

- *Deviated septum*: a severe shift of the nasal septum from the midline

## CAUSES

- May be acquired or congenital:
  - Trauma
  - Birth defects

## CLINICAL MANIFESTATIONS

- Occlusion of 1 side, either partial or complete, producing difficulty in breathing or blocked air flow on that side
- May also cause:
  - Sinusitis
  - Epistaxis
  - Nasal congestion

## TREATMENT

- May be treated by septoplasty

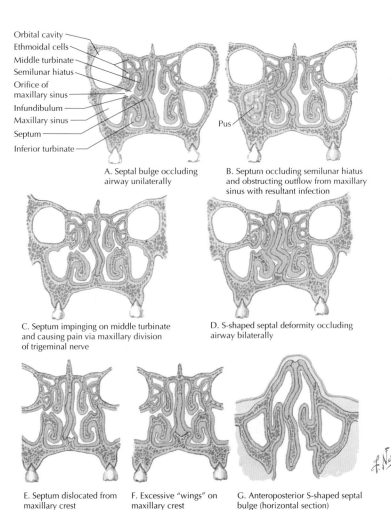

Orbital cavity
Ethmoidal cells
Middle turbinate
Semilunar hiatus
Orifice of maxillary sinus
Infundibulum
Maxillary sinus
Septum
Inferior turbinate

Pus

A. Septal bulge occluding airway unilaterally

B. Septum occluding semilunar hiatus and obstructing outflow from maxillary sinus with resultant infection

C. Septum impinging on middle turbinate and causing pain via maxillary division of trigeminal nerve

D. S-shaped septal deformity occluding airway bilaterally

E. Septum dislocated from maxillary crest

F. Excessive "wings" on maxillary crest

G. Anteroposterior S-shaped septal bulge (horizontal section)

**Figure 11-25**

- *Rhinitis*: an inflammation of the mucosa of the nasal cavity that results in:
  - Nasal congestion
  - Sneezing
  - Rhinorrhea
  - Nasal itching
- May involve the eyes, ears, sinuses, and throat and cause headaches
- Most commonly caused by allergic rhinitis

## ALLERGIC RHINITIS

- Can be associated with nasal polyps, deviated septum, and asthma
- Caused by an allergen inducing an immunoglobulin E (IgE)-mediated response on the mast cells
- Because mast cells are located on the nasal mucosa, an allergen can bind to the mast cell, resulting in the release of histamines, prostaglandins, cytokines, and leukotrienes
- Typically treated with decongestants, antihistamines, and steroids

### Mechanism of Type 1 (Immediate) Hypersensitivity

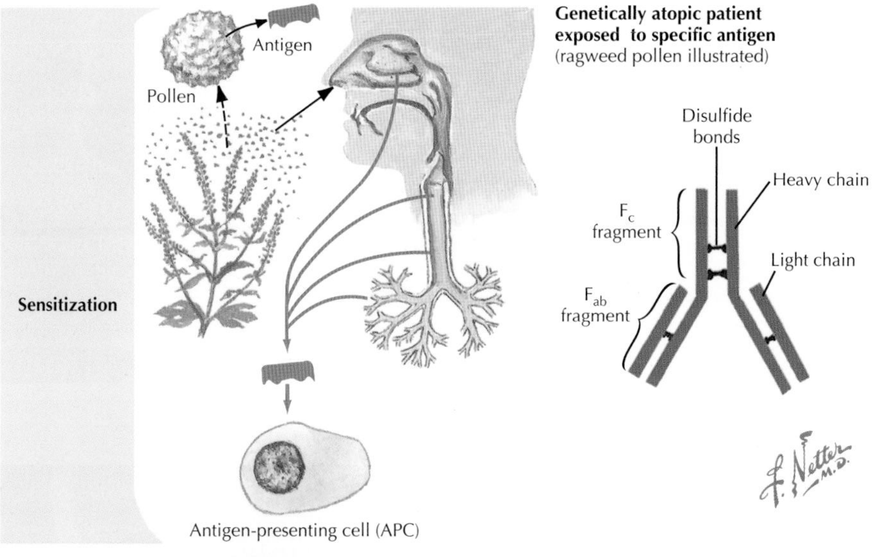

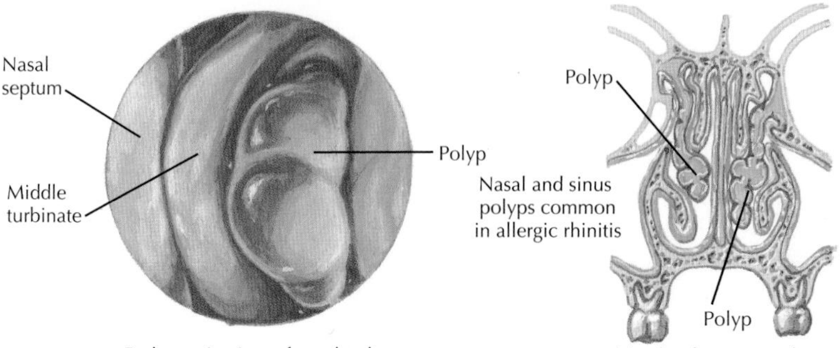

Genetically atopic patient exposed to specific antigen (ragweed pollen illustrated)

Antigen

Pollen

Sensitization

Antigen-presenting cell (APC)

Disulfide bonds

Heavy chain

F<sub>c</sub> fragment

Light chain

F<sub>ab</sub> fragment

Nasal septum

Middle turbinate

Polyp

Polyp

Nasal and sinus polyps common in allergic rhinitis

Polyp

Endoscopic view of nasal polyp protruding from middle meatus

Nasal polyps most often bilateral in allergic sinusitis

**Figure 11-26**

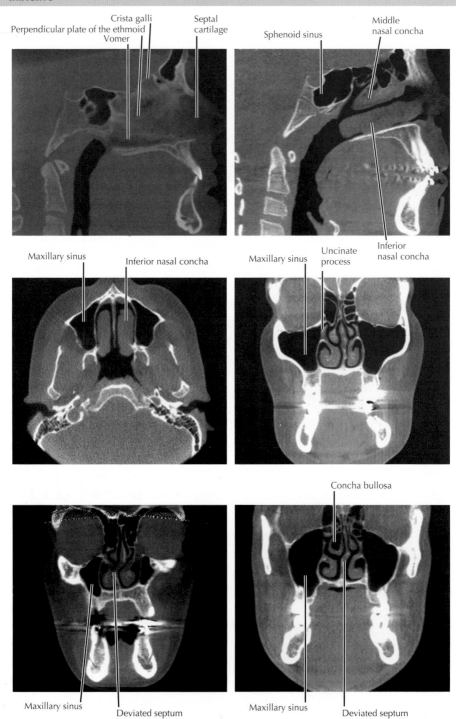

**Figure 11-27**

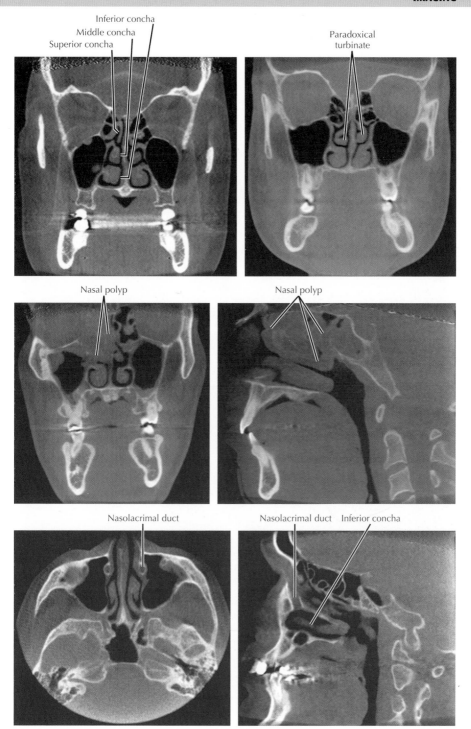

**Figure 11-28**

- The *paranasal sinuses* are invaginations from the nasal cavity that drain into spaces associated with the lateral nasal wall
- There are 4 paranasal sinuses:
  - Frontal
  - Maxillary
  - Ethmoid
  - Sphenoid
- Each paranasal sinus is named after the bone in which it is located
- Each is lined by a respiratory epithelium (pseudostratified columnar epithelium with cilia)
- Morphology of the sinuses is highly variable

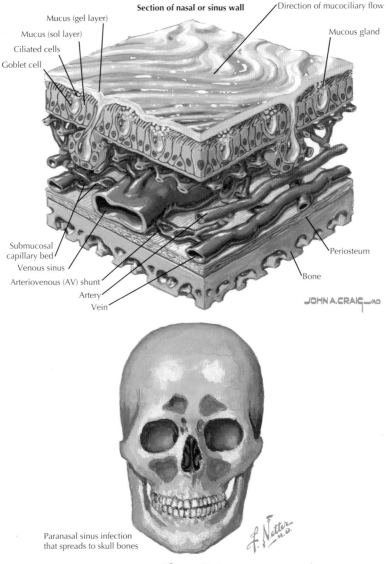

Section of nasal or sinus wall

Direction of mucociliary flow

Mucus (gel layer)

Mucus (sol layer)

Ciliated cells

Goblet cell

Mucous gland

Submucosal capillary bed

Venous sinus

Arteriovenous (AV) shunt

Artery

Vein

Periosteum

Bone

JOHN A. CRAIG—AD

Paranasal sinus infection that spreads to skull bones

**Figure 12-1**

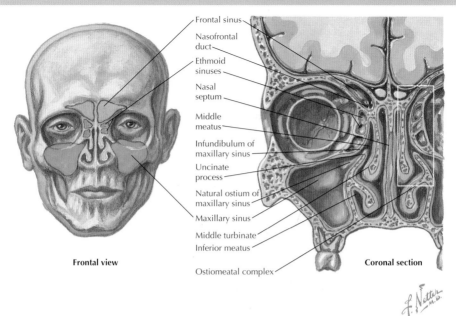

Frontal sinus
Nasofrontal duct
Ethmoid sinuses
Nasal septum
Middle meatus
Infundibulum of maxillary sinus
Uncinate process
Natural ostium of maxillary sinus
Maxillary sinus
Middle turbinate
Inferior meatus
Ostiomeatal complex

**Frontal view**

**Coronal section**

**Figure 12-2**

| FEATURES OF THE PARANASAL SINUSES | | | | |
|---|---|---|---|---|
| **Sinus** | **Location** | **Comment** | **Artery** | **Nerve** |
| Frontal | Within frontal bone | Flattened triangular shape<br>Manifests as a small outpouching at birth | Ophthalmic branches | Ophthalmic division of the trigeminal n. |
| Maxillary | Within maxillary bone | Pyramidal shape<br>Small sinus is present at birth | Maxillary branches | Maxillary division of the trigeminal n. |
| Ethmoid | Within ethmoid bone | 3 to 18 irregularly shaped cells<br>Small sinus is present at birth | Ophthalmic and maxillary branches | Ophthalmic and maxillary divisions of the trigeminal n. |
| Sphenoid | Within sphenoid bone | Cuboid shape<br>No pneumatization at birth | | |

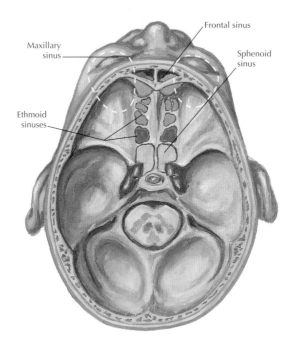

Frontal sinus

Sphenoid
sinus

Maxillary
sinus

Ethmoid
sinuses

**Superior view**

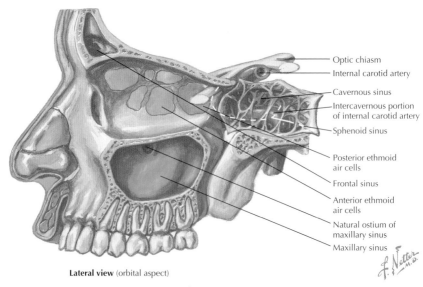

Optic chiasm

Internal carotid artery

Cavernous sinus

Intercavernous portion
of internal carotid artery

Sphenoid sinus

Posterior ethmoid
air cells

Frontal sinus

Anterior ethmoid
air cells

Natural ostium of
maxillary sinus

Maxillary sinus

**Lateral view** (orbital aspect)

**Figure 12-3**

- All paranasal sinuses drain into the nasal cavity
- Different sinuses serve as drainage conduits for different regions

| SUMMARY OF PARANASAL SINUS DRAINAGE | | |
|---|---|---|
| **Region Drained** | **Location** | **Structure(s) Drained** |
| Sphenoethmoidal recess | Superior to the superior concha | Sphenoid sinus |
| Superior meatus | Inferior to the superior concha | Posterior ethmoid sinus |
| Middle meatus | Inferior to the middle concha | Anterior ethmoid sinus Middle ethmoid sinus Maxillary sinus Frontal sinus |
| Inferior meatus | Inferior to the inferior concha | Nasolacrimal duct |

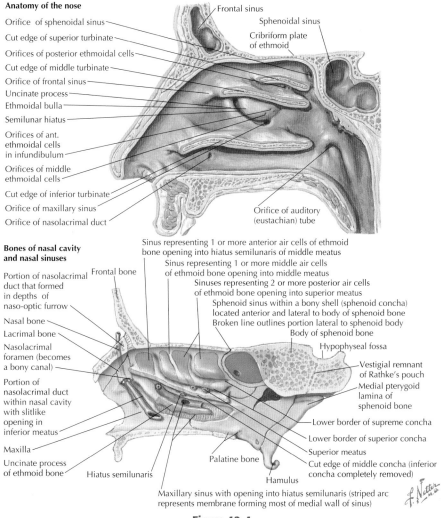

**Anatomy of the nose**

Orifice of sphenoidal sinus
Cut edge of superior turbinate
Orifices of posterior ethmoidal cells
Cut edge of middle turbinate
Orifice of frontal sinus
Uncinate process
Ethmoidal bulla
Semilunar hiatus
Orifices of ant. ethmoidal cells in infundibulum
Orifices of middle ethmoidal cells
Cut edge of inferior turbinate
Orifice of maxillary sinus
Orifice of nasolacrimal duct

Frontal sinus
Sphenoidal sinus
Cribriform plate of ethmoid

Orifice of auditory (eustachian) tube

**Bones of nasal cavity and nasal sinuses**

Portion of nasolacrimal duct that formed in depths of naso-optic furrow
Nasal bone
Lacrimal bone
Nasolacrimal foramen (becomes a bony canal)
Portion of nasolacrimal duct within nasal cavity with slitlike opening in inferior meatus
Maxilla
Uncinate process of ethmoid bone

Frontal bone
Hiatus semilunaris

Sinus representing 1 or more anterior air cells of ethmoid bone opening into hiatus semilunaris of middle meatus
Sinus representing 1 or more middle air cells of ethmoid bone opening into middle meatus
Sinuses representing 2 or more posterior air cells of ethmoid bone opening into superior meatus
Sphenoid sinus within a bony shell (sphenoid concha) located anterior and lateral to body of sphenoid bone
Broken line outlines portion lateral to sphenoid body
Body of sphenoid bone
Hypophyseal fossa
Vestigial remnant of Rathke's pouch
Medial pterygoid lamina of sphenoid bone
Lower border of supreme concha
Lower border of superior concha
Superior meatus
Cut edge of middle concha (inferior concha completely removed)

Palatine bone
Hamulus

Maxillary sinus with opening into hiatus semilunaris (striped arc represents membrane forming most of medial wall of sinus)

**Figure 12-4**

- The 2 *frontal sinuses* typically are asymmetric
- Usually not present at birth, or there is a small outpouching
- The most common of the paranasal sinuses to undergo aplasia
- Is the last paranasal sinus to begin to pneumatize—beginning around the 2nd year
- Usually well developed by the age of 7 or 8 years
- A prime expansion in size occurs when the 1st deciduous molars erupt and another when the permanent molars begin to appear at about age 6
- The adult frontal sinus has 2 extensions:
  - Frontal—which extends superiorly into the frontal bone in the region of the forehead
  - Orbital—which extends posteriorly into the frontal bone over the medial part of the orbit
- Drainage varies; may drain in front of, above, or into the ethmoidal infundibulum
- Primary lymphatic drainage is to the submandibular lymph nodes
- The frontal sinus receives its nerve supply from branches of the ophthalmic division of the trigeminal nerve

RELATIONS OF SINUS

- *Superior*: anterior cranial fossa and contents
- *Inferior*: orbit, anterior ethmoidal sinuses, nasal cavity
- *Anterior*: forehead, superciliary arches
- *Posterior*: anterior cranial fossa and contents
- *Medial*: other frontal sinus

LOCATION OF OSTIUM

- Middle meatus

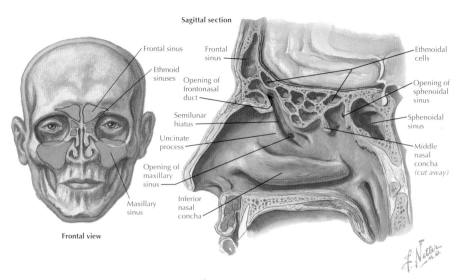

**Figure 12-5**

| Artery | Source | Course |
|---|---|---|
| Anterior ethmoid | Ophthalmic a. (from the internal carotid a.) | Enters the anterior ethmoid foramen with the nerve to pass through the canal |
| | | At this location, it supplies the anterior and middle ethmoid air cells and the frontal sinus |
| Supraorbital | | Branches from the ophthalmic a. when crossing the optic n. |
| | | Ascends medial to both the levator palpebrae superioris and the superior rectus mm. |
| | | At this location, it runs with the supraorbital n. and is found between the levator palpebrae superioris m. and the periosteum of the orbit |
| | | Travels to the supraorbital foramen (notch) |
| | | At the level of the supraorbital margin, it supplies the frontal sinus |

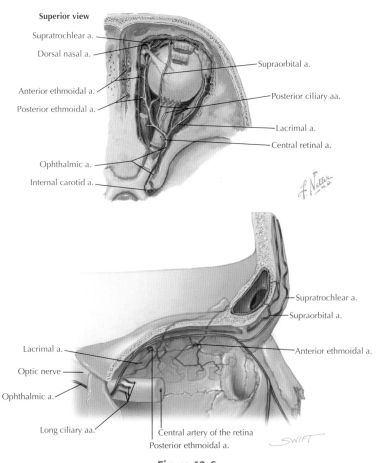

**Figure 12-6**

| Nerve | Source | Course |
|-------|--------|--------|
| Supraorbital | Ophthalmic division of the trigeminal n. | Passes between the levator palpebrae superioris m. and periosteum of the orbit |
| | | Continues anteriorly to the supraorbital foramen (notch) |
| | | At the level of the supraorbital margin, it sends nerve supply to the frontal sinus |

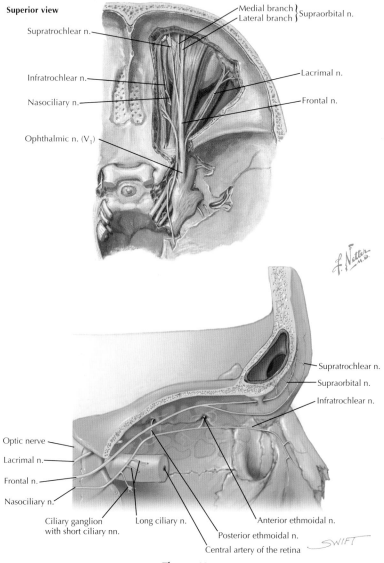

Superior view

Supratrochlear n.

Infratrochlear n.

Nasociliary n.

Ophthalmic n. (V₁)

Medial branch
Lateral branch } Supraorbital n.

Lacrimal n.

Frontal n.

Supratrochlear n.

Supraorbital n.

Infratrochlear n.

Optic nerve

Lacrimal n.

Frontal n.

Nasociliary n.

Ciliary ganglion with short ciliary nn.

Long ciliary n.

Anterior ethmoidal n.

Posterior ethmoidal n.

Central artery of the retina

**Figure 12-7**

Eyes Frontal sinus

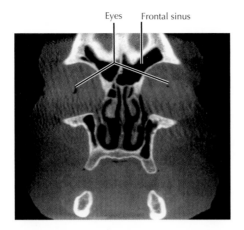

Frontal sinus

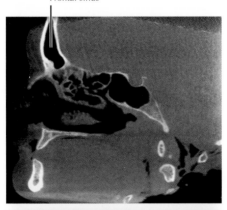

Frontal sinus

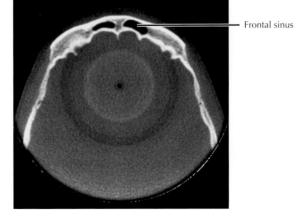

**Figure 12-8**

- Ethmoid sinuses form within the ethmoid as many individual air cells
- Anatomically they are located between the superior portion of the nasal cavity and the orbit, and the surrounding bone is very thin
- From 3 to 18 total ethmoid air cells may be present on each side
- Divided into an anterior and a posterior group, or into anterior, middle, and posterior groups, by different authors
- The most anterior ethmoid sinus is called the agger nasi
- The ethmoidal bulla, which protrudes from the lateral wall of the nasal cavity, represents the largest group of ethmoidal air cells
- The most posterior group of ethmoidal air cells is closely related to the orbit
- Ethmoid air cells may invade any of the other 3 sinuses
- The middle ethmoid air cells produce the swelling on the lateral wall of the middle meatus called the ethmoid bulla
- Primary lymphatic drainage is to the submandibular lymph nodes for the anterior and middle ethmoid sinuses, and the retropharyngeal lymph nodes for the posterior ethmoid sinus

## RELATIONS OF SINUS

- *Superior*: anterior cranial fossa and contents, frontal bone with sinus
- *Medial*: nasal cavity
- *Lateral*: orbit

## LOCATION OF OSTIUM

- *Anterior*: middle meatus (frontonasal duct or ethmoidal infundibulum)
- *Middle:* middle meatus (on or above ethmoid bulla)
- *Posterior*: superior meatus

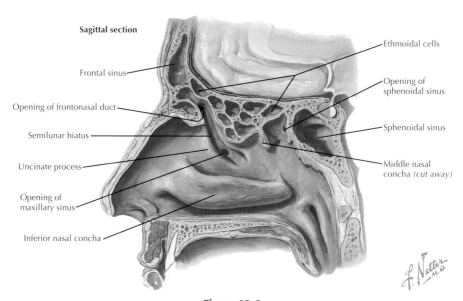

Sagittal section

Frontal sinus

Opening of frontonasal duct

Semilunar hiatus

Uncinate process

Opening of maxillary sinus

Inferior nasal concha

Ethmoidal cells

Opening of sphenoidal sinus

Sphenoidal sinus

Middle nasal concha *(cut away)*

**Figure 12-9**

**Horizontal section**

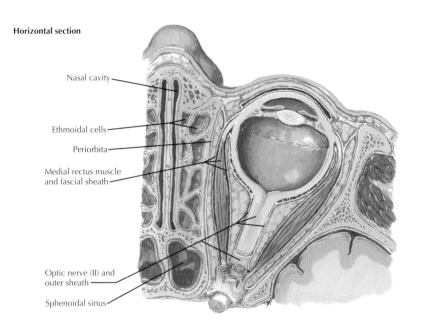

Nasal cavity

Ethmoidal cells

Periorbita

Medial rectus muscle
and fascial sheath

Optic nerve (II) and
outer sheath

Sphenoidal sinus

**Frontal section**

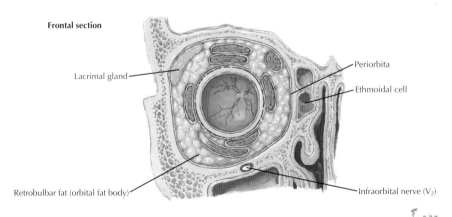

Lacrimal gland

Periorbita

Ethmoidal cell

Retrobulbar fat (orbital fat body)

Infraorbital nerve (V₂)

**Figure 12-10**

| Artery | Source | Course |
|--------|--------|--------|
| Anterior ethmoid | Ophthalmic a. (from the internal carotid) | Enters the anterior ethmoid foramen with the nerve to pass though the canal |
| | | There it supplies the anterior and middle ethmoid air cells and sometimes the frontal sinus |
| Posterior ethmoid | | Passes through the posterior ethmoid foramen to enter the canal |
| | | There it supplies the posterior ethmoid air cells and sphenoid sinus |
| Posterior lateral nasal branches | Sphenopalatine a. (from the maxillary a. from the external carotid a.) | Anastomose with the ethmoidal arteries to help supply the ethmoid air cells and sphenoid sinus |

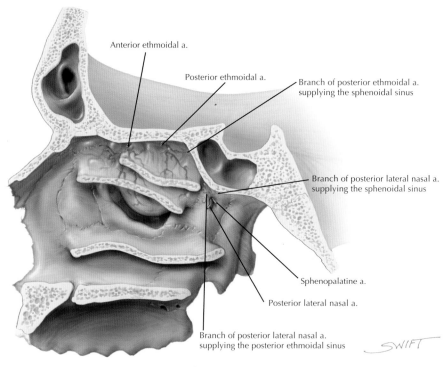

Anterior ethmoidal a.

Posterior ethmoidal a.

Branch of posterior ethmoidal a. supplying the sphenoidal sinus

Branch of posterior lateral nasal a. supplying the sphenoidal sinus

Sphenopalatine a.

Posterior lateral nasal a.

Branch of posterior lateral nasal a. supplying the posterior ethmoidal sinus

SWIFT

**Figure 12-11**

| Nerve | Source | Course |
|---|---|---|
| Anterior ethmoid | Nasociliary n. on the medial wall of the orbit (from the ophthalmic division of the trigeminal n.) | Enters the anterior ethmoid foramen and travels through the canal to enter the anterior cranial fossa<br><br>While descending toward the nasal cavity, it provides innervation to the anterior and middle ethmoid air cells |
| Posterior ethmoid | | Enters the posterior ethmoid foramen to supply the posterior ethmoid air cells<br><br>Also innervates the sphenoid sinus at this location |
| Posterior lateral superior nasal | Pterygopalatine ganglion in the pterygopalatine fossa (from the maxillary division of the trigeminal n.) | Passes through the sphenopalatine foramen to enter the nasal cavity<br><br>Branches supply the posterior ethmoid air cells at this location |

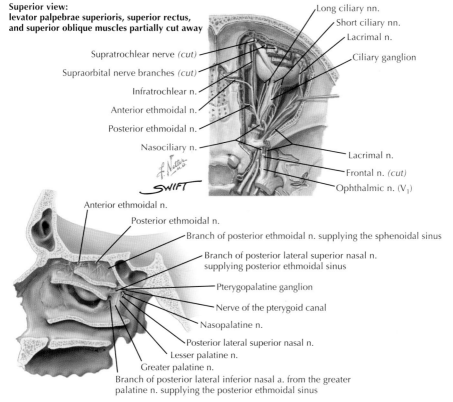

Superior view:
**levator palpebrae superioris, superior rectus, and superior oblique muscles partially cut away**

Supratrochlear nerve *(cut)*
Supraorbital nerve branches *(cut)*
Infratrochlear n.
Anterior ethmoidal n.
Posterior ethmoidal n.
Nasociliary n.

Long ciliary nn.
Short ciliary nn.
Lacrimal n.
Ciliary ganglion

Lacrimal n.
Frontal n. *(cut)*
Ophthalmic n. (V₁)

Anterior ethmoidal n.
Posterior ethmoidal n.
Branch of posterior ethmoidal n. supplying the sphenoidal sinus
Branch of posterior lateral superior nasal n. supplying posterior ethmoidal sinus
Pterygopalatine ganglion
Nerve of the pterygoid canal
Nasopalatine n.
Posterior lateral superior nasal n.
Lesser palatine n.
Greater palatine n.
Branch of posterior lateral inferior nasal a. from the greater palatine n. supplying the posterior ethmoidal sinus

**Figure 12-12**

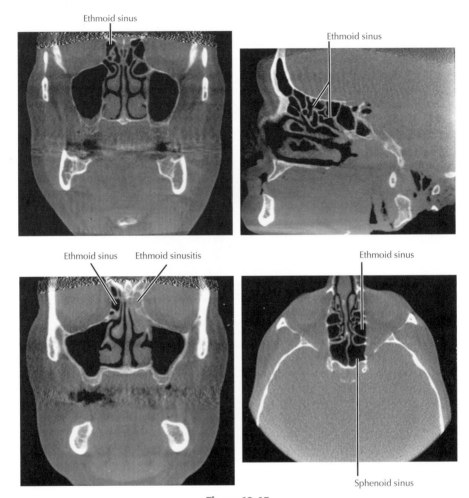

**Figure 12-13**

- The *maxillary sinus* (also referred to as the antrum of Highmore) is a large pyramidal cavity that is present at birth
- Pneumatization occurs rapidly during the early years, with the floor of the sinus being superior to the unerupted permanent teeth
- As the permanent teeth erupt into the oral cavity, the maxillary sinus pneumatizes into the alveolar bone
- The epithelium of the maxillary sinus is often called the Schneiderian membrane in clinical texts
- Because the floor of the adult maxillary sinus typically is in close proximity to the roots of the maxillary molars and premolars, it is not uncommon for a maxillary sinus infection to manifest as tooth pain (via referred pain)
- The maxillary sinus tends to be more prone to sinus infections because the ostium is located at the superior part of the sinus
- The maxillary sinus is thin-walled and may be divided by septa
- Primary lymphatic drainage is to the submandibular lymph nodes

RELATIONS OF SINUS

- *Superior*: orbit, infraorbital nerve and vessels
- *Inferior*: roots of molars and premolars
- *Medial*: nasal cavity
- *Lateral and anterior*: cheek
- *Posterior*: infratemporal fossa, pterygopalatine fossa and contents

LOCATION OF OSTIUM

- Middle meatus

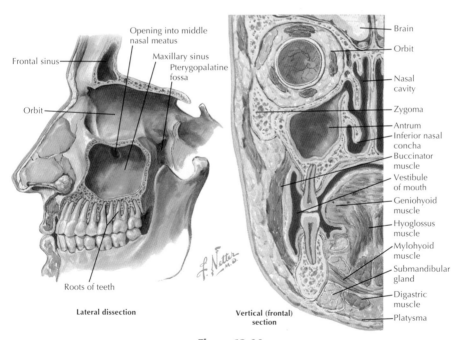

**Figure 12-14**

| Artery | Source | Course |
|--------|--------|--------|
| Anterior superior alveolar | Maxillary a. from the external carotid a. | Arises from the infraorbital a. of the maxillary a. after it passes through the inferior orbital fissure and into the infraorbital canal<br><br>Descends via the alveolar canals to supply the sinus |
| Middle superior alveolar | | When present, it arises from the infraorbital a. of the maxillary a. after passing through the inferior orbital fissure and into the infraorbital canal<br><br>Descends via the alveolar canals to supply the sinus |
| Posterior superior alveolar | | Arises from the 3rd part of the maxillary a. before the maxillary a. enters the pterygopalatine fossa<br><br>Enters the infratemporal surface of the maxilla to supply the sinus |

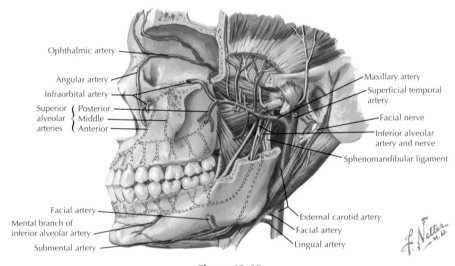

**Figure 12-15**

| Nerve | Source | Course |
|-------|--------|--------|
| Anterior superior alveolar | Infraorbital n., which is the continuation of the maxillary division of the trigeminal n. | Branches from the infraorbital n. as it travels in the infraorbital canal<br><br>As it descends to form the superior dental plexus, it innervates part of the maxillary sinus |
| Middle superior alveolar | | When present, it branches from the infraorbital n. as it travels in the infraorbital canal<br><br>As it descends to form the superior dental plexus, it innervates part of the maxillary sinus |
| Posterior superior alveolar | Maxillary division of the trigeminal n. | Arises in the pterygopalatine fossa<br><br>Travels laterally through the pterygomaxillary fissure to enter the infratemporal fossa<br><br>Enters the infratemporal surface of the maxilla<br><br>As it descends to form the superior dental plexus, it innervates part of the maxillary sinus |

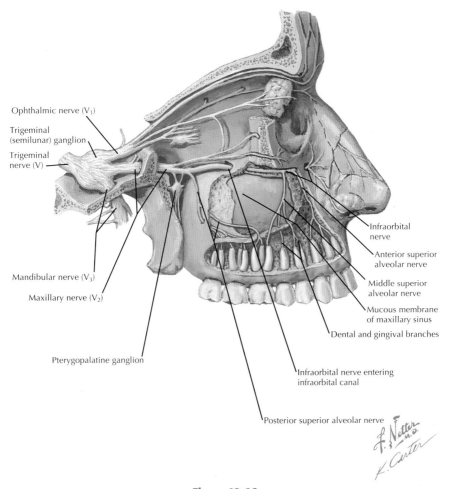

Ophthalmic nerve (V₁)

Trigeminal (semilunar) ganglion

Trigeminal nerve (V)

Mandibular nerve (V₃)

Maxillary nerve (V₂)

Pterygopalatine ganglion

Infraorbital nerve

Anterior superior alveolar nerve

Middle superior alveolar nerve

Mucous membrane of maxillary sinus

Dental and gingival branches

Infraorbital nerve entering infraorbital canal

Posterior superior alveolar nerve

**Figure 12-16**

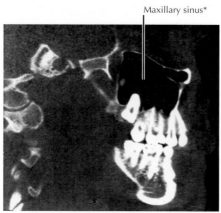

Maxillary sinus*

*Root of 3rd maxillary molar protruding into sinus*

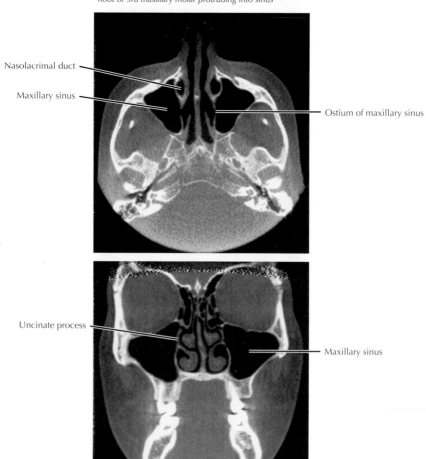

Nasolacrimal duct

Maxillary sinus

Ostium of maxillary sinus

Uncinate process

Maxillary sinus

**Figure 12-17**

- The *sphenoid sinus* consists of 2 large, irregularly shaped cavities
- Separated by an irregular septum
- Pneumatization begins around 7 to 8 months after birth
- Sphenoid sinus anatomy is important in transsphenoidal approaches to the pituitary gland
- Primary lymphatic drainage is to the retropharyngeal lymph nodes

## RELATIONS OF SINUS

- *Superior*: hypophyseal fossa, pituitary gland, optic chiasm
- *Inferior*: nasopharynx, pterygoid canal
- *Medial*: other sphenoid bone
- *Lateral*: cavernous sinus, internal carotid artery, cranial nerves III, IV, $V_1$, $V_2$, and VI
- *Anterior*: nasal cavity

## LOCATION OF OSTIUM

- Sphenoethmoidal recess

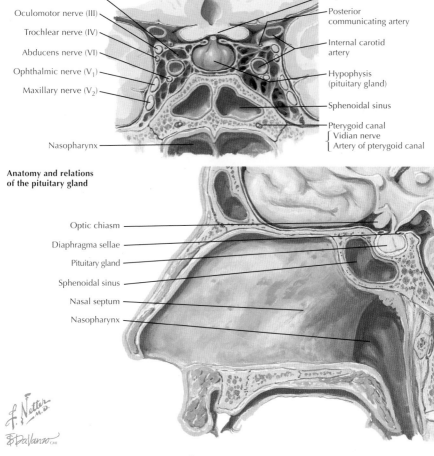

Coronal section through cavernous sinus

Cavernous sinus
Oculomotor nerve (III)
Trochlear nerve (IV)
Abducens nerve (VI)
Ophthalmic nerve ($V_1$)
Maxillary nerve ($V_2$)
Nasopharynx

Optic chiasm
Posterior communicating artery
Internal carotid artery
Hypophysis (pituitary gland)
Sphenoidal sinus
Pterygoid canal
{ Vidian nerve
{ Artery of pterygoid canal

Anatomy and relations of the pituitary gland

Optic chiasm
Diaphragma sellae
Pituitary gland
Sphenoidal sinus
Nasal septum
Nasopharynx

**Figure 12-18**

| Artery | Source | Course |
|--------|--------|--------|
| Posterior ethmoid | Ophthalmic a. (from the internal carotid a.) | Passes through the posterior ethmoid foramen to enter the canal <br> There it supplies the sphenoid sinus and the posterior ethmoid air cells |
| Posterior lateral nasal branches | Sphenopalatine a. from the maxillary a. (from the external carotid a.) | These branches anastomose with the ethmoidal arteries to help supply the sphenoid sinus and the ethmoid air cells |

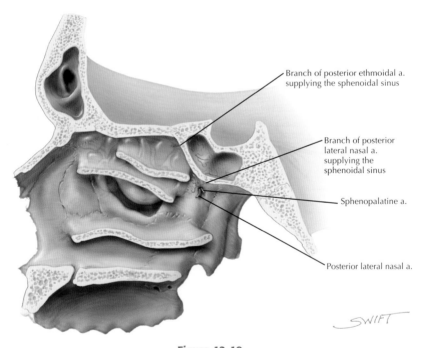

Branch of posterior ethmoidal a. supplying the sphenoidal sinus

Branch of posterior lateral nasal a. supplying the sphenoidal sinus

Sphenopalatine a.

Posterior lateral nasal a.

**Figure 12-19**

| Nerve | Source | Course |
|-------|--------|--------|
| Posterior ethmoid | Ophthalmic division of the trigeminal n. | A branch of the nasociliary n. that lies on the medial wall of the orbit |
| | | Enters the posterior ethmoid foramen to supply the sphenoid sinus |
| | | Also innervates the posterior ethmoid air cell at this location |
| Orbital branch from the pterygopalatine ganglion | Maxillary division of the trigeminal n. | Orbital branches arising from the pterygopalatine ganglion enter the orbit through the inferior orbital fissure |
| | | Some of these branches supply the sphenoid sinus at this location, but this is mainly for secretomotor function |

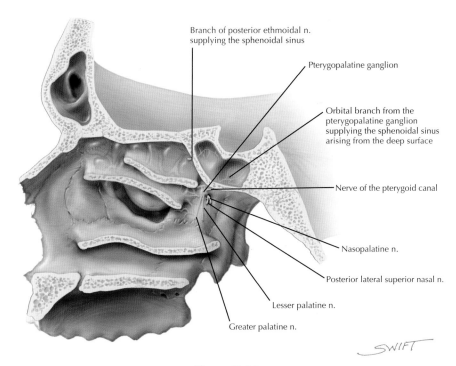

Branch of posterior ethmoidal n. supplying the sphenoidal sinus

Pterygopalatine ganglion

Orbital branch from the pterygopalatine ganglion supplying the sphenoidal sinus arising from the deep surface

Nerve of the pterygoid canal

Nasopalatine n.

Posterior lateral superior nasal n.

Lesser palatine n.

Greater palatine n.

**Figure 12-20**

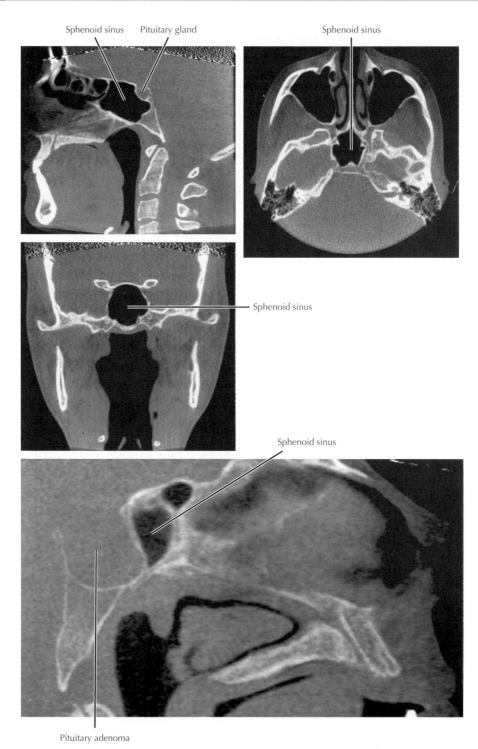

**Figure 12-21**

- *Sinusitis*: an inflammation of the membrane of the sinus cavities caused by infections (by bacteria or viruses) or noninfectious means (such as allergy)
- 2 types of sinusitis: acute and chronic
- Common clinical manifestations include sinus congestion, discharge, pressure, face pain, headaches

## ACUTE SINUSITIS

- The most common form of sinusitis
- Typically caused by a cold that results in inflammation of the sinus membranes
- Normally resolves in 1 to 2 weeks
- Sometimes a secondary bacterial infection may settle in the passageways after a cold; bacteria normally located in the area (*Streptococcus pneumoniae* and *Haemophilus influenzae*) may then begin to increase, producing an acute bacterial sinusitis

## CHRONIC SINUSITIS

- An infection of the sinuses that is present for longer than 1 month and requires longer-duration medical therapy
- Typically either chronic bacterial sinusitis or chronic noninfectious sinusitis
- Chronic bacterial sinusitis is treated with antibiotics
- Chronic noninfectious sinusitis often is treated with steroids (topical or oral) and nasal washes

## LOCATIONS

- Maxillary: the most common location for sinusitis; associated with all of the common signs and symptoms but also results in tooth pain, usually in the molar region
- Sphenoid: rare, but in this location can result in problems with the pituitary gland, cavernous sinus syndrome, and meningitis
- Frontal: usually associated with pain over the forehead and possibly fever; rare complications include osteomyelitis
- Ethmoid: potential complications include meningitis and orbital cellulitis

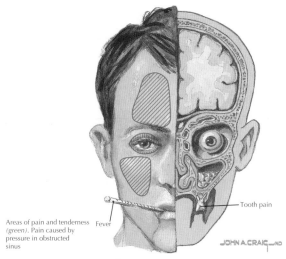

Tooth pain

Areas of pain and tenderness *(green)*. Pain caused by pressure in obstructed sinus    Fever

JOHN A. CRAIG—AD

**Figure 12-22**

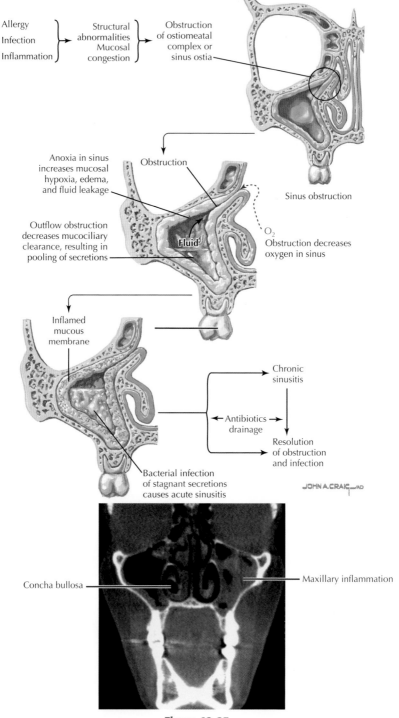

Allergy
Infection
Inflammation → Structural abnormalities Mucosal congestion → Obstruction of ostiomeatal complex or sinus ostia

Sinus obstruction

Anoxia in sinus increases mucosal hypoxia, edema, and fluid leakage

Obstruction

Outflow obstruction decreases mucociliary clearance, resulting in pooling of secretions

Fluid

O₂ Obstruction decreases oxygen in sinus

Inflamed mucous membrane

Chronic sinusitis

← Antibiotics → drainage

Resolution of obstruction and infection

Bacterial infection of stagnant secretions causes acute sinusitis

JOHN A.CRAIG—AD

Concha bullosa

Maxillary inflammation

**Figure 12-23**

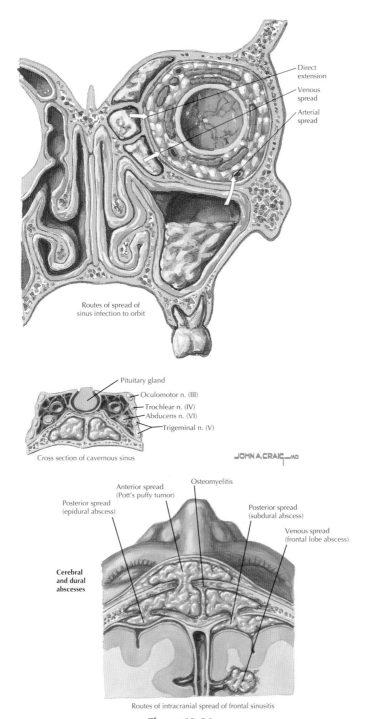

Direct
extension

Venous
spread

Arterial
spread

Routes of spread of
sinus infection to orbit

Pituitary gland

Oculomotor n. (III)

Trochlear n. (IV)

Abducens n. (VI)

Trigeminal n. (V)

Cross section of cavernous sinus

JOHN A.CRAIG—AD

Anterior spread
(Pott's puffy tumor)

Osteomyelitis

Posterior spread
(epidural abscess)

Posterior spread
(subdural abscess)

Venous spread
(frontal lobe abscess)

Cerebral
and dural
abscesses

Routes of intracranial spread of frontal sinusitis

**Figure 12-24**

FRONTAL SINUS OBLITERATION

- In a *frontal sinus obliteration* procedure, the frontal sinus is completely removed to treat problematic cases of frontal sinus infection, osteomyelitis, and trauma
- Once the sinus is opened, all of the sinus membrane is removed with a burr; otherwise, any remaining membrane may form a mucocele
- The remaining area often is filled with adipose tissue from the patient because it is thought to impede regrowth of the mucoperiosteum

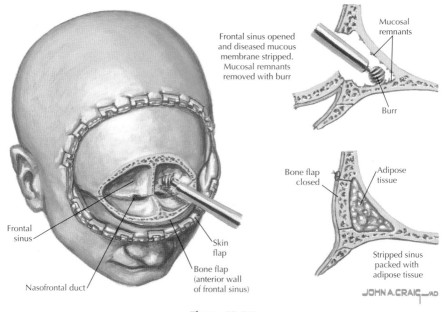

**Figure 12-25**

CALDWELL-LUC PROCEDURE

- The intraoral *Caldwell-Luc procedure* allows direct entry into the maxillary sinus
- Also provides access to the ethmoid sinus
- The maxillary sinus is entered through the canine fossa above the maxillary premolar teeth
- The maxillary antrum is opened, the sinus membrane is stripped, and an additional antrostomy is made between the maxillary sinus and the inferior meatus

*Conditions Treated*

- The antrostomy allows drainage of the maxillary sinus into the nasal cavity
- With the advent of functional endoscopic sinus surgery for antrostomies, the Caldwell-Luc procedure often is used for exposure and removal of tumors
- Used to be commonly performed to treat chronic maxillary sinusitis
- Was also used for procedures such as removal of benign tumors and foreign bodies, access to the pterygopalatine fossa, and closure of dental fistulas into the maxillary sinus

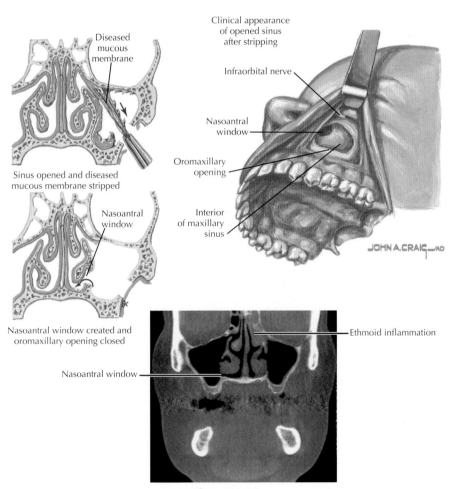

Diseased mucous membrane

Clinical appearance of opened sinus after stripping

Infraorbital nerve

Nasoantral window

Oromaxillary opening

Sinus opened and diseased mucous membrane stripped

Nasoantral window

Interior of maxillary sinus

JOHN A.CRAIG_AD

Nasoantral window created and oromaxillary opening closed

Ethmoid inflammation

Nasoantral window

**Figure 12-26**

MAXILLARY IMPLANTS

- Placement of *maxillary implants* is a common dental procedure to add fixed maxillary teeth to the oral cavity
- Patient should be in relatively good health
- Patient must have sufficient bone in a location suitable for placement of an implant
- It is becoming more common to use bone grafting before the surgical implant is placed
- Bone grafts to provide adequate bed for implants may be harvested from the body or as allografts, or may be supplied as xenografts or synthetic bone substitutes

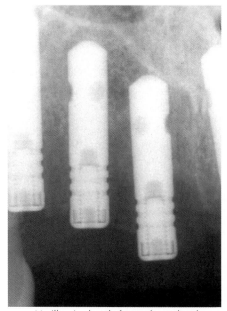

Maxillary implants before teeth are placed

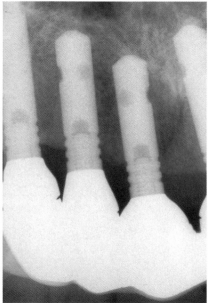

Maxillary implants after teeth are placed on the implant

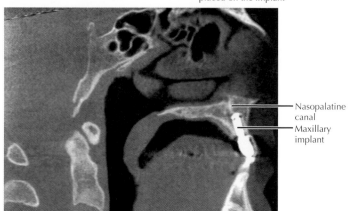

Nasopalatine canal

Maxillary implant

**Figure 12-27**

## SINUS LIFT PROCEDURE

- A *sinus lift procedure* is also called maxillary sinus augmentation
- It is a surgical procedure important for maxillary dental implants
- When teeth are lost, the alveolar bone is resorbed, which can affect neighboring teeth
- Additionally, when posterior teeth are lost (maxillary premolars and molars), the sinus will pneumatize, with reduction in the amount of bone available in those areas
- Because a dental implant relies heavily on osseointegration of the implant into the bone, if there is not enough bone to allow osseointegration, a dental implant will fail
- The goal of the procedure is to increase the amount of bone, to allow for proper osseointegration
- For this surgical procedure:
  - The sinus membrane needs to be carefully elevated from the floor of the maxilla
  - Bone graft material is placed onto the maxilla, the sinus membrane is allowed to rest on the bone graft material, and the access site is closed
  - Great care is needed to prevent perforation of the sinus membrane
- The presence of septa within the maxillary sinus complicates the surgery because the sinus membrane tends to attach more firmly to the bone at the septa

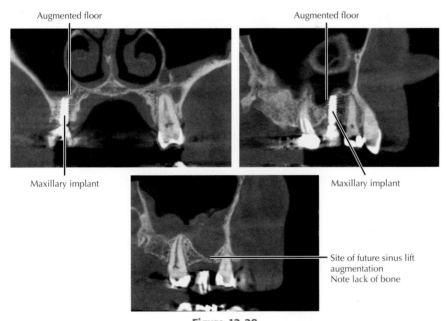

Augmented floor

Augmented floor

Maxillary implant

Maxillary implant

Site of future sinus lift augmentation
Note lack of bone

**Figure 12-28**

FUNCTIONAL ENDOSCOPIC SINUS SURGERY

- In *functional endoscopic sinus surgery,* an endoscope is inserted into the nose to view the nasal cavity and sinuses, thereby eliminating an external incision
- Often performed as an outpatient procedure
- Provides increased visualization of the area, making it easier to remove diseased tissue and leave a greater amount of normal tissue intact
- Standard surgical treatment for sinusitis for people whose chronic sinus problems do not respond to medical therapy
- Also used for removal of polyps, mucoceles, tumors, and foreign bodies and for control of epistaxis

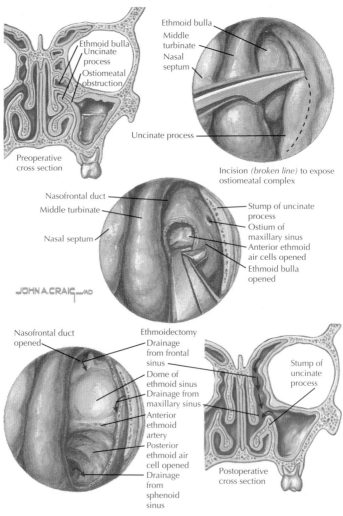

**Figure 12-29**

- *Oral cavity*: the space located between the lips and cheeks on the external surface to the palatoglossal fold on the internal surface
- The oral cavity is important in mastication, tasting, and talking
- The area of the oral cavity can be divided into:
  - Vestibule—the area between the teeth and lips or cheek
  - Oral cavity proper—the area located internal to the teeth
- Posteriorly, the oral cavity is continuous with the oropharynx
- The hard palate and the soft palate are important boundaries within the oral cavity
- The tongue is a major structure located on the oral cavity floor
- All of the major salivary glands (parotid, submandibular, and sublingual) and minor salivary glands (lingual, palatal, buccal, and labial) empty into the oral cavity
- The muscles of the oral cavity include those of the mouth, cheeks, tongue,* and soft palate

Waldeyer's ring is the anatomical name for the ring of lymphatic tissue in the pharynx and oral cavity:
- Lingual tonsil (posterior 1/3rd of tongue)
- Palatine tonsil (oropharynx)
- Tubal tonsil (nasopharynx)
- Pharyngeal tonsil (nasopharynx)

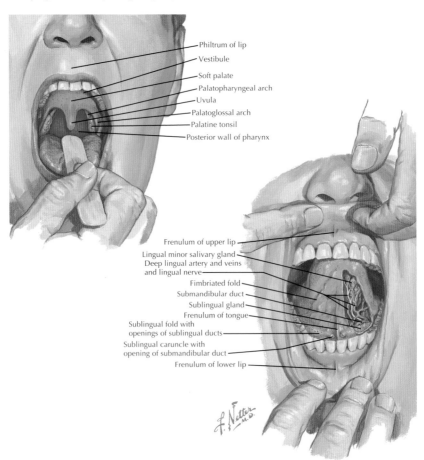

**Figure 13-1**

*The muscles of the tongue are covered in Chapter 14.

| Structure | Comments |
|-----------|----------|
| Lips | Divided into an upper and a lower lip that surround the opening of the oral cavity |
| | Both lips have a muscular "skeleton" composed of the orbicularis oris m. |
| | Upper lip is separated from the cheek by the nasolabial groove |
| | Lower lip is separated from the chin by the labiomental groove |
| | Upper and lower lips meet at the labial commissures |
| | *Vermilion zone*—the red area of the lip that is clearly demarcated from the skin of the face at the vermilion border and is lined by a thinly keratinized layer of stratified squamous epithelium which changes upon transition to the mucous membrane of the oral cavity; also known as the red zone |
| | *Philtrum*—the depressed area located between the base of the nose and the vermilion border of the upper lip |
| | Many mucus-secreting labial glands are located within the submucosal layer of the lips at the area of transition to mucous membrane of the oral cavity, which is nonkeratinized stratified squamous epithelium |
| | *Vestibule*—the region between the lips or cheeks and the teeth |
| | The fold of tissue created by the vestibule between the lip and teeth is called the vestibular or mucolabial fold |
| | As the vestibular fold reflects on the alveolar bone holding the teeth, the mucous membrane abruptly changes into the gingiva |
| | Within the vestibular fold are bands of tissue known as labial frenula |
| | The labial frenula are pronounced at the maxillary and mandibular midline as the upper and lower frenula, respectively |
| | Other accessory frenula also are located in the vestibule |
| Cheek | Located between the labial commissure and the mucosa overlying the ramus of the mandible |
| | Has a muscular "skeleton" composed of the buccinator m. |
| | Many mucus-secreting glands, known as buccal glands, are located within the submucosal layer of the inside of the cheeks, which is lined by mucous membrane of the oral cavity (nonkeratinized stratified squamous epithelium) |
| | Vestibule continues from the region between the lips and teeth posteriorly, to be located between the cheek and the teeth |
| | The fold of tissue created by the vestibule between the lip and the teeth is called the vestibular or mucobuccal fold |
| | The retromolar region is the only area in which the vestibule and the oral cavity proper communicate |
| | The parotid duct drains into the oral cavity at the parotid papilla, located along the mucous membrane of the cheek opposite the 2nd maxillary molar |
| | Fordyce spots, ectopic sebaceous glands found in the mucosa of the cheeks appearing as yellowish spots, can be observed in the cheek |

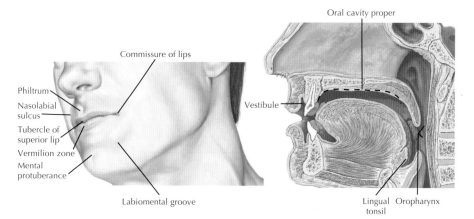

Oral cavity proper

Commissure of lips

Philtrum
Nasolabial sulcus
Tubercle of superior lip
Vermilion zone
Mental protuberance

Vestibule

Labiomental groove

Lingual tonsil   Oropharynx

*Figure 13-2*

| ARTERIAL SUPPLY | | |
|---|---|---|
| **Artery** | **Source** | **Comments** |
| Superior labial branch of the facial | Facial a. off the external carotid a. | Supplies the structures associated with the upper lip<br><br>Gives rise to the septal branch that travels to the nasal septum |
| Superior labial branch of the infraorbital | Infraorbital a. off the maxillary a. | A continuation of the 3rd part of the maxillary a.<br><br>1 of the 3 terminal branches of the infraorbital a., along with the inferior palpebral branch and the nasal branch<br><br>Accompanied by the nerve and vein of the same name<br><br>Helps supply the upper lip |
| Inferior labial branch of the facial | Facial a. off the external carotid a. | Supplies the structures associated with the lower lip |
| Mental | Inferior alveolar a. | A terminal branch from the inferior alveolar a., which arises from the 1st part of the maxillary a.<br><br>Emerges from the mental foramen to supply the chin region |
| Buccal | Maxillary a. | A branch of the 2nd part of the maxillary a.<br><br>A small artery that runs obliquely in an anterior direction between the medial pterygoid and the insertion of the temporalis m. until it reaches the outer surface of the buccinator m. to supply that muscle and the face |

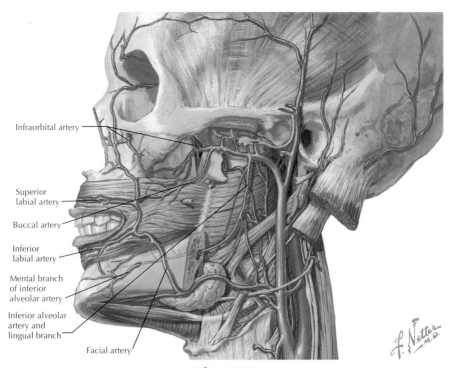

Infraorbital artery

Superior labial artery

Buccal artery

Inferior labial artery

Mental branch of inferior alveolar artery

Inferior alveolar artery and lingual branch

Facial artery

**Figure 13-3**

| VENOUS DRAINAGE | |
| --- | --- |
| **Vein** | **Comments** |
| Superior labial branch of the facial | Drains the upper lip and joins the facial v. |
| Inferior labial branch of the facial | Drains the lower lip and joins the facial v. |
| Mental | Drains the chin and lower lip and joins the pterygoid plexus of veins |
| Buccal | Drains the cheek and joins the pterygoid plexus of veins |

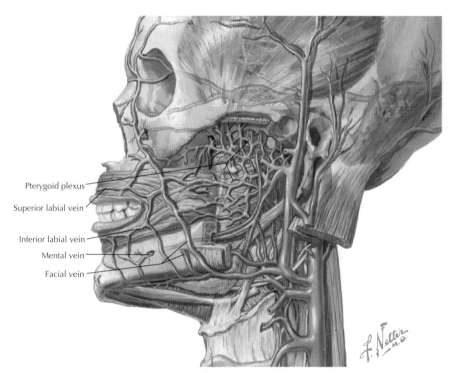

Pterygoid plexus
Superior labial vein
Inferior labial vein
Mental vein
Facial vein

**Figure 13-4**

| Muscle | Origin | Insertion | Actions | Nerve | Comments |
|---|---|---|---|---|---|
| Orbicularis oris | *Bone*: anterior midline of the maxilla and mandible<br><br>*Muscular*: angle of the mouth where fibers blend with levator anguli oris, depressor anguli oris, zygomaticus major, and risorius mm. | Skin along the mouth | Closes lips<br><br>Protrusion of lips<br><br>Pursing of lips | Facial (buccal and mandibular branches) | Sphincter of the mouth<br><br>Muscle fibers encircle the mouth |
| Buccinator | Pterygomandibular raphe<br><br>Alveolar margins of the maxilla and mandible | Some fibers blend and provide origin for the orbicularis oris<br><br>Some fibers blend into the upper and lower lips | Aids in mastication, keeping the bolus between cheek and teeth<br><br>Helps forcibly expel air<br><br>Helps create a sucking action | Facial (buccal branch) | Creates the framework of the cheek |

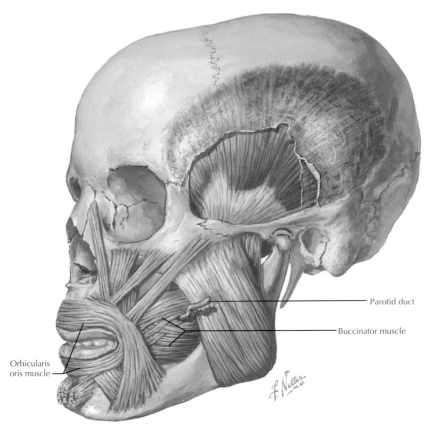

Parotid duct

Buccinator muscle

Orbicularis oris muscle

**Figure 13-5**

| SENSORY INNERVATION | | |
|---|---|---|
| **Nerve** | **Source** | **Course** |
| • All sensory innervation to the skin of this region is supplied by the trigeminal n. | | |
| Superior labial branch of the infraorbital | Infraorbital n. (a continuation of the maxillary division of the trigeminal n.) | 1 of the 3 terminal branches of the infraorbital n., along with the inferior palpebral and the nasal, as it exits onto the face via the infraorbital foramen<br><br>Supplies the skin of the upper lip |
| Mental | Inferior alveolar n. | 1 of the 2 terminal branches of the inferior alveolar n.<br><br>Emerges through the mental foramen of the mandible in the region of the 2nd mandibular premolar<br><br>Supplies the skin of the lower lip, chin, and facial gingiva as far posteriorly as the 2nd mandibular premolar |
| Buccal branch of the mandibular division of the trigeminal | Mandibular division of the trigeminal n. | Passes anteriorly between the 2 heads of the lateral pterygoid m.<br><br>Descends inferiorly along the lower part of the temporalis m. to emerge from deep to the anterior border of the masseter m.<br><br>Supplies the skin over the buccinator m. before passing through it to supply the mucous membrane lining its inner surface and the gingiva along the mandibular molars |

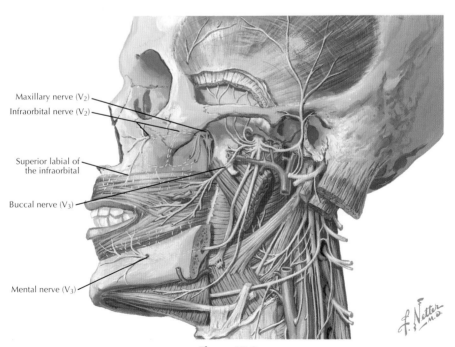

Maxillary nerve (V₂)
Infraorbital nerve (V₂)

Superior labial of the infraorbital

Buccal nerve (V₃)

Mental nerve (V₃)

**Figure 13-6**

| Boundary | Structure |
|----------|-----------|
| Superior | Hard palate |
| Posterosuperior | Soft palate |
| Lateral | Cheeks |
| Inferior | The floor of the oral cavity (which is located along the lingual border of the mandible, forming a horseshoe-shaped region) |

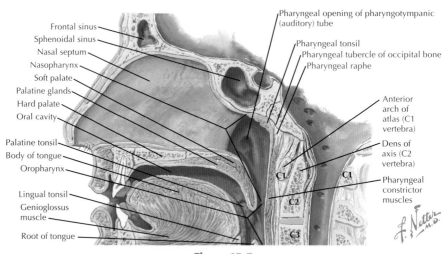

**Figure 13-7**

- The superior border (or roof) of the oral cavity is the hard palate, comprising the anterior 2/3 of the entire palate
- Separates the oral cavity from the nasal cavity
- Composed of:
  - Palatal process of the maxilla
  - Horizontal process of the palatine
- In the anterior midline, an incisive foramen is located on the right and left sides that transmits the terminal branches of the nasopalatine nerve and sphenopalatine vessels
- In the posterolateral region of the hard palate, the greater and lesser palatine foramina are located on the right and left sides; these openings transmit the greater and lesser palatine nn. and vessels
- The bones of the hard palate are covered by a thick mucous membrane, known as masticatory mucosa (keratinized stratified squamous epithelium)
- The mucous membrane has a small elevation in the anterior midline called the incisive papilla that overlies the incisive foramen
- The mucous membrane in the anterior region is tightly attached to the underlying palatal process of the maxilla
- The mucous membrane in the anterior region is frequently avulsed from the palatal process of the maxilla during the administration of a Nasopalatine nerve block
- Moving posteriorly from the incisive papilla, the mucous membrane has a thick midline palatal raphe
- Lateral transverse ridges called transverse rugae (plicae) are located along the mucous membrane of the hard palate
- Deep to the mucous membrane of the hard palate are numerous mucus-secreting glands called palatal (palatine) glands

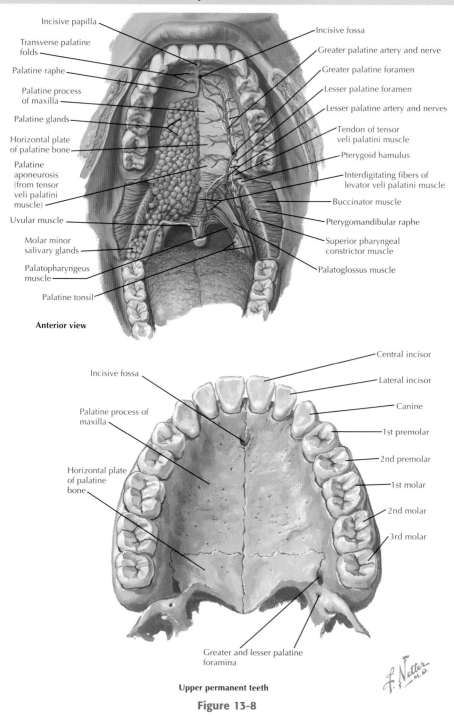

Incisive papilla

Transverse palatine folds

Palatine raphe

Palatine process of maxilla

Palatine glands

Horizontal plate of palatine bone

Palatine aponeurosis (from tensor veli palatini muscle)

Uvular muscle

Molar minor salivary glands

Palatopharyngeus muscle

Palatine tonsil

Incisive fossa

Greater palatine artery and nerve

Greater palatine foramen

Lesser palatine foramen

Lesser palatine artery and nerves

Tendon of tensor veli palatini muscle

Pterygoid hamulus

Interdigitating fibers of levator veli palatini muscle

Buccinator muscle

Pterygomandibular raphe

Superior pharyngeal constrictor muscle

Palatoglossus muscle

**Anterior view**

Incisive fossa

Palatine process of maxilla

Horizontal plate of palatine bone

Central incisor

Lateral incisor

Canine

1st premolar

2nd premolar

1st molar

2nd molar

3rd molar

Greater and lesser palatine foramina

**Upper permanent teeth**

**Figure 13-8**

- The posterosuperior border of the oral cavity is the soft palate
- The soft palate is the continuation of the palate posteriorly and makes up approximately 1/3 of the entire palate
- The soft palate separates the oral cavity from the oropharynx
- An abundance of mucus-secreting palatal glands, which are continuous with the hard palate, are located in the soft palate
- The soft palate has 3 margins:
  - Anteriorly, it is continuous with the hard palate at the vibrating line
  - Posterolaterally, it forms the superior portion of the palatoglossal and palatopharyngeal folds
  - Posteriorly, the uvula hangs in the center of the posterior free margin
- The thick palatine aponeurosis forms the foundation of the soft palate
- The soft palate is composed of 5 muscles:
  - Musculus uvulae
  - Tensor veli palatini
  - Levator veli palatini
  - Palatopharyngeus
  - Palatoglossus (sometimes considered in the grouping of tongue muscles)
- The soft palate helps close off the nasopharynx during deglutition by forming a seal at the fold of Passavant

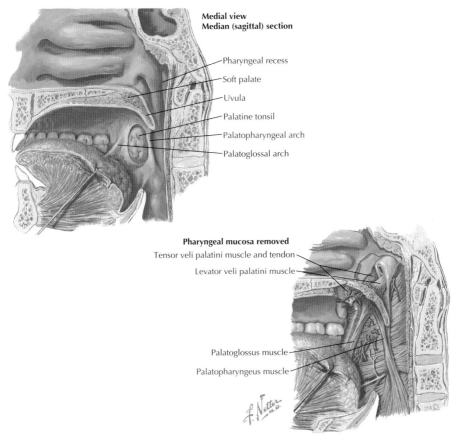

Medial view
Median (sagittal) section

Pharyngeal recess

Soft palate

Uvula

Palatine tonsil

Palatopharyngeal arch

Palatoglossal arch

Pharyngeal mucosa removed

Tensor veli palatini muscle and tendon

Levator veli palatini muscle

Palatoglossus muscle

Palatopharyngeus muscle

**Figure 13-9**

| MUSCLES OF THE SOFT PALATE | | | | | |
|---|---|---|---|---|---|
| **Muscle** | **Origin** | **Insertion** | **Actions** | **Nerve Supply** | **Comment** |
| Tensor veli palatini | Cartilaginous part of the auditory tube<br>Scaphoid fossa of the sphenoid | Palatine aponeurosis | Pulls the soft palate laterally, which broadens it | Mandibular division of the trigeminal n. | The tendon of the tensor veli palatini m. wraps around the pterygoid hamulus |
| Musculus uvulae | Posterior nasal spine<br>Palatine aponeurosis | Fibers insert into the mucosa of the uvula | Retracts uvula<br>Pulls uvula in a posterosuperior direction | Pharyngeal plexus (the motor portion of this plexus is formed by the pharyngeal branch of the vagus n.) | May be bifid |
| Levator veli palatini | Cartilaginous portion of the auditory tube<br>Petrous portion of the temporal bone | Palatine aponeurosis<br>Fibers also insert into the muscle of the opposite side | Elevates soft palate<br>Pulls soft palate posterosuperiorly which acts to help close the nasopharynx | | The levator veli palatini m. passes through an aperture superior to the superior constrictor m. |
| Palatopharyngeus | Posterior border of hard palate<br>Palatine aponeurosis | Posterior border of the lamina of the thyroid cartilage | Elevates the pharynx and larynx<br>Acts to help close the nasopharynx | | Grouped either with soft palate muscles or with muscles of the pharynx |
| Palatoglossus | Palatine aponeurosis (oral surface) | Lateral aspect of the tongue where some fibers intermix with the transverse m. and some along the dorsal surface of the tongue | Elevation of the root of the tongue<br>Narrows the oropharyngeal isthmus for deglutition | | Grouped either with extrinsic muscles of the tongue or with muscles of the soft palate |

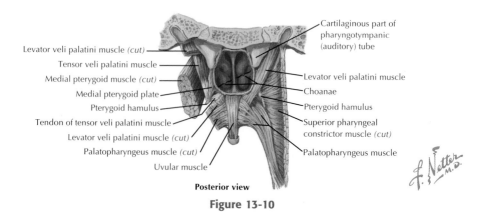

Levator veli palatini muscle *(cut)*
Tensor veli palatini muscle
Medial pterygoid muscle *(cut)*
Medial pterygoid plate
Pterygoid hamulus
Tendon of tensor veli palatini muscle
Levator veli palatini muscle *(cut)*
Palatopharyngeus muscle *(cut)*
Uvular muscle

Cartilaginous part of pharyngotympanic (auditory) tube
Levator veli palatini muscle
Choanae
Pterygoid hamulus
Superior pharyngeal constrictor muscle *(cut)*
Palatopharyngeus muscle

Posterior view

**Figure 13-10**

**Section through cartilaginous part of pharyngotympanic (auditory) tube, with tube closed**

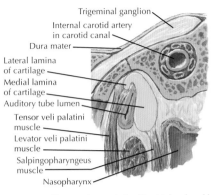

Trigeminal ganglion

Internal carotid artery in carotid canal

Dura mater

Lateral lamina of cartilage

Medial lamina of cartilage

Auditory tube lumen

Tensor veli palatini muscle

Levator veli palatini muscle

Salpingopharyngeus muscle

Nasopharynx

Pharyngotympanic (auditory) tube closed by elastic recoil of cartilage, tissue turgidity, and tension of salpingopharyngeus muscles

**Section through cartilaginous part of pharyngotympanic (auditory) tube, with tube open**

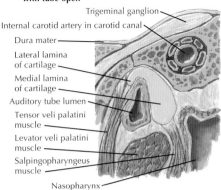

Trigeminal ganglion

Internal carotid artery in carotid canal

Dura mater

Lateral lamina of cartilage

Medial lamina of cartilage

Auditory tube lumen

Tensor veli palatini muscle

Levator veli palatini muscle

Salpingopharyngeus muscle

Nasopharynx

Lumen opened chiefly when attachment of tensor veli palatini muscle pulls wall of tube laterally during swallowing

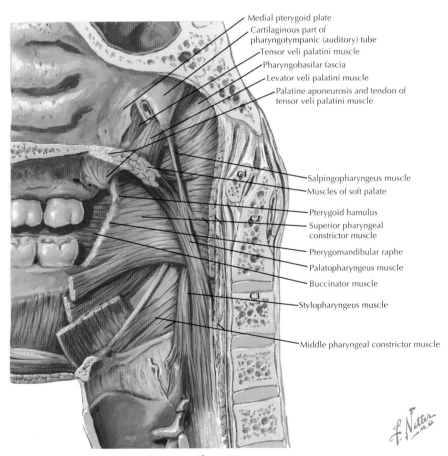

Medial pterygoid plate

Cartilaginous part of pharyngotympanic (auditory) tube

Tensor veli palatini muscle

Pharyngobasilar fascia

Levator veli palatini muscle

Palatine aponeurosis and tendon of tensor veli palatini muscle

C1

C2

C3

Salpingopharyngeus muscle

Muscles of soft palate

Pterygoid hamulus

Superior pharyngeal constrictor muscle

Pterygomandibular raphe

Palatopharyngeus muscle

Buccinator muscle

Stylopharyngeus muscle

Middle pharyngeal constrictor muscle

**Figure 13-11**

- The lateral border of the oral cavity extends anteriorly from the labial commissure, posteriorly to the ramus of the mandible
- Superior limit of the cheek is the maxillary vestibule; inferior limit is the mandibular vestibule
- Mucous membrane of the cheek is stratified squamous epithelium
- Fordyce spots are ectopic sebaceous glands that may be observed on the inner surface of the cheek
- Parotid papilla is located in the cheek opposite the maxillary 2nd molar
- Pterygomandibular raphe is located in the posterior portion and serves as a landmark for the pterygomandibular space for inferior alveolar nerve blocks

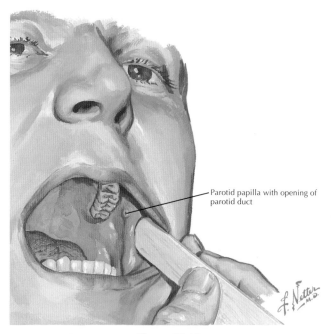

Parotid papilla with opening of parotid duct

**Figure 13-12**

- The inferior border is the floor of the oral cavity
- It is located along the lingual border of the mandible forming a horseshoe-shaped region
- The mylohyoid m. serves as the sling of the floor of the oral cavity and structures superior to it are the major contents
- The largest structure is the tongue and related musculature
- Please see Chapter 14 on the tongue for a detailed explanation of the musculature of the tongue

| Structure | Comments |
|---|---|
| Tongue | Largest structure in the floor (see Chapter 14) |
| Lingual frenulum | A midline fold of tissue located at the base of the tongue and extends along the inferior surface of the tongue |
| Mucous membrane | Stratified squamous epithelium that extends from the tongue to the mandible |
| Sublingual papilla | A swelling located on both sides of the lingual frenulum at the base of the tongue<br>Continuous with the sublingual folds overlying the sublingual glands on the floor of the oral cavity<br>Marks the entrance of the saliva from the submandibular glands into the oral cavity |
| Submandibular duct | Lies along the sublingual gland under the mucosa |
| Lingual n. | Crosses the submandibular duct passing lateral, inferior, and medial to the duct to reach the tongue and supply general sensation to the anterior 2/3 |
| Plica fimbriata | Fimbriated folds located lateral to the lingual frenulum |
| Mylohyoid m. | Forms the muscular sling of the floor of the oral cavity<br>Passes from the mylohyoid line of the mandible to the opposite mylohyoid m. in the midline at the mylohyoid raphe and attaches posteriorly to the hyoid bone |
| Geniohyoid mm. | Lie superior to the mylohyoid mm.<br>Attach from the inferior genial tubercles of the mandible to the hyoid bone |

| MUSCLES OF THE FLOOR OF THE ORAL CAVITY | | | | | |
|---|---|---|---|---|---|
| **Muscle** | **Origin** | **Insertion** | **Actions** | **Nerve Supply** | **Comment** |
| Mylohyoid | Mylohyoid line of the mandible | Mylohyoid raphe<br>Body of the hyoid bone | Raises the floor of the oral cavity<br>Can elevate the hyoid bone | Mylohyoid n. from the inferior alveolar branch of the mandibular division of the trigeminal n. | Forms the sling of the oral cavity |
| Geniohyoid | Inferior genial tubercle | Body of the hyoid bone | Elevates the hyoid bone | C1 ventral ramus, which follows the hypoglossal n. | Superior to the mylohyoid m. |

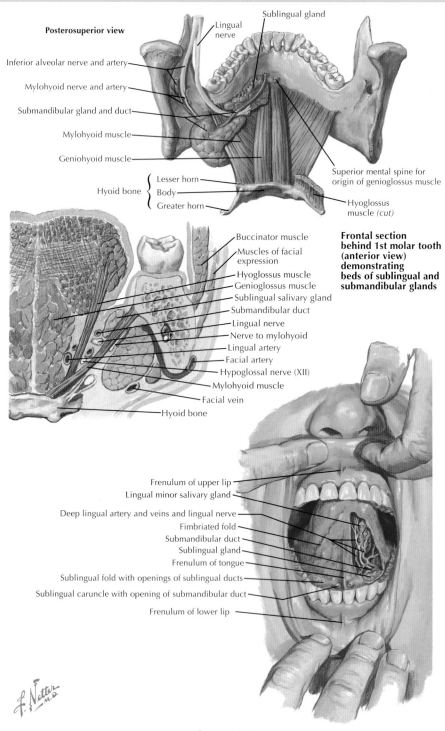

**Posterosuperior view**

Sublingual gland

Lingual nerve

Inferior alveolar nerve and artery

Mylohyoid nerve and artery

Submandibular gland and duct

Mylohyoid muscle

Geniohyoid muscle

Hyoid bone { Lesser horn / Body / Greater horn

Superior mental spine for origin of genioglossus muscle

Hyoglossus muscle *(cut)*

Buccinator muscle

Muscles of facial expression

Hyoglossus muscle

Genioglossus muscle

Sublingual salivary gland

Submandibular duct

Lingual nerve

Nerve to mylohyoid

Lingual artery

Facial artery

Hypoglossal nerve (XII)

Mylohyoid muscle

Facial vein

Hyoid bone

**Frontal section behind 1st molar tooth (anterior view) demonstrating beds of sublingual and submandibular glands**

Frenulum of upper lip

Lingual minor salivary gland

Deep lingual artery and veins and lingual nerve

Fimbriated fold

Submandibular duct

Sublingual gland

Frenulum of tongue

Sublingual fold with openings of sublingual ducts

Sublingual caruncle with opening of submandibular duct

Frenulum of lower lip

**Figure 13-13**

- Teeth are hard structures attached to the jaws and involved primarily in eating
- 2 arches contain the teeth:
  - Maxillary arch
  - Mandibular arch
- Humans have 2 sets of teeth during a lifetime:
  - Deciduous teeth—the primary dentition
  - Permanent teeth—the secondary dentition
- Between the ages of 6 and 12 years, there is a mixed dentition, in which both primary and permanent teeth are present in the oral cavity at the same time

## DECIDUOUS TEETH

- There are 20 total deciduous teeth: 2 incisors, 1 canine, and 2 molars in each of the 4 quadrants of the oral cavity
- The primary dentition is represented by the formula $I\frac{2}{2}C\frac{1}{1}M\frac{2}{2}$, which specifies the total number of teeth (10) on each side of the oral cavity
- No deciduous teeth are present at birth; however, by the 3rd year of life, all 20 deciduous teeth have erupted

## PERMANENT TEETH

- There are 32 total permanent teeth: 2 incisors, 1 canine, 2 premolars, and 3 molars in each of the 4 quadrants of the oral cavity
- The permanent dentition is represented by the formula $I\frac{2}{2}C\frac{1}{1}P\frac{2}{2}M\frac{3}{3}$, which specifies the total number of teeth (16) on each side of the oral cavity
- The 1st permanent tooth to erupt into the oral cavity normally is the mandibular 1st molar
  - This eruption occurs at about 6 years of age
  - It erupts distal to the primary dentition
- The primary teeth eventually are replaced by the permanent teeth
- The replacement teeth are termed succedaneous teeth

| SURFACES OF A TOOTH | |
|---|---|
| Labial | The surface of the anterior teeth that is closest to the lip |
| Buccal | The surface of the posterior teeth that is closest to the cheek |
| Facial | Used as a synonym for labial or buccal |
| Lingual | Opposite the tongue in the mandibular arch and opposite the hard palate of the maxillary arch |
| Mesial | Closest to the midline of the dental arch |
| Distal | Farthest from the midline of the dental arch |
| Occlusal | Used for chewing in posterior teeth |
| Incisal | The cutting edge of anterior teeth |

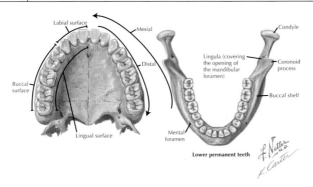

Labial surface · Mesial · Condyle · Distal · Lingula (covering the opening of the mandibular foramen) · Coronoid process · Buccal surface · Buccal shelf · Lingual surface · Mental foramen · Lower permanent teeth

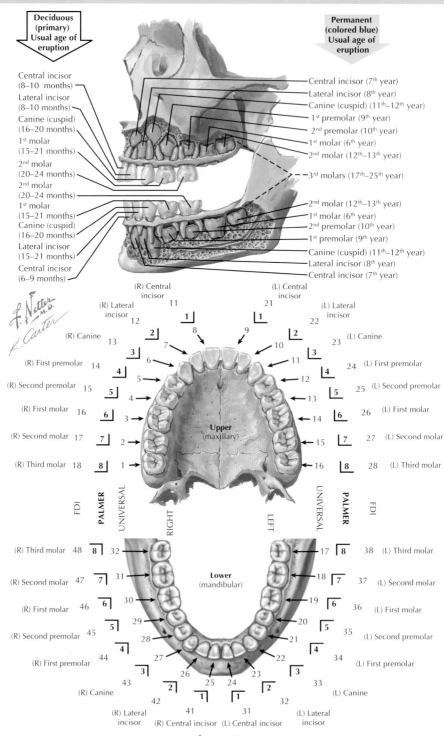

**Figure 13-14**

| Crown | *Anatomic crown*: the portion of the tooth that has a surface of enamel |
|---|---|
| | *Clinical crown*: the portion of the tooth that is exposed within the oral cavity |
| Root | *Anatomic root*: the portion of the tooth that has a surface of cementum |
| | *Clinical root*: the portion of the tooth that is entrenched within the maxilla or mandible and is not exposed to the oral cavity |
| Apex of the root | The end tip of the root, which also is the location of a small aperture at the point of each root, which provides an entrance for the neurovascular connective tissue into the pulp cavity |
| Cervical line | The anatomic demarcation between the crown and the root |
| | It often is termed the cementoenamel junction (CEJ) |
| Enamel | The hard, shiny surface of the anatomic crown |
| | The hardest portion of the tooth |
| | Made of small hexagonal rods, called enamel prisms, that are parallel to one another |
| Cementum | A thin, dull layer on the surface of the anatomic root |
| | Similar in structure and chemical composition to bone |
| | With age, cementum increases in thickness |
| Dentin | The hard tissue that underlies both the enamel and cementum and constitutes the major portion of the tooth |
| | A modification of osseous tissue |
| | Composed of a number of dental tubules (small wavy and branching tubes) that are located in a dense matrix |
| Cusp | An elevation on the occlusal surface of molars and premolars that makes up a divisional part of the tooth |
| | The incisal edge of canines is referred to as a cusp and is used for prehension (grasping and tearing) of food |
| Pulp cavity | Contains the dental pulp (highly neurovascular connective tissue) |
| | Separated into the *pulp chamber*, located in the coronal portion of the tooth, and the *pulp canal*, located in the root portion of the tooth |
| Cingulum | A convex elevation that is located on the lingual surface of the crowns of anterior teeth just incisal to the CEJ |

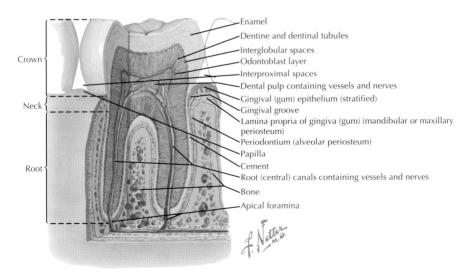

**Figure 13-15**

- There are 32 permanent teeth in the oral cavity:
  - 16 maxillary teeth
  - 16 mandibular teeth
- To aid the clinician in effective discussion of specific teeth, a dental notation system is required
- The major dental notation systems are:
  - FDI World Dental Federation Notation System
  - Palmer Notation System
  - Universal Numbering System
- In the United States, the most commonly used system is the Universal Numbering System
- In the Universal Numbering System, the numbering begins with the right 3rd maxillary molar as number 1, continuing over to the left 3rd maxillary molar as number 16, then moving to the mandibular arch with the left 3rd mandibular molar as number 17 and continuing over to the right 3rd mandibular molar as number 32

| MAXILLARY INCISORS | | | | |
|---|---|---|---|---|
| **Tooth** | **Crown** | **Surfaces** | **Root(s)** | **Comments** |
| Central incisor | The widest of all of the anterior teeth, nearly as wide as it is long<br><br>*Cingulum*: well developed | From a labial view, the distal surface is more convex than the mesial surface<br><br>*Mamelons*: 3 elevations on the incisal edge of anterior teeth that denote centers of formation<br><br>Observed in central incisors before they are worn away during function | 1 conical root that is triangular in cross section | Incisors are cutting teeth |
| Lateral incisor | More narrow than the central incisor in a mesial-to-distal measurement | *Labial surface*: convex<br><br>*Incisal edges* on the mesial and distal surfaces: more convex than central incisors<br><br>*Mamelons*: tend to be less prominent on the lateral incisor<br><br>*Lingual surface*: more concave than on the central incisors<br><br>*Mesial and distal marginal ridges* more prominent than central incisor and typically demonstrate a lingual pit | 1 conical root that is oval in cross section | |

| MAXILLARY CANINE | | | | |
|---|---|---|---|---|
| **Tooth** | **Crown** | **Surfaces** | **Root(s)** | **Comments** |
| Canine | *Cingulum*: prominent | *Labial surface*: convex<br>*Incisal edge*: rounded into a cusp that displays a mesial and distal cusp ridge<br>*Lingual surface*: exhibits a strong ridge from the cusp tip to the cingulum, which divides the lingual surface into a mesial and a distal fossa | 1 long and conical root that is rectangular in cross section, with depressions on the mesial and distal surfaces | Also called cuspid; longest tooth in the oral cavity<br>Prehensile tooth |

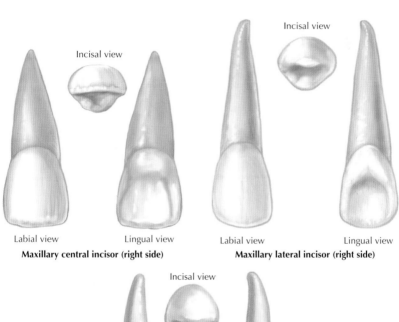

Incisal view

Labial view      Lingual view
**Maxillary central incisor (right side)**

Incisal view

Labial view      Lingual view
**Maxillary lateral incisor (right side)**

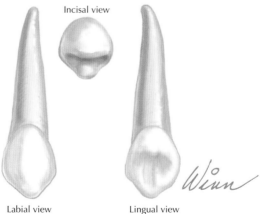

Incisal view

Labial view      Lingual view
**Maxillary canine (right side)**

**Figure 13-16**

| MAXILLARY PREMOLARS | | | | |
|---|---|---|---|---|
| **Tooth** | **Crown** | **Surfaces** | **Root(s)** | **Comments** |
| 1st premolar | Shorter than the anterior teeth<br><br>Wider in a facial-lingual dimension than in a mesial-distal dimension | Has a lingual and a facial cusp<br><br>*Facial surface*: convex<br><br>*Facial cusp*: long and similar in appearance to the cusp of the canine<br><br>*Lingual cusp*: shorter than the facial cusp and positioned mesial of the mesial distal midline<br><br>Displays a mesial marginal developmental groove | Usually 2 roots—a facial and a lingual root | Often referred to as bicuspid teeth, but a more accepted designation would be premolar teeth<br><br>Prehensile tooth |
| 2nd premolar | Not as angular in shape as the 1st premolar | *Facial surface*: convex<br><br>Has a lingual and a facial cusp<br><br>*Facial cusp*: not as sharp as the facial cusp of the 1st premolar<br><br>*Lingual cusp*: nearly equal in size and similar in shape to the facial cusp | Usually 1 root | Occlusal surface contains supplemental grooves, which gives it a wrinkled appearance<br><br>Supplements the molars in function |

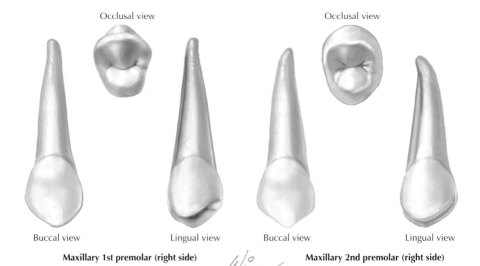

Occlusal view             Occlusal view

Buccal view     Lingual view     Buccal view     Lingual view

**Maxillary 1st premolar (right side)**      **Maxillary 2nd premolar (right side)**

**Figure 13-17**

| MAXILLARY MOLARS | | | | |
|---|---|---|---|---|
| **Tooth** | **Crown** | **Surfaces** | **Root(s)** | **Comments** |
| • The molar teeth are used for crushing and chewing | | | | |
| 1st molar | Larger in a facial-lingual dimension than it is in a mesial-distal dimension<br>From an occlusal view, the crown is rhomboidal in form | 5 cusps:<br>• Mesiobuccal cusp<br>• Distobuccal cusp<br>• Mesiolingual cusp<br>• Distolingual cusp<br>• 5th cusp: present on the lingual surface of the mesiolingual cusp and termed the cusp of Carabelli | 3 roots:<br>• Mesiobuccal root<br>• Distobuccal root (smallest)<br>• Lingual root (largest) | Usually the largest of the molar teeth |
| 2nd molar | Supplements the 1st molar in function 2 forms:<br>• Resembles the 1st molar with a more extreme rhomboidal form<br>• A heart-shaped form with a poorly developed distolingual cusp | 4 cusps:<br>• Mesiobuccal cusp<br>• Distobuccal cusp<br>• Mesiolingual cusp<br>• Distolingual cusp (sometimes absent)<br>There is no 5th cusp | 3 roots:<br>• Mesiobuccal root<br>• Distobuccal root<br>• Lingual root | Smaller than the 1st molar |
| 3rd molar | Great variation in the crown (it may resemble the 1st or 2nd molar) | 3-cusp form is more common:<br>• Mesiobuccal cusp<br>• Distobuccal cusp<br>• Mesiolingual cusp | 3 roots:<br>• Mesiobuccal root<br>• Distobuccal root<br>• Lingual root<br>The roots usually are fused, functioning as 1 large root | Variable in size<br>Often extracted as a preventive measure |

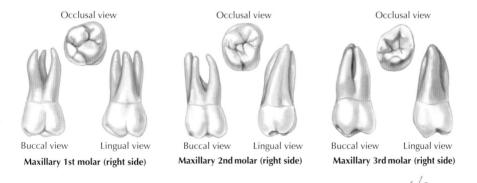

Occlusal view     Occlusal view     Occlusal view

Buccal view   Lingual view    Buccal view   Lingual view    Buccal view   Lingual view

**Maxillary 1st molar (right side)**    **Maxillary 2nd molar (right side)**    **Maxillary 3rd molar (right side)**

**Figure 13-18**

| MANDIBULAR CANINE | | | | |
|---|---|---|---|---|
| **Tooth** | **Crown** | **Surfaces** | **Root(s)** | **Comments** |
| Canine | Longer than the maxillary canine<br><br>*Cingulum*: not as prominent as on the maxillary canine | *Incisal edge*: rounded into a cusp<br><br>*Mamelons*: not usually located on canine teeth<br><br>*Mesial surface* of crown and root: relatively straight, without much convexity | 1 long and conical root | Also called cuspids<br><br>Smaller and more symmetric than the maxillary canine |

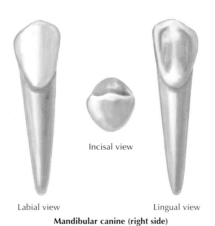

Incisal view

Labial view                    Lingual view
**Mandibular canine (right side)**

*Winn*

**Figure 13-19**

| MANDIBULAR INCISORS | | | | |
|---|---|---|---|---|
| Tooth | Crown | Surfaces | Root(s) | Comments |
| Central incisor | 2/3 the width of the maxillary central incisor<br><br>Appears bilaterally symmetric<br><br>*Cingulum*: small and poorly developed | *Labial surface:* convex<br><br>*Lingual surface:* concave<br><br>*Mamelons:* observed in central incisors before wear<br><br>*Lingual fossa:* poorly developed | 1 root that is flattened and is wide in a facial-lingual direction | Incisors are cutting teeth |
| Lateral incisor | Not bilaterally symmetric | *Labial surface:* convex<br><br>*Lingual fossa:* poorly developed | 1 root similar in shape to the central incisor | When viewed from the incisal aspect, the crown appears twisted distally on the root<br><br>Incisors are cutting teeth |

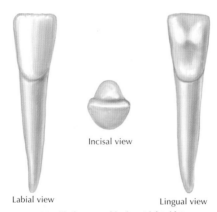

Labial view    Lingual view

Incisal view

**Mandibular central incisor (right side)**

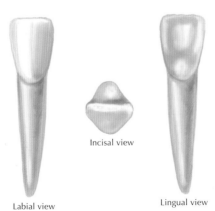

Labial view    Lingual view

Incisal view

**Mandibular lateral incisor (right side)**

*Winn*

**Figure 13-20**

| MANDIBULAR PREMOLARS | | | | |
|---|---|---|---|---|
| **Tooth** | **Crown** | **Surfaces** | **Root(s)** | **Comments** |
| 1st premolar | Diamond-shaped | *Facial surface*: convex<br>Has a lingual and a buccal cusp<br>• Buccal cusp—well developed<br>• Lingual cusp—small and not well developed<br>Displays a mesial lingual developmental groove | 1 root that is oval in cross section, with a slight lingual taper | The smallest of the premolar teeth |
| 2nd premolar | Convex | Demonstrates either of 2 occlusal schemes:<br>• A 2-cusp form, with a facial and a lingual cusp<br>• A 3-cusp form, with 2 lingual cusps and a single facial cusp—predominant form<br>Facial and lingual surfaces are convex<br>*Facial cusp* is not as sharp as that of the 1st premolar<br>*Lingual cusp(s)* are smaller than the facial cusp | 1 root that is oval in cross section, with a slight lingual taper | Differs in appearance from the 1st premolar<br>Much larger than the 1st premolar |

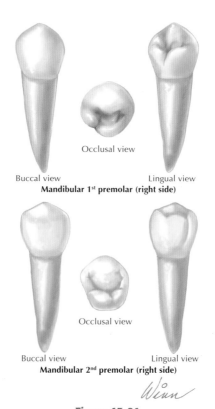

Occlusal view

Buccal view        Lingual view
**Mandibular 1ˢᵗ premolar (right side)**

Occlusal view

Buccal view        Lingual view
**Mandibular 2ⁿᵈ premolar (right side)**

**Figure 13-21**

| MANDIBULAR MOLARS | | | | |
|---|---|---|---|---|
| **Tooth** | **Crown** | **Surfaces** | **Root(s)** | **Comments** |
| 1st molar | Wider in a mesial-distal dimension than in a facial-lingual length | 5 cusps:<br>• Mesiobuccal cusp (largest)<br>• Distobuccal cusp<br>• Distal cusp (smallest)<br>• Mesiolingual cusp<br>• Distolingual cusp | 2 roots:<br>• Mesial root (containing 2 pulp canals)<br>• Distal root (containing 1 pulp canal) | Used for crushing and chewing |
| 2nd molar | Normally the 2nd molar is smaller than the 1st molar | 4 cusps:<br>• Mesiobuccal cusp<br>• Distobuccal cusp<br>• Mesiolingual cusp<br>• Distolingual cusp | 2 roots:<br>• Mesial root (containing 2 pulp canals)<br>• Distal root (containing 1 pulp canal) | Supplements the 1st molar in function |
| 3rd molar | Development is similar to that of the 2nd molar | 4 cusps of variable shape and size | 2 roots:<br>• Mesial root<br>• Distal root<br>Roots are often fused | Variable, but not as variable as the maxillary 3rd molar<br>Often the smallest of the molar teeth<br>Often extracted as a preventive measure |

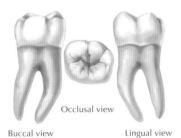

Occlusal view

Buccal view          Lingual view

**Mandibular 1st molar (right side)**

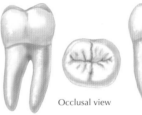

Occlusal view

Buccal view          Lingual view

**Mandibular 2nd molar (right side)**

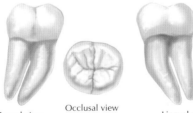

Occlusal view

Buccal view          Lingual view

**Mandibular 3rd molar (right side)**

**Figure 13-22**

| ARTERIAL SUPPLY OF THE PALATE | | |
|---|---|---|
| **Artery** | **Source** | **Course** |
| Maxillary | External carotid a. | Gives rise to a series of branches; 3 supply the palate:<br>• Sphenopalatine<br>• Greater palatine<br>• Lesser palatine<br>Gives rise to 3 branches that supply the maxillary arch:<br>• Anterior superior alveolar<br>• Middle superior alveolar<br>• Posterior superior alveolar<br>Gives rise to 1 branch that supplies the mandibular arch:<br>• Inferior alveolar |
| *Sphenopala-tine* | 3rd part of the maxillary a. | Enters the nasal cavity after passing through the sphenopalatine foramen<br>On entering the nasal cavity, gives rise to the posterior superior nasal branches:<br>• Posterior superior lateral branch<br>• Posterior superior medial branch, which continues along the nasal septum to enter the hard palate via the incisive canal |
| *Greater palatine* | Descending palatine a. from the 3rd part of the maxillary a. | A branch of the descending palatine a. that travels in the palatine canal<br>Within the canal, the descending palatine a. splits into the:<br>• Lesser palatine a.<br>• Greater palatine a.<br>The greater palatine a. exits the greater palatine foramen and passes anteriorly toward the incisive foramen to supply the hard palate gingiva, mucosa, and palatal glands and anastomose with the terminal branch of the sphenopalatine a., which exits the incisive foramen |
| *Lesser palatine* | Descending palatine a. from the 3rd part of the maxillary a. | A branch of the descending palatine a. that travels in the palatine canal<br>Within the canal, the descending palatine a. splits into the:<br>• Greater palatine a.<br>• Lesser palatine a.<br>Lesser palatine a. supplies the soft palate and palatine tonsil |
| Facial | External carotid a. | Arises in the carotid triangle of the neck<br>Passes superiorly immediately deep to the posterior belly of the digastric m. and the stylohyoid m.<br>Passes along the submandibular gland, giving rise to the submental a., which helps supply the gland<br>Passes superiorly over the body of the mandible at the masseter |
| *Ascending palatine* | Facial a. | Supplies the soft palate<br>Ascends between the styloglossus and stylopharyngeus mm. along the side of the pharynx<br>Divides near the levator veli palatini m.<br>A branch follows the levator veli palatini, supplying the soft palate and the palatine glands<br>A 2nd branch pierces the superior constrictor m. to supply the palatine tonsil and auditory tube<br>Anastomoses with the ascending pharyngeal and tonsillar aa. |
| Ascending pharyngeal | External carotid a. | Arises in the carotid triangle of the neck<br>Lies deep to the other branches of the external carotid a. and under the stylopharyngeus m.<br>Gives rise to pharyngeal, inferior tympanic, posterior meningeal, and palatine branches<br>The palatine branch passes over the superior constrictor m. and sends branches to the soft palate, tonsil, and auditory tube |

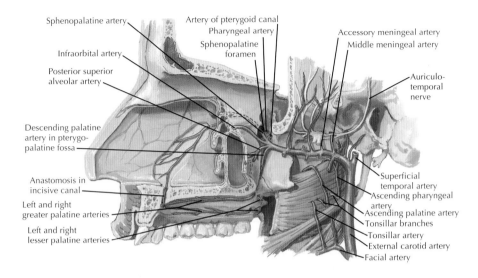

Sphenopalatine artery

Infraorbital artery

Posterior superior alveolar artery

Descending palatine artery in pterygo-palatine fossa

Anastomosis in incisive canal

Left and right greater palatine arteries

Left and right lesser palatine arteries

Artery of pterygoid canal
Pharyngeal artery
Sphenopalatine foramen

Accessory meningeal artery
Middle meningeal artery

Auriculo-temporal nerve

Superficial temporal artery
Ascending pharyngeal artery
Ascending palatine artery
Tonsillar branches
Tonsillar artery
External carotid artery
Facial artery

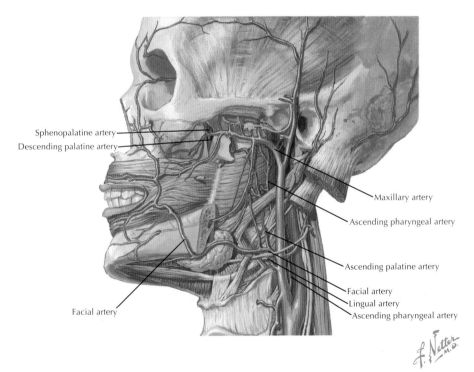

Sphenopalatine artery
Descending palatine artery

Maxillary artery

Ascending pharyngeal artery

Ascending palatine artery

Facial artery
Lingual artery
Ascending pharyngeal artery

Facial artery

**Figure 13-23**

| ARTERIAL SUPPLY OF THE FLOOR OF THE ORAL CAVITY | | |
| --- | --- | --- |
| **Artery** | **Source** | **Course** |
| Facial | External carotid a. | Arises in the carotid triangle of the neck |
| | | Passes superiorly immediately deep to the posterior belly of the digastric m. and the stylohyoid m. |
| | | Passes along the submandibular gland, giving rise to the submental a. that helps supply the gland |
| | | Passes superiorly over the body of the mandible at the masseter m. |
| *Ascending palatine* | Facial a. | Supplies the soft palate |
| | | Ascends between the styloglossus and stylopharyngeus mm. along the side of the pharynx |
| | | Divides near the levator veli palatini m. |
| | | A branch follows the levator veli palatini, supplying the soft palate and the palatine glands |
| | | A 2nd branch pierces the superior constrictor m. to supply the palatine tonsil and auditory tube |
| | | Anastomoses with the ascending pharyngeal and tonsillar aa. |
| *Submental* | Facial a. | Arises in the submandibular triangle of the neck |
| | | Supplies the submandibular gland and surrounding muscles |
| Lingual | External carotid a. | Passes superiorly and medially toward the hyoid bone |
| | | Curves inferiorly and anteriorly, forming a loop that lies on the middle constrictor m. and is passed superficially by the hypoglossal n. |
| | | Passes deep to the posterior belly of the digastric m. and the stylohyoid m., traveling anteriorly |
| | | Passes deep to the hyoglossus m. and ascends along the tongue |
| | | Gives rise to dorsal lingual branches, a sublingual branch, and the deep lingual branch |
| | | Sublingual branch begins at the anterior margin of the hyoglossus and travels anteriorly between the genioglossus and mylohyoideus mm. to supply the sublingual gland, surrounding muscles, and mucous membrane of the oral cavity and gingiva |
| | | Deep lingual branch passes anteriorly under the surface of the tongue, then anastomoses with the opposite deep lingual a. at the tip of the tongue |

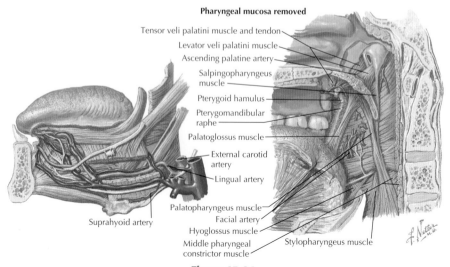

**Pharyngeal mucosa removed**

Tensor veli palatini muscle and tendon
Levator veli palatini muscle
Ascending palatine artery
Salpingopharyngeus muscle
Pterygoid hamulus
Pterygomandibular raphe
Palatoglossus muscle
External carotid artery
Lingual artery
Palatopharyngeus muscle
Suprahyoid artery
Facial artery
Hyoglossus muscle
Middle pharyngeal constrictor muscle
Stylopharyngeus muscle

**Figure 13-24**

| ARTERIAL SUPPLY OF THE MAXILLARY AND MANDIBULAR TEETH | | |
|---|---|---|
| **Artery** | **Source** | **Course** |
| Maxillary | External carotid a. | Gives rise to 3 branches that form a plexus to supply the maxillary arch:<br>• Anterior superior alveolar<br>• Middle superior alveolar<br>• Posterior superior alveolar<br>• Gives rise to 1 branch that supplies the mandibular arch:<br>• Inferior alveolar |
| Maxillary Teeth | | |
| Anterior superior alveolar | Infraorbital a. (of the maxillary a.) | Arises after the infraorbital a. passes through the inferior orbital fissure and into the infraorbital canal<br>Descends via the alveolar canals to supply part of the maxillary arch<br>Supplies the maxillary sinus and the anterior teeth |
| Middle superior alveolar | Infraorbital a. | May or may not be present<br>If present, arises from the infraorbital a. of the maxillary after it passes through the inferior orbital fissure and into the infraorbital canal<br>Descends via the alveolar canals to supply the maxillary sinus and supplies the plexus at the canine |
| Posterior superior alveolar | 3rd part of the maxillary a. | Arises before the maxillary a. enters the pterygopalatine fossa<br>Enters the infratemporal surface of the maxilla to supply the maxillary sinus, premolars, and molars |
| Mandibular Teeth | | |
| Inferior alveolar | 3rd part of the maxillary a. | Descends inferiorly following the inferior alveolar n. to enter the mandibular foramen<br>Terminates into the mental and incisive aa. at the region of the 2nd premolar<br>Supplies all of the mandibular teeth |
| *Mental* | Inferior alveolar a. | Supplies the labial gingiva of the anterior teeth |
| *Incisive* | Inferior alveolar a. | Supplies the anterior teeth |

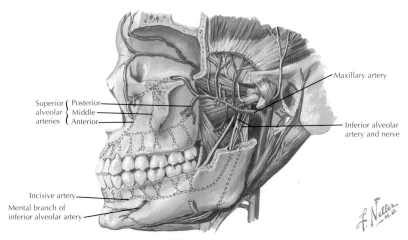

Superior alveolar arteries { Posterior / Middle / Anterior }

Maxillary artery

Inferior alveolar artery and nerve

Incisive artery

Mental branch of inferior alveolar artery

**Figure 13-25**

| VENOUS DRAINAGE OF THE PALATE AND FLOOR OF THE ORAL CAVITY ||
| Vein | Course |
| --- | --- |
| Greater palatine | Connect to the pterygoid plexus |
| Lesser palatine | |
| Sphenopalatine | |
| Lingual | Receives tributaries from the deep lingual vv. on the ventral surface, and dorsal lingual vv. from the dorsal surface of the tongue |
| | Passes with the lingual a., deep to the hyoglossus m., and ends in the internal jugular v. |
| | The vena comitans nervi hypoglossi, or accompanying vein of the hypoglossal n., begins at the apex of the tongue and may either join the lingual v. or accompany the hypoglossal n. and enter the common facial v., which empties into the internal jugular v. |
| Submental | Anastomoses with the branches of the lingual v. and the inferior alveolar v. |
| | Parallels the submental a. on the superficial surface of the mylohyoid m. |
| | Ends in the facial v. |
| Pharyngeal plexus | Located along the lateral pterygoid m. |
| | Most of the vessels in the infratemporal fossa and oral cavity drain into the pterygoid plexus |
| | Connected to the cavernous sinus, the pterygoid plexus of veins, and the facial v. |
| | Valveless |
| | Eventually drains into the maxillary v. |
| VENOUS DRAINAGE OF THE TEETH ||
| Vein | Course |
| Anterior superior alveolar | Drain onto the pterygoid plexus of veins |
| Middle superior alveolar | |
| Posterior superior alveolar | |
| Inferior alveolar | |

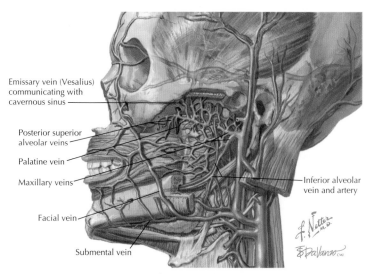

Emissary vein (Vesalius) communicating with cavernous sinus

Posterior superior alveolar veins

Palatine vein

Maxillary veins

Facial vein

Submental vein

Inferior alveolar vein and artery

**Figure 13-26**

- The oral cavity receives its sensory innervation from branches of the maxillary and mandibular divisions of the trigeminal nerve

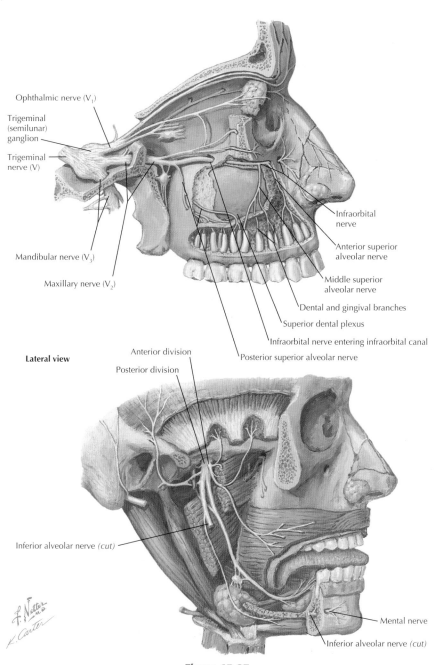

Ophthalmic nerve (V₁)

Trigeminal (semilunar) ganglion

Trigeminal nerve (V)

Infraorbital nerve

Anterior superior alveolar nerve

Mandibular nerve (V₃)

Maxillary nerve (V₂)

Middle superior alveolar nerve

Dental and gingival branches

Superior dental plexus

Infraorbital nerve entering infraorbital canal

**Lateral view**

Anterior division

Posterior division

Posterior superior alveolar nerve

Inferior alveolar nerve *(cut)*

Mental nerve

Inferior alveolar nerve *(cut)*

**Figure 13-27**

| MAXILLARY TEETH | | |
|---|---|---|
| **Nerve** | **Source** | **Course** |
| Maxillary | Trigeminal n. | Sensory in function |
| | | Travels along the lateral wall of the cavernous sinus |
| | | Passes from the middle cranial fossa into the pterygopalatine fossa via the foramen rotundum |
| | | Within the pterygopalatine fossa, it gives rise to 4 branches: |
| | | • Infraorbital (continuation of the maxillary) |
| | | • Ganglionic |
| | | • Posterior superior alveolar |
| | | • Zygomatic |
| | | The infraorbital n. gives rise to 2 branches that form a plexus with the posterior superior alveolar to supply the maxillary arch: |
| | | • Anterior superior alveolar |
| | | • Middle superior alveolar |
| *Infraorbital* | Continuation of the maxillary division of the trigeminal n. | Passes through the inferior orbital fissure to enter the orbit |
| | | Passes anteriorly through the infraorbital groove and infraorbital canal and exits onto the face via the infraorbital foramen |
| | | Once the infraorbital n. exits onto the face, it divides into 3 terminal branches: |
| | | • Nasal—supplies the ala of the nose |
| | | • Inferior palpebral—supplies the skin of the lower eyelid |
| | | • Superior labial—supplies the skin of the upper lip |
| • *Anterior superior alveolar* | Infraorbital n. as it travels in the infraorbital canal | As it descends to form the superior dental plexus, it innervates part of the maxillary sinus and generally the incisors and canines |
| • *Middle superior alveolar* | | A variable nerve |
| | | As it descends to form the superior dental plexus, it innervates part of the maxillary sinus and the premolars and possibly the mesiobuccal root of the 1st molar |
| *Posterior superior alveolar* | Maxillary n. in the pterygopalatine fossa | Travels laterally through the pterygomaxillary fissure to enter the infratemporal fossa |
| | | Enters the infratemporal surface of the maxilla |
| | | As it descends to form the superior dental plexus, it innervates part of the maxillary sinus and the molars, with the possible exception of the mesiobuccal root of the 1st molar |

| MANDIBULAR TEETH | | |
|---|---|---|
| **Nerve** | **Source** | **Course** |
| Mandibular | Trigeminal n. | This division has motor function in addition to sensory function<br><br>The largest of the 3 divisions of the trigeminal n.<br><br>Created by a large sensory and a small motor root that unite just after passing through the foramen ovale to enter the infratemporal fossa<br><br>Immediately gives rise to a meningeal branch and divides into an anterior and a posterior division<br><br>Anterior division is smaller and mainly motor, with 1 sensory branch (buccal):<br>• Masseteric<br>• Anterior and posterior deep temporal<br>• Medial pterygoid<br>• Lateral pterygoid<br>• Buccal<br><br>Posterior division is larger and mainly sensory, with 1 motor branch (mylohyoid):<br>• Auriculotemporal<br>• Lingual<br>• Inferior alveolar<br>• Mylohyoid |
| *Inferior alveolar* | The largest branch of the mandibular division | Descends, following the inferior alveolar a. inferior to the lateral pterygoid and, last, between the sphenomandibular ligament and the ramus of the mandible until it enters the mandibular foramen, where it terminates as the mental and incisive nn. in the area of the 2nd premolar<br><br>Innervates all mandibular teeth (via inferior alveolar and incisive nn.), periodontal ligaments (via inferior alveolar and incisive nn.), and the gingiva from the premolars anteriorly to the midline (via the mental branch) |
| • *Mental* | Inferior alveolar n. | Supplies the chin, lip, and facial gingiva and mucosa from the 2nd premolar anteriorly |
| • *Incisive* | | Supplies the teeth and periodontal ligaments from the 1st premolar anteriorly (depends on the location of the branching of the inferior alveolar n. into the incisive and mental nn.) |

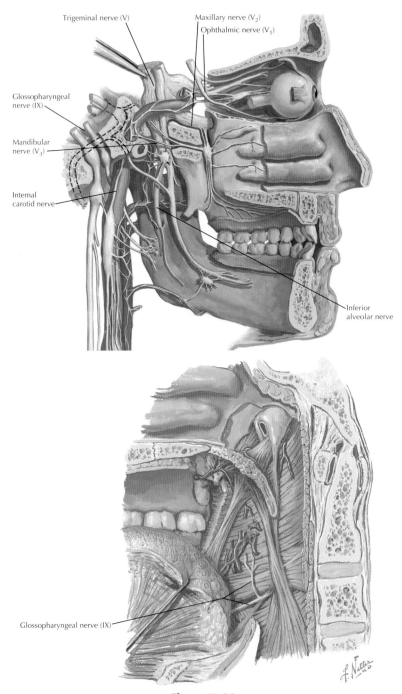

Trigeminal nerve (V)

Maxillary nerve (V₂)

Ophthalmic nerve (V₁)

Glossopharyngeal nerve (IX)

Mandibular nerve (V₃)

Internal carotid nerve

Inferior alveolar nerve

Glossopharyngeal nerve (IX)

**Figure 13-28**

| Nerve | Source | Course |
|-------|--------|--------|
| Lingual | Mandibular division of the trigeminal n. | Lies inferior to the lateral pterygoid and medial nn. and anterior to the inferior alveolar n. within the infratemporal fossa |
| | | The chorda tympani branch of the facial n. also joins the posterior part of the lingual n. |
| | | Passes between the medial pterygoid m. and the ramus of the mandible to pass obliquely to enter the oral cavity, bounded by the superior pharyngeal constrictor m., the medial pterygoid, and the mandible |
| | | Enters the oral cavity lying against the lingual tuberosity of the mandible |
| | | The submandibular ganglion is suspended from the lingual n. at the posterior border of the hyoglossus |
| | | Continues anteriorly and passes on the lateral surface of the hyoglossus |
| | | Passes from the lateral side, inferiorly, and medially to the submandibular duct to reach the mucosa of the tongue |
| | | Supplies general somatic afferent (GSA) fibers to the mucous membrane and papilla of the anterior 2/3 of the tongue and gingiva and mucosa on the lingual side of the mandibular teeth |
| Glossopharyngeal | Medulla oblongata | Passes through the jugular foramen with the vagus and accessory nn. |
| | | As it passes through the foramen, it passes between the internal carotid a. and the internal jugular v. |
| | | Continues to pass inferiorly and travels posterior to the stylopharyngeus m. |
| | | Passes anteriorly with the stylopharyngeus m. and travels between the superior and middle constrictor mm. to be located by the palatine tonsils |
| | | Small lingual branches arise from it and distribute GSA fibers to the mucous membrane of the posterior 1/3 of the tongue, in addition to the pillars of the fauces |
| | | In addition, small lingual branches arise from it and distribute special visceral afferent (SVA) fibers to the taste buds in the mucous membrane of the posterior 1/3 of the tongue and the circumvallate papillae |
| Internal laryngeal | Superior laryngeal branch of the vagus n. | Vagus n. branches from the medulla oblongata and passes through the jugular foramen with the glossopharyngeal and accessory nn. |
| | | As the vagus n. passes through the foramen, it passes between the internal carotid a. and the internal jugular v. |
| | | A series of nerves branch from the vagus in the neck, including the superior laryngeal n. |
| | | Superior laryngeal n. travels inferiorly posterior to the internal carotid a. and on the side of the pharynx and divides into the internal and external laryngeal nn. |
| | | Internal laryngeal n. passes inferiorly to the larynx and passes through the thyrohyoid membrane along with the superior laryngeal vessels |
| | | Branches of the internal laryngeal n. distribute the GSA fibers to the base of the tongue at the epiglottic region and to the mucous membranes of the larynx as far inferiorly as the false vocal folds |
| | | In addition, the branches distribute SVA fibers to the taste buds scattered at the base of the tongue at the epiglottic region |

*Continued on next page*

| Nerve | Source | Course |
|---|---|---|
| Chorda tympani | Facial n. in the tympanic cavity | Carries the preganglionic parasympathetic fibers to the submandibular ganglion and taste fibers to the anterior 2/3 of the tongue<br>Passes anteriorly to enter the tympanic cavity and lies along the tympanic membrane and malleus until exiting the petrotympanic fissure<br>Once it exits the petrotympanic fissure, the chorda tympani joins the posterior border of the lingual n.<br>The lingual n. is distributed to the anterior 2/3 of the tongue and the SVA fibers from the chorda tympani travel to the taste buds in this region |

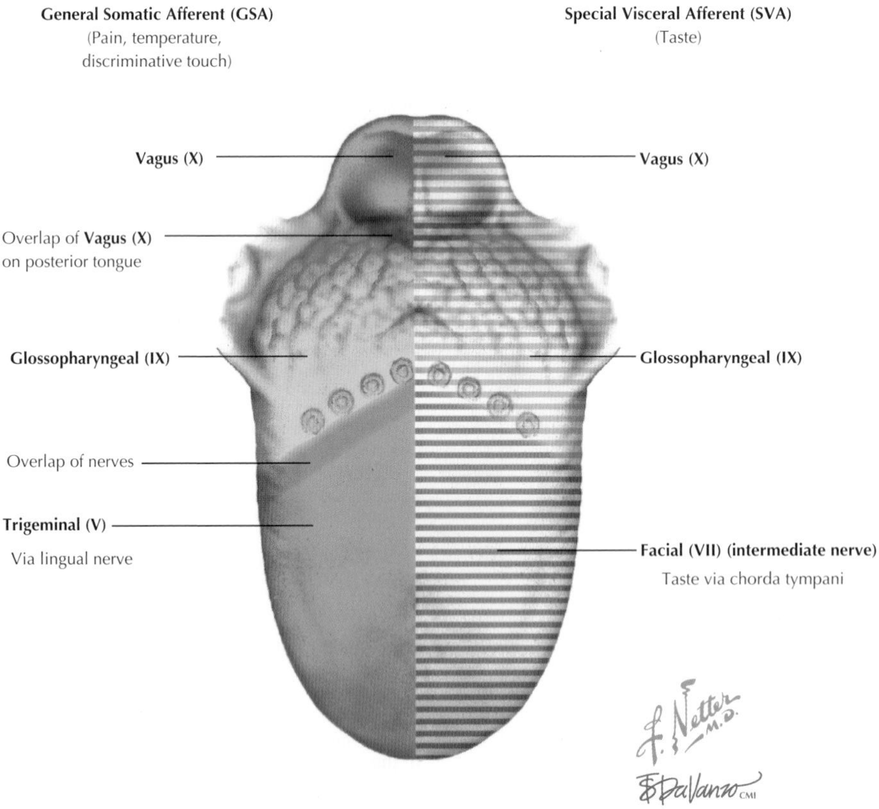
General Somatic Afferent (GSA)
(Pain, temperature, discriminative touch)
Special Visceral Afferent (SVA)
(Taste)
Vagus (X)
Vagus (X)
Overlap of Vagus (X) on posterior tongue
Glossopharyngeal (IX)
Glossopharyngeal (IX)
Overlap of nerves
Trigeminal (V)
Via lingual nerve
Facial (VII) (intermediate nerve)
Taste via chorda tympani
F. Netter M.D.
DaVanzo CMI

**Figure 13-29**

| Nerve | Source | Course |
|---|---|---|
| Maxillary | Trigeminal n. | Sensory in function<br><br>Travels along the lateral wall of the cavernous sinus<br><br>Passes from the middle cranial fossa into the pterygopalatine fossa via the foramen rotundum<br><br>Within the pterygopalatine fossa, it gives rise to 4 branches:<br><br>• Infraorbital (considered the continuation of the maxillary)<br>• Ganglionic<br>• Posterior superior alveolar<br>• Zygomatic<br><br>The infraorbital passes through the inferior orbital fissure to enter the orbit and passes anteriorly through the infraorbital groove and canal and exits onto the face via the infraorbital foramen<br><br>Once the infraorbital n. exits onto the face, it divides into 3 terminal branches:<br><br>• Nasal—supplies the ala of the nose<br>• Inferior palpebral—supplies the skin of the lower eyelid<br>• Superior labial—supplies the skin of the upper lip; 3 of its branches form a plexus to supply the maxillary arch:<br>  • Anterior superior alveolar<br>  • Middle superior alveolar<br>  • Posterior superior alveolar |
| *Nasopalatine* | Maxillary division of the trigeminal n. via the pterygopalatine ganglion in the pterygopalatine fossa | Passes through the sphenopalatine foramen to enter the nasal cavity<br><br>Passes along the superior portion of the nasal cavity to the nasal septum, where it travels anteroinferiorly to the incisive canal supplying the septum<br><br>Once entering the oral cavity, it provides sensory innervation to the palatal gingiva and mucosa from the area anterior to the premolars |
| *Greater palatine* | | Passes through the palatine canal to enter the hard palate via the greater palatine foramen<br><br>Provides sensory innervation to the palatal gingiva and mucosa from the premolars to the posterior border of the hard palate |
| *Lesser palatine* | | Passes through the palatine canal to enter the hard palate via the lesser palatine foramen<br><br>Provides sensory innervation to the soft palate |
| Glossopharyngeal | Medulla oblongata | Passes through the jugular foramen with the vagus and accessory nn.<br><br>As it passes through the foramen, it passes between the internal carotid a. and internal jugular v.<br><br>Continues to pass inferiorly and travels posterior to the stylopharyngeus m.<br><br>Passes anteriorly with the stylopharyngeus and travels between the superior and middle constrictor mm. to be located by the palatine tonsils<br><br>Small lingual branches arise from it and distribute general somatic afferent fibers to the mucous membrane of the posterior 1/3 of the tongue, in addition to the pillars of the fauces |

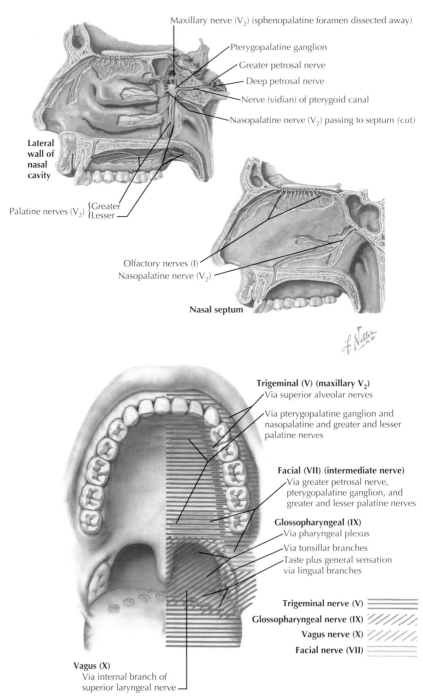

Maxillary nerve (V₂) (sphenopalatine foramen dissected away)

Pterygopalatine ganglion

Greater petrosal nerve

Deep petrosal nerve

Nerve (vidian) of pterygoid canal

Nasopalatine nerve (V₂) passing to septum *(cut)*

**Lateral wall of nasal cavity**

Palatine nerves (V₂) {Greater {Lesser

Olfactory nerves (I)
Nasopalatine nerve (V₂)

**Nasal septum**

**Trigeminal (V) (maxillary V₂)**
Via superior alveolar nerves

Via pterygopalatine ganglion and nasopalatine and greater and lesser palatine nerves

**Facial (VII) (intermediate nerve)**
Via greater petrosal nerve, pterygopalatine ganglion, and greater and lesser palatine nerves

**Glossopharyngeal (IX)**
Via pharyngeal plexus

Via tonsillar branches

Taste plus general sensation via lingual branches

**Trigeminal nerve (V)**
**Glossopharyngeal nerve (IX)**
**Vagus nerve (X)**
**Facial nerve (VII)**

**Vagus (X)**
Via internal branch of superior laryngeal nerve

**Figure 13-30**

- There are 3 pairs of major salivary glands:
  - Parotid gland
  - Submandibular gland
  - Sublingual gland
- They secrete saliva into the oral cavity to aid in the digestion, mastication, and deglutition of food
- Saliva is mucous or serous in consistency
- Many minor salivary glands are ubiquitously distributed throughout the oral mucosa of the oral cavity

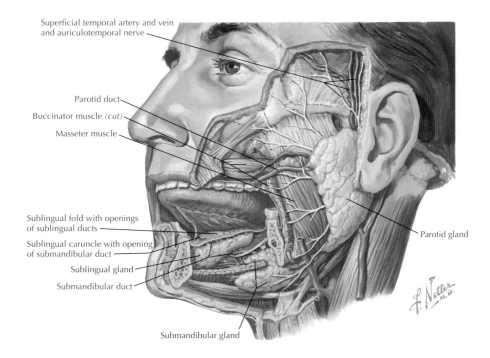

Superficial temporal artery and vein and auriculotemporal nerve

Parotid duct

Buccinator muscle *(cut)*

Masseter muscle

Sublingual fold with openings of sublingual ducts

Sublingual caruncle with opening of submandibular duct

Sublingual gland

Submandibular duct

Parotid gland

Submandibular gland

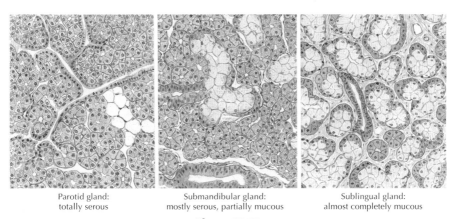

Parotid gland:
totally serous

Submandibular gland:
mostly serous, partially mucous

Sublingual gland:
almost completely mucous

**Figure 13-31**

| FEATURES OF THE MAJOR SALIVARY GLANDS | | | |
|---|---|---|---|
| **Gland** | **Duct** | **Comment** | **Autonomic Innervation** |
| Parotid | Parotid duct (Stensen's duct) | The largest salivary gland<br><br>Pyramidal in shape, with up to 5 processes (or extensions)<br><br>Saliva created by the parotid is serous<br><br>Facial n. splits the parotid gland into a superficial lobe and a deep lobe, which are connected by an isthmus<br><br>The parotid duct (Stensen's duct) forms within the deep lobe and passes from the anterior border of the gland across the masseter m. superficially, through the buccinator m. into the oral cavity opposite the 2nd maxillary molar | Glossopharyngeal n. |
| Submandibular | Submandibular duct (Wharton's duct) | 2nd largest salivary gland<br><br>A mixed salivary gland, secreting both serous and mucous saliva, but predominantly serous-secreting<br><br>Wraps around the posterior border of the mylohyoid m., to be located in the submandibular triangle of the neck and the floor of the oral cavity<br><br>The part of the submandibular gland located in the submandibular triangle is referred to as the superficial portion and is surrounded by the investing layer of deep cervical fascia<br><br>Facial a. crosses between the submandibular gland and the mandible before giving off the submental a., while the facial v. normally lies superficial to the gland<br><br>Deep portion of the submandibular gland lies in the oral cavity between the hyoglossus m. and the mandible and ends at the posterior border of the sublingual gland<br><br>The submandibular duct lies along the sublingual gland and empties into the oral cavity at the sublingual papilla | Facial n. |
| Sublingual | Numerous small ducts opening along the sublingual fold | Smallest of the 3 major salivary glands<br><br>A mixed salivary gland, secreting both mucous and serous saliva, but predominantly mucus-secreting<br><br>Located in the oral cavity between the mucosa of the oral cavity and the mylohyoid m.<br><br>Creates a sublingual fold in the floor of the oral cavity<br><br>Lies between the sublingual fossa of the mandible and the genioglossus m. of the tongue<br><br>The submandibular duct lies on the sublingual gland<br><br>Bartholin's duct, a common duct that drains the anterior part of the gland in the region of the sublingual papilla, may be present | |

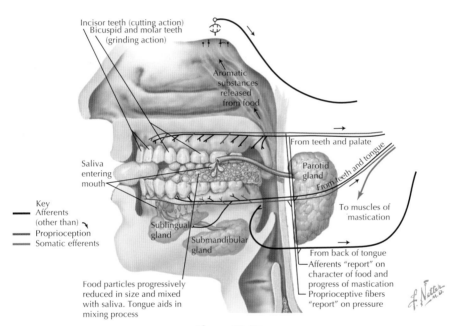

Incisor teeth (cutting action)
Bicuspid and molar teeth (grinding action)

Aromatic substances released from food

From teeth and palate

From teeth and tongue

Parotid gland

Saliva entering mouth

To muscles of mastication

**Key**
Afferents (other than)
Proprioception
Somatic efferents

Sublingual gland

Submandibular gland

From back of tongue
Afferents "report" on character of food and progress of mastication
Proprioceptive fibers "report" on pressure

Food particles progressively reduced in size and mixed with saliva. Tongue aids in mixing process

**Figure 13-32**

| PARASYMPATHETICS OF THE PAROTID GLAND | | | |
|---|---|---|---|
| **Type of Neuron** | **Name of Cell Body** | **Characteristics of Cell Body** | **Course of the Neuron** |
| Preganglionic neuron | Inferior salivatory nucleus | A collection of nerve cell bodies located in the medulla | Preganglionic parasympathetic fibers arise from the inferior salivatory nucleus in the medulla<br><br>Travel through the glossopharyngeal n. and exit the jugular foramen<br><br>Gives rise to the tympanic branch of cranial n. IX, which reenters the skull via the tympanic canaliculus<br><br>The tympanic branch of IX forms the tympanic plexus along the promontory of the ear<br><br>The plexus re-forms as the lesser petrosal n., typically exiting the foramen ovale to enter the infratemporal fossa<br><br>Lesser petrosal n. joins the otic ganglion |
| Postganglionic neuron | Otic ganglion | A collection of nerve cell bodies located inferior to the foramen ovale, medial to the mandibular division of the trigeminal | Postganglionic parasympathetic fibers arise in the otic ganglion<br><br>These fibers travel to the auriculotemporal branch of the trigeminal n.<br><br>Auriculotemporal n. travels to parotid gland<br><br>Postganglionic parasympathetic fibers innervate the:<br>• Parotid gland |

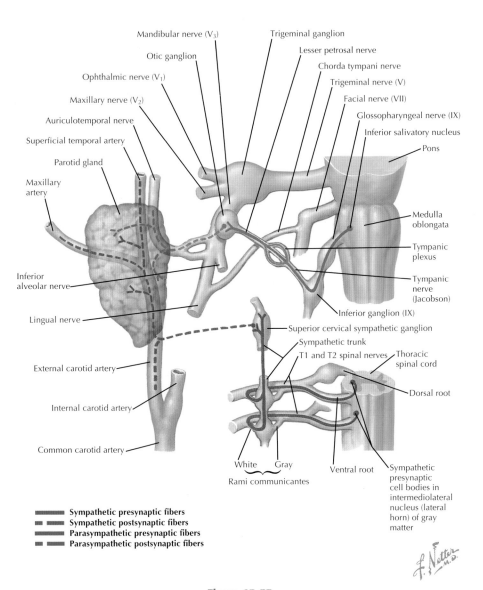

Figure 13-33

| PARASYMPATHETICS OF THE SUBMANDIBULAR, SUBLINGUAL, AND MINOR SALIVARY GLANDS | | | |
|---|---|---|---|
| **Type of Neuron** | **Name of Cell Body** | **Characteristics of Cell Body** | **Course of the Neuron** |
| Preganglionic neuron | Superior salivatory nucleus | A collection of nerve cell bodies located in the pons<br><br>Travel through the nervus intermedius of the facial n. into the internal acoustic meatus<br><br>In the facial canal, the facial n. gives rise to 2 parasympathetic branches:<br>• Greater petrosal n.<br>• Chorda tympani n. | **Greater Petrosal Nerve**<br>Exits along the hiatus for the greater petrosal n. toward the foramen lacerum, where it joins the deep petrosal n. (sympathetics) to form the nerve of the pterygoid canal (vidian n.)<br>Vidian n. passes through the pterygoid canal and enters the pterygopalatine fossa, where it joins with the pterygopalatine ganglion<br>**Chorda Tympani Nerve**<br>Exits the petrotympanic fissure to enter the infratemporal fossa, where it joins the lingual n.<br>Preganglionic fibers travel with the lingual n. into the floor of the oral cavity, where it joins with the submandibular ganglion |
| Postganglionic neuron | Pterygopalatine ganglion | A collection of nerve cell bodies located in the pterygopalatine fossa<br><br>Postganglionic parasympathetic fibers that arise in the pterygopalatine ganglion are distributed to the ophthalmic and maxillary divisions of the trigeminal n. to the:<br>• Lacrimal gland<br>• Nasal glands<br>• Palatine glands<br>• Pharyngeal glands<br>• Paranasal sinus glands | **Ophthalmic and Maxillary Division Distribution**<br>Postganglionic fibers travel along the zygomatic branch of the maxillary division for a short distance to enter the orbit<br>A short communicating branch joins the lacrimal n. of the ophthalmic division of the trigeminal n.<br>These fibers innervate:<br>• Lacrimal gland, to cause the secretion of tears<br>**Maxillary Division Distribution**<br>Postganglionic fibers travel along the maxillary division of the trigeminal n. to be distributed along its branches that are located in the nasal cavity, oral cavity, and pharynx (e.g., nasopalatine, greater palatine)<br>These fibers innervate:<br>• Nasal glands<br>• Palatine glands<br>• Pharyngeal glands<br>• Paranasal sinus glands |
| | Submandibular ganglion | A collection of nerve cell bodies in the oral cavity<br><br>Suspended from the lingual n. at the posterior border of the mylohyoid m. immediately superior to the deep portion of the submandibular gland | Postganglionic parasympathetic fibers arise in the submandibular ganglion and are distributed to the:<br>• Submandibular gland<br>• Sublingual gland |

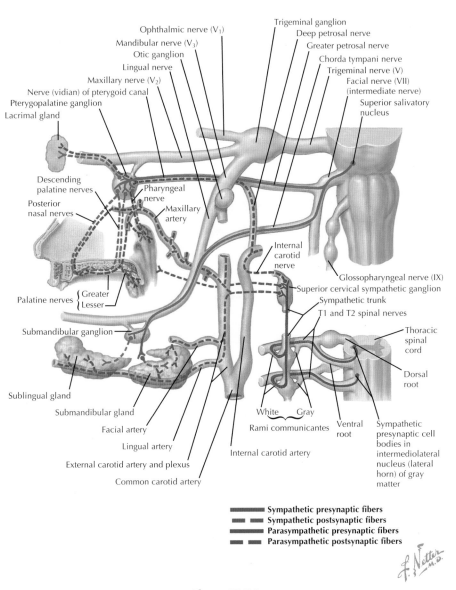

Ophthalmic nerve (V₁)
Mandibular nerve (V₃)
Otic ganglion
Lingual nerve
Maxillary nerve (V₂)
Nerve (vidian) of pterygoid canal
Pterygopalatine ganglion
Lacrimal gland

Trigeminal ganglion
Deep petrosal nerve
Greater petrosal nerve
Chorda tympani nerve
Trigeminal nerve (V)
Facial nerve (VII)
(intermediate nerve)
Superior salivatory
nucleus

Descending
palatine nerves
Posterior
nasal nerves

Pharyngeal
nerve
Maxillary
artery

Internal
carotid
nerve

Glossopharyngeal nerve (IX)
Superior cervical sympathetic ganglion
Sympathetic trunk
T1 and T2 spinal nerves

Palatine nerves { Greater
Lesser

Submandibular ganglion

Thoracic
spinal
cord

Dorsal
root

Sublingual gland

Submandibular gland
Facial artery
Lingual artery
External carotid artery and plexus
Common carotid artery

White    Gray
Rami communicantes

Internal carotid artery

Ventral
root

Sympathetic
presynaptic cell
bodies in
intermediolateral
nucleus (lateral
horn) of gray
matter

▬▬▬ Sympathetic presynaptic fibers
▬ ▬ Sympathetic postsynaptic fibers
▬▬▬ Parasympathetic presynaptic fibers
▬ ▬ Parasympathetic postsynaptic fibers

**Figure 13-34**

- *Gingivitis*: an inflammation of the gingiva that occurs when bacteria accumulate between the teeth and gingiva
- In addition to the inflammation, the gums may demonstrate irritation and bleeding
- When plaque (composed of bacteria, food debris, and saliva) is deposited on the teeth, it can form tartar if it is not removed
- Plaque and tartar cause irritation to the gingiva, and the bacteria (and their toxins) further irritate the gingiva, leading to bleeding and swelling
- If gingivitis remains untreated, it may progress to more serious gingival diseases, such as periodontitis
- Long-term untreated gingivitis may lead to damage of bone and loss of teeth
- Risk factors for gingivitis include poor dental hygiene, pregnancy, diabetes, illness, and human immunodeficiency virus (HIV) infection

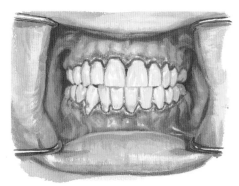

Marginal gingivitis

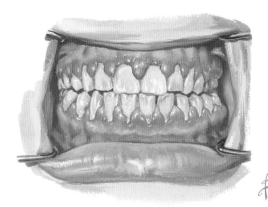

Hypertrophic gingivitis

**Figure 13-35**

- *Dental caries* (tooth decay), leading to "cavities," are caused by bacteria in the oral cavity
- The bacteria convert foods into acids and help form plaque (made of bacteria, food debris, and saliva), which is deposited on the teeth
- Plaque that is not removed from the teeth can mineralize to form tartar
- Plaque is most prominent on difficult-to-reach teeth, such as the posterior molars
- Acids formed in the plaque begin to erode the enamel on the surface of the tooth, causing a "cavity"
- If not treated, the cavity grows in size, with onset of pain as the nerves and blood vessels of the affected teeth become irritated
- Consuming foods rich in sugar and starch increases the risk of dental caries
- Dental caries can be detected on routine dental examinations
- The damage associated with dental caries cannot be repaired by the affected tooth, which now must be restored
- Fluoride is used to reduce the risk of dental caries by inhibiting demineralization and promoting remineralization of tooth structure
- Saliva helps promote the remineralization process; medications that decrease salivary flow (such as anticholinergics) promote dental caries

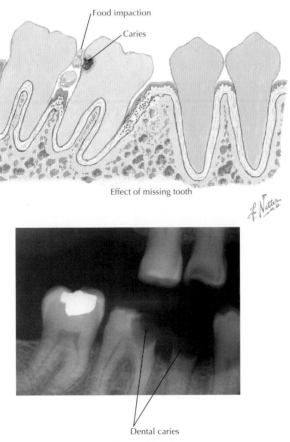

Food impaction

Caries

Effect of missing tooth

Dental caries

**Figure 13-36**

- *Torus*: a nonpathologic bony elevation that occurs in the oral cavity
- The presence of a torus does not impede eating or verbal communication but can cause difficulty in the application of a dental appliance, such as a denture
- 2 major types:
  - Palatine–a downgrowth of bone in the midline of the hard palate
  - Mandibular–an outgrowth of bone that occurs on the lingual surface of the mandible
- A torus does not require treatment unless it interferes with normal function or application of dental appliances

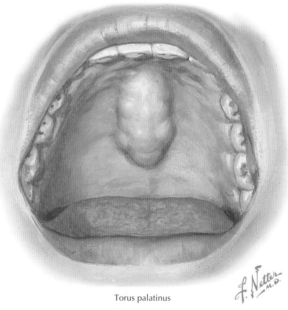

Torus palatinus

**Figure 13-37**

- *Mucocele*: a mucous cyst that results from obstruction of the ducts of minor salivary glands (this lesion also can be associated with blockage of the major salivary glands)
- Often caused by trauma to the duct system
- Usually located on the lingual aspect of the lip
- These lesions contain mucin and granulation tissue
- Persistent mucoceles often are excised

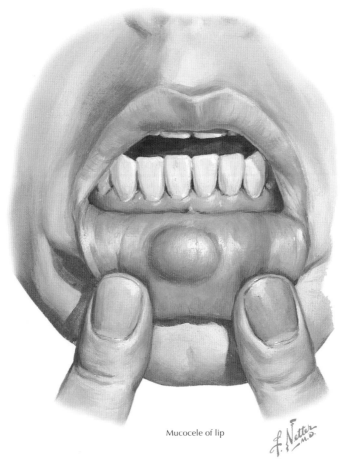

Mucocele of lip

**Figure 13-38**

- *Herpes simplex* is the most common cause of viral stomatitis
- Caused by exposure to herpes simplex virus type 1 (HSV-1)
- HSV-1 usually affects the regions above the waist, causing fever blisters
- Most affected people acquire the infection as a child
- During the primary infection with HSV-1, multiple vesicles appear on the lips, gingiva, hard palate, and tongue
- These vesicles rupture, producing ulcers that heal in 7 to 10 days
- After initial exposure, the virus is transported along a retrograde path into the trigeminal ganglion, where it stays inactive and does not replicate
- Episodes may recur
- Some recurrence triggers:
  - Stress
  - Fever
  - Anxiety
  - Exposure to the sun
  - Suppressed immune system
- Infection can be spread through contact with infected lips
- Systemic administration of antiviral agents, such as acyclovir, decreases the duration of the recurrent episodes

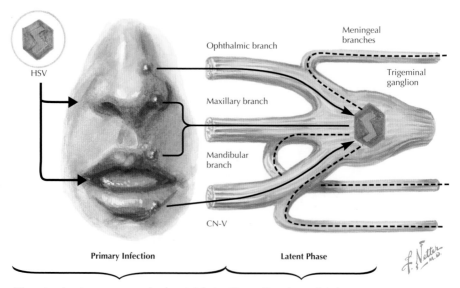

| Primary Infection | Latent Phase |
|---|---|
| Virus enters via cutaneous or mucosal surfaces to infect sensory or autonomic nerve endings with transport to cell bodies in ganglia. | Virus replicates in ganglia before establishing latent phase. |

**Figure 13-39**

- *Tonsillitis*: an inflammation of the tonsils, the lymph nodes located in the oral cavity and pharynx
- There are 3 sets of tonsils:
  - Pharyngeal (adenoids)
  - Palatine (between the palatoglossal and palatopharyngeal arches)
  - Lingual (on posterior 1/3 of the tongue)
- These 3 sets of tonsils form Waldeyer's ring
- Symptoms of tonsillitis:
  - Sore throat
  - Dysphagia
  - Fever
  - Headache
- Tonsillitis often is caused by a virus or bacterium
- When caused by a bacterial infection, it may be treated by antibiotics
- If necessary, a tonsillectomy is performed to remove the tonsils. Palatine tonsils are removed in a tonsillectomy (although the pharyngeal tonsils also may be removed at the same time, especially if they are obstructing nasal breathing)

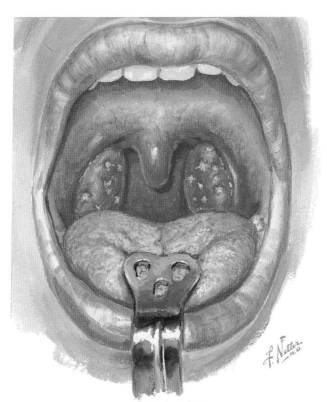

Acute follicular tonsillitis

**Figure 13-40**

- *Sialolithiasis* is a condition in which stones or calculi form in the salivary glands or ducts
- Greater than 80% of sialoliths are of submandibular gland origin
- More common in men than in women
- When saliva diminishes in flow, it is easier for stones or calculi to form
- Certain medications, such as anticholinergics, diminish salivary flow, making the patient more susceptible to the formation of sialoliths
- Treatment includes conservative methods such as hydration and warm compresses and more specific approaches ranging from antibiotics to surgical intervention
- Other treatments include shock-wave lithotripsy and endoscopic intracorporeal laser lithotripsy to fracture the sialolith into smaller pieces to pass

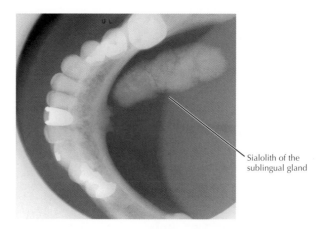

Sialolith of the
sublingual gland

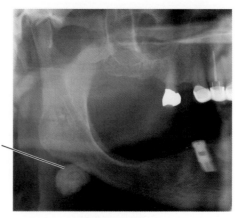

Sialolith of the
submandibular gland

**Figure 13-41**

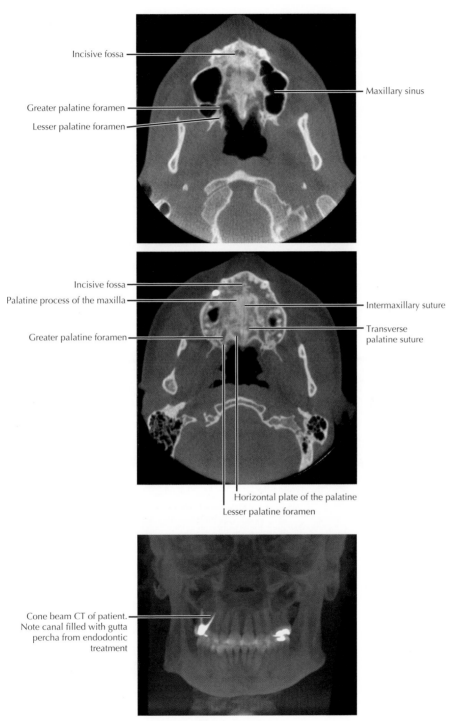

Incisive fossa

Greater palatine foramen

Lesser palatine foramen

Maxillary sinus

Incisive fossa

Palatine process of the maxilla

Greater palatine foramen

Intermaxillary suture

Transverse
palatine suture

Horizontal plate of the palatine

Lesser palatine foramen

Cone beam CT of patient.
Note canal filled with gutta
percha from endodontic
treatment

**Figure 13-42**

**Dental Procedures and Findings**

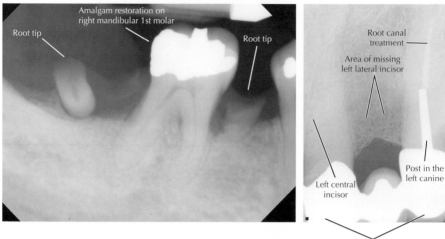

Root tip

Amalgam restoration on
right mandibular 1st molar

Root tip

Root canal
treatment

Area of missing
left lateral incisor

Post in the
left canine

Left central
incisor

Bridge between the left central incisor
and the left canine (with a post)

**Panoramic X-rays**

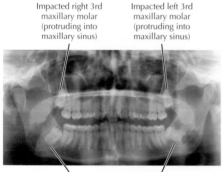

Impacted right 3rd
maxillary molar
(protruding into
maxillary sinus)

Impacted left 3rd
maxillary molar
(protruding into
maxillary sinus)

Mandibular
Condyle   fossa

Maxillary
sinus

Caries on left 3rd
maxillary molar

Impacted right 3rd
mandibular molar

Impacted left 3rd
mandibular molar

Mental
foramen

Mandibular
canal

**Maxillary and Mandibular Radiographs**

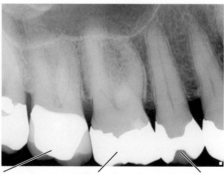

2nd maxillary molar
(porcelain fused to
metal crown – PFM)

1st maxillary molar (with
metallic restoration)

2nd maxillary premolar
(with metallic restoration)

**Figure 13-43**

**Maxillary and Mandibular Radiographs**

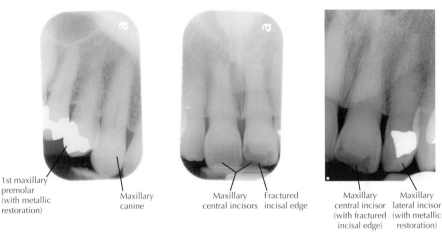

1st maxillary premolar (with metallic restoration)

Maxillary canine

Maxillary central incisors

Fractured incisal edge

Maxillary central incisor (with fractured incisal edge)

Maxillary lateral incisor (with metallic restoration)

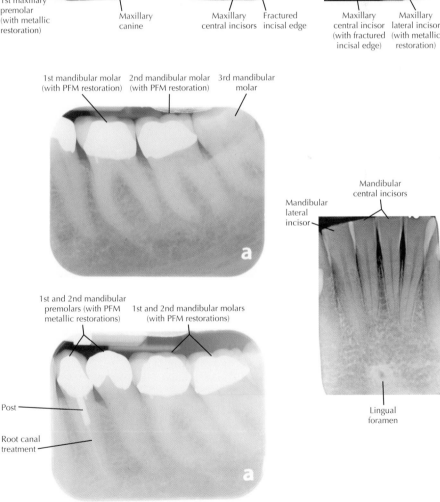

1st mandibular molar (with PFM restoration)

2nd mandibular molar (with PFM restoration)

3rd mandibular molar

Mandibular central incisors

Mandibular lateral incisor

1st and 2nd mandibular premolars (with PFM metallic restorations)

1st and 2nd mandibular molars (with PFM restorations)

Post

Root canal treatment

Lingual foramen

**Figure 13-44**

- *Tongue*: a muscular structure in the oral cavity, divided into 2 parts:
  - Oral (presulcal), movable part—the anterior 2/3 of the tongue
  - Pharyngeal (postsulcal), nonmovable part—the posterior 1/3 of the tongue
- The sulcus terminalis, a V-shaped groove immediately posterior to the circumvallate papilla, separates the oral part from the pharyngeal part of the tongue
- The foramen cecum, which was the initial development site for the thyroid gland, is located at the tip (or angle) of the V
- Median fibrous septum separates the tongue into halves

## FUNCTIONS

- Mastication
- Taste
- Talking
- Deglutition

## APPEARANCE

- The tongue typically is pink and covered with numerous small bumps called papilla
- Change in color or texture may reflect health problems:
  - Leukoplakia
  - Squamous cell carcinoma
  - Nutritional deficiencies
- An unusual appearance of the tongue may represent a benign harmless condition:
  - Fissured tongue
  - Black hairy tongue
  - Geographic tongue

## MUSCLE TYPES

- *Extrinsic*—move the tongue as an anatomic structure
- *Intrinsic*—change the tongue's shape

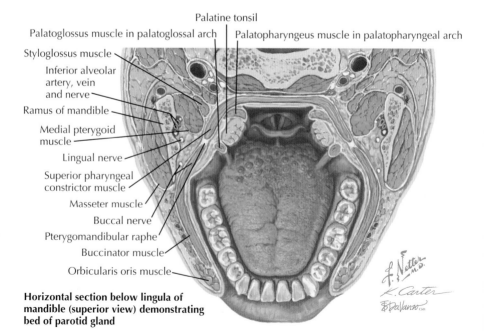

Palatine tonsil

Palatoglossus muscle in palatoglossal arch

Palatopharyngeus muscle in palatopharyngeal arch

Styloglossus muscle

Inferior alveolar artery, vein and nerve

Ramus of mandible

Medial pterygoid muscle

Lingual nerve

Superior pharyngeal constrictor muscle

Masseter muscle

Buccal nerve

Pterygomandibular raphe

Buccinator muscle

Orbicularis oris muscle

**Horizontal section below lingula of mandible (superior view) demonstrating bed of parotid gland**

**Figure 14-1**

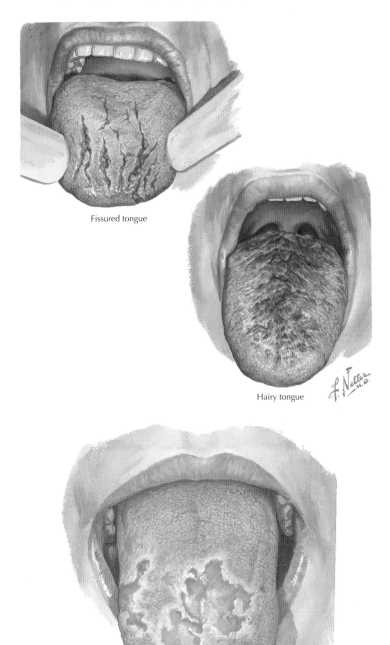

Fissured tongue

Hairy tongue

Geographic tongue

**Figure 14-2**

| ORAL PART (PRESULCAL) |
|---|
| • The oral part of the tongue is also known as the anterior 2/3 of the tongue |
| • Develops from the 2 lateral lingual swellings and tuberculum impar of the 1st pharyngeal arch—thus mucosa is innervated by the nerve of the 1st arch, which is the trigeminal nerve (lingual n.) |
| • Has a dorsal and a ventral surface |

| Dorsal Surface |
|---|
| • The mucosa is keratinized stratified squamous epithelium |
| • Is bounded posteriorly by the sulcus terminalis |

| Structures | Comments |
|---|---|
| Median sulcus | A groove that travels anteriorly in the midline |
| | Represents the location of the median septum that divides the tongue in halves |
| | The septum is thicker posteriorly but thinner anteriorly |
| Papillae—there are 4 types of papillae on the dorsal surface of the tongue: | Papillae are raised projections that increase the surface area |
| • Filiform—lack taste buds | 5 basic types of taste are differentiated by the taste buds: |
|   Most numerous type of papillae | • *Bitter* |
|   Have thick keratin on epithelium | • *Salt* |
| • Fungiform—have taste buds that receive taste innervation from the facial nerve (chorda tympani branch) | • *Sweet* |
|   Scattered throughout the dorsum of the oral part | • *Sour* |
|   Lack keratin on the epithelium | • *Umami* |
| • Foliate—have taste buds that receive taste innervation from the facial nerve (chorda tympani branch) | |
|   Are located on the sides of the tongue in 4 to 5 folds immediately anterior to the palatoglossal fold | |
|   Lack keratin on the epithelium | |
| • Circumvallate—have taste buds that receive taste innervation from the glossopharyngeal nerve | |
|   Generally a nonkeratinized epithelium | |
|   Lie in a row immediately anterior to the sulcus terminalis | |
| Glands | There are numerous mucous and serous glands on the dorsal surface |

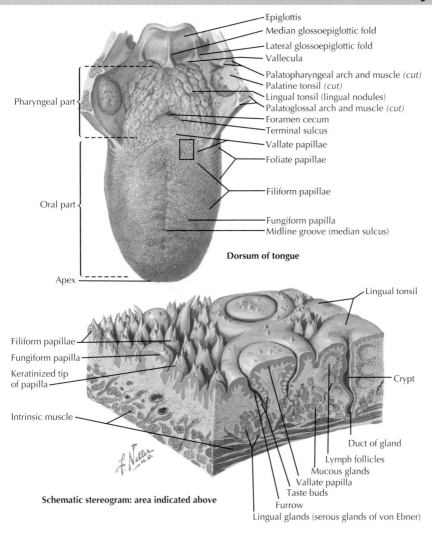

Epiglottis
Median glossoepiglottic fold
Lateral glossoepiglottic fold
Vallecula
Palatopharyngeal arch and muscle *(cut)*
Palatine tonsil *(cut)*
Lingual tonsil (lingual nodules)
Palatoglossal arch and muscle *(cut)*
Foramen cecum
Terminal sulcus
Vallate papillae
Foliate papillae
Filiform papillae
Fungiform papilla
Midline groove (median sulcus)

Pharyngeal part

Oral part

Apex

**Dorsum of tongue**

Lingual tonsil
Filiform papillae
Fungiform papilla
Keratinized tip of papilla
Intrinsic muscle
Crypt
Duct of gland
Lymph follicles
Mucous glands
Vallate papilla
Taste buds
Furrow
Lingual glands (serous glands of von Ebner)

**Schematic stereogram: area indicated above**

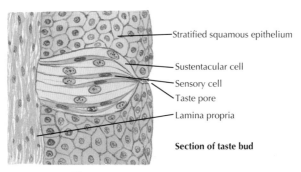

Stratified squamous epithelium
Sustentacular cell
Sensory cell
Taste pore
Lamina propria

**Section of taste bud**

**Figure 14-3**

TONGUE **403**

| Ventral Surface | |
| --- | --- |
| • The mucosa is nonkeratinized stratified squamous epithelium | |
| **Structures** | **Comments** |
| Lingual frenulum | A midline fold of tissue<br>Connects the ventral surface of the tongue to the floor of the oral cavity |
| Sublingual papilla | A swelling on both sides of the lingual frenulum at the tongue base<br>Marks the entrance of saliva from the submandibular glands into the oral cavity<br>Continuous with the sublingual folds overlying the sublingual glands on the floor of the oral cavity |
| Plica fimbriata | Fimbriated folds<br>Lateral to the lingual frenulum |
| Deep lingual veins | Can be observed through the mucosa between the plica fimbriata and the lingual frenulum |

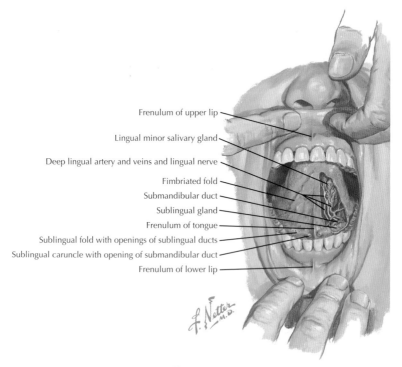

Frenulum of upper lip

Lingual minor salivary gland

Deep lingual artery and veins and lingual nerve

Fimbriated fold

Submandibular duct

Sublingual gland

Frenulum of tongue

Sublingual fold with openings of sublingual ducts

Sublingual caruncle with opening of submandibular duct

Frenulum of lower lip

**Figure 14-4**

| PHARYNGEAL PART (POSTSULCAL) |
|---|

- The pharyngeal part of the tongue is also known as the posterior 1/3 of the tongue
- Develops from the hypobranchial eminence of the 3rd pharyngeal arch—thus mucosa is innervated by the nerve of the 3rd arch (the glossopharyngeal nerve)
- The area immediately posterior to the palatoglossal folds (also called the anterior pillar of the fauces) is the oropharynx
- Has a dorsal surface only
- Does not possess any papilla

| Dorsal Surface |
|---|

- The mucosa is nonkeratinized stratified squamous epithelium

| Structures | Comments |
|---|---|
| Lingual tonsils | Large nodules of lymphatic tissue<br>Cover the pharyngeal surface of the tongue |
| Glossoepiglottic folds | Mucous membrane of nonkeratinized stratified squamous epithelium from the pharyngeal part and lateral wall of pharynx that reflects onto the anterior epiglottis, forming:<br>• Median glossoepiglottic fold<br>• 2 lateral glossoepiglottic folds<br>The median glossoepiglottic fold is bordered by a depression on each side:<br>• Vallecula<br>Connect the posterior portion of the pharyngeal part of the tongue with the epiglottis of the larynx |

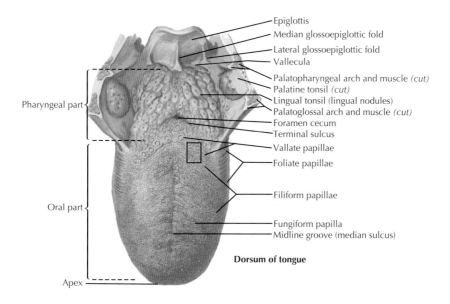

Epiglottis
Median glossoepiglottic fold
Lateral glossoepiglottic fold
Vallecula
Palatopharyngeal arch and muscle *(cut)*
Palatine tonsil *(cut)*
Lingual tonsil (lingual nodules)
Palatoglossal arch and muscle *(cut)*
Foramen cecum
Terminal sulcus
Vallate papillae
Foliate papillae
Filiform papillae
Fungiform papilla
Midline groove (median sulcus)

Pharyngeal part

Oral part

Apex

**Dorsum of tongue**

| Muscle | Origin | Insertion | Actions | Nerve | Comment |
|--------|--------|-----------|---------|-------|---------|
| Genioglossus | Superior genial tubercle of the mandible | Superior fibers fan into the entire ventral surface of the tongue while intermixing with the intrinsic muscles) Intermediate fibers fan posteriorly in attach to the posterior tongue Inferior fibers insert into the body of the hyoid via an aponeurosis | Protrusion of the tongue *Bilaterally*—the 2 muscles will depress the central portion of the tongue, which makes the dorsal surface concave *Unilaterally*—makes the tongue deviate to the contralateral side | Hypoglossal n. | The lingual a. is located between the genioglossus and hyoglossus mm. |
| Hyoglossus | Greater cornu and anterior portion of the body of the hyoid | Lateral portion of the tongue between the styloglossus m. and the inferior longitudinal m. | Depresses the tongue | | The lingual n., hypoglossal n., and submandibular duct are located on the lateral surface of the hyoglossus m. Some authors describe the chondroglossus as a separate muscle or as part of the hyoglossus |
| Styloglossus | Anterolateral portion near the apex of the styloid process Stylomandibular ligament | Longitudinal portion inserts into the dorsolateral part of the tongue to intermix with the inferior longitudinal m. Oblique portion inserts into the dorsolateral portion of the tongue to intermix with the hyoglossus m. | Retrusion of the tongue Elevation of the tongue | | Smallest of the extrinsic tongue muscles |
| Palatoglossus | Palatine aponeurosis (oral surface) | Lateral side of the tongue where some fibers intermix with the transverse m. and some along the dorsal surface of the tongue | Elevation of the root of the tongue Narrows the oropharyngeal isthmus for deglutition | Pharyngeal plexus (the motor portion of this plexus is formed by the pharyngeal branch of the vagus n.) | Grouped as either an extrinsic tongue muscle of the tongue or a muscle of the soft palate |

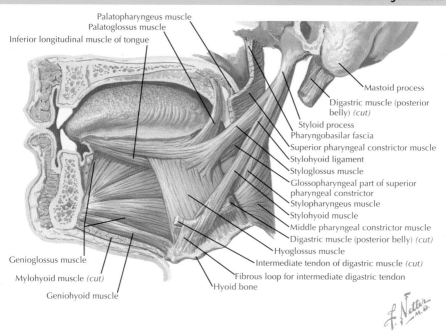

Palatopharyngeus muscle
Palatoglossus muscle
Inferior longitudinal muscle of tongue

Mastoid process
Digastric muscle (posterior belly) (cut)
Styloid process
Pharyngobasilar fascia
Superior pharyngeal constrictor muscle
Stylohyoid ligament
Styloglossus muscle
Glossopharyngeal part of superior pharyngeal constrictor
Stylopharyngeus muscle
Stylohyoid muscle
Middle pharyngeal constrictor muscle
Digastric muscle (posterior belly) (cut)
Hyoglossus muscle
Intermediate tendon of digastric muscle (cut)
Fibrous loop for intermediate digastric tendon
Hyoid bone

Genioglossus muscle
Mylohyoid muscle (cut)
Geniohyoid muscle

**Figure 14-5**

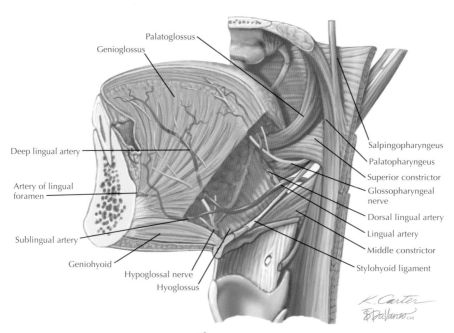

Palatoglossus
Genioglossus

Salpingopharyngeus
Palatopharyngeus
Superior constrictor
Glossopharyngeal nerve
Dorsal lingual artery
Lingual artery
Middle constrictor
Stylohyoid ligament

Deep lingual artery

Artery of lingual foramen

Sublingual artery

Geniohyoid
Hypoglossal nerve
Hyoglossus

**Figure 14-6**

| Muscle | Origin | Insertion | Actions | Nerve | Comment |
|---|---|---|---|---|---|
| Superior longitudinal | Median septum<br>Submucous layer near epiglottis | Lingual margins | Shortens<br>Curls the tongue's apex and lateral margins *upward,* which makes the dorsal surface *concave* | Hypoglossal n. | Located immediately deep to the mucous membrane of the tongue's dorsal surface |
| Inferior longitudinal | Root of the tongue<br>Body of the hyoid | Apex of the tongue | Shortens<br>Curls the tongue's apex *downward,* which makes the dorsal surface *convex* | | Runs the length of the tongue between the hyoglossus and genioglossus mm. |
| Transverse | Median septum | Fibrous tissue in the submucosa of the lingual margins<br>Some fibers intermix with palatoglossus | Narrows<br>Lengthens | | Runs the width of the tongue |
| Vertical | Submucosa of dorsal surface of tongue | Submucosa of ventral surface of tongue | Broadens<br>Flattens | | Runs from the dorsal to the ventral tongue surface |

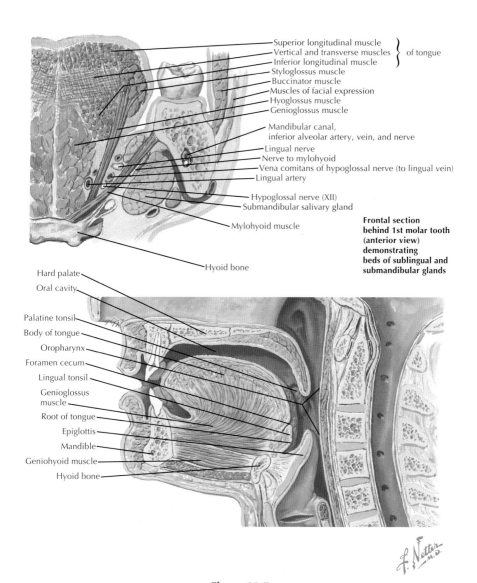

Superior longitudinal muscle ⎫
Vertical and transverse muscles ⎬ of tongue
Inferior longitudinal muscle ⎭
Styloglossus muscle
Buccinator muscle
Muscles of facial expression
Hyoglossus muscle
Genioglossus muscle

Mandibular canal,
inferior alveolar artery, vein, and nerve
Lingual nerve
Nerve to mylohyoid
Vena comitans of hypoglossal nerve (to lingual vein)
Lingual artery

Hypoglossal nerve (XII)
Submandibular salivary gland

Mylohyoid muscle

**Frontal section
behind 1st molar tooth
(anterior view)
demonstrating
beds of sublingual and
submandibular glands**

Hyoid bone

Hard palate
Oral cavity

Palatine tonsil
Body of tongue
Oropharynx
Foramen cecum
Lingual tonsil
Genioglossus
muscle
Root of tongue
Epiglottis
Mandible
Geniohyoid muscle
Hyoid bone

**Figure 14-7**

| TYPES OF SENSORY NERVE SUPPLY | | |
|---|---|---|
| **Type** | **Function** | **Nerves** |
| General somatic afferent (GSA) | Pain, temperature, discriminative touch | Trigeminal (via lingual), glossopharyngeal, and vagus (via internal laryngeal), to innervate the mucosa |
| Special visceral afferent (SVA) | Taste | Facial (via chorda tympani), glossopharyngeal, and vagus (via internal laryngeal), to innervate the taste buds |

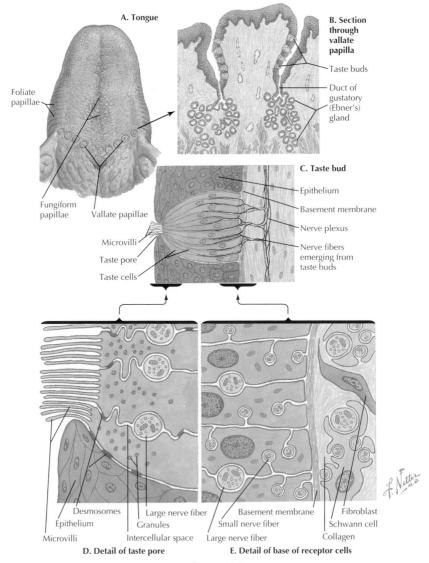

**A. Tongue**

Foliate papillae

Fungiform papillae

Vallate papillae

**B. Section through vallate papilla**

Taste buds

Duct of gustatory (Ebner's) gland

**C. Taste bud**

Epithelium

Basement membrane

Nerve plexus

Nerve fibers emerging from taste buds

Microvilli

Taste pore

Taste cells

Desmosomes

Epithelium

Microvilli

Large nerve fiber

Granules

Intercellular space

Basement membrane

Small nerve fiber

Large nerve fiber

Fibroblast

Schwann cell

Collagen

**D. Detail of taste pore**

**E. Detail of base of receptor cells**

**Figure 14-8**

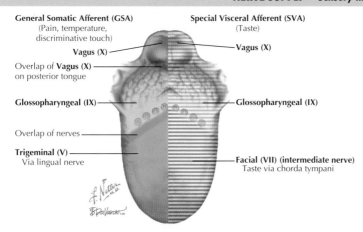

General Somatic Afferent (GSA)
(Pain, temperature, discriminative touch)

Special Visceral Afferent (SVA)
(Taste)

Vagus (X)

Vagus (X)

Overlap of **Vagus (X)** on posterior tongue

Glossopharyngeal (IX)

Glossopharyngeal (IX)

Overlap of nerves

Trigeminal (V)
Via lingual nerve

Facial (VII) (intermediate nerve)
Taste via chorda tympani

**Figure 14-9**

| GENERAL SENSORY INNERVATION (GENERAL SOMATIC AFFERENT) | | |
|---|---|---|
| **Nerve** | **Source** | **Course** |
| Lingual | Mandibular division of the trigeminal n. | Lies inferior to the lateral pterygoid m. and medial and anterior to the inferior alveolar nn. within the infratemporal fossa<br>Chorda tympani branch of the facial n. joins its posterior part<br>Lingual n. passes between the medial pterygoid m. and the ramus of the mandible to pass obliquely, entering the oral cavity bounded by the superior pharyngeal constrictor m., the medial pterygoid, and the mandible<br>Enters the oral cavity lying along the lingual tuberosity of the mandible<br>The submandibular ganglion is suspended from the lingual n. at the posterior border of the hyoglossus m.<br>Continues anteriorly and passes onto the lateral surface of the hyoglossus<br>Passes from the lateral side inferiorly and medial to the submandibular duct to reach the mucosa of the tongue<br>Supplies GSA fibers to the epithelium and papillae of the tongue's anterior 2/3, mucosa along the floor of the oral cavity (linguoalveolar ridge), and gingiva on the lingual aspect of the mandibular teeth |
| Glossopharyngeal | Arises as a cranial nerve from the medulla oblongata | Passes through the jugular foramen with the vagus and accessory nn.<br>Within the foramen, it passes between the internal carotid a. and the internal jugular v.<br>Continues inferiorly and posteriorly relative to the stylopharyngeus m.<br>Passes anteriorly with the stylopharyngeus m. and travels between the superior and middle constrictor mm. to become located by the palatine tonsils<br>Small lingual branches distribute GSA fibers to the epithelium of the tongue's posterior 1/3, in addition to the fauces |
| Internal laryngeal | Superior laryngeal branch of the vagus n. | Vagus n. branches from the medulla oblongata and passes through the jugular foramen with the glossopharyngeal and accessory nn.<br>Within the foramen, it passes between the internal carotid a. and the internal jugular v.<br>A series of nerves branch from the vagus in the neck, including the superior laryngeal n., which travels inferiorly posterior to the internal carotid a. on the side of the pharynx and divides into the internal and external laryngeal nn.<br>The internal laryngeal n. passes inferior to the larynx and passes through the thyrohyoid membrane with the superior laryngeal vv.<br>Distributes GSA fibers to the tongue's base at the epiglottic region and the mucous membranes of the larynx as far inferiorly as the false vocal folds |

| SPECIAL SENSORY INNERVATION  (SPECIAL VISCERAL AFFERENT) | | |
|---|---|---|
| **Nerve** | **Source** | **Course** |
| Chorda tympani | Facial n. in the tympanic cavity | Carries preganglionic parasympathetic fibers to the submandibular ganglion and taste fibers to the anterior 2/3 of the tongue |
| | | Passes anteriorly to enter the tympanic cavity and lies along the tympanic membrane and malleus until exiting the petrotympanic fissure |
| | | Joins the posterior border of the lingual n. |
| | | Lingual n. is distributed to the anterior 2/3 of the tongue, and the SVA fibers from the chorda tympani travel to the taste buds in this region |
| Glossopharyngeal | Arises as a cranial nerve from the medulla oblongata | Passes through the jugular foramen with the vagus and accessory nn. |
| | | Within the foramen, it passes between the internal carotid a. and the internal jugular v. |
| | | Continues inferiorly and travels posterior to the stylopharyngeus m. |
| | | Passes anteriorly with the stylopharyngeus m. and travels between the superior and middle constrictor mm., to be located by the palatine tonsils |
| | | Small lingual branches distribute SVA fibers to the taste buds in the mucous membrane of the tongue's posterior 1/3 and the circumvallate papilla |
| Internal laryngeal | Superior laryngeal branch of the vagus n. | Vagus n. branches from the medulla oblongata and passes through the jugular foramen with the glossopharyngeal and accessory nn. |
| | | Within the foramen, it passes between the internal carotid a. and the internal jugular v. |
| | | A series of nerves branch from the vagus in the neck, including the superior laryngeal n., which travels inferiorly posterior to the internal carotid on the side of the pharynx and divides into the internal and external laryngeal nn. |
| | | The internal laryngeal n. passes inferior to the larynx and passes through the thyrohyoid membrane with the superior laryngeal vv. |
| | | Distributes SVA fibers to the taste buds scattered at the base of the tongue at the epiglottic region |

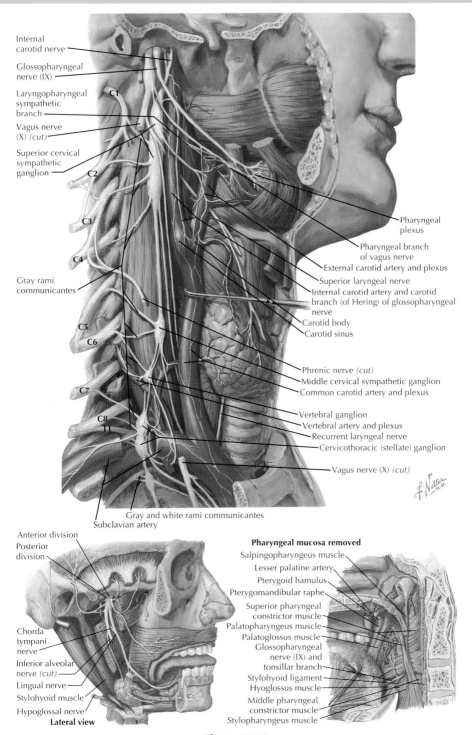

Internal
carotid nerve

Glossopharyngeal
nerve (IX)

Laryngopharyngeal
sympathetic
branch

Vagus nerve
(X) *(cut)*

Superior cervical
sympathetic
ganglion

C1

C2

C3

C4

Gray rami
communicantes

C5
C6

C7

C8
T1

Gray and white rami communicantes
Subclavian artery

Pharyngeal
plexus

Pharyngeal branch
of vagus nerve

External carotid artery and plexus

Superior laryngeal nerve

Internal carotid artery and carotid
branch (of Hering) of glossopharyngeal
nerve

Carotid body

Carotid sinus

Phrenic nerve *(cut)*

Middle cervical sympathetic ganglion

Common carotid artery and plexus

Vertebral ganglion

Vertebral artery and plexus

Recurrent laryngeal nerve

Cervicothoracic (stellate) ganglion

Vagus nerve (X) *(cut)*

Anterior division

Posterior
division

Chorda
tympani
nerve

Inferior alveolar
nerve *(cut)*

Lingual nerve

Stylohyoid muscle

Hypoglossal nerve

**Lateral view**

**Pharyngeal mucosa removed**

Salpingopharyngeus muscle

Lesser palatine artery

Pterygoid hamulus

Pterygomandibular raphe

Superior pharyngeal
constrictor muscle

Palatopharyngeus muscle

Palatoglossus muscle

Glossopharyngeal
nerve (IX) and
tonsillar branch

Stylohyoid ligament

Hyoglossus muscle

Middle pharyngeal
constrictor muscle

Stylopharyngeus muscle

**Figure 14-10**

| Nerve | Source | Course |
|---|---|---|
| Hypoglossal | Arises as a series of rootlets from the medulla oblongata and passes through the hypoglossal canal | Travels inferiorly and is located between the internal carotid a. and the internal jugular v. |
| | | Passes anteriorly as it wraps around the occipital a. |
| | | Passes superficial to the external carotid and the loop of the lingual a. in its anterior path |
| | | Passes deep to the posterior belly of the digastric and the stylohyoid m. and lies superficial to the hyoglossus m. with the accompanying vein of the hypoglossal n. |
| | | Passes deep to the mylohyoid m. and continues anteriorly in the genioglossus m. |
| | | Muscular branches supply: |
| | | • All intrinsic tongue muscles |
| | | • Hyoglossus m. |
| | | • Styloglossus m. |
| | | • Genioglossus m. |
| Pharyngeal plexus | Pharyngeal plexus (the motor portion of this plexus is formed by the pharyngeal branch of the vagus n.) | Arises from the upper part of the inferior ganglion of the vagus n. |
| | | Lies along the upper border of the middle constrictor m., where it forms the pharyngeal plexus |
| | | Motor branches from the plexus are distributed to the muscles of the pharynx and soft palate (with the exception of the tensor veli palatini m.) |
| | | In the tongue, it innervates: |
| | | • Palatoglossus m. |

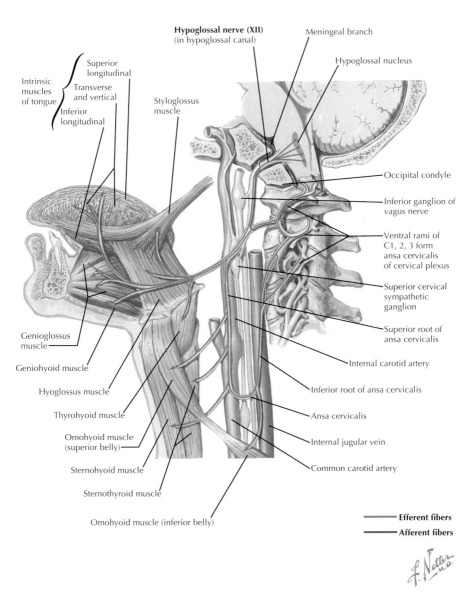

Hypoglossal nerve (XII)
(in hypoglossal canal)

Meningeal branch

Hypoglossal nucleus

Intrinsic muscles of tongue

Superior longitudinal

Transverse and vertical

Inferior longitudinal

Styloglossus muscle

Occipital condyle

Inferior ganglion of vagus nerve

Ventral rami of C1, 2, 3 form ansa cervicalis of cervical plexus

Superior cervical sympathetic ganglion

Superior root of ansa cervicalis

Genioglossus muscle

Geniohyoid muscle

Hyoglossus muscle

Thyrohyoid muscle

Omohyoid muscle (superior belly)

Sternohyoid muscle

Sternothyroid muscle

Omohyoid muscle (inferior belly)

Internal carotid artery

Inferior root of ansa cervicalis

Ansa cervicalis

Internal jugular vein

Common carotid artery

Efferent fibers

Afferent fibers

**Figure 14-11**

| Artery | Source | Course |
|---|---|---|
| Lingual | External carotid a. within the carotid triangle | Passes superiorly and medially (obliquely) toward the greater cornu of the hyoid bone and makes a loop by passing anteriorly and inferiorly while traveling superficial to the middle constrictor m. |
| | | While forming a loop, the artery is crossed superficially by the hypoglossal n. |
| | | Passes deep to the posterior belly of the digastric m. and the stylohyoid m. as it travels anteriorly, where it gives off a suprahyoid branch that travels on the superior surface of the hyoid bone, supplying the muscles in that area |
| | | The lingual a. passes deep to the hyoglossus m. and travels anteriorly between it and the genioglossus m. |
| | | After passing deep to the hyoglossus, 2 to 3 small dorsal lingual aa. are given off at the posterior border of the hyoglossus. |
| | | The lingual a. continues to pass anteriorly and gives off the sublingual branch at the anterior border of the hyoglossus |
| | | The deep lingual a., the terminal branch or continuation of the lingual a. once the sublingual a. is given off, travels superiorly to reach the tongue's ventral surface |
| *Dorsal lingual* | Lingual | After passing deep to the hyoglossus, 2 to 3 small dorsal lingual aa. are given off at the posterior border of the hyoglossus; they pass in a superior direction to the posterior 1/3 of the dorsum of the tongue and provide vascular supply to the mucous membrane in this region, the palatoglossal arch, the palatine tonsil, the epiglottis, and the surrounding soft palate |
| *Deep lingual* | | The deep lingual a., the terminal branch or continuation of the lingual a. once the sublingual a. is given off, travels superiorly to reach the tongue's ventral surface |
| | | Located between the inferior longitudinal m. of the tongue and the mucous membrane, the deep lingual a. is accompanied by branches of the lingual n., and it anastomoses with its counterpart from the other side |
| *Sublingual* | | The sublingual branch arises at the anterior border of the hyoglossus |
| | | The sublingual a. passes anteriorly between the genioglossus and mylohyoid mm. to the sublingual gland and provides vascular supply to the gland and the muscles and mucosa in the area |
| | | Typically has 2 branches of significance: |
| | | • Branch that passes mylohyoid to anastomose with submental a. |
| | | • Branch that passes deep to the gingiva to anastomose with branch from contralateral side |
| | | • At this anastomosis, typically 1 branch (although may be multiple branches) arises to enter a small lingual foramen superior to the genial tubercles in the posterior midline |
| Submental | A branch of the facial a. from the external carotid a. | Given off at the submandibular gland, travels anteriorly superficial to the mylohyoid m. |
| | | Anastomoses with a branch from the sublingual branch of the lingual a. to help supply the tongue |
| Tonsillar | | While ascending superiorly along the lateral side of the pharynx, it passes into and supplies the superior constrictor m. until reaching the palatine tonsil and root of the tongue |
| Ascending pharyngeal | External carotid a. | The smallest branch arising from the external carotid a. |
| | | Ascends superiorly between the lateral aspect of the pharynx and the internal carotid a. |
| | | Has branches supplying the palatine tonsil that anastomose with tonsillar branch of facial and dorsal lingual branches at root of the tongue |

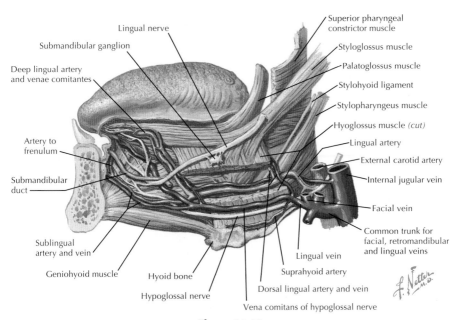

**Figure 14-12**

Lingual nerve

Submandibular ganglion

Deep lingual artery and venae comitantes

Artery to frenulum

Submandibular duct

Sublingual artery and vein

Geniohyoid muscle

Hyoid bone

Hypoglossal nerve

Vena comitans of hypoglossal nerve

Dorsal lingual artery and vein

Suprahyoid artery

Lingual vein

Superior pharyngeal constrictor muscle

Styloglossus muscle

Palatoglossus muscle

Stylohyoid ligament

Stylopharyngeus muscle

Hyoglossus muscle *(cut)*

Lingual artery

External carotid artery

Internal jugular vein

Facial vein

Common trunk for facial, retromandibular and lingual veins

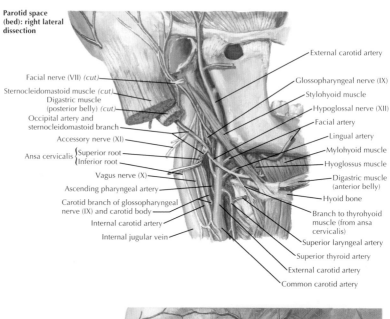

Parotid space
(bed): right lateral
dissection

External carotid artery

Facial nerve (VII) *(cut)*

Glossopharyngeal nerve (IX)

Sternocleidomastoid muscle *(cut)*
Digastric muscle
(posterior belly) *(cut)*

Stylohyoid muscle
Hypoglossal nerve (XII)

Occipital artery and
sternocleidomastoid branch

Facial artery

Accessory nerve (XI)

Lingual artery

Ansa cervicalis {Superior root
{Inferior root

Mylohyoid muscle

Hyoglossus muscle

Vagus nerve (X)

Digastric muscle
(anterior belly)

Ascending pharyngeal artery

Hyoid bone

Carotid branch of glossopharyngeal
nerve (IX) and carotid body

Branch to thyrohyoid
muscle (from ansa
cervicalis)

Internal carotid artery

Internal jugular vein

Superior laryngeal artery

Superior thyroid artery

External carotid artery

Common carotid artery

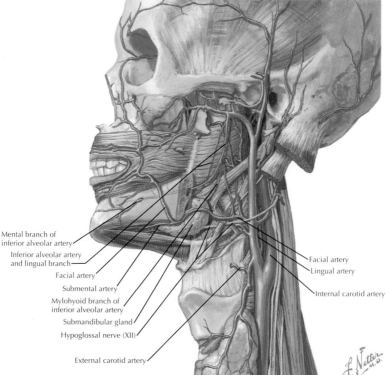

Mental branch of
inferior alveolar artery

Inferior alveolar artery
and lingual branch

Facial artery

Submental artery

Facial artery

Lingual artery

Mylohyoid branch of
inferior alveolar artery

Internal carotid artery

Submandibular gland

Hypoglossal nerve (XII)

External carotid artery

**Figure 14-13**

| Vein | Course |
|------|--------|
| Lingual | Receives tributaries from the deep lingual vv. on the ventral surface, and the dorsal lingual vv. from the dorsal surface |
| | Passes with the lingual a., deep to the hyoglossus m., and ends in the internal jugular v. |
| | The vena comitans nervi hypoglossi, or accompanying vein of the hypoglossal n., begins at the tongue's apex and may either join the lingual v. or accompany the hypoglossal n. and enter the common facial v., which empties into the internal jugular |
| Submental | Anastomoses with the branches of the lingual v. |
| | Parallels the submental a. on the superficial surface of the mylohyoid m. and ends in the facial v. |

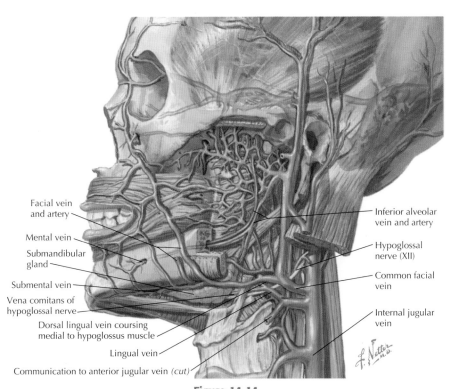

**Figure 14-14**

- *Ankyloglossia*: condition in which the lingual frenulum is restricted because of an increase in tissue, leading to reduced tongue mobility
- Also known as tongue-tie

PRESENTATIONS

- Tongue may not be capable of protrusion beyond the incisors
- Tongue may not be capable of touching the palate
- Tongue may have a **V**-shaped notch at its tip or may appear bilobed on protrusion

COMPLICATIONS

- Causes problems for babies who breastfeed
- If the tongue cannot clear the oral cavity of food, caries, periodontal disease, and halitosis can result
- If condition is severe, can cause a speech impediment

TREATMENT

- If necessary, the lingual frenulum may be cut (frenectomy)

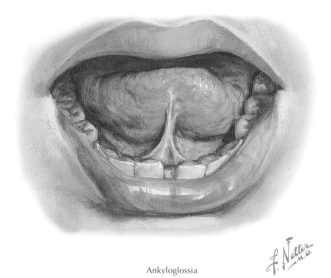

Ankyloglossia

**Figure 14-15**

- *Hypoglossal nerve lesions* paralyze the tongue on 1 side
- On protrusion, the tongue deviates to the ipsilateral (same) or contralateral side, depending on the lesion site

## LOWER MOTOR NEURON LESION

- Lesions to the hypoglossal nerve cause paralysis on the ipsilateral side:
  - Tongue deviates to the paralyzed side on protrusion (the paralyzed muscles will lag, causing the tip to deviate)
  - Musculature atrophies on the paralyzed side
  - Tongue fasciculations occur on the paralyzed side
  - *Example*: With a neck wound that cuts the right hypoglossal nerve, the tongue deviates to the right on protrusion, and the right half of the tongue will later demonstrate atrophy and fasciculations

## UPPER MOTOR NEURON LESION

- Causes paralysis on the contralateral side:
  - Tongue deviates to the side *opposite* the lesion
  - Musculature atrophies on side *opposite* the lesion
  - *Example*: After a stroke on the right side of the brain that affects the right upper motor neurons, the tongue deviates to the left on protrusion, and the left half of the tongue will atrophy

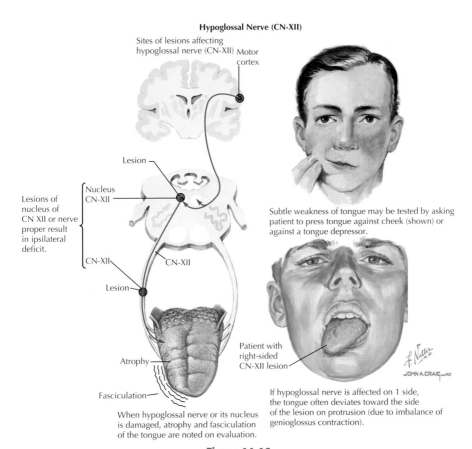

**Hypoglossal Nerve (CN-XII)**

Sites of lesions affecting hypoglossal nerve (CN-XII) Motor cortex

Lesion

Nucleus CN-XII

Lesions of nucleus of CN XII or nerve proper result in ipsilateral deficit.

CN-XII

CN-XII

Lesion

Atrophy

Fasciculation

When hypoglossal nerve or its nucleus is damaged, atrophy and fasciculation of the tongue are noted on evaluation.

Subtle weakness of tongue may be tested by asking patient to press tongue against cheek (shown) or against a tongue depressor.

Patient with right-sided CN-XII lesion

If hypoglossal nerve is affected on 1 side, the tongue often deviates toward the side of the lesion on protrusion (due to imbalance of genioglossus contraction).

**Figure 14-16**

- *Squamous cell carcinoma* accounts for most cancers of the oral cavity
- In the tongue, usually located on the anterolateral aspect
- Alcohol and tobacco use are risk factors
- Premalignant lesions, such as erythroplasia and leukoplakia, should be identified, because early diagnosis and treatment are paramount for long-term survival
- Radiographic imaging helps reveal the tumor's extent and location
- Staging of the tumor guides prognosis

TREATMENT

- Excision or radiation therapy, or possibly in combination with chemotherapy
- If lesion is detected early, excision may suffice
- With later tumor stages, a 2nd primary squamous cell carcinoma must be excluded

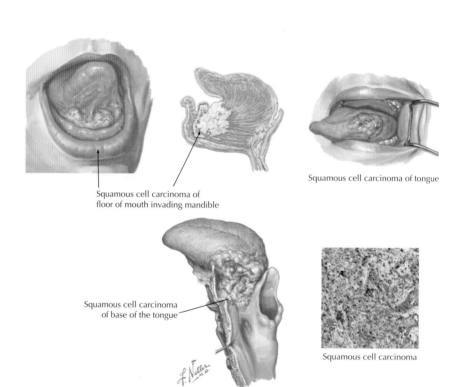

Squamous cell carcinoma of floor of mouth invading mandible

Squamous cell carcinoma of tongue

Squamous cell carcinoma of base of the tongue

Squamous cell carcinoma

**Figure 14-17**

- *Leukoplakia*: a common premalignant condition of the oral cavity involving the formation of white spots on the mucous membranes of the tongue and inside the mouth
- Hairy leukoplakia is a type observed in persons with compromised immune systems
- Risk factors:
  - Tobacco use
  - Alcohol use
  - Human immunodeficiency virus (HIV) infection
  - Epstein-Barr virus infection
- Although a precancerous lesion, it may not progress to oral cancer

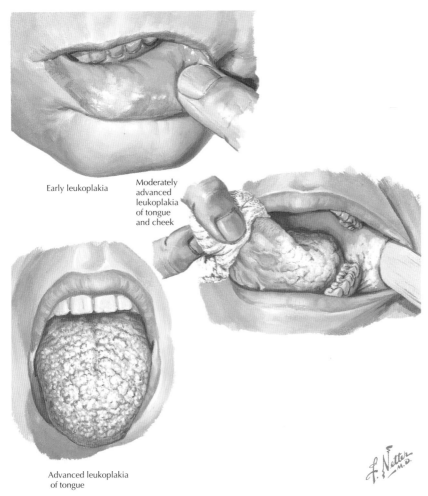

Early leukoplakia

Moderately advanced leukoplakia of tongue and cheek

Advanced leukoplakia of tongue

**Figure 14-18**

- *Pharynx*: 5-inch muscular tube from base of the skull (posterior portion of the body of the sphenoid bone and basilar portion of the occipital bone) to the lower border of the cricoid cartilage (C6), where it is continuous with the esophagus
- Is funnel-shaped
- Posterior portion of the pharynx lies against the prevertebral fascia
- The retropharyngeal and parapharyngeal spaces surround the pharynx
- Lies posterior to the nasal and oral cavities and the larynx and thus is divided into 3 parts:
  - Nasopharynx
  - Oropharynx
  - Laryngopharynx
- Responsible for properly conducting food to the esophagus and air to the lungs
- Composed of:
  - 3 constrictor muscles
  - 3 longitudinal muscles
  - Cartilaginous part of the pharyngotympanic tube
  - Soft palate
- The wall of the pharynx has 5 layers:
  - Mucous membrane—the innermost layer
  - Submucosa
  - Pharyngobasilar fascia—the fibrous layer attached to the skull anchoring the pharynx
  - Muscular—3 inner longitudinal and 3 outer circular (constrictor) muscles that overlap such that the superior constrictor is the innermost, whereas the inferior constrictor is the outermost muscle
  - Buccopharyngeal fascia—loose layer of connective tissue continuous with the fascia over the buccinator and pharyngeal muscles, and the location of the pharyngeal plexus of nerves and the pharyngeal plexus of veins

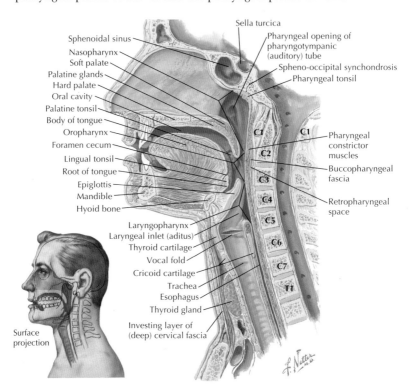

**Figure 15-1**

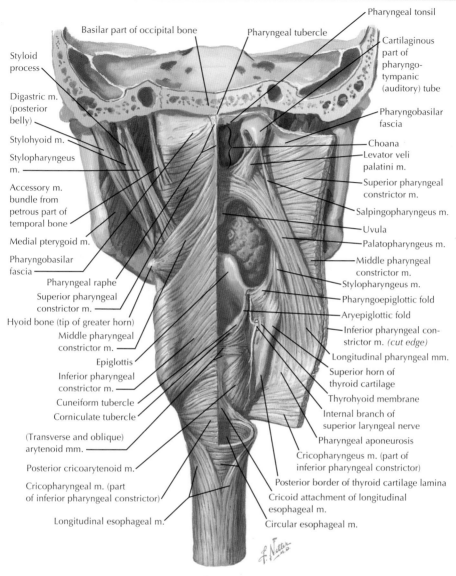

**Figure 15-2**

- Waldeyer's ring is the anatomical name for the ring of lymphatic tissue in the pharynx and oral cavity:
  - Lingual tonsil (posterior 1/3rd of tongue)
  - Palatine tonsil (oropharynx)
  - Tubal tonsil (nasopharynx)
  - Pharyngeal tonsil (nasopharynx)

## NASOPHARYNX

| Boundaries | Major Anatomic Features | Comments | Vertebral Level |
|---|---|---|---|
| *Roof*—posterior portion of the body of the sphenoid bone and basilar portion of the occipital bone<br><br>*Floor*—soft palate (upper surface)<br><br>*Anterior*—choanae of the nasal cavity<br><br>*Posterior*—mucosa covering superior constrictor<br><br>*Lateral*—mucosa covering superior constrictor | Ostium of the auditory tube opens into the nasopharynx<br><br>Torus tubarius is an elevation formed by the base of the cartilaginous portion of the auditory tube, which lies superior to the ostium of the tube<br><br>Torus levatorius is an elevation of mucous membrane that lies over the levator veli palatini m.<br><br>Salpingopharyngeal fold is mucous membrane that lies over the salpingopharyngeus m., connecting the torus tubarius to the lateral wall of the pharynx<br><br>Pharyngeal recess is located posterior to the salpingopharyngeal fold and contains the pharyngeal tonsil (adenoid)<br><br>Pharyngeal tonsil (adenoid) is mucosa-associated lymphatic tissue (MALT) located along the midline<br><br>Tubal tonsils are MALT located posterior to the opening of each auditory tube and are considered by some authors to be extensions of the pharyngeal tonsil<br><br>Nasopharynx epithelium:<br><br>• *Anterior*—pseudostratified columnar with cilia in anterior portion near nasal cavity<br><br>• *Posterior*—stratified squamous nonkeratinized in posterior portion | Has a respiratory function<br><br>The auditory tube connects the middle ear with the nasopharynx, which helps equalize air pressure on both sides of the tympanic membrane<br><br>The cartilaginous portion of the auditory tube normally is closed, except during deglutition and yawning<br><br>The auditory tube allows spread of infections between the middle ear and the nasopharynx<br><br>The roof and walls tend to be firm and do not close during muscular contraction of the pharyngeal and palatal muscles | C1 (and dens of C2) |

## OROPHARYNX

| Boundaries | Major Anatomic Features | Comment | Vertebral Level |
|---|---|---|---|
| *Superior*—nasopharynx<br><br>*Inferior*—superior border of epiglottis<br><br>*Anterior*—palatoglossal fold of the oral cavity (oropharyngeal isthmus)<br><br>*Posterior*—mucosa covering the superior and middle constrictor mm.<br><br>*Lateral*—mucosa covering the superior and middle constrictor mm. | Palatine tonsils are located in the oropharynx between the palatoglossal and palatopharyngeal folds (tonsillar sinus)<br><br>Palatopharyngeal fold is an elevation of mucous membrane that lies over the palatopharyngeal m.<br><br>Epiglottic vallecula is the depression immediately posterior to the root of the tongue<br><br>Oropharynx epithelium is stratified squamous nonkeratinized | Has a respiratory and a digestive function | C2-C3 |

## LARYNGOPHARYNX

| Boundaries | Major Anatomic Features | Comment | Vertebral Level |
|---|---|---|---|
| *Superior*—oropharynx<br>*Inferior*—inferior border of cricoid cartilage (where becomes continuous with esophagus)<br>*Anterior*—larynx<br>*Posterior*—mucosa covering middle and inferior constrictor mm.<br>*Lateral*—mucosa covering middle and inferior constrictor mm. | Piriform recess is a small depression located on the lateral wall of the laryngopharyngeal cavity on either side of the entrance to the larynx<br><br>Laryngopharynx epithelium is stratified squamous nonkeratinized | Communicates with the larynx<br><br>The piriform recess is a potential location for objects to become lodged | C4-C6 |

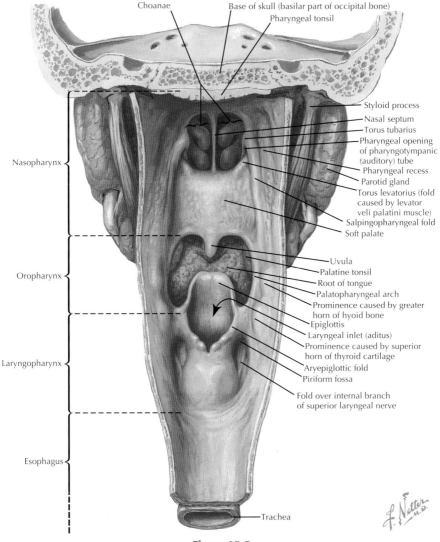

Figure 15-3

| Muscle | Origin | Insertion | Actions | Nerve Supply |
|---|---|---|---|---|
| Superior constrictor | Pterygoid hamulus<br>Pterygomandibular raphe<br>Retromolar trigone of mandible<br>Side of tongue | Pharyngeal tubercle<br>Pharyngeal raphe | Constricts the *upper* portion of the pharynx | Pharyngeal plexus (the motor portion of this plexus is formed by the pharyngeal branch of the vagus n.) |
| Middle constrictor | Stylohyoid lig.<br>Lesser cornu of hyoid<br>Greater cornu of hyoid | Pharyngeal raphe | Constricts the *middle* portion of the pharynx | |
| Inferior constrictor (divided by some authors into:<br>• Thyropharyngeus<br>• Cricopharyngeus) | Oblique line of thyroid cartilage<br>Side of cricoid cartilage | | Constricts the *lower* portion of the pharynx | Pharyngeal plexus (the motor portion of this plexus is formed by the pharyngeal branch of the vagus n.)<br>External laryngeal n. of the vagus (also helps supply the cricopharyngeus portion of the inferior constrictor)<br>Recurrent laryngeal n. of the vagus (also helps supply the cricopharyngeus portion of the inferior constrictor) |
| Palatopharyngeus | Posterior border of hard palate<br>Palatine aponeurosis | Posterior border of the lamina of the thyroid cartilage | Elevates pharynx<br>Helps close the nasopharynx | Pharyngeal plexus (the motor portion of this plexus is formed by the pharyngeal branch of the vagus n.) |
| Salpingopharyngeus | Cartilage of auditory tube | | Elevates the upper and lateral portions of the pharynx | |
| Stylopharyngeus | Medial aspect of base of styloid process | | Elevates pharynx<br>Expands the sides of the pharynx | Glossopharyngeal n. |

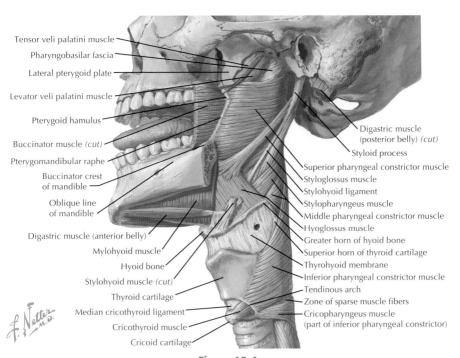

Tensor veli palatini muscle

Pharyngobasilar fascia

Lateral pterygoid plate

Levator veli palatini muscle

Pterygoid hamulus

Buccinator muscle *(cut)*

Pterygomandibular raphe

Buccinator crest of mandible

Oblique line of mandible

Digastric muscle (anterior belly)

Mylohyoid muscle

Hyoid bone

Stylohyoid muscle *(cut)*

Thyroid cartilage

Median cricothyroid ligament

Cricothyroid muscle

Cricoid cartilage

Digastric muscle (posterior belly) *(cut)*

Styloid process

Superior pharyngeal constrictor muscle

Styloglossus muscle

Stylohyoid ligament

Stylopharyngeus muscle

Middle pharyngeal constrictor muscle

Hyoglossus muscle

Greater horn of hyoid bone

Superior horn of thyroid cartilage

Thyrohyoid membrane

Inferior pharyngeal constrictor muscle

Tendinous arch

Zone of sparse muscle fibers

Cricopharyngeus muscle (part of inferior pharyngeal constrictor)

**Figure 15-4**

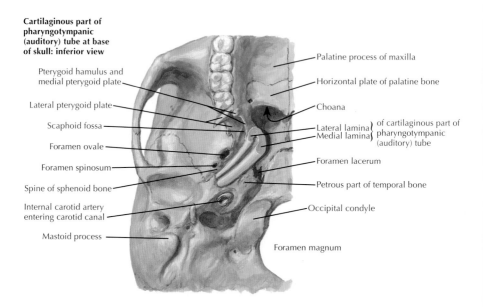

**Cartilaginous part of pharyngotympanic (auditory) tube at base of skull: inferior view**

Pterygoid hamulus and medial pterygoid plate

Lateral pterygoid plate

Scaphoid fossa

Foramen ovale

Foramen spinosum

Spine of sphenoid bone

Internal carotid artery entering carotid canal

Mastoid process

Palatine process of maxilla

Horizontal plate of palatine bone

Choana

Lateral lamina }
Medial lamina } of cartilaginous part of pharyngotympanic (auditory) tube

Foramen lacerum

Petrous part of temporal bone

Occipital condyle

Foramen magnum

**Section through cartilaginous part of pharyngotympanic (auditory) tube, with tube closed**

Trigeminal ganglion

Internal carotid artery in carotid canal

Dura mater

Lateral lamina of cartilage

Medial lamina of cartilage

Auditory tube lumen

Tensor veli palatini muscle

Levator veli palatini muscle

Salpingopharyngeus muscle

Nasopharynx

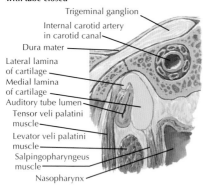

Pharyngotympanic (auditory) tube closed by elastic recoil of cartilage, tissue turgidity, and tension of salpingopharyngeus muscles

**Section through cartilaginous part of pharyngotympanic (auditory) tube, with tube open**

Trigeminal ganglion

Internal carotid artery in carotid canal

Dura mater

Lateral lamina of cartilage

Medial lamina of cartilage

Auditory tube lumen

Tensor veli palatini muscle

Levator veli palatini muscle

Salpingopharyngeus muscle

Nasopharynx

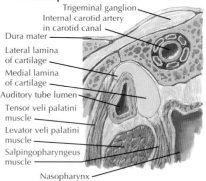

Lumen opened chiefly when attachment of tensor veli palatini muscle pulls wall of tube laterally during swallowing

**Figure 15-5**

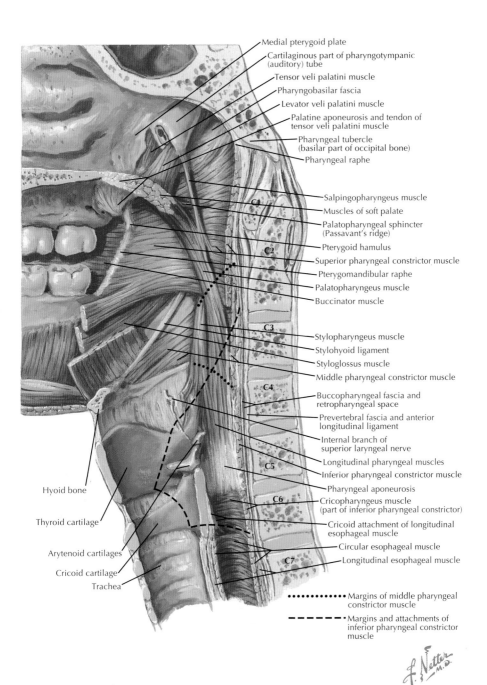

Medial pterygoid plate
Cartilaginous part of pharyngotympanic (auditory) tube
Tensor veli palatini muscle
Pharyngobasilar fascia
Levator veli palatini muscle
Palatine aponeurosis and tendon of tensor veli palatini muscle
Pharyngeal tubercle (basilar part of occipital bone)
Pharyngeal raphe

Salpingopharyngeus muscle
Muscles of soft palate
Palatopharyngeal sphincter (Passavant's ridge)
Pterygoid hamulus
Superior pharyngeal constrictor muscle
Pterygomandibular raphe
Palatopharyngeus muscle
Buccinator muscle

Stylopharyngeus muscle
Stylohyoid ligament
Styloglossus muscle
Middle pharyngeal constrictor muscle
Buccopharyngeal fascia and retropharyngeal space
Prevertebral fascia and anterior longitudinal ligament
Internal branch of superior laryngeal nerve
Longitudinal pharyngeal muscles
Inferior pharyngeal constrictor muscle
Pharyngeal aponeurosis
Cricopharyngeus muscle (part of inferior pharyngeal constrictor)
Cricoid attachment of longitudinal esophageal muscle
Circular esophageal muscle
Longitudinal esophageal muscle

Hyoid bone
Thyroid cartilage
Arytenoid cartilages
Cricoid cartilage
Trachea

•••••••••••••Margins of middle pharyngeal constrictor muscle
– – – – – – – Margins and attachments of inferior pharyngeal constrictor muscle

Figure 15-6

- The overlapping arrangement of the 3 constrictor muscles leaves 4 potential apertures in the pharyngeal musculature
- Anatomic structures enter and exit the pharynx through these potential apertures

| OVERVIEW OF POTENTIAL APERTURES | |
|---|---|
| **Location** | **Anatomic Structures That Pass Through** |
| Between base of the skull and the superior constrictor m. | Auditory tube<br>Levator veli palatini m.<br>Ascending pharyngeal a.<br>Ascending palatine a. |
| Between the superior and middle constrictor mm. | Stylopharyngeus m.<br>Glossopharyngeal n.<br>Tonsillar branch of the ascending palatine a.<br>Stylohyoid lig. |
| Between the middle and inferior constrictor mm. | Internal laryngeal n.<br>Superior laryngeal a. and v. |
| Inferior to the inferior constrictor m. | Recurrent laryngeal n.<br>Inferior laryngeal a. and v. |

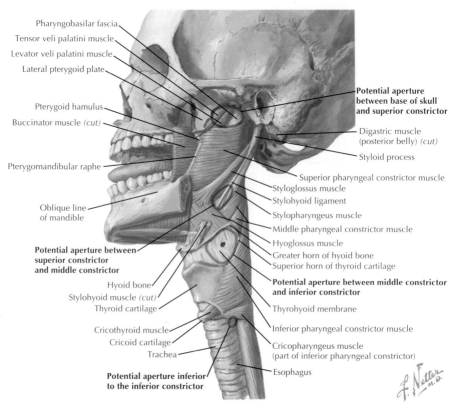

Pharyngobasilar fascia
Tensor veli palatini muscle
Levator veli palatini muscle
Lateral pterygoid plate

Pterygoid hamulus
Buccinator muscle *(cut)*

Pterygomandibular raphe

Oblique line
of mandible

**Potential aperture between
superior constrictor
and middle constrictor**

Hyoid bone
Stylohyoid muscle *(cut)*
Thyroid cartilage

Cricothyroid muscle
Cricoid cartilage
Trachea

**Potential aperture inferior
to the inferior constrictor**

Potential aperture
between base of skull
and superior constrictor

Digastric muscle
(posterior belly) *(cut)*
Styloid process

Superior pharyngeal constrictor muscle
Styloglossus muscle
Stylohyoid ligament
Stylopharyngeus muscle
Middle pharyngeal constrictor muscle
Hyoglossus muscle
Greater horn of hyoid bone
Superior horn of thyroid cartilage

**Potential aperture between middle constrictor
and inferior constrictor**

Thyrohyoid membrane

Inferior pharyngeal constrictor muscle

Cricopharyngeus muscle
(part of inferior pharyngeal constrictor)

Esophagus

**Figure 15-7**

| Artery | Source | Course |
|---|---|---|
| Ascending pharyngeal | The posterior portion of the external carotid a. near the bifurcation of the common carotid a. | The smallest branch arising from the external carotid a.<br>Ascends superiorly between the lateral aspect of the pharynx and the internal carotid a.<br>*Has 2 major sets of branches:*<br>• Pharyngeal—a series of 3 small branches that supplies the stylopharyngeus and the middle and inferior constrictor mm.<br>• Palatine—supplies the superior constrictor, palatine tonsil, soft palate, and auditory tube |
| Ascending palatine | Facial a. | Ascends superiorly along the lateral side of the pharynx, typically between the stylopharyngeus and the styloglossus mm.<br>Passes through the aperture between the base of the skull and the superior constrictor m. to supply it and the soft palate |
| Tonsillar | | While ascending superiorly along the lateral side of the pharynx, it passes into and supplies the superior constrictor m. until reaching the palatine tonsil and root of the tongue |
| Pharyngeal | The 3rd part of the maxillary a. in the pterygopalatine fossa | Passes posteriorly with the pharyngeal n. into the pharyngeal canal<br>Emerges to supply the superior portion of the nasopharynx and the auditory tube |
| Artery of the pterygoid canal | The 3rd part of the maxillary a. in the pterygopalatine fossa | Passes posteriorly into the pterygoid canal, accompanying the nerve of the pterygoid canal (vidian n.)<br>Helps supply the auditory tube |
| Lesser palatine | Descending palatine a. from the 3rd part of the maxillary a. | A branch of the descending palatine a. that travels in the palatine canal<br>Within the canal, the descending palatine a. splits into the:<br>• Greater palatine a.<br>• Lesser palatine a.<br>Lesser palatine a. supplies the soft palate and palatine tonsil |
| Superior thyroid | The 1st branch of the external carotid a. | Passes inferiorly along the inferior constrictor m., providing small muscular branches as it descends to supply the thyroid gland |
| Inferior thyroid | Thyrocervical trunk | Has a series of muscular branches that supply the pharynx |

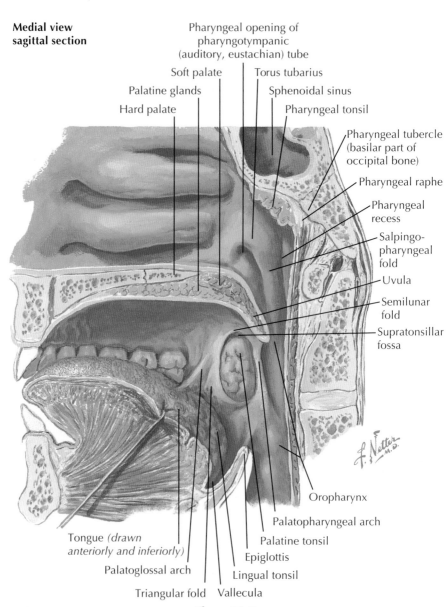

**Medial view
sagittal section**

Pharyngeal opening of
pharyngotympanic
(auditory, eustachian) tube

Soft palate

Torus tubarius

Palatine glands

Sphenoidal sinus

Hard palate

Pharyngeal tonsil

Pharyngeal tubercle
(basilar part of
occipital bone)

Pharyngeal raphe

Pharyngeal
recess

Salpingo-
pharyngeal
fold

Uvula

Semilunar
fold

Supratonsillar
fossa

Oropharynx

Palatopharyngeal arch

Palatine tonsil

Tongue (drawn
anteriorly and inferiorly)

Epiglottis

Palatoglossal arch

Lingual tonsil

Triangular fold   Vallecula

**Figure 15-8**

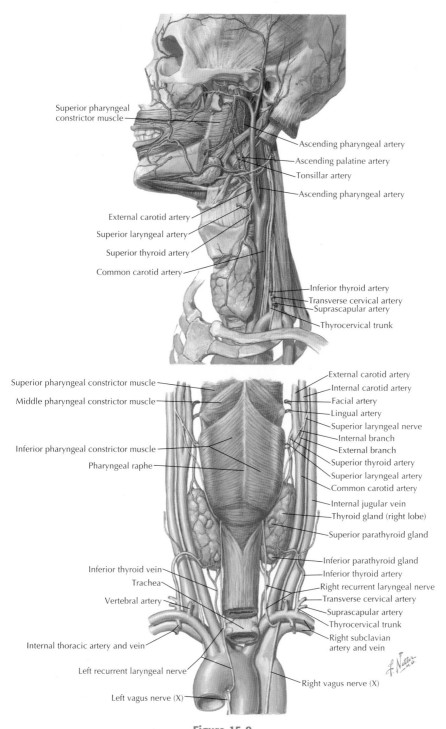

Superior pharyngeal constrictor muscle

Ascending pharyngeal artery
Ascending palatine artery
Tonsillar artery
Ascending pharyngeal artery

External carotid artery
Superior laryngeal artery
Superior thyroid artery
Common carotid artery

Inferior thyroid artery
Transverse cervical artery
Suprascapular artery
Thyrocervical trunk

External carotid artery
Internal carotid artery
Facial artery
Lingual artery
Superior laryngeal nerve
Internal branch
External branch
Superior thyroid artery
Superior laryngeal artery
Common carotid artery
Internal jugular vein
Thyroid gland (right lobe)
Superior parathyroid gland

Superior pharyngeal constrictor muscle
Middle pharyngeal constrictor muscle

Inferior pharyngeal constrictor muscle
Pharyngeal raphe

Inferior parathyroid gland
Inferior thyroid artery
Right recurrent laryngeal nerve
Transverse cervical artery
Suprascapular artery
Thyrocervical trunk
Right subclavian artery and vein

Inferior thyroid vein
Trachea
Vertebral artery

Internal thoracic artery and vein

Left recurrent laryngeal nerve

Left vagus nerve (X)

Right vagus nerve (X)

**Figure 15-9**

| Vein | Course |
|------|--------|
| Pharyngeal plexus | Located on the outer surface of the pharynx in the buccopharyngeal fascia |
| | Gives rise to pharyngeal vv., which drain into the internal jugular v. and also into the pterygoid plexus of veins along the lateral pterygoid m. |
| | The pharyngeal vv. also may drain into the facial, lingual, or superior thyroid v. |

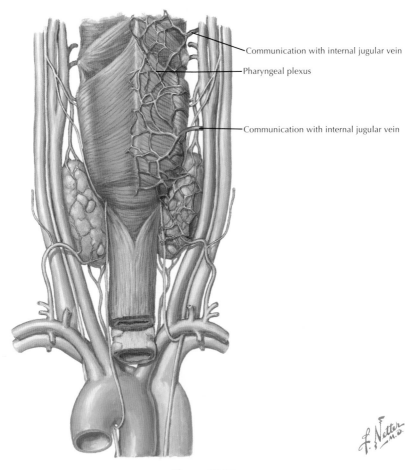

Communication with internal jugular vein

Pharyngeal plexus

Communication with internal jugular vein

**Figure 15-10**

- Supplies a majority of the motor and sensory innervation to the pharynx
- Is located on the lateral aspect of the middle constrictor muscle
- Composed of:
  - Pharyngeal branch of the glossopharyngeal nerve
  - Pharyngeal branch of the vagus nerve
  - Sympathetic fibers (laryngopharyngeal branches) from the superior cervical ganglion (postganglionic fibers)

### Pharyngeal Plexus

| Nerve | Function | Course | Sensory | Motor |
|---|---|---|---|---|
| Pharyngeal branch of the glossopharyngeal | The major branch of the glossopharyngeal n. that contributes to the pharyngeal plexus<br><br>Sensory | 3 or 4 filaments unite to form 1 pharyngeal branch opposite the middle constrictor m.<br><br>This branch, along with the pharyngeal branch of the vagus and laryngopharyngeal branches from the sympathetics, forms the pharyngeal plexus | Sensory branches contributing to the plexus perforate the pharyngeal muscles and supply its mucous membranes (mainly oropharynx and laryngopharynx region) | |
| Pharyngeal branch of the vagus | The major branch of the vagus n. that contributes to the pharyngeal plexus<br><br>Motor | Arises from the upper part of the inferior ganglion of the vagus n.<br><br>Lies along the upper border of the middle constrictor m., where it forms the pharyngeal plexus<br><br>From the plexus, the motor branches are distributed to the pharyngeal and soft palate muscles (with the exception of the stylopharyngeus m. and tensor veli palatini m.) | | Superior constrictor, middle constrictor, inferior constrictor, palatopharyngeus, salpingopharyngeus mm. |
| Sympathetic fibers (laryngopharyngeal branches) from the superior cervical ganglion | Vasomotor | A series of laryngopharyngeal branches pass along the lateral side of the middle constrictor m. | | Vasomotor |

- N.B.—some authors still describe the cranial root of the accessory n. as a component of the pharyngeal plexus—however, literature regarding the cranial root is controversial and many authors argue that what is described as the cranial root of the accessory n. is actually part of the vagus n. because the fibers arise from the nucleus ambiguus.

| Nerve | Function | Course | Sensory | Motor |
|-------|----------|--------|---------|-------|
| Recurrent laryngeal branch of the vagus | A small contributor to the motor innervation of the muscles of the pharynx<br><br>Provides significant innervation to the larynx | Branch of the vagus n.<br><br>Wraps around the aorta posterior to the ligamentum arteriosum on the left side<br><br>Wraps around the right subclavian a. on the right side<br><br>Ascends on the lateral aspect of the trachea until reaching the pharynx, where it passes deep to the inferior constrictor to reach the larynx | | Part of the inferior constrictor m. (cricopharyngeus portion) |
| External laryngeal n. | A small contributor to the motor innervation of the muscles of the pharynx<br><br>Provides innervation to the cricothyroid m. | A branch of the superior laryngeal n. that branches from the vagus n.<br><br>Descends posterior to the sternohyoid, traveling with the superior thyroid a.<br><br>Lies along the inferior constrictor m.<br><br>Passes deep to the inferior constrictor m. to travel anteriorly to the cricothyroid m. | | Part of the inferior constrictor m. (cricopharyngeus portion) |
| Pharyngeal | A small sensory nerve | Arises from the maxillary division of the trigeminal in the pterygopalatine fossa<br><br>Passes posteriorly through the pharyngeal canal with the artery to enter the nasopharynx | Supplies sensory fibers to the nasopharynx and the auditory tube | |

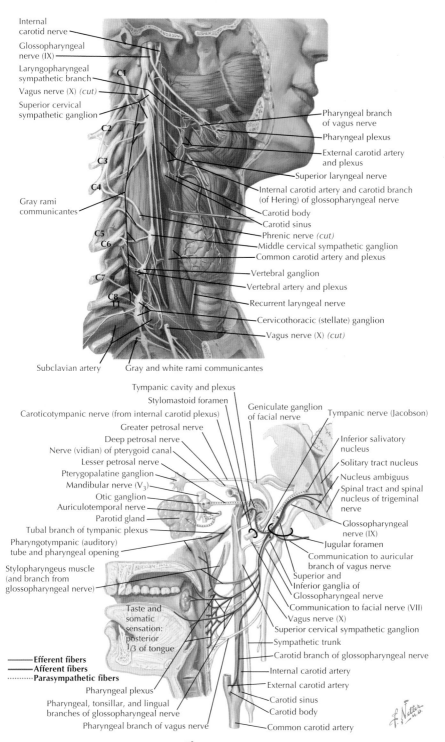

Internal carotid nerve

Glossopharyngeal nerve (IX)

Laryngopharyngeal sympathetic branch

Vagus nerve (X) *(cut)*

Superior cervical sympathetic ganglion

C1

C2

C3

C4

Gray rami communicantes

C5
C6

C7

C8
T1

Subclavian artery

Gray and white rami communicantes

Pharyngeal branch of vagus nerve

Pharyngeal plexus

External carotid artery and plexus

Superior laryngeal nerve

Internal carotid artery and carotid branch (of Hering) of glossopharyngeal nerve

Carotid body

Carotid sinus

Phrenic nerve *(cut)*

Middle cervical sympathetic ganglion

Common carotid artery and plexus

Vertebral ganglion

Vertebral artery and plexus

Recurrent laryngeal nerve

Cervicothoracic (stellate) ganglion

Vagus nerve (X) *(cut)*

Tympanic cavity and plexus

Stylomastoid foramen

Caroticotympanic nerve (from internal carotid plexus)

Greater petrosal nerve

Deep petrosal nerve

Nerve (vidian) of pterygoid canal

Lesser petrosal nerve

Pterygopalatine ganglion

Mandibular nerve (V₃)

Otic ganglion

Auriculotemporal nerve

Parotid gland

Tubal branch of tympanic plexus

Pharyngotympanic (auditory) tube and pharyngeal opening

Stylopharyngeus muscle (and branch from glossopharyngeal nerve)

Taste and somatic sensation: posterior ⅓ of tongue

Geniculate ganglion of facial nerve

Tympanic nerve (Jacobson)

Inferior salivatory nucleus

Solitary tract nucleus

Nucleus ambiguus

Spinal tract and spinal nucleus of trigeminal nerve

Glossopharyngeal nerve (IX)

Jugular foramen

Communication to auricular branch of vagus nerve

Superior and Inferior ganglia of Glossopharyngeal nerve

Communication to facial nerve (VII)

Vagus nerve (X)

Superior cervical sympathetic ganglion

Sympathetic trunk

Carotid branch of glossopharyngeal nerve

Internal carotid artery

External carotid artery

Carotid sinus

Carotid body

Common carotid artery

——— **Efferent fibers**
——— **Afferent fibers**
·········· **Parasympathetic fibers**

Pharyngeal plexus

Pharyngeal, tonsillar, and lingual branches of glossopharyngeal nerve

Pharyngeal branch of vagus nerve

**Figure 15-11**

- *Deglutition*, or swallowing, is a combination of voluntary and involuntary muscular contractions to move a bolus of food from the oral cavity to the esophagus
- Deglutition begins when the tip of the tongue is placed into contact with the anterior portion of the palate and the bolus is pushed posteriorly
- The soft palate begins to elevate, and Passavant's ridge starts to form in the posterior wall of the pharynx and moves closer to the soft palate
- As more of the tongue is pushed against the hard palate, the bolus is moved into the oropharynx, and the soft palate makes contact with Passavant's ridge to close off the nasopharynx from the oropharynx
- Once the bolus reaches the epiglottic vallecula, the hyoid and larynx are elevated and the tip of the epiglottis is tipped down slightly over the laryngeal aditus
- A "stripping wave" is created on the posterior wall of the pharynx to help move the bolus
- Bolus splits into 2 streams that flow on either side of the epiglottis and unite to enter the esophagus
- The soft palate is pulled down by the palatopharyngeus muscles and the pressure of the wave from the movement of the bolus, while the stripping wave continues to help move the bolus from the oropharynx
- The cricopharyngeal portion of the inferior constrictor relaxes to help the bolus enter the esophagus
- Laryngeal vestibule and rima glottidis are closed to prevent the bolus from entering the larynx
- Stripping wave empties the last of the bolus from the epiglottic vallecula, and the major portion of the bolus is already in the esophagus
- All structures return to their initial position as the stripping wave moves into the esophagus

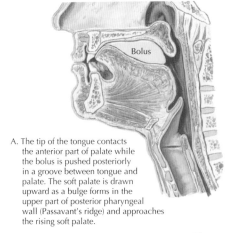

A. The tip of the tongue contacts the anterior part of palate while the bolus is pushed posteriorly in a groove between tongue and palate. The soft palate is drawn upward as a bulge forms in the upper part of posterior pharyngeal wall (Passavant's ridge) and approaches the rising soft palate.

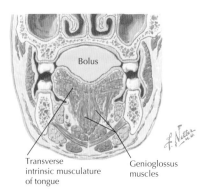

Transverse intrinsic musculature of tongue

Genioglossus muscles

B. The bolus lies in a groove on the dorsal surface of the tongue created by contraction of genioglossus and transverse intrinsic mm.

**Figure 15-12**

*Figure continued on next page*

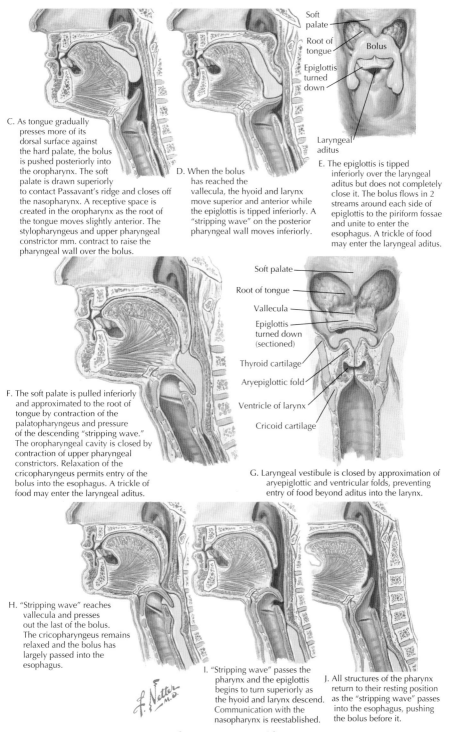

C. As tongue gradually presses more of its dorsal surface against the hard palate, the bolus is pushed posteriorly into the oropharynx. The soft palate is drawn superiorly to contact Passavant's ridge and closes off the nasopharynx. A receptive space is created in the oropharynx as the root of the tongue moves slightly anterior. The stylopharyngeus and upper pharyngeal constrictor mm. contract to raise the pharyngeal wall over the bolus.

D. When the bolus has reached the vallecula, the hyoid and larynx move superior and anterior while the epiglottis is tipped inferiorly. A "stripping wave" on the posterior pharyngeal wall moves inferiorly.

Soft palate
Root of tongue
Bolus
Epiglottis turned down
Laryngeal aditus

E. The epiglottis is tipped inferiorly over the laryngeal aditus but does not completely close it. The bolus flows in 2 streams around each side of epiglottis to the piriform fossae and unite to enter the esophagus. A trickle of food may enter the laryngeal aditus.

Soft palate
Root of tongue
Vallecula
Epiglottis turned down (sectioned)
Thyroid cartilage
Aryepiglottic fold
Ventricle of larynx
Cricoid cartilage

F. The soft palate is pulled inferiorly and approximated to the root of tongue by contraction of the palatopharyngeus and pressure of the descending "stripping wave." The oropharyngeal cavity is closed by contraction of upper pharyngeal constrictors. Relaxation of the cricopharyngeus permits entry of the bolus into the esophagus. A trickle of food may enter the laryngeal aditus.

G. Laryngeal vestibule is closed by approximation of aryepiglottic and ventricular folds, preventing entry of food beyond aditus into the larynx.

H. "Stripping wave" reaches vallecula and presses out the last of the bolus. The cricopharyngeus remains relaxed and the bolus has largely passed into the esophagus.

I. "Stripping wave" passes the pharynx and the epiglottis begins to turn superiorly as the hyoid and larynx descend. Communication with the nasopharynx is reestablished.

J. All structures of the pharynx return to their resting position as the "stripping wave" passes into the esophagus, pushing the bolus before it.

**Figure 15-12, cont'd**

- *Pharyngitis* is an inflammation of the pharynx often caused by an upper respiratory infection
- The most common symptom is a sore throat (although often accompanied by a cough)
- Pharyngitis also can cause the tonsils to enlarge and become inflamed, leading to tonsillitis

### ETIOLOGY

- Various etiologic agents may cause infection associated with pharyngitis:
  - Viral
    - Adenovirus
    - Herpes simplex virus
    - Epstein-Barr virus (infectious mononucleosis)
    - Influenza virus
    - Rhinovirus
  - Bacterial
    - *Corynebacterium diphtheriae* (diphtheria)
    - *Streptococcus* (peritonsillar abscess, "strep throat")
  - Fungal
    - *Candida albicans* (oral thrush)

### TREATMENT

- Most treatment is symptomatic
- Bacterial and fungal pharyngitis respond well to antibiotics and antifungals

**Infections of Pharynx**

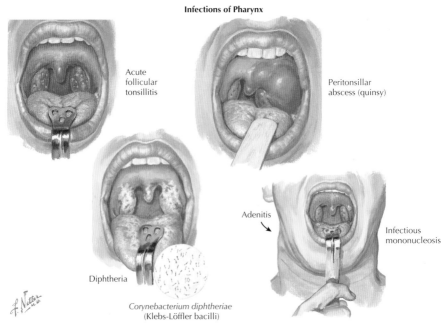

Acute follicular tonsillitis

Peritonsillar abscess (quinsy)

Adenitis

Infectious mononucleosis

Diphtheria

*Corynebacterium diphtheriae* (Klebs-Löffler bacilli)

**Figure 15-13**

- *Larynx*: connection between the pharynx and the trachea
- Prevents foreign bodies from entering the airways
- Designed for the production of sound (phonation)
- Is mobile during deglutition
- Located in the midline opposite the 3rd to the 6th cervical vertebrae (C3 to C6)
- Shorter in women and children
- Prepubescent larynx is similar in size in females and males
- After the onset of puberty, the larynx in males enlarges significantly
- Formed by 9 cartilages: 3 paired and 3 unpaired
- Vallecula is a depression in the mucosa between the pharyngeal portion of the tongue and the anterior border of the epiglottis
- Laryngeal epithelium is primarily pseudostratified columnar with cilia, except:
  - Anterior surface along the epiglottis—stratified squamous nonkeratinized
  - True vocal cord—stratified squamous nonkeratinized
- Regions of the larynx:
  - Vestibule (supraglottic)—from the laryngeal inlet to the vestibular folds
  - Ventricle—from the vestibular fold to the vocal fold
  - Infraglottic (subglottic)—from vocal folds to the inferior border of the cricoid cartilage

## RELATIONS OF THE LARYNX

- *Anterolateral*—infrahyoid muscles, platysma
- *Lateral*—lobes of the thyroid gland, carotid sheath
- *Posterior*—it forms the anterior wall of the laryngopharynx
- *Superior*—base of tongue and vallecula
- *Inferior*—trachea

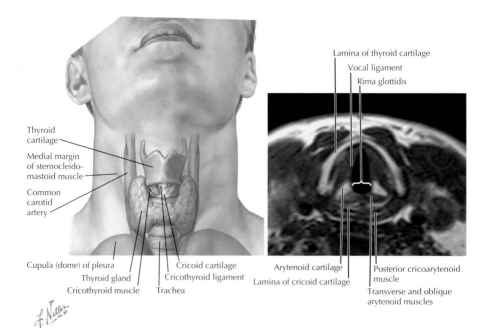

Figure 16-1

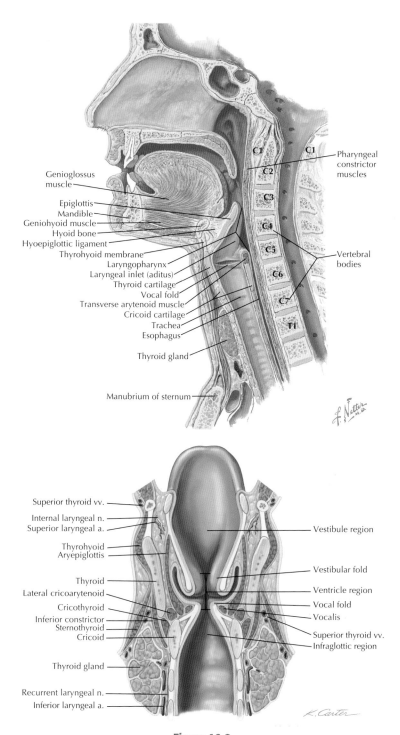

**Figure 16-2**

| Cartilage | Cartilage Type | Paired | Comments |
|-----------|---------------|--------|----------|
| Thyroid | Hyaline | No | Largest of the laryngeal cartilages |
| | | | Connects to the hyoid bone via the thyrohyoid membrane, which allows the internal laryngeal n. and superior laryngeal vessels to pass through to enter the larynx |
| | | | Lies between C4 and C6 |
| Cricoid | | | Only complete ring of cartilage in the respiratory system |
| | | | Signet in shape |
| | | | Both intrinsic and extrinsic laryngeal muscles attach to the cricoid |
| | | | Lies at C6 |
| Arytenoid | Hyaline (majority of arytenoid cartilage) | Yes | Forms framework of the true vocal cord |
| | Elastic (only the apex and small portion of vocal process) | | |
| Epiglottis | Elastic | No | Helps prevent foreign bodies from entering the larynx |
| Corniculate (minor) | | Yes | Minor cartilages that lie in the aryepiglottic fold |
| Cuneiform (minor) | | | |

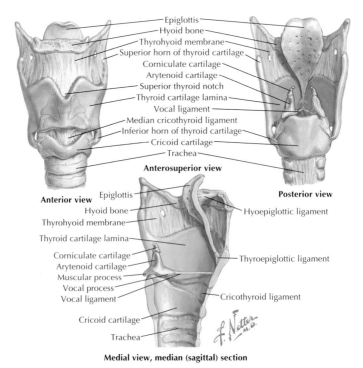

Epiglottis
Hyoid bone
Thyrohyoid membrane
Superior horn of thyroid cartilage
Corniculate cartilage
Arytenoid cartilage
Superior thyroid notch
Thyroid cartilage lamina
Vocal ligament
Median cricothyroid ligament
Inferior horn of thyroid cartilage
Cricoid cartilage
Trachea
**Anterosuperior view**

**Posterior view**

**Anterior view**
Epiglottis
Hyoid bone
Thyrohyoid membrane
Thyroid cartilage lamina
Corniculate cartilage
Arytenoid cartilage
Muscular process
Vocal process
Vocal ligament
Cricoid cartilage
Trachea

Hyoepiglottic ligament
Thyroepiglottic ligament
Cricothyroid ligament

**Medial view, median (sagittal) section**

**Figure 16-3**

| Anatomic Feature | Comments |
|---|---|
| 2 lateral laminae | 2 plates that meet at an acute angle in the anterior midline |
| Laryngeal prominence | Also known as the Adam's apple<br>Formed by the fusion of the 2 lateral lamina<br>The fusion of the 2 lateral lamina forms an angle that is more acute in males (90 degrees) than females (120 degrees)<br>Larger in males than in females |
| Thyroid notch | Superior portion of the laryngeal prominence, which forms a V shape |
| Superior tubercle | Superior border of the oblique line |
| Oblique line | Attachment for sternothyroid, thyrohyoid, and inferior constrictor mm. (extrinsic muscles of the larynx) |
| Inferior tubercle | Inferior border of the oblique line |
| Superior horn | Provides lateralmost attachment for the thyrohyoid membrane |
| Inferior horn | Articulates with the cricoid to form the cricothyroid joint |

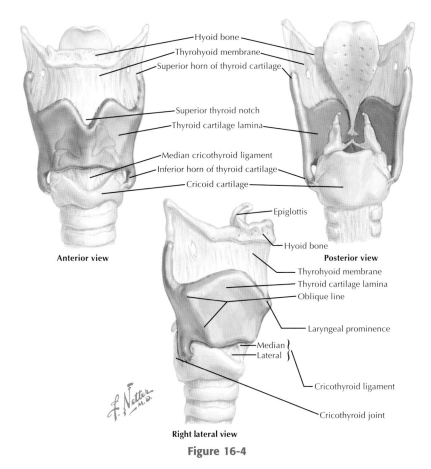

Anterior view

- Hyoid bone
- Thyrohyoid membrane
- Superior horn of thyroid cartilage
- Superior thyroid notch
- Thyroid cartilage lamina
- Median cricothyroid ligament
- Inferior horn of thyroid cartilage
- Cricoid cartilage

Posterior view

- Epiglottis
- Hyoid bone
- Thyrohyoid membrane
- Thyroid cartilage lamina
- Oblique line
- Laryngeal prominence
- Median
- Lateral
- Cricothyroid ligament
- Cricothyroid joint

Right lateral view

**Figure 16-4**

| Anatomic Feature | Comments |
|---|---|
| Arch (anteriorly) | 6 mm height<br>Narrow<br>Cricothyroid m. attaches to the arch<br>Inferior portion of the inferior constrictor m. (cricopharyngeus) attaches to the arch posterior to the cricothyroid m. |
| Lamina (posteriorly) | 2 to 3 cm in height<br>Posterior cricoarytenoid m. attaches to the lamina |
| Superior border (on the lamina) | Articulates with the arytenoid cartilage to form the cricoarytenoid joint |
| Inferior border (on the lamina) | Articulates with the inferior cornu of the thyroid cartilage to form the cricothyroid joint |

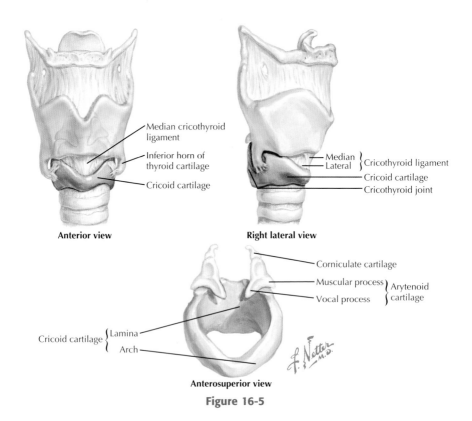

Median cricothyroid ligament
Inferior horn of thyroid cartilage
Cricoid cartilage

**Anterior view**

Median
Lateral } Cricothyroid ligament
Cricoid cartilage
Cricothyroid joint

**Right lateral view**

Corniculate cartilage
Muscular process } Arytenoid
Vocal process } cartilage

Cricoid cartilage { Lamina
Arch

**Anterosuperior view**

**Figure 16-5**

| Anatomic Feature | Comments |
|---|---|
| Divided into: | Are paired<br>Each arytenoid cartilage has:<br>• 3 surfaces (anterolateral, posterior, medial)<br>• Apex<br>• Base (with 2 processes) |
| *Apex* | Apex is the superior extension of the arytenoid cartilage<br>Corniculate cartilage articulates with the apex<br>Apex is composed of elastic cartilage |
| *Base* | Base is the larger broad surface that articulates with the cricoid cartilage<br>• Has a *muscular* process (lateral process) that extends laterally and provides for muscular attachment<br>• Has a *vocal* process (anterior process) that extends anteriorly and gives rise to the true vocal cord<br>Composed of hyaline cartilage (except a small portion of the vocal process)<br>Base articulates with cricoid to form the cricoarytenoid joint<br>Arytenoid cartilage can dislocate between the base and cricoid cartilages as a complication from instrumentation of the airway |

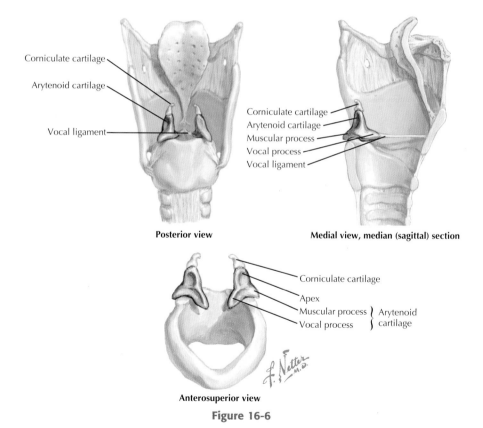

Corniculate cartilage
Arytenoid cartilage
Vocal ligament

**Posterior view**

Corniculate cartilage
Arytenoid cartilage
Muscular process
Vocal process
Vocal ligament

**Medial view, median (sagittal) section**

Corniculate cartilage
Apex
Muscular process } Arytenoid
Vocal process    } cartilage

**Anterosuperior view**

**Figure 16-6**

| Anatomic Feature | Comment |
|---|---|
| Epiglottic tubercle | Pear-shaped |
| | Connected to the thyroid cartilage by the thyroepiglottic ligament |
| | Connected to the hyoid bone by the hyoepiglottic ligament |
| | During deglutition (as the hyoid bone and remainder of larynx elevates), the epiglottis is positioned in a posterior direction, diverting food and liquid from the laryngeal inlet |
| | The mucosa covering the anterior surface of the epiglottis is stratified squamous nonkeratinized epithelium |
| | The mucosa covering the posterior surface of the epiglottis is pseudostratified columnar epithelium with cilia |

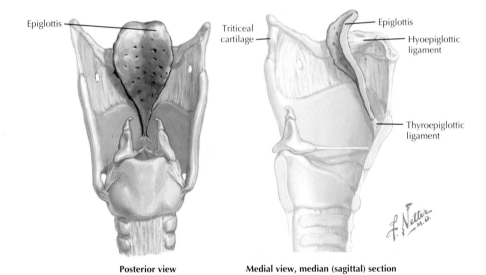

Posterior view    Medial view, median (sagittal) section

**Figure 16-7**

| Cartilage | Comments |
|-----------|----------|
| Corniculate | Lies on the apex of the arytenoid cartilage<br>Helps support the aryepiglottic fold |
| Cuneiform | Lies superior to the corniculate cartilage<br>Helps support the aryepiglottic fold |
| Triticeal | Small piece of elastic cartilage that lies in the posterior border of the thyrohyoid membrane |

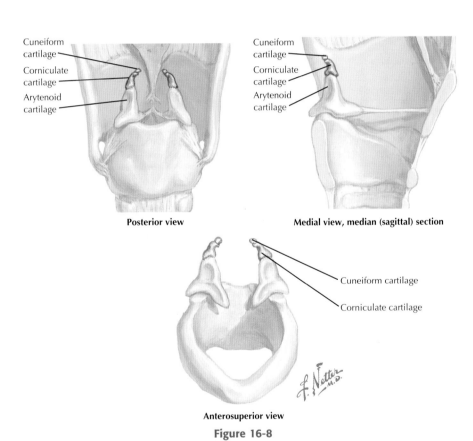

Posterior view

Medial view, median (sagittal) section

Anterosuperior view

Figure 16-8

| Joint | Comments |
|---|---|
| Cricothyroid joint | Located between the inferior cornu of the thyroid cartilage and the inferior border of the lamina of the cricoid cartilage<br>Synovial joint<br>Allows rotation between thyroid and cricoid cartilages |
| Cricoarytenoid joint | Located between the superior border of the lamina of the cricoid cartilage and the base of the arytenoid cartilage<br>Synovial joint<br>2 movements occur:<br>• Rotation<br>• Gliding<br>Medial rotation and medial gliding occur together to close the rima glottidis<br>Lateral rotation and lateral gliding occur together to open the rima glottidis |

## Major Extrinsic Membranes and Ligaments

| Ligament | Location | Comments |
|---|---|---|
| Thyrohyoid membrane | Thyroid cartilage to hyoid bone | Allows passage of the internal laryngeal n. and superior laryngeal a. and v. |
| Thyroepiglottic ligament | Thyroid cartilage to epiglottis | Holds epiglottis to the thyroid cartilage |
| Hyoepiglottic ligament | Hyoid bone to the epiglottis | Holds epiglottis to the hyoid bone |
| Cricotracheal ligament | Cricoid cartilage to trachea | Attaches the cricoid cartilage to the first tracheal ring<br>May be used in establishing an emergency airway |

## Major Intrinsic Membranes and Ligaments

| Ligament | Location | Comments |
|---|---|---|
| Vocal ligament | Arytenoid (vocal process) to thyroid cartilage | Help form *true* vocal cord |
| Conus elasticus<br>*Divided into:* | | Also known as the cricovocal or cricothyroid membrane |
| *Lateral part of conus elasticus* | *Superior*—thyroid, vocal lig., arytenoid (vocal process)<br>*Inferior*—upper border of cricoid | Lateral part of the conus elasticus is bilateral<br>Help form true vocal cord |
| *Medial part of conus elasticus (also called median cricothyroid ligament)* | Cricoid cartilage to thyroid cartilage | Primary site for establishing an emergency airway |
| Quadrangular membrane | Arytenoid to epiglottis | Help form *false* vocal cord |
| Vestibular ligament | Free edge of the inferior border of the quadrangular membrane | |

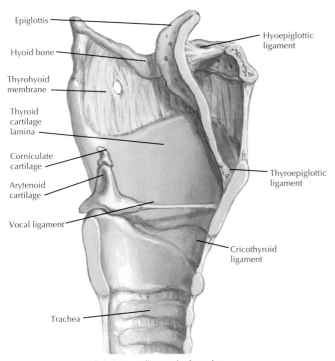

Epiglottis

Hyoid bone

Thyrohyoid membrane

Thyroid cartilage lamina

Corniculate cartilage

Arytenoid cartilage

Vocal ligament

Trachea

Hyoepiglottic ligament

Thyroepiglottic ligament

Cricothyroid ligament

**Medial view, median (sagittal) section**

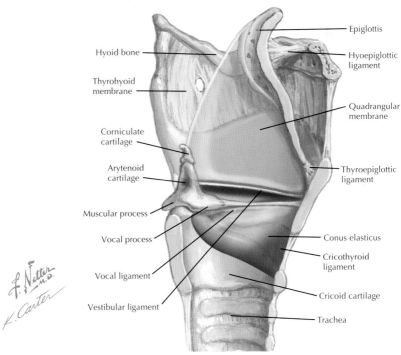

Hyoid bone

Thyrohyoid membrane

Corniculate cartilage

Arytenoid cartilage

Muscular process

Vocal process

Vocal ligament

Vestibular ligament

Epiglottis

Hyoepiglottic ligament

Quadrangular membrane

Thyroepiglottic ligament

Conus elasticus

Cricothyroid ligament

Cricoid cartilage

Trachea

**Figure 16-9**

| Muscle | Origin | Insertion | Action | Nerve Supply |
|--------|--------|-----------|--------|--------------|
| Cricothyroid | Arch of cricoid | Lamina and inferior cornu of thyroid | Increases (lengthens) tension on vocal ligaments | External laryngeal n. |
| Thyroarytenoid | Angle of thyroid cartilage | Arytenoid (vocal process) | Decreases (relaxes) tension on vocal ligaments | Recurrent laryngeal n. |
| (Vocalis—inferior fibers of the thyroarytenoid) | | | Decreases (relaxes) tension on the posterior part of the vocal ligaments | |
| Posterior cricoarytenoid | Lamina of cricoid | Arytenoid (muscular process) | Opens rima glottidis | |
| Lateral cricoarytenoid | Arch of cricoid (lateral portion) | | Closes rima glottidis | |
| Transverse arytenoid | Arytenoid (muscular process) | Opposite arytenoid (muscular process) | | |
| Oblique arytenoid | | Opposite arytenoid (apex) | | |
| Aryepiglotticus | Arytenoid (apex) | Epiglottis | Helps close laryngopharyngeal opening | |
| Thyroepiglotticus | Thyroid lamina | | | |

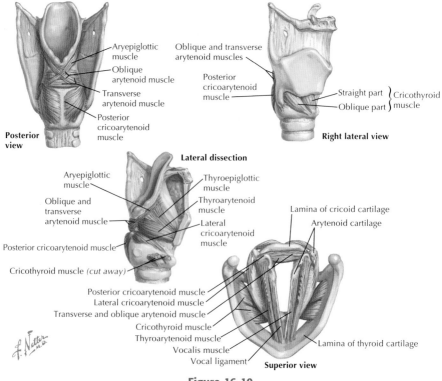

**Figure 16-10**

| SUMMARY OF MUSCLE ACTIONS | | | |
|---|---|---|---|
| Altering the Rima Glottidis | | Altering Tension on the Vocal Cords | |
| **Muscle** | **Action** | **Muscle** | **Action** |
| Posterior cricoarytenoid | *Opens* the rima glottidis | Cricothyroid | *Increasing* tension |
| Transverse arytenoids<br>Oblique arytenoids<br>Lateral cricoarytenoid | *Close* the rima glottidis | Thyroarytenoid | *Decreasing* tension |

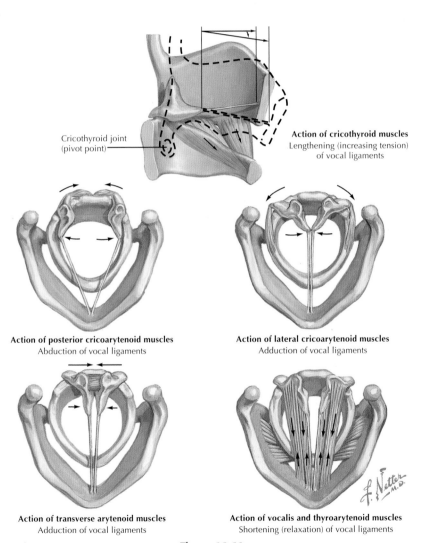

Cricothyroid joint (pivot point)

**Action of cricothyroid muscles**
Lengthening (increasing tension)
of vocal ligaments

**Action of posterior cricoarytenoid muscles**
Abduction of vocal ligaments

**Action of lateral cricoarytenoid muscles**
Adduction of vocal ligaments

**Action of transverse arytenoid muscles**
Adduction of vocal ligaments

**Action of vocalis and thyroarytenoid muscles**
Shortening (relaxation) of vocal ligaments

**Figure 16-11**

| Artery | Source | Course |
|--------|--------|--------|
| Superior laryngeal | Superior thyroid a., which arises from the external carotid a. | Passes through the thyrohyoid membrane with the internal laryngeal n. to enter the deep surface of the larynx |
| Inferior laryngeal | Inferior thyroid a., which arises from the thyrocervical trunk | Passes superiorly on the trachea to reach the posterior border of the larynx<br><br>Lies immediately deep to the inferior constrictor m. traveling beside the recurrent laryngeal n. |

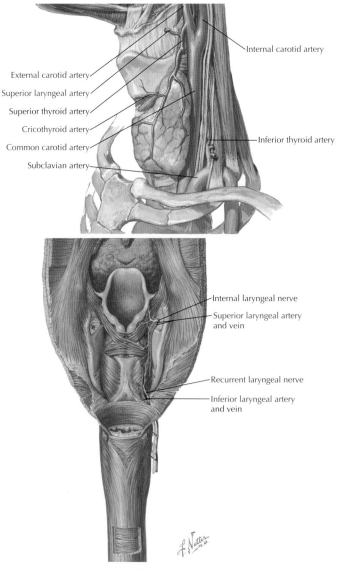

**Figure 16-12**

| Vein | Course |
|------|--------|
| Superior laryngeal | Begins in the deep surface of the superior part of the larynx |
| | Passes with the superior laryngeal a. and the internal laryngeal n. |
| | Passes through the thyrohyoid membrane to lie on the superficial surface of the larynx |
| | Drains into the superior thyroid v., which drains into the internal jugular v. |
| Inferior laryngeal | Arises within the deep surface of the inferior part of the larynx |
| | Passes with the inferior laryngeal a. and the recurrent laryngeal n. |
| | Passes inferiorly deep to the inferior constrictor to exit the larynx |
| | Drains into the inferior thyroid v., which drains into the brachiocephalic vv. |

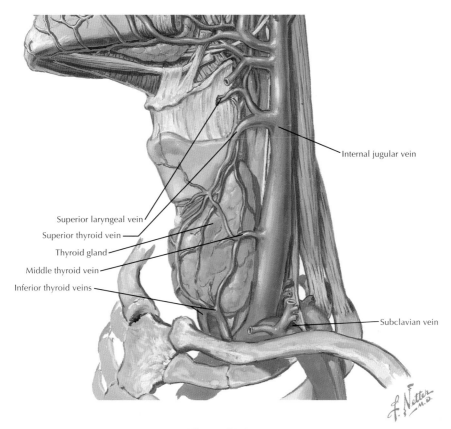

**Figure 16-13**

| Nerve | Type | Sensory Target | Muscle(s) Innervated | Comments |
|---|---|---|---|---|
| External laryngeal | Motor | | Cricothyroid | Branch of superior laryngeal nerve from the vagus |
| Internal laryngeal | Sensory | Mucosa above the vocal folds | | Branch of superior laryngeal nerve from the vagus<br><br>Carries afferent fibers responsible for the cough reflex |
| Recurrent laryngeal | Sensory and motor | Mucosa below the vocal folds | Thyroarytenoid<br>Posterior cricoarytenoid<br>Lateral cricoarytenoid<br>Transverse arytenoid<br>Oblique arytenoid<br>Aryepiglotticus<br>Thyroepiglotticus | Branch of the vagus<br>Wraps around the aorta posterior to the ligamentum arteriosum on the left side<br>Wraps around the right subclavian artery on the right side<br>Ascends on the lateral aspect of the trachea until reaching the pharynx, where it passes deep to the inferior constrictor to reach the larynx |

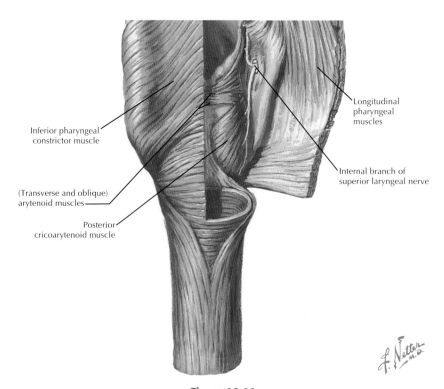

Inferior pharyngeal constrictor muscle

(Transverse and oblique) arytenoid muscles

Posterior cricoarytenoid muscle

Longitudinal pharyngeal muscles

Internal branch of superior laryngeal nerve

**Figure 16-14**

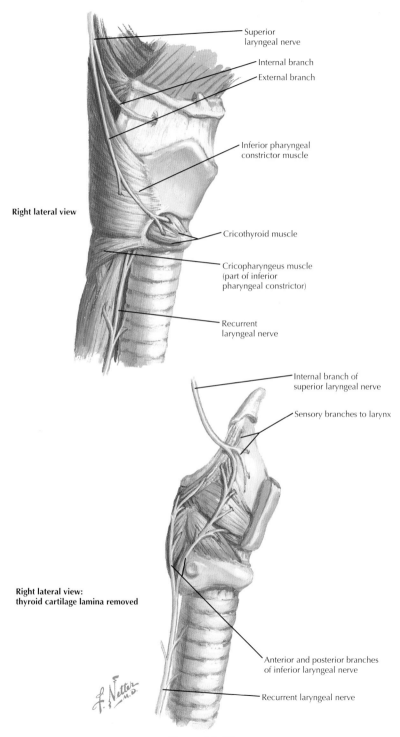

Superior
laryngeal nerve

Internal branch

External branch

Inferior pharyngeal
constrictor muscle

Right lateral view

Cricothyroid muscle

Cricopharyngeus muscle
(part of inferior
pharyngeal constrictor)

Recurrent
laryngeal nerve

Internal branch of
superior laryngeal nerve

Sensory branches to larynx

Right lateral view:
thyroid cartilage lamina removed

Anterior and posterior branches
of inferior laryngeal nerve

Recurrent laryngeal nerve

**Figure 16-15**

- *Cricothyrotomy*: a procedure for establishing an emergency airway when other methods are unsuitable
- Once the anatomy of the larynx is identified, the procedure can be performed with 2 incisions:
  - Incision through the skin
  - Incision through the cricothyroid membrane
- The correct location for the incision is easiest to find by identifying the thyroid notch on the thyroid cartilage
- By sliding the examining finger in an inferior direction, the groove between the thyroid and cricoid cartilages can be located
- A 3-cm vertical incision is made through the skin, and the thyrohyoid membrane is located
- A small midline incision is made, and a tracheostomy tube is inserted to establish an airway

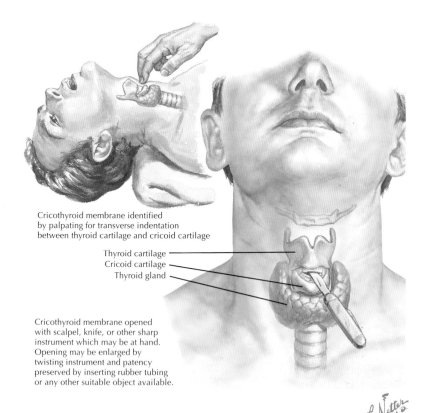

Cricothyroid membrane identified
by palpating for transverse indentation
between thyroid cartilage and cricoid cartilage

Thyroid cartilage
Cricoid cartilage
Thyroid gland

Cricothyroid membrane opened
with scalpel, knife, or other sharp
instrument which may be at hand.
Opening may be enlarged by
twisting instrument and patency
preserved by inserting rubber tubing
or any other suitable object available.

**Figure 16-16**

- *Laryngitis*: an inflammation of the vocal cords in the larynx that typically does not persist longer than 7 days
- Characterized by a weak and hoarse voice, sore throat, and cough
- Most common cause is a viral infection, although it may be caused by a bacterial infection
- Can also be caused by excessive yelling (such as cheering at a sporting event) and smoking
- Because most cases of laryngitis are viral in nature, antibiotics generally are not used as treatment

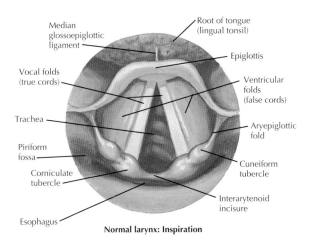

Median glossoepiglottic ligament

Root of tongue (lingual tonsil)

Epiglottis

Vocal folds (true cords)

Ventricular folds (false cords)

Trachea

Aryepiglottic fold

Piriform fossa

Cuneiform tubercle

Corniculate tubercle

Interarytenoid incisure

Esophagus

**Normal larynx: Inspiration**

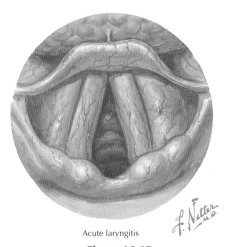

Acute laryngitis

**Figure 16-17**

- The vagus nerve provides all of the motor and sensory innervation to the larynx
- The superior laryngeal nerve divides into the internal laryngeal (sensory) and external laryngeal (motor to the cricothyroid)
- The recurrent laryngeal provides sensory and motor innervation to the remainder of the muscles of the larynx
- Lesions of the recurrent laryngeal nerve result in a paralysis of the ipsilateral vocal fold
- This problem usually manifests clinically as hoarseness with an ineffective cough
- Common causes include:
  - Thyroid tumors
  - Neck tumors
  - Cerebrovascular accident (stroke)
  - Lung tumors
  - Surgery
  - Thyroiditis
- The voice also may be affected in Parkinson's disease and myasthenia gravis

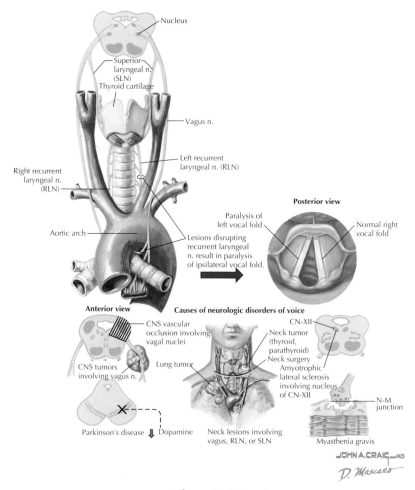

**Figure 16-18**

- *Fascia*: a band of connective tissue that surrounds structures (such as enveloping muscles), giving rise to potential tissue spaces and pathways that allow infection to spread

## SUPERFICIAL FASCIA

- Immediately deep to the skin
- Contains fat

## DEEP FASCIA

- Deep to the superficial fascia
- Aids muscle movements
- Provides passageways for nerves and vessels
- Provides attachment for some muscles
- In the neck, it is divided into *4 regions*:
  - Visceral region
  - Musculoskeletal region
  - 2 neurovascular compartments
- Also divided into *4 layers*:
  - Superficial layer of deep cervical fascia (investing layer of deep cervical fascia)
  - Middle layer of deep cervical fascia
  - Deep layer of deep cervical fascia
  - Carotid sheath (composed of the contributions of all 3 layers of deep cervical fascia)
- There is no deep fascia in the face, which allows free spread of fluid

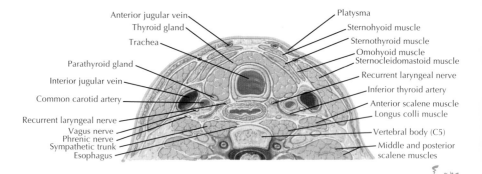

**Figure 17-1**

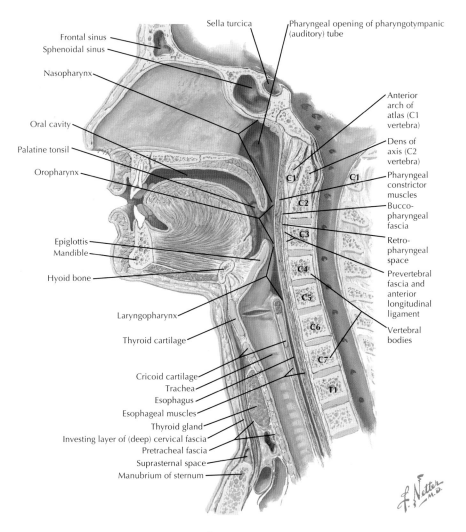

Frontal sinus
Sphenoidal sinus
Nasopharynx
Oral cavity
Palatine tonsil
Oropharynx
Epiglottis
Mandible
Hyoid bone
Laryngopharynx
Thyroid cartilage
Cricoid cartilage
Trachea
Esophagus
Esophageal muscles
Thyroid gland
Investing layer of (deep) cervical fascia
Pretracheal fascia
Suprasternal space
Manubrium of sternum

Sella turcica
Pharyngeal opening of pharyngotympanic (auditory) tube

Anterior arch of atlas (C1 vertebra)
Dens of axis (C2 vertebra)
Pharyngeal constrictor muscles
Bucco-pharyngeal fascia
Retro-pharyngeal space
Prevertebral fascia and anterior longitudinal ligament
Vertebral bodies

C1
C2
C3
C4
C5
C6
C7
T1

C1

**Figure 17-2**

- Superficial fascia lies deep to the skin and contains the cutaneous vessels and nerves
- In the neck, the platysma muscle lies within the superficial fascia
- Has a variable amount of adipose tissue, depending on the individual patient
- Superficial fascia has fibrous septa which can help localize infections

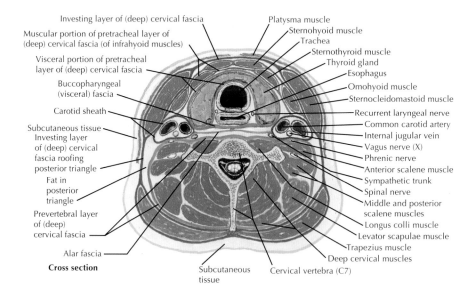

Investing layer of (deep) cervical fascia
Muscular portion of pretracheal layer of (deep) cervical fascia (of infrahyoid muscles)
Visceral portion of pretracheal layer of (deep) cervical fascia
Buccopharyngeal (visceral) fascia
Carotid sheath
Subcutaneous tissue
Investing layer of (deep) cervical fascia roofing posterior triangle
Fat in posterior triangle
Prevertebral layer of (deep) cervical fascia
Alar fascia
**Cross section**

Platysma muscle
Sternohyoid muscle
Trachea
Sternothyroid muscle
Thyroid gland
Esophagus
Omohyoid muscle
Sternocleidomastoid muscle
Recurrent laryngeal nerve
Common carotid artery
Internal jugular vein
Vagus nerve (X)
Phrenic nerve
Anterior scalene muscle
Sympathetic trunk
Spinal nerve
Middle and posterior scalene muscles
Longus colli muscle
Levator scapulae muscle
Trapezius muscle
Deep cervical muscles

Subcutaneous tissue
Cervical vertebra (C7)

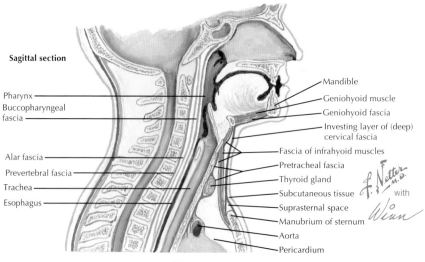

**Sagittal section**

Pharynx
Buccopharyngeal fascia
Alar fascia
Prevertebral fascia
Trachea
Esophagus

Mandible
Geniohyoid muscle
Geniohyoid fascia
Investing layer of (deep) cervical fascia
Fascia of infrahyoid muscles
Pretracheal fascia
Thyroid gland
Subcutaneous tissue
Suprasternal space
Manubrium of sternum
Aorta
Pericardium

**Figure 17-3**

| SUPERFICIAL LAYER OF DEEP CERVICAL FASCIA | | | |
|---|---|---|---|
| Layer | Location | Attachment | Comments |
| Superficial layer of deep cervical fascia (also known as the investing layer of deep cervical fascia) | Immediately deep to the superficial fascia<br><br>Encircles the neck completely<br><br>When the layer approaches the sternocleidomastoid and trapezius mm., it splits to lie on the superficial and deep surfaces | *Anterior*—chin, hyoid, sternum<br><br>*Posterior*—spinous process of cervical vertebra and the ligamentum nuchae<br><br>*Superior*—external occipital protuberance, superior nuchal line, mastoid process, inferior border of the zygomatic arch, inferior border of the mandible from the angle to the midline<br><br>*Inferior*—sternum (splitting into anterior and posterior parts), clavicle, acromion of the scapula | Forms the roof of the posterior triangle<br><br>In the area between the mastoid process and the angle of the mandible, this layer forms the deep portion of the parotid fascia (evidence supports that the superficial portion is continuous with the platysma fascia and is classified as part of the superficial muscular aponeurotic system [SMAS], although some claim the superficial portion is also from the superficial layer of deep cervical fascia)<br><br>Helps define the masticator space |

| MIDDLE LAYER OF DEEP CERVICAL FASCIA (sometimes collectively referred to as the Pretracheal fascia) | | | |
|---|---|---|---|
| Layer | Location | Attachment | Comments |
| Muscular portion: *(Infrahyoid fascia)* | Completely surrounds the strap muscles of the neck | *Superior*—hyoid bone and thyroid cartilage<br><br>*Inferior*—sternum | Is continuous across the midline |
| Visceral portion: *(Pretracheal layer of fascia)* | Deep to the superficial layer of deep cervical fascia | *Superior*—larynx<br><br>*Inferior*—fibrous pericardium in the superior mediastinum of the thorax | Forms a covering around the visceral structures in the neck, such as the thyroid gland, esophagus, and trachea |
| Visceral portion: *(Buccopharyngeal fascia)* | Deep to the superficial layer of deep cervical fascia posterior to the pharynx | *Superior*—base of the skull<br><br>*Inferior*—superior mediastinum where the middle layer of deep cervical fascia joins the alar fascia | Continuous with the pretracheal layer of fascia posterior to the pharynx and the esophagus |

| DEEP LAYER OF DEEP CERVICAL FASCIA (sometimes collectively referred to as the Prevertebral fascia) | | | |
|---|---|---|---|
| Layer | Location | Attachment | Comments |
| Prevertebral layer of fascia | Completely encircles the cervical portion of the vertebral column with its associated pre- and postvertebral muscles | *Superior*—base of skull<br><br>*Inferior*—coccyx | Forms the floor of the posterior triangle<br><br>Encloses the vertebral muscles<br><br>Forms the axillary sheath |
| Alar fascia | An anterior slip of prevertebral fascia found between the middle layer of deep cervical fascia and prevertebral layers of deep cervical fascia | *Superior*—base of skull<br><br>*Inferior*—merges with visceral portion of the middle layer of deep cervical fascia at about the level of T2 | Separates the retropharyngeal space from the danger space |

| COMBINATION OF ALL 3 LAYERS | | | |
|---|---|---|---|
| Layer | Location | Attachment | Comments |
| Carotid sheath | In the neck between the investing layer, pretracheal layer, and the prevertebral layer | *Superior*—base of skull<br><br>*Inferior*—merges with connective tissue around arch of the aorta | Contains the internal or common carotid a., internal jugular v., and vagus n. (parts of the ansa cervicalis tend to be found with the carotid sheath) |

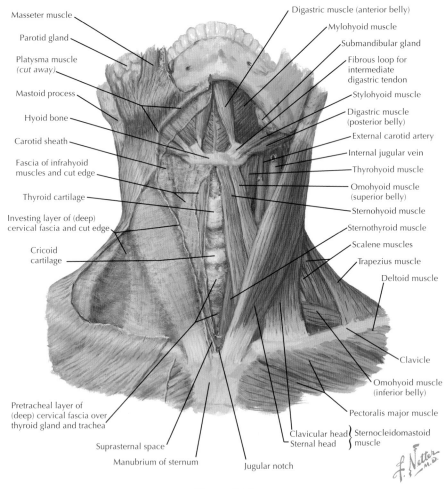

Masseter muscle
Parotid gland
Platysma muscle (cut away)
Mastoid process
Hyoid bone
Carotid sheath
Fascia of infrahyoid muscles and cut edge
Thyroid cartilage
Investing layer of (deep) cervical fascia and cut edge
Cricoid cartilage
Pretracheal layer of (deep) cervical fascia over thyroid gland and trachea
Suprasternal space
Manubrium of sternum

Digastric muscle (anterior belly)
Mylohyoid muscle
Submandibular gland
Fibrous loop for intermediate digastric tendon
Stylohyoid muscle
Digastric muscle (posterior belly)
External carotid artery
Internal jugular vein
Thyrohyoid muscle
Omohyoid muscle (superior belly)
Sternohyoid muscle
Sternothyroid muscle
Scalene muscles
Trapezius muscle
Deltoid muscle
Clavicle
Omohyoid muscle (inferior belly)
Pectoralis major muscle
Clavicular head } Sternocleidomastoid
Sternal head } muscle
Jugular notch

**Figure 17-4**

- Layers of fascia "create" potential fascial spaces
- All are filled by loose areolar connective tissue
- Infections or other inflammatory conditions spread by the path of least resistance to reach the fascial spaces
- Most odontogenic infections are caused by endogenous bacteria
- Spread typically is between contiguous fascial layers, but bacteria release enzymes that cause cellular lysis, allowing spread between fascia spaces that are not continuous
- The hyoid bone is the most important anatomic structure in the neck that limits the spread of infection
- Most are divided into spaces in relation to the hyoid bone:
  - Suprahyoid
  - Infrahyoid
  - Entire length of the neck
- In dentistry, fascial spaces are classified according to mode of spread of odontogenic infections
- Thus fascial spaces are designated as either *primary,* with infection occurring by direct spread from involved tissue, or *secondary,* with infection occurring by continued spread from another space
- A commonly accepted classification is:
  - Primary maxillary spaces:
    - Canine
    - Buccal (bridges between maxillary and mandibular regions)
    - Infratemporal
  - Primary mandibular spaces:
    - Submandibular
    - Submental
    - Sublingual
    - Buccal (bridges between maxillary and mandibular regions)
  - Secondary spaces:
    - Masticator (pterygomandibular, submasseteric, temporal)
    - Lateral pharyngeal
    - Retropharyngeal
    - Parotid
    - Prevertebral
- Some of the fascial spaces are directly continuous with other fascial spaces, whereas others will communicate if infections break through 1 of the walls of a space

Horizontal section below lingula of mandible (superior view) demonstrating bed of parotid gland

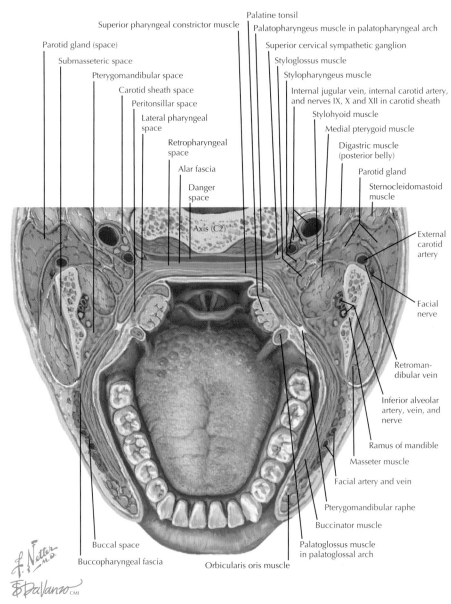

Superior pharyngeal constrictor muscle
Palatine tonsil
Palatopharyngeus muscle in palatopharyngeal arch
Parotid gland (space)
Superior cervical sympathetic ganglion
Submasseteric space
Styloglossus muscle
Pterygomandibular space
Stylopharyngeus muscle
Carotid sheath space
Internal jugular vein, internal carotid artery, and nerves IX, X and XII in carotid sheath
Peritonsillar space
Stylohyoid muscle
Lateral pharyngeal space
Medial pterygoid muscle
Retropharyngeal space
Digastric muscle (posterior belly)
Alar fascia
Parotid gland
Danger space
Sternocleidomastoid muscle
Axis (C2)
External carotid artery
Facial nerve
Retromandibular vein
Inferior alveolar artery, vein, and nerve
Ramus of mandible
Masseter muscle
Facial artery and vein
Pterygomandibular raphe
Buccinator muscle
Buccal space
Palatoglossus muscle in palatoglossal arch
Buccopharyngeal fascia
Orbicularis oris muscle

**Figure 17-5**

| Space | Location | Direct Communications | Comments and Potential for Infection |
|---|---|---|---|
| Buccal | *Lateral*–skin and superficial fascia<br>*Medial*–buccinator<br>*Superior*–zygomatic process<br>*Inferior*–mandible<br>*Anterior*–mouth<br>*Posterior*–masseter | Buccal space communicates with:<br>• Canine space<br>• Pterygomandibular space<br>• Infratemporal space<br>• Submasseteric space<br>• Lateral pharyngeal space | Dental infections of the maxillary and mandibular molars |
| Canine | *Superior*–levator labii superioris<br>*Inferior*–levator anguli oris | Canine space communicates with:<br>• Buccal space | Dental infections of the maxillary canine or maxillary 1st premolar<br>Infections can erode superiorly toward the orbit, in which case they can travel via the inferior ophthalmic vein into the cavernous sinus |
| Infratemporal | *Superior*–infratemporal surface of greater wing of sphenoid<br>*Inferior*–lateral pterygoid<br>*Lateral*–temporalis<br>*Medial*–lateral pterygoid plate<br>*Anterior*–maxilla<br>*Posterior*–lateral pterygoid | Infratemporal space communicates with:<br>• Buccal space<br>• Pterygomandibular space | Dental infections are rare in the infratemporal space<br>When they occur, they usually are the result of maxillary 3rd molar infection<br>Infections in this area are in close proximity to the pterygoid plexus and can travel to the cavernous sinus |
| Submaxillary (also called submandibular, but then is confused with the smaller submandibular part) | *Anterior* and *lateral*–mandible<br>*Posterior*–hyoid bone<br>*Superior*–mucosa of the floor of the oral cavity and the tongue<br>*Inferior*–superficial layer of deep cervical fascia | Submaxillary space communicates with:<br>• Lateral pharyngeal space | The anterior part of the peripharyngeal spaces, which create a ring around the pharynx (the retropharyngeal and lateral pharyngeal spaces are the other components)<br>Divided into 3 parts:<br>• Sublingual space<br>• Submandibular space<br>• Submental space |
| *Sublingual* | Between the mucosa and the mylohyoid m.<br>*Anterior* and *lateral*–mandible<br>*Posterior*–muscles along the base of the tongue<br>*Superior*–mucosa of the floor of the oral cavity and the tongue<br>*Inferior*–mylohyoid m. | Sublingual space communicates with:<br>• Lateral pharyngeal space<br>• Submandibular space | Contains the:<br>• Hypoglossal n.<br>• Lingual n.<br>• Sublingual gland<br>• Deep part of the submandibular gland<br>• Submandibular duct<br>Dental infections from the mandibular premolars and molars may spread to the sublingual space |

*Continued on next page*

| Space | Location | Direct Communications | Comments and Potential for Infection |
|---|---|---|---|
| *Submandibular* | Between the mylohyoid m. and the superficial layer of deep cervical fascia<br><br>On the superficial surface of the mylohyoid between the anterior and posterior bellies of the digastric m. and the mandible | Submandibular space communicates with:<br>• Lateral pharyngeal space<br>• Sublingual space<br>• Submental space | Contains the:<br>• Submandibular gland<br>• Anterior digastric m.<br>Continuous with the sublingual space along the posterior free border of the mylohyoid m.<br>Because the roots of the 1st, 2nd, and 3rd molars are inferior to the attachment of the mylohyoid on the mandible, dental infections of these teeth may pass into the submandibular space, which is continuous with the lateral pharyngeal space<br>Corresponds to the area of the submandibular triangle |
| *Submental* | Between the mylohyoid m. and the superficial layer of deep cervical fascia<br><br>Bounded laterally by the anterior digastric m. | Submental space communicates with:<br>• Submandibular space | The submental space is an anterior extension of the submandibular space<br>Corresponds to the area of the submental triangle<br>Infections of mandibular anterior teeth may pass into the submental space |
| Lateral pharyngeal (also called the parapharyngeal space) | On the lateral aspect of the pharynx, continuous with the retropharyngeal space posteriorly and the submandibular space anteriorly<br><br>Extends from the base of the skull to the hyoid bone<br><br>Extends in an anterosuperior direction to the pterygomandibular raphe<br><br>Bounded medially by the middle layer of deep cervical fascia (buccopharyngeal fascia) covering the superior constrictor m. of the pharynx and laterally by the superficial layer of deep cervical fascia covering the medial pterygoid m. and the deep portion of the parotid gland | Lateral pharyngeal space communicates with:<br>• Submandibular space<br>• Retropharyngeal space<br>• Pterygomandibular space<br>• Peritonsillar space | Very susceptible to the spread of infections from the teeth, jaws, and pharynx, including the nasopharynx, adenoids, and tonsils<br>Infections of mandibular 3rd molars may spread to this space<br>Tonsillar infections may spread to this space<br>Tumors of the lateral pharyngeal space also will spread through the space |

*Continued on next page*

| Space | Location | Direct Communications | Comments and Potential for Infection |
|---|---|---|---|
| Masticator | Formed when the superficial layer of deep cervical fascia splits to enclose the ramus of the mandible and overlies the masseter m. on the lateral surface and the medial pterygoid m. and the lower portion of the temporalis m. on the medial surface | Masticator space communicates with:<br>• Infratemporal space<br>• Pterygomandibular space<br>• Submasseteric space<br>• Temporal space | Contains the:<br>• Masseter m.<br>• Medial pterygoid m.<br>• Lateral pterygoid m.<br>• Lower portion (insertion) of the temporalis m.<br>• Contents of the pterygomandibular space<br>Is the collective space that can be divided into the:<br>• Pterygomandibular<br>• Submasseteric<br>• Temporal |
| *Pterygomandibular* | *Medial*—medial pterygoid<br>*Lateral*—mandible<br>*Superior*—lateral pterygoid<br>*Posterior*—parotid gland<br>*Anterior*—buccal space | Pterygomandibular space communicates with:<br>• Submasseteric space<br>• Temporal space<br>• Buccal space | Dental infections that travel to this space are from mandibular 3rd molars or mandibular 2nd molars<br>Contents include:<br>• Inferior alveolar n., a., and v.<br>• Sphenomandibular ligament |
| *Submasseteric* | *Anterior*—masseter<br>*Posterior*—parotid gland<br>*Lateral*—masseter<br>*Medial*—mandible<br>*Superior*—zygomatic arch<br>*Inferior*—mandible (inferior attachment of masseter) | Submasseteric space communicates with:<br>• Pterygomandibular space<br>• Buccal space | Dental infections in this space are rare<br>Usually the result of an infection of an impacted mandibular 3rd molar |
| *Temporal* | Formed when the superficial layer of deep cervical fascia encloses the temporalis m. | Temporal space communicates with:<br>• Infratemporal space<br>• Pterygomandibular space (subdivision of masticator space) | Can be further subdivided into a superficial and a deep space |
| Peritonsillar | *Anterior*—palatoglossal fold<br>*Posterior*—palatopharyngeal fold<br>*Medial*—palatine tonsil capsule<br>*Lateral*—superior constrictor m. | Peritonsillar space communicates with:<br>• Lateral pharyngeal space | Located within the wall of the pharynx<br>Infections of the peritonsillar space may extend into the lateral pharyngeal space |
| Parotid gland [space] | Formed when the superficial layer of deep cervical fascia encloses the parotid gland as a capsule | No direct communication | The parotid fascia is weaker on the medial side, and infections of this space can break through the fascia to enter the lateral pharyngeal space |
| Submandibular gland [space] | Formed when the superficial layer of deep cervical fascia encloses the submandibular gland as a capsule | No direct communication | The inner layer of the capsule is weaker, and infections of this space tend to break through the fascia to this side |

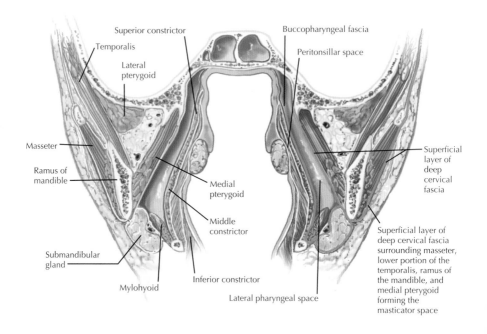

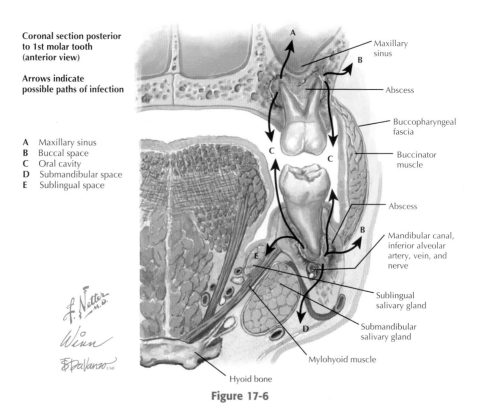

Coronal section posterior
to 1st molar tooth
(anterior view)

Arrows indicate
possible paths of infection

A   Maxillary sinus
B   Buccal space
C   Oral cavity
D   Submandibular space
E   Sublingual space

**Figure 17-6**

| Space | Location | Direct Communications | Comments and Potential for Infection |
|-------|----------|----------------------|--------------------------------------|
| Pretracheal (anterior visceral) | *Superior*—larynx<br>*Inferior*—superior mediastinum<br>Completely surrounds the trachea and also contains the thyroid and esophagus | No direct communication | Usually infections spread to the pretracheal space only by puncturing the esophagus anteriorly or by a perforation in the retropharyngeal space |

## Fascial Spaces Traversing the Length of the Neck

| Space | Location | Direct Communication | Comments and Potential for Infection |
|-------|----------|---------------------|--------------------------------------|
| Superficial | Between the superficial fascia and the superficial layer of deep cervical fascia<br>Surrounds the platysma m. | Superficial space communicates with:<br>• Superficial fascia of face | Infections are superficial and often observed early |
| Retropharyngeal | Posterior to the buccopharyngeal layer of the middle layer of cervical fascia covering the pharynx and esophagus, and anterior to the alar fascia<br>Extends from the base of the skull to about the level of T2, where the 2 layers of fascia fuse<br>The inferior portion of the retropharyngeal space (posterior to the esophagus) is sometimes called the retrovisceral space | Retropharyngeal space communicates with:<br>• Lateral pharyngeal space | Infections in this space often are the result of infections in Waldeyer's ring that spread to the retropharyngeal lymph nodes<br>Other nasal and pharyngeal infections may spread to the retropharyngeal space<br>Dental infections that traverse the lateral pharyngeal space can travel to the retropharyngeal space<br>Cellulitis or abscess may eventually result<br>Retropharyngeal infections may continue to spread posteriorly into the danger space |
| "Danger space" | Posterior to the alar fascia (and fascia where the alar fascia and middle layer of the cervical fascia fuse) and anterior to the prevertebral fascia<br>Extends from the base of the skull to the diaphragm | Not directly continuous with another fascial space<br>Danger space is continuous with mediastinum | Via the superior mediastinum, it allows infection to spread into the thorax |
| Prevertebral | Between the prevertebral fascia and the vertebral column | Not directly continuous with another space | Closed off superiorly, laterally, and inferiorly, so spread of infections in this space is not common |
| Carotid sheath | A potential space is created by the carotid sheath<br>Bounded superiorly by the skull base, inferiorly it merges with connective tissue around the aortic arch | Not directly continuous with another space<br>However, infections from surrounding areas may erode into carotid sheath | Infections from visceral spaces may enter and pass within the carotid sheath |

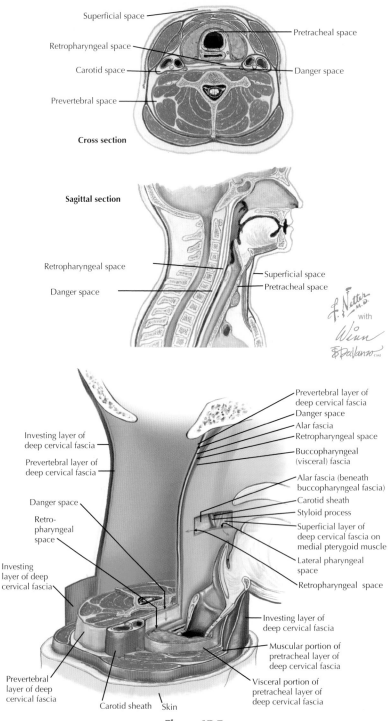

**Cross section**

Superficial space
Pretracheal space
Retropharyngeal space
Carotid space
Danger space
Prevertebral space

**Sagittal section**

Retropharyngeal space
Danger space
Superficial space
Pretracheal space

Prevertebral layer of deep cervical fascia
Danger space
Alar fascia
Retropharyngeal space
Buccopharyngeal (visceral) fascia
Investing layer of deep cervical fascia
Prevertebral layer of deep cervical fascia
Alar fascia (beneath buccopharyngeal fascia)
Carotid sheath
Styloid process
Danger space
Retro-pharyngeal space
Superficial layer of deep cervical fascia on medial pterygoid muscle
Lateral pharyngeal space
Investing layer of deep cervical fascia
Retropharyngeal space
Investing layer of deep cervical fascia
Muscular portion of pretracheal layer of deep cervical fascia
Prevertebral layer of deep cervical fascia
Visceral portion of pretracheal layer of deep cervical fascia
Carotid sheath    Skin

**Figure 17-7**

- *Ludwig's angina*: a severe cellulitis due to bacterial infection (usually from *Streptococcus, Actinomyces, Prevotella, Fusobacterium,* or *Staphylococcus*) in the floor of the oral cavity under the tongue
- Often begins in the sublingual and submandibular spaces after infection of the premolar teeth or, more commonly, molar teeth (such as an abscess of a mandibular molar), because their roots extend inferior to the mylohyoid line of the mandible
- May follow the planes of the fascial spaces to spread in the neck
- May cause sufficient neck swelling to block the airway
- More common in children
- Antibiotic therapy, incision of the neck to drain the infection, and excision of the infected tooth are the possible treatments

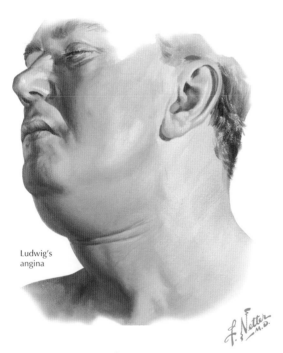

Ludwig's angina

**Figure 17-8**

- *Abscesses* may spread via the fascial planes of the neck to become more serious, such as in Ludwig's angina

## DENTOALVEOLAR ABSCESS (PERIAPICAL ABSCESS)

- An acute lesion characterized by localization of pus in the structures surrounding the apex of a tooth
- May originate in the dental pulp and be secondary to dental caries with erosion of enamel and dentin, or to traumatic injury to tooth, allowing bacteria to invade the dental pulp
- Resulting pulpitis can progress to necrosis as bacteria invade the surrounding alveolar bone, causing formation of a local abscess

## PERIODONTAL ABSCESS

- Typically involves the supporting structures of the teeth, such as the periodontal ligaments and alveolar bone, leading to formation of a local abscess

## PERICORONITIS

- An inflammation around the crown of a tooth from an infection of the gingiva, leading to formation of an abscess
- Most commonly affected tooth is a partially erupted 3rd mandibular molar

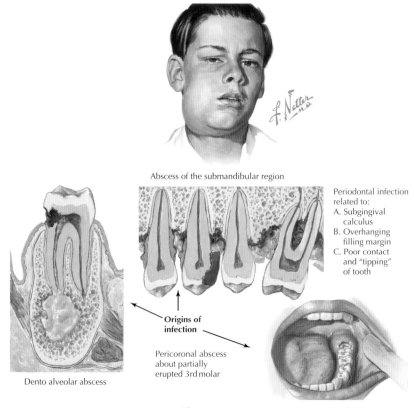

Abscess of the submandibular region

Periodontal infection related to:
A. Subgingival calculus
B. Overhanging filling margin
C. Poor contact and "tipping" of tooth

**Origins of infection**

Pericoronal abscess about partially erupted 3rd molar

Dento alveolar abscess

**Figure 17-9**

- *Cervical emphysema*: presence of gas deep to the skin, which may be iatrogenic (e.g., from surgery) or secondary to trauma or infection
- Some causes include fractures of the head and neck, introduction of air from a high-speed dental drill, and surgical procedures such as root canals and extractions of mandibular 3rd molars
- In the head and neck, cervical emphysema can spread along the fascial planes
- May be benign or fatal, depending on severity or pattern of spread

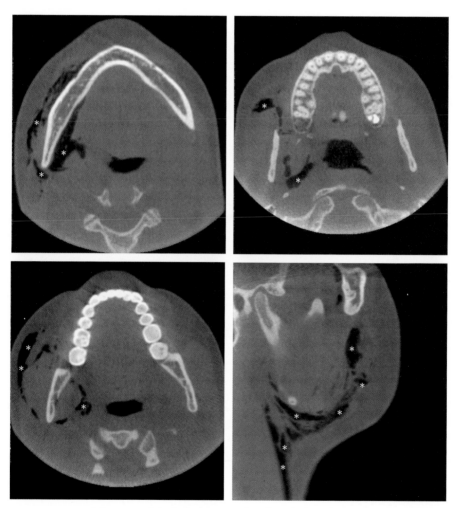

\* Presence of air displaying extension of cervical emphysema

**Figure 17-10**

- Dual functions:
  - Maintains the balance of the body (vestibular)
  - Perceives sound (auditory)
- 3 divisions:
  - External ear
  - Middle ear
  - Inner ear

EXTERNAL EAR

- The most superficial portion of the ear, the external ear includes the auricle, external acoustic meatus, and the tympanic membrane
- Helps gather sound and direct it to the tympanic membrane

MIDDLE EAR

- Transmits sound vibrations from the tympanic membrane to the inner ear via the ear ossicles: malleus, incus, and stapes
- Mainly within the petrous portion of the temporal bone
- General shape resembles a biconcave lens
- Composed of the tympanic cavity that connects anteriorly with the nasopharynx via the auditory tube and the mastoid air cells posteriorly
- Tympanic cavity contains the ear ossicles (malleus, incus, and stapes), muscles (tensor tympani and stapedius muscles), nerves (chorda tympani, tympanic branch of the glossopharyngeal nerve, and lesser petrosal nerve), and tympanic plexus (parasympathetics from the glossopharyngeal nerve plus sympathetics from the superior cervical ganglion via the carotid plexus)

INNER EAR

- Vestibular and auditory structures, which are filled with fluid, make up the inner ear:
  - Auditory portion (cochlea) is stimulated by the movement of the fluid
  - Vestibular portion (utricle, saccule, and semicircular canals) is stimulated by fluid movement within these chambers
- Consists of a membranous labyrinth that lies within an osseous labyrinth
- The receptors for auditory and vestibular function are located within the membranous labyrinth
- Fluids located in the membranous labyrinth (endolymph) and osseous labyrinth (perilymph) stimulate the auditory and vestibular receptors
- The vestibulocochlear nerve enters the internal ear via the internal acoustic meatus

**Frontal section**

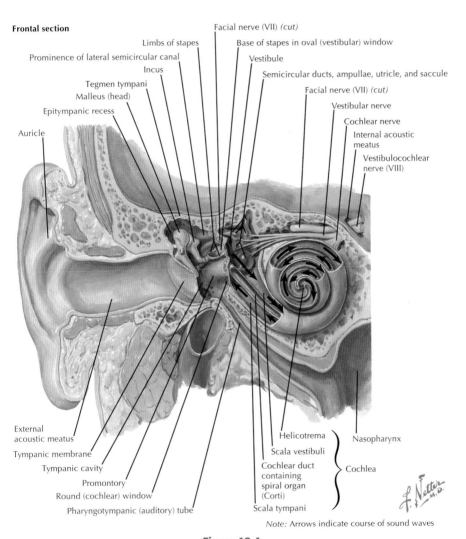

Facial nerve (VII) *(cut)*

Limbs of stapes

Base of stapes in oval (vestibular) window

Prominence of lateral semicircular canal

Vestibule

Incus

Semicircular ducts, ampullae, utricle, and saccule

Tegmen tympani

Facial nerve (VII) *(cut)*

Malleus (head)

Vestibular nerve

Epitympanic recess

Cochlear nerve

Auricle

Internal acoustic meatus

Vestibulocochlear nerve (VIII)

External acoustic meatus

Helicotrema

Nasopharynx

Tympanic membrane

Scala vestibuli

Tympanic cavity

Cochlear duct containing spiral organ (Corti)

Cochlea

Promontory

Round (cochlear) window

Scala tympani

Pharyngotympanic (auditory) tube

*Note:* Arrows indicate course of sound waves

**Figure 18-1**

**Section through turn of cochlea**

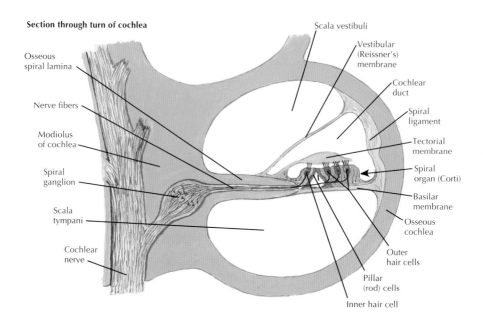

Osseous spiral lamina

Nerve fibers

Modiolus of cochlea

Spiral ganglion

Scala tympani

Cochlear nerve

Scala vestibuli

Vestibular (Reissner's) membrane

Cochlear duct

Spiral ligament

Tectorial membrane

Spiral organ (Corti)

Basilar membrane

Osseous cochlea

Outer hair cells

Pillar (rod) cells

Inner hair cell

**Superior projection of right bony labyrinth on floor of skull**

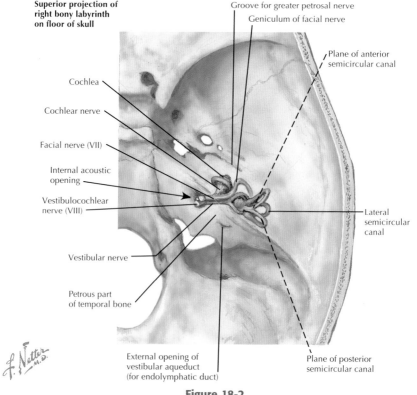

Groove for greater petrosal nerve

Geniculum of facial nerve

Plane of anterior semicircular canal

Cochlea

Cochlear nerve

Facial nerve (VII)

Internal acoustic opening

Vestibulocochlear nerve (VIII)

Vestibular nerve

Petrous part of temporal bone

Lateral semicircular canal

External opening of vestibular aqueduct (for endolymphatic duct)

Plane of posterior semicircular canal

**Figure 18-2**

| Structure | Comments |
|---|---|
| Auricle | An irregularly shaped structure made of elastic cartilage and skin<br>Superior portion has a skeleton of elastic cartilage<br>Inferior portion is known as the lobule, and has no cartilage<br>*Helix*: the outermost curved rim of the auricle, continues anteriorly to blend with the head at the crus helix<br>*Antihelix*: the portion of cartilage that follows along the helix from the inside<br>*Scaphoid fossa*: the depressed area between the helix and the antihelix<br>*Concha*: demarcated by the antihelix, it is the depressed area that leads to the external acoustic meatus<br>*Tragus*: extends from the face into the concha<br>*Antitragus*: extends from the inferior portion of the antihelix into the concha and is separated from the tragus by the intertragic notch |
| External acoustic meatus | The passageway connecting the concha of the auricle to the tympanic membrane<br>Covered by skin rich in sebaceous and cerumen-secreting glands<br>About 2.5 cm in length<br>*Lateral 1/3*: cartilaginous, extends into the temporal bone<br>*Medial 2/3*: osseous, formed by the tympanic, squamous, and petrous portions of the temporal bone |
| Tympanic membrane | The most medial portion of the external ear that separates it from the middle ear<br>Lies in a groove on the tympanic part of the temporal bone<br>A thin, semitransparent, 3-layered membrane:<br>• *External layer*—derived from skin; composed of stratified squamous epithelium<br>• *Middle layer*—fibrous, with fibers attaching to the malleus<br>• *Inner layer*—continuous with the mucous membrane of the middle ear cavity; composed of columnar epithelium with cilia<br>Anterior and posterior malleolar folds lie on the superior portion of the tympanic membrane<br>Tense and loose portions are called the pars tensa and pars flaccida, respectively |

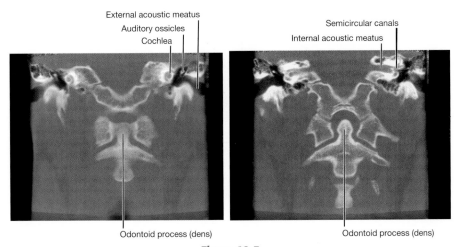

External acoustic meatus
Auditory ossicles
Cochlea

Semicircular canals
Internal acoustic meatus

Odontoid process (dens)                    Odontoid process (dens)

**Figure 18-3**

**Right auricle (pinna)**

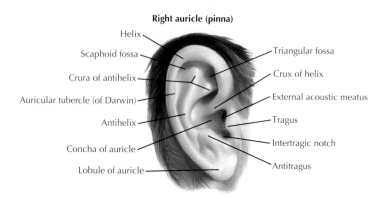

Helix

Scaphoid fossa

Crura of antihelix

Auricular tubercle (of Darwin)

Antihelix

Concha of auricle

Lobule of auricle

Triangular fossa

Crux of helix

External acoustic meatus

Tragus

Intertragic notch

Antitragus

**Otoscopic view of right tympanic membrane**

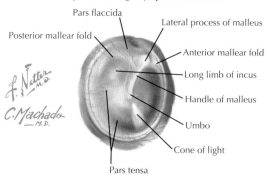

Pars flaccida

Posterior mallear fold

Lateral process of malleus

Anterior mallear fold

Long limb of incus

Handle of malleus

Umbo

Cone of light

Pars tensa

**Coronal oblique section of external acoustic meatus and middle ear (tympanic cavity)**

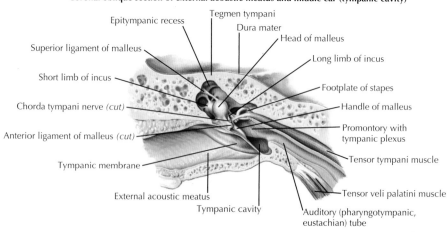

Epitympanic recess

Tegmen tympani

Dura mater

Head of malleus

Superior ligament of malleus

Long limb of incus

Short limb of incus

Footplate of stapes

Chorda tympani nerve *(cut)*

Handle of malleus

Anterior ligament of malleus *(cut)*

Promontory with tympanic plexus

Tympanic membrane

Tensor tympani muscle

External acoustic meatus

Tensor veli palatini muscle

Tympanic cavity

Auditory (pharyngotympanic, eustachian) tube

**Figure 18-4**

| Boundary | Comments |
|---|---|
| Roof | Made by the tegmen tympani, separating the middle ear from the temporal lobe of the middle cranial fossa |
| Floor | Thin bone separates the middle ear from the internal jugular v.<br>Tympanic canaliculus, located in the floor of the middle ear; allows the tympanic branch of the glossopharyngeal n. to enter the middle ear |
| Anterior wall | *Auditory tube*: located in the middle ear's anterior wall; connects the middle ear with the nasopharynx; equilibrates pressure on either side of the tympanic membrane, and allows proper drainage of the middle ear<br>Lesser petrosal n. exits the middle ear through the anterior wall<br>Postganglionic sympathetic nerve fibers from the internal carotid a. pass through the anterior wall to enter the middle ear |
| Posterior wall | *Facial canal*: passes superoinferiorly immediately posterior to the middle ear until it terminates at the stylomastoid foramen<br>*Mastoid antrum*: located in the superior portion of the posterior wall near the junction with the roof of the middle ear<br>*Pyramid*: a hollow projection from the posterior wall; contains the tendon of the stapedius m.<br>Posterior cranial fossa and sigmoid sinus are located posterior to the posterior wall |
| Medial wall | The medial wall separates the middle ear from the inner ear<br>*Promontory*: a large protuberance created by the cochlea of the inner ear<br>In the superior portion of the medial wall is a protuberance formed by the lateral semicircular canal<br>Inferior to the lateral semicircular canal on the opposite side of the medial wall is the horizontal portion of the facial canal<br>*Fenestra vestibuli* (oval window—where the footplate of the stapes is located) and *fenestra cochleae* (round window—an opening covered by a membrane): located in a superior-inferior relationship on the medial wall posterior to the promontory<br>Tendon of the tensor tympani m. enters the middle ear through the medial wall |
| Lateral wall | The lateral wall separates the middle ear from the external ear; mainly created by the tympanic membrane, with the malleus attached to the membrane at the umbo<br>*Epitympanic recess*: the region superior to the tympanic membrane that houses portions of the malleus and incus<br>Chorda tympani n. lies along the tympanic membrane and malleus until exiting the petrotympanic fissure |

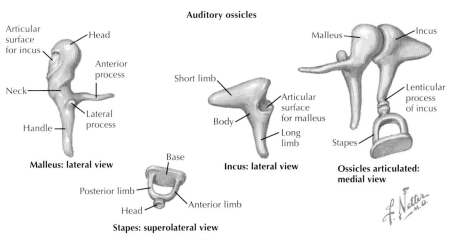

**Auditory ossicles**

Articular surface for incus

Head

Anterior process

Neck

Lateral process

Handle

**Malleus: lateral view**

Short limb

Body

Base

Articular surface for malleus

Long limb

**Incus: lateral view**

Posterior limb

Head

Anterior limb

**Stapes: superolateral view**

Malleus

Incus

Lenticular process of incus

Stapes

**Ossicles articulated: medial view**

**Figure 18-5**

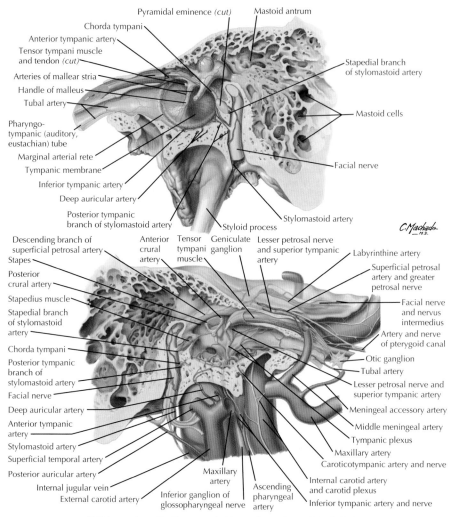

Pyramidal eminence *(cut)*

Mastoid antrum

Chorda tympani

Anterior tympanic artery

Tensor tympani muscle and tendon *(cut)*

Arteries of mallear stria

Handle of malleus

Tubal artery

Pharyngo-tympanic (auditory, eustachian) tube

Marginal arterial rete

Tympanic membrane

Inferior tympanic artery

Deep auricular artery

Posterior tympanic branch of stylomastoid artery

Stapedial branch of stylomastoid artery

Mastoid cells

Facial nerve

Stylomastoid artery

Styloid process

Descending branch of superficial petrosal artery

Stapes

Posterior crural artery

Stapedius muscle

Stapedial branch of stylomastoid artery

Chorda tympani

Posterior tympanic branch of stylomastoid artery

Facial nerve

Deep auricular artery

Anterior tympanic artery

Stylomastoid artery

Superficial temporal artery

Posterior auricular artery

Internal jugular vein

External carotid artery

Anterior crural artery

Tensor tympani muscle

Geniculate ganglion

Lesser petrosal nerve and superior tympanic artery

Labyrinthine artery

Superficial petrosal artery and greater petrosal nerve

Facial nerve and nervus intermedius

Artery and nerve of pterygoid canal

Otic ganglion

Tubal artery

Lesser petrosal nerve and superior tympanic artery

Meningeal accessory artery

Middle meningeal artery

Tympanic plexus

Maxillary artery

Caroticotympanic artery and nerve

Internal carotid artery and carotid plexus

Inferior tympanic artery and nerve

Maxillary artery

Ascending pharyngeal artery

Inferior ganglion of glossopharyngeal nerve

**Right tympanic cavity after removal of tympanic membrane (lateral view)**

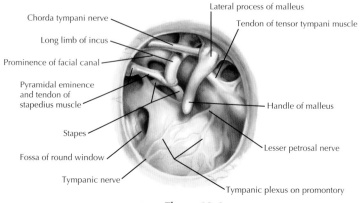

Lateral process of malleus

Chorda tympani nerve

Tendon of tensor tympani muscle

Long limb of incus

Prominence of facial canal

Pyramidal eminence and tendon of stapedius muscle

Handle of malleus

Stapes

Lesser petrosal nerve

Fossa of round window

Tympanic nerve

Tympanic plexus on promontory

**Figure 18-6**

| Structure | Description |
|---|---|
| Osseous labyrinth | Located in the petrous portion of the temporal bone |
| | Surrounds the membranous labyrinth and contains perilymph |
| | Connects to the middle ear via the fenestra vestibuli and the fenestra cochleae |
| | Divided into 3 parts: vestibule, cochlea, and semicircular canals |
| *Vestibule* | The middle portion of the osseous labyrinth, it contains the saccule and utricle of the membranous labyrinth |
| | Contains an opening for the vestibular aqueduct containing the endolymphatic duct |
| *Cochlea* | Anterior portion of the osseous labyrinth contains the cochlear duct of the membranous labyrinth |
| | Like a seashell, it spirals around a central point (the modiolus), which carries branches of the cochlear n. to the cochlear duct, for $2\frac{3}{4}$ turns, getting progressively smaller while approaching its apex |
| | As the cochlea spirals, the spiral lamina is raised from the modiolus |
| | Within the spiral lamina, the cochlear duct lies between the scala vestibuli and the scala tympani |
| | Scala vestibuli and scala tympani are continuous at the helicotrema at the apex |
| | An opening for the aqueduct of the cochlea allows perilymph to drain into the cerebrospinal fluid |
| *Semicircular canals* | The posterior portion of the osseous labyrinth |
| | 3 *semicircular canals*: anterior, posterior, and lateral |
| | *Ampulla*: a dilated end of each |
| | Anterior and posterior semicircular canals have a common crus |
| Membranous labyrinth | Located within the osseous labyrinth; contains endolymph |
| | Divided into 4 parts: cochlear duct, saccule, utricle, and semicircular ducts |
| *Cochlear duct* | A spiral structure located within the cochlea |
| | Begins at a blind end of the cochlea at the apex and ends where it joins the saccule via the ductus reuniens |
| | Triangular in shape, with a base created by the endosteum of the canal known as the spiral ligament and the stria vascularis |
| | Roof is formed by the vestibular membrane that separates the cochlear duct from the scala vestibuli |
| | Floor is formed by the basilar membrane, on which lies the organ of Corti; separates the duct from the scala tympani |
| *Saccule* | A small structure located within the vestibule of the osseous labyrinth |
| | Connected to the utricle via the utriculosaccular duct and the endolymphatic duct |
| | Sensory receptors (the maculae) are located in the saccule |
| *Utricle* | Located within the vestibule of the osseous labyrinth |
| | Sensory receptors (maculae) are located in the utricle |
| *Semicircular ducts* | Correspond to the semicircular canals of the osseous labyrinth (anterior, posterior, and lateral) |
| | Open into the utricle via 5 openings |
| | Sensory receptors known as crista are located in the ampullae of the semicircular ducts |

**Right membranous labyrinth with nerves: posteromedial view**

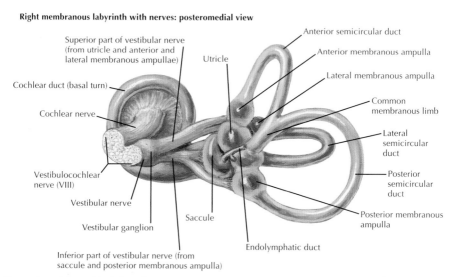

Superior part of vestibular nerve
(from utricle and anterior and
lateral membranous ampullae)

Anterior semicircular duct

Anterior membranous ampulla

Utricle

Lateral membranous ampulla

Cochlear duct (basal turn)

Cochlear nerve

Common
membranous limb

Lateral
semicircular
duct

Vestibulocochlear
nerve (VIII)

Posterior
semicircular
duct

Vestibular nerve

Saccule

Posterior membranous
ampulla

Vestibular ganglion

Endolymphatic duct

Inferior part of vestibular nerve (from
saccule and posterior membranous ampulla)

**Bony and membranous labyrinths: schema**

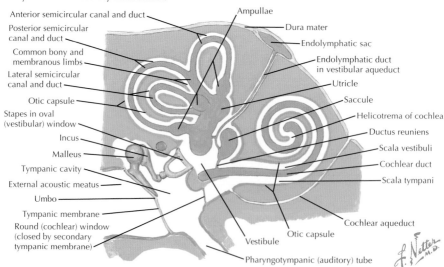

Anterior semicircular canal and duct

Ampullae

Dura mater

Posterior semicircular
canal and duct

Endolymphatic sac

Common bony and
membranous limbs

Endolymphatic duct
in vestibular aqueduct

Lateral semicircular
canal and duct

Utricle

Otic capsule

Saccule

Stapes in oval
(vestibular) window

Helicotrema of cochlea

Incus

Ductus reuniens

Malleus

Scala vestibuli

Tympanic cavity

Cochlear duct

External acoustic meatus

Scala tympani

Umbo

Tympanic membrane

Cochlear aqueduct

Round (cochlear) window
(closed by secondary
tympanic membrane)

Otic capsule

Vestibule

Pharyngotympanic (auditory) tube

**Figure 18-7**

**Membranous labyrinth within bony labyrinth** (path of sound waves)

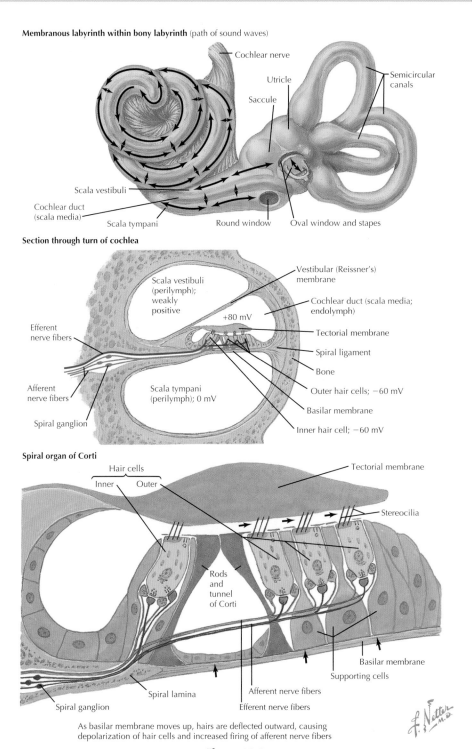

Cochlear nerve

Utricle

Saccule

Semicircular canals

Scala vestibuli

Cochlear duct (scala media)

Scala tympani

Round window

Oval window and stapes

**Section through turn of cochlea**

Scala vestibuli (perilymph); weakly positive

+80 mV

Vestibular (Reissner's) membrane

Cochlear duct (scala media; endolymph)

Tectorial membrane

Spiral ligament

Bone

Efferent nerve fibers

Afferent nerve fibers

Spiral ganglion

Scala tympani (perilymph); 0 mV

Outer hair cells; −60 mV

Basilar membrane

Inner hair cell; −60 mV

**Spiral organ of Corti**

Hair cells

Inner    Outer

Tectorial membrane

Stereocilia

Rods and tunnel of Corti

Basilar membrane

Supporting cells

Spiral lamina

Afferent nerve fibers

Spiral ganglion

Efferent nerve fibers

As basilar membrane moves up, hairs are deflected outward, causing depolarization of hair cells and increased firing of afferent nerve fibers

**Figure 18-8**

| Muscle | Origin | Insertion | Actions | Nerve Supply |
|---|---|---|---|---|
| Tensor tympani | Bony canal at auditory tube<br>Cartilaginous part of auditory tube<br>Greater wing of the sphenoid | Handle of the malleus | Tenses the tympanic membrane and helps dampen sound vibrations | Mandibular division of the trigeminal n. |
| Stapedius | Pyramid on posterior wall of the tympanic cavity | Neck of the stapes | Dampens excessive sound vibrations | Stapedius branch of the facial n. |

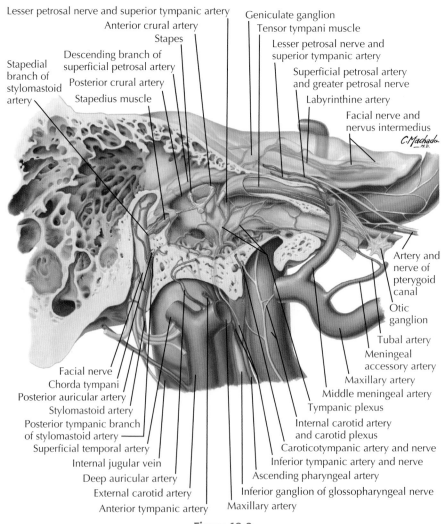

**Figure 18-9**

| Nerve | Source | Course |
|---|---|---|
| Great auricular | Cervical plexus, formed by contributions of C2 and C3 ventral rami | After passing posterior to the sternocleidomastoid m. at Erb's point, it ascends along the sternocleidomastoid, dividing into anterior and posterior branches<br><br>The posterior branch innervates the skin over the mastoid process, the posterior portion of the auricle, and the concha and lobule |
| Lesser occipital | Cervical plexus, formed by contributions from C2 ventral ramus | After passing posterior to the sternocleidomastoid m. at Erb's point, it ascends posterior to the sternocleidomastoid along the posterior portion of the head<br><br>Continues on the head posterior to the auricle<br><br>Supplies the skin posterior to the auricle |
| Auriculotemporal | Posterior part of the mandibular division of the trigeminal n. | Normally arises by 2 roots, between which the middle meningeal a. passes<br><br>Runs posteriorly just inferior to the lateral pterygoid m. and continues to the medial aspect of the neck of the mandible<br><br>Turns superiorly with the superficial temporal vessels between the auricle and condyle of the mandible deep to the parotid gland<br><br>On exiting the parotid gland, ascends over the zygomatic arch<br><br>Innervates the skin in the region of the tragus, crus helix, anterior portion of the external acoustic meatus, and outer surface of the tympanic membrane |
| Auricular branch of the vagus | Superior ganglion of the vagus n. | Travels posterior to the internal jugular v. and passes along the temporal bone<br><br>Crosses the facial canal superior to the stylomastoid foramen<br><br>Enters the mastoid canaliculus between the mastoid process and the tympanic part of the temporal bone and gives rise to 2 branches:<br>• 1 branch joins the posterior auricular branch of the facial n.<br>• The 2nd branch innervates the skin of the back of the auricle and the posterior portion of the external acoustic meatus |
| Tympanic branch of glossopharyngeal | Branches from the inferior ganglion of the vagus n., located in the petrous portion of the temporal bone | Passes superiorly through the tympanic canaliculus to enter the middle ear<br><br>In the middle ear, it divides into branches that form part of the tympanic plexus<br><br>Tympanic plexus gives rise to:<br>• Preganglionic parasympathetic fibers to the parotid gland<br>• Postganglionic sympathetic fibers to the parotid gland<br>• Sensory fibers to the middle ear cavity, including the tympanic membrane and auditory tube (mainly from the tympanic branch of the glossopharyngeal n.) |

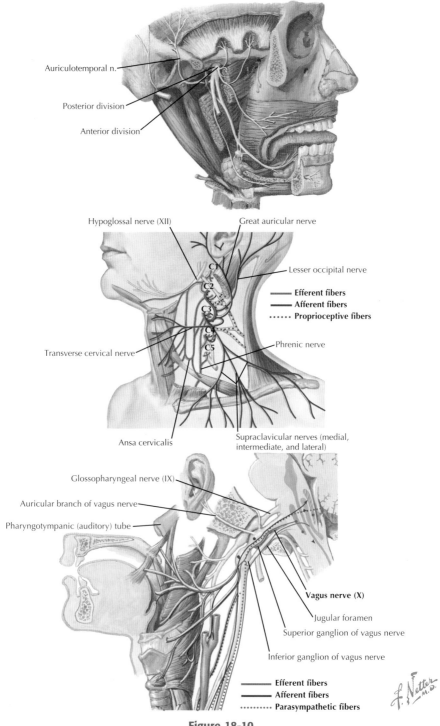

Auriculotemporal n.

Posterior division

Anterior division

Hypoglossal nerve (XII)

Great auricular nerve

C1

C2

C3

C4

C5

Lesser occipital nerve

Efferent fibers
Afferent fibers
Proprioceptive fibers

Transverse cervical nerve

Phrenic nerve

Ansa cervicalis

Supraclavicular nerves (medial,
intermediate, and lateral)

Glossopharyngeal nerve (IX)

Auricular branch of vagus nerve

Pharyngotympanic (auditory) tube

**Vagus nerve (X)**

Jugular foramen

Superior ganglion of vagus nerve

Inferior ganglion of vagus nerve

Efferent fibers
Afferent fibers
Parasympathetic fibers

**Figure 18-10**

| Nerve | Source | Course |
|-------|--------|--------|
| Tympanic plexus | Formed by the:<br>• Tympanic branch of the glossopharyngeal n. (arises from the inferior ganglion located in the petrous portion of the temporal bone)<br>• Caroticotympanic nn. (arise from the carotid plexus on the internal carotid a.) | Tympanic branch of the glossopharyngeal n. passes superiorly through the tympanic canaliculus to enter the middle ear<br>In the middle ear, it divides into branches that form the tympanic plexus<br>Caroticotympanic nn. join the tympanic branch of the glossopharyngeal n.<br>Tympanic plexus gives rise to:<br>• Preganglionic parasympathetic fibers to the parotid gland<br>• Postganglionic sympathetic fibers to the parotid gland<br>• Sensory fibers to the middle ear cavity, including the tympanic membrane and auditory tube (mainly from the tympanic branch of the glossopharyngeal) |
| Facial | Cranial n. VII has multiple motor and sensory functions<br>Created by:<br>• Nervus intermedius, which contains the sensory fibers and the parasympathetic fibers<br>• Motor portion that innervates the muscles derived from the 2nd pharyngeal arch | Nervus intermedius and motor portions—enter the internal acoustic meatus of the temporal bone<br>Facial n. then passes through the facial canal until it exits the stylomastoid foramen, initially traveling horizontally along the outside of the medial wall of the middle ear; then it bends posteriorly and inferiorly to the middle ear<br>Where the nerve changes direction is in the geniculate ganglion; here the greater petrosal n. is given off to travel anteriorly toward the pterygopalatine fossa<br>Within the facial canal, the nerve gives rise to the nerve to the stapedius m. and the chorda tympani n.<br>Chorda tympani passes anteriorly along the tympanic membrane and the malleus until it exits via the petrotympanic fissure<br>Chorda tympani carries preganglionic parasympathetic fibers to the submandibular ganglion of the oral cavity, and taste fibers to the anterior 2/3 of the tongue<br>Stapedius n. innervates the stapedius m. |

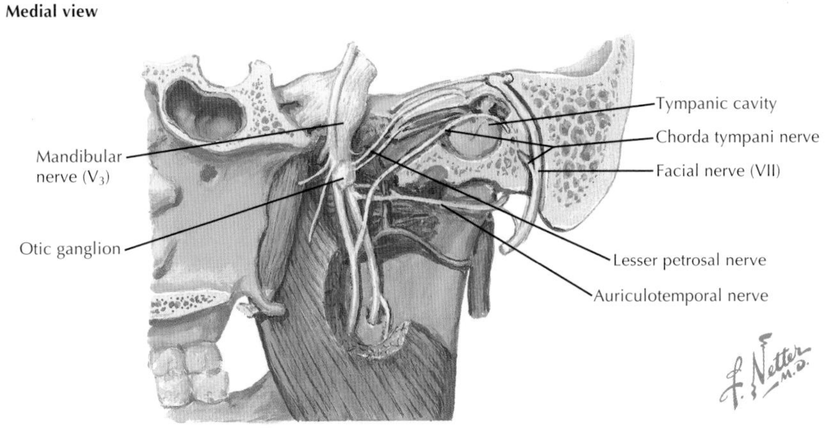

**Medial view**

Figure 18-11

| Nerve | Source | Course |
|-------|--------|--------|
| Vestibulocochlear | Also called cranial n. VIII, it emerges between the pons and the medulla oblongata | Enters the internal acoustic meatus with the facial n.<br>Within the internal acoustic meatus, it divides into vestibular branches and the cochlear branch |
| Vestibular | The vestibular portion has nerve cell bodies in the vestibular ganglion (Scarpa's ganglion) | Divides into superior and inferior branches:<br>• Superior vestibular branch innervates the maculae of the saccule and utricle and the ampulla of the anterior and lateral semicircular ducts<br>• Inferior vestibular branch innervates the macula of the saccule and the ampulla of the posterior semicircular duct |
| Cochlear | The cochlear portion has nerve cell bodies in the spiral ganglion | Utilizes the spiral ganglion within the modiolus to pass to the organ of Corti |

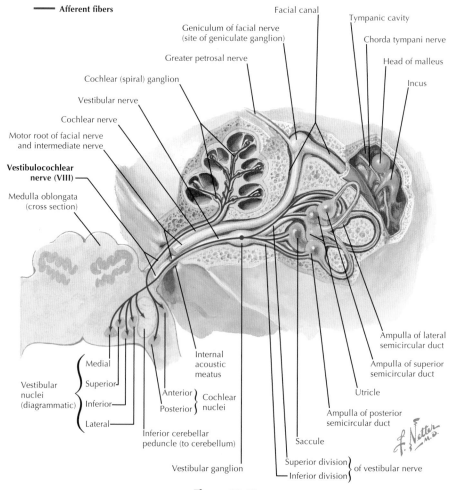

Figure 18-12

| Artery | Source | Course |
|--------|--------|--------|
| Superficial temporal | A terminal branch of the external carotid a. that arises within the parotid gland | Within the parotid gland, it gives off a transverse facial a.<br><br>Emerges from the superior part of the parotid gland immediately posterior to the temporomandibular joint and anterior to the external auditory meatus<br><br>Passes superficial to the root of the zygomatic arch just anterior to the auriculotemporal n. and the auricle<br><br>While passing superiorly, it gives off branches that supply the auricle and the external acoustic meatus |
| Posterior auricular | External carotid a. within the parotid gland | Passes superiorly between the mastoid process and cartilage of the ear<br><br>During its path to anastomose with the superficial temporal and the occipital aa., it supplies the auricle and external acoustic meatus<br><br>A stylomastoid branch arises from the posterior auricular and enters the stylomastoid foramen to supply the internal surface of the tympanic membrane |
| Deep auricular | A branch of the maxillary a. (1 of the terminal branches of the external carotid a.)<br><br>Arises in the same area as the anterior tympanic a. | Lies in the parotid gland, posterior to the temporomandibular joint, where it supplies that joint<br><br>Passes into the external acoustic meatus to supply it; then supplies the outer surface of the tympanic membrane |
| Anterior tympanic | A branch of the maxillary a. (1 of the terminal branches of the external carotid a.) | Given off in the same area as for the deep auricular a.<br><br>Passes superiorly immediately posterior to the temporomandibular joint<br><br>Enters the tympanic cavity through the petrotympanic fissure<br><br>Aids in supplying the inner surface of the tympanic membrane |

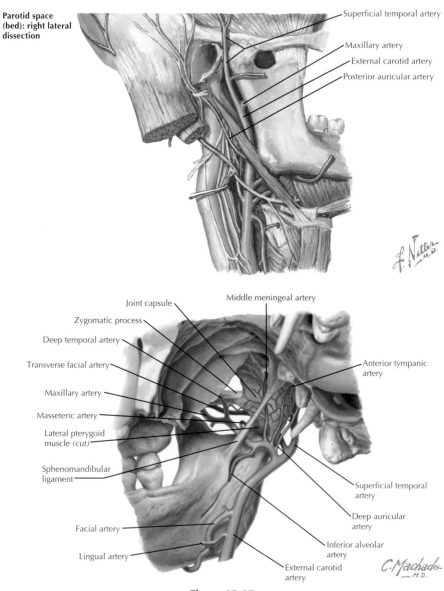

**Parotid space (bed): right lateral dissection**

Superficial temporal artery

Maxillary artery

External carotid artery

Posterior auricular artery

Joint capsule

Zygomatic process

Deep temporal artery

Transverse facial artery

Maxillary artery

Masseteric artery

Lateral pterygoid muscle *(cut)*

Sphenomandibular ligament

Facial artery

Lingual artery

Middle meningeal artery

Anterior tympanic artery

Superficial temporal artery

Deep auricular artery

Inferior alveolar artery

External carotid artery

**Figure 18-13**

| Artery | Source | Course |
|---|---|---|
| Posterior auricular | External carotid a. within the parotid gland | Passes superiorly between the mastoid process cartilage of the ear<br><br>During its path to anastomose with the superficial temporal and the occipital aa., it supplies the auricle and external acoustic meatus<br><br>A stylomastoid branch arises from the posterior auricular a. and enters the stylomastoid foramen to supply the internal surface of the tympanic membrane |
| Anterior tympanic | Maxillary a. (1 of the terminal branches of the external carotid a.) | Given off in the same area as for the deep auricular a.<br><br>Passes superiorly immediately posterior to the temporomandibular joint<br><br>Enters the tympanic cavity through the petrotympanic fissure<br><br>Aids in supplying the outer surface of the tympanic membrane and the anterior portion of the tympanic cavity |
| Inferior tympanic | Ascending pharyngeal a. of the external carotid a. | Ascends deep to the other branches of the external carotid a. and more superiorly to the stylopharyngeus m.<br><br>Passes into the middle ear through the petrous portion of the temporal bone<br><br>Helps supply the medial wall of the tympanic cavity |
| Superior tympanic | Middle meningeal a. of the maxillary a. | Arises from the middle meningeal a. immediately after passing through the foramen spinosum within the middle cranial fossa<br><br>Passes in the canal of the tensor tympani m. to help supply the tensor tympani and its bony canal |
| Caroticotympanic branch of the internal carotid | Internal carotid a. | Passes into the tympanic cavity through an aperture in the carotid canal<br><br>Helps supply the middle ear |

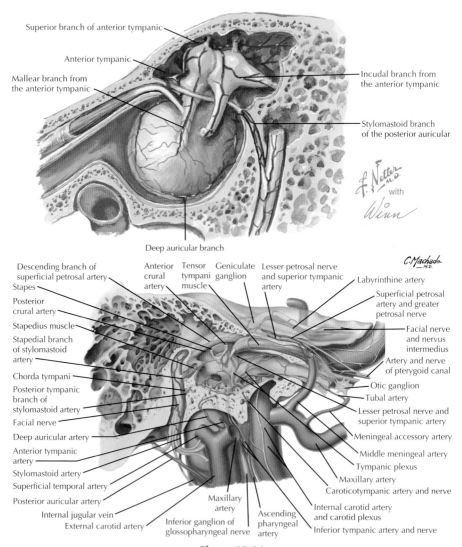

Superior branch of anterior tympanic

Anterior tympanic

Mallear branch from the anterior tympanic

Incudal branch from the anterior tympanic

Stylomastoid branch of the posterior auricular

Deep auricular branch

Descending branch of superficial petrosal artery

Stapes

Posterior crural artery

Stapedius muscle

Stapedial branch of stylomastoid artery

Chorda tympani

Posterior tympanic branch of stylomastoid artery

Facial nerve

Deep auricular artery

Anterior tympanic artery

Stylomastoid artery

Superficial temporal artery

Posterior auricular artery

Internal jugular vein

External carotid artery

Anterior crural artery

Tensor tympani muscle

Geniculate ganglion

Lesser petrosal nerve and superior tympanic artery

Maxillary artery

Inferior ganglion of glossopharyngeal nerve

Ascending pharyngeal artery

Labyrinthine artery

Superficial petrosal artery and greater petrosal nerve

Facial nerve and nervus intermedius

Artery and nerve of pterygoid canal

Otic ganglion

Tubal artery

Lesser petrosal nerve and superior tympanic artery

Meningeal accessory artery

Middle meningeal artery

Tympanic plexus

Caroticotympanic artery and nerve

Internal carotid artery and carotid plexus

Inferior tympanic artery and nerve

**Figure 18-14**

| Artery | Source | Course |
|--------|--------|--------|
| Labyrinthine | Basilar a., which gives rise to the circle of Willis | Passes through the internal acoustic meatus, where it further divides into cochlear and vestibular branches that supply the cochlear and vestibular structures |
| Posterior auricular | External carotid a. within the parotid gland | Passes superiorly between the mastoid process and cartilage of the ear |
| | | Anastomoses with the superficial temporal and the occipital aa. |
| | | A stylomastoid branch arises from the posterior auricular a., enters the stylomastoid foramen, and continues to the inner ear |
| | | During its path to anastomose with the superficial temporal and the occipital aa., it supplies the auricle and external acoustic meatus |
| | | Stylomastoid branch supplies the internal surface of the tympanic membrane and the posterior portion of the tympanic cavity; then helps supply the inner ear |

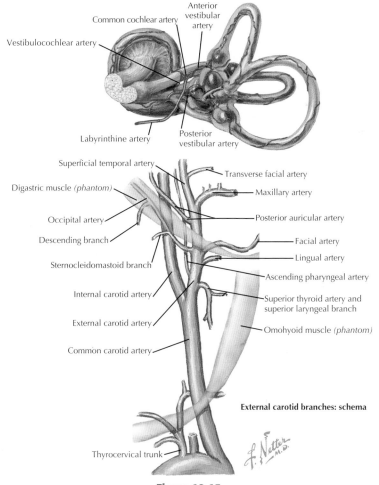

**Figure 18-15**

### Venous Drainage of the External Ear

| Vein | Comments |
|------|----------|
| Superficial temporal | Descends posterior to the zygomatic root of the temporal bone alongside the auriculotemporal n. to enter the substance of the parotid gland<br>Unites with the maxillary v. to form the retromandibular v.<br>Along its path, receives tributaries from the auricle |
| Posterior auricular | Arises from a plexus of veins created by the occipital and superficial temporal vv.<br>Descends posterior to the auricle to unite with the posterior division of the retromandibular v. to form the external jugular v.<br>Along its path, receives blood from the stylomastoid branch of the posterior auricular v., which drains the auricle, external acoustic meatus, and tympanic membrane |
| Maxillary | A short vein, sometimes paired, formed by the convergence of the tributaries of the pterygoid plexus<br>Enters the substance of the parotid gland, traveling posteriorly between the sphenomandibular lig. and the neck of the mandible<br>Unites with the superficial temporal v. to form the retromandibular v.<br>Helps drain blood from the external acoustic meatus and tympanic membrane |
| Pterygoid plexus | An extensive network of veins that parallels the 2nd and 3rd parts of the maxillary a.<br>Receives branches that correspond to the same branches of the maxillary a.<br>Tributaries eventually converge to form a short maxillary v.<br>Communicates with the cavernous sinus, pharyngeal venous plexus, and facial vein via the deep facial v. and ophthalmic vv.<br>Helps drain the external acoustic meatus |
| Transverse sinus | 1 of the deep venous sinuses that helps drain the brain<br>Aids in receiving blood from the tympanic membrane |

### Venous Drainage of the Middle Ear

| Vein | Comments |
|------|----------|
| Pterygoid plexus | An extensive network of veins that parallels the 2nd and 3rd parts of the maxillary a.<br>Receives branches that correspond to the same branches of the maxillary a.<br>Tributaries eventually converge to form a short maxillary v.<br>Communicates with the cavernous sinus, pharyngeal venous plexus, and facial vein via the deep facial v. and ophthalmic vv.<br>Helps drain the tympanic cavity |
| Superior petrosal sinus | 1 of the deep venous sinuses that helps drain the brain, running along the superior margin of the petrous portion of the temporal bone<br>Aids in receiving blood from the tympanic cavity |

### Venous Drainage of the Inner Ear

| Vein | Comments |
|------|----------|
| Labyrinthine | Begins in the cochlear and vestibular structures and passes medially through the internal acoustic meatus alongside the labyrinthine a.<br>Drains into the superior petrosal sinus |

Lateral projection of right membranous labyrinth

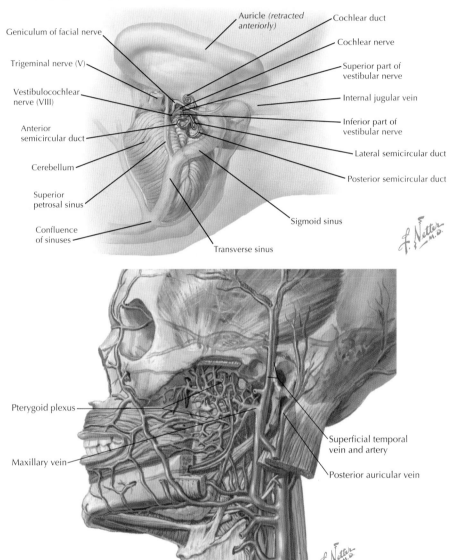

Geniculum of facial nerve

Trigeminal nerve (V)

Vestibulocochlear nerve (VIII)

Anterior semicircular duct

Cerebellum

Superior petrosal sinus

Confluence of sinuses

Auricle *(retracted anteriorly)*

Cochlear duct

Cochlear nerve

Superior part of vestibular nerve

Internal jugular vein

Inferior part of vestibular nerve

Lateral semicircular duct

Posterior semicircular duct

Sigmoid sinus

Transverse sinus

Pterygoid plexus

Maxillary vein

Superficial temporal vein and artery

Posterior auricular vein

**Figure 18-16**

- *Acute otitis externa*: infection or inflammation of the auricle and external auditory canal located in the external ear, causing ear pain (otalgia)
- Also called "swimmer's ear"
- 2 major bacteria are involved: *Staphylococcus aureus* and *Pseudomonas aeruginosa*

PATHOGENESIS

- Excess water from swimming removes some of the ceruminous wax that lines the external auditory canal
- Because the wax helps maintain a healthy canal, loss of the wax predisposes the canal to bacterial infections

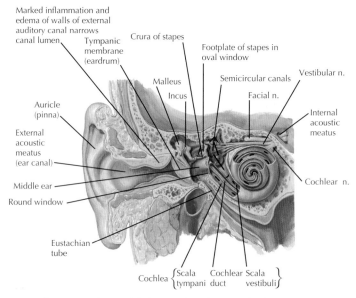

In otitis externa, inflammation, edema, and discharge are limited to external auditory canal and its walls

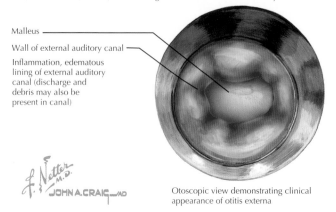

Otoscopic view demonstrating clinical appearance of otitis externa

**Figure 18-17**

- *Acute otitis media*: an inflammation of the middle ear cavity
- More common in children
- 2 major bacteria are involved: *Streptococcus pneumoniae* and *Haemophilus influenzae*

PATHOGENESIS

- Often results from auditory tube dysfunction
- Because the auditory tube allows drainage from the tympanic cavity into the nasopharynx, any blockage leads to a buildup of fluid in the tympanic cavity
- When the fluid sits in the tympanic cavity, it predisposes the region to a bacterial infection
- The resulting inflammation leads to ear pain (otalgia) and often diminished hearing

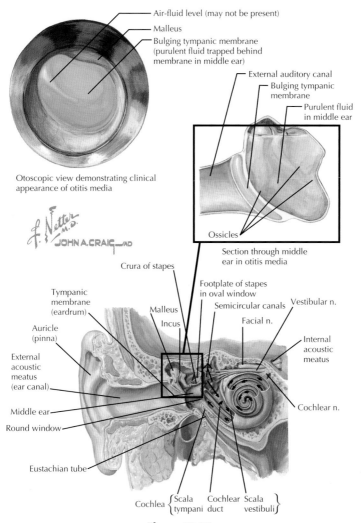

Air-fluid level (may not be present)

Malleus

Bulging tympanic membrane
(purulent fluid trapped behind
membrane in middle ear)

External auditory canal

Bulging tympanic
membrane

Purulent fluid
in middle ear

Otoscopic view demonstrating clinical
appearance of otitis media

Ossicles

Section through middle
ear in otitis media

Crura of stapes

Footplate of stapes
in oval window

Tympanic
membrane
(eardrum)

Malleus

Incus

Semicircular canals

Vestibular n.

Facial n.

Auricle
(pinna)

External
acoustic
meatus
(ear canal)

Internal
acoustic
meatus

Middle ear

Cochlear n.

Round window

Eustachian tube

Cochlea { Scala
tympani   Cochlear
duct   Scala
vestibuli }

**Figure 18-18**

- *Mastoiditis*: a bacterial infection of the mastoid air cells
- More common in children than in adults

PATHOGENESIS

- Although less common since the advent of antibiotics, formerly it often occurred as a complication of acute otitis media, when infection spread from the middle ear cavity to the mastoid air cells
- Once within the mastoid air cells, the infection can lead to inflammation and destruction of the mastoid bone
- Because of the infection's location, it may lead to partial (or total) hearing loss, damage to the mastoid bone, or formation of an epidural abscess, or it may spread to involve the brain

TREATMENT

- Can be difficult because medications cannot readily reach the mastoid air cells
- In some cases, a mastoidectomy may be performed to drain the mastoid if antibiotic therapy is not successful
- A myringotomy (creating an opening in the middle ear cavity through the tympanic membrane) is performed to drain the ear in acute otitis media

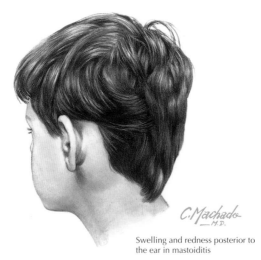

Swelling and redness posterior to
the ear in mastoiditis

**Figure 18-19**

# EYE AND ORBIT

- *Orbit*: a pyramid-shaped bony recess in the anterior part of the skull, lined by periosteum called the periorbital fascia
- Contents include:
  - Eye—organ associated with vision
  - Extrinsic muscles
  - Optic nerve
  - Oculomotor nerve
  - Ciliary ganglion
  - Trochlear nerve
  - Ophthalmic division of the trigeminal nerve
  - Abducens nerve
  - Ophthalmic artery and branches
  - Superior and inferior ophthalmic veins
  - Lacrimal apparatus
  - Much fatty tissue

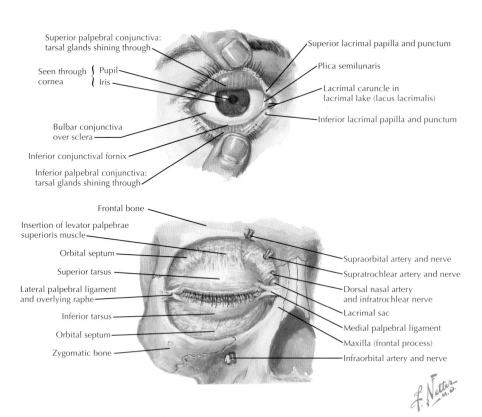

Superior palpebral conjunctiva: tarsal glands shining through

Seen through cornea { Pupil / Iris

Bulbar conjunctiva over sclera

Inferior conjunctival fornix

Inferior palpebral conjunctiva: tarsal glands shining through

Superior lacrimal papilla and punctum

Plica semilunaris

Lacrimal caruncle in lacrimal lake (lacus lacrimalis)

Inferior lacrimal papilla and punctum

Frontal bone

Insertion of levator palpebrae superioris muscle

Orbital septum

Superior tarsus

Lateral palpebral ligament and overlying raphe

Inferior tarsus

Orbital septum

Zygomatic bone

Supraorbital artery and nerve

Supratrochlear artery and nerve

Dorsal nasal artery and infratrochlear nerve

Lacrimal sac

Medial palpebral ligament

Maxilla (frontal process)

Infraorbital artery and nerve

**Figure 19-1**

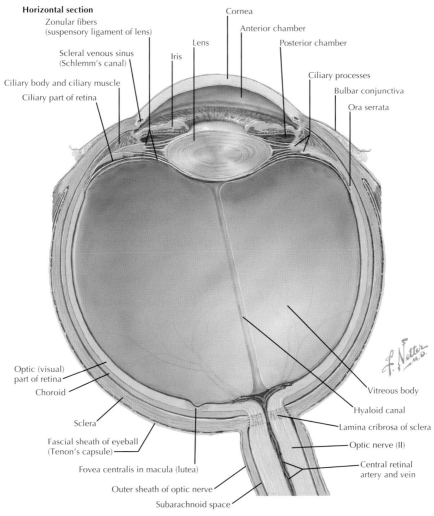

**Horizontal section**

Zonular fibers (suspensory ligament of lens)

Scleral venous sinus (Schlemm's canal)

Iris

Lens

Cornea

Anterior chamber

Posterior chamber

Ciliary processes

Bulbar conjunctiva

Ora serrata

Ciliary body and ciliary muscle

Ciliary part of retina

Optic (visual) part of retina

Choroid

Sclera

Fascial sheath of eyeball (Tenon's capsule)

Fovea centralis in macula (lutea)

Outer sheath of optic nerve

Subarachnoid space

Vitreous body

Hyaloid canal

Lamina cribrosa of sclera

Optic nerve (II)

Central retinal artery and vein

**Figure 19-2**

| Opening | Bony Boundaries | Structures Passing Through Opening |
|---------|-----------------|-----------------------------------|
| Optic canal | Lesser wing of the sphenoid | Optic n.<br>Ophthalmic a. (branch of internal carotid a.) |
| Superior orbital fissure | Between the:<br>• Greater wing of the sphenoid, and<br>• Lesser wing of the sphenoid | 3 major branches of ophthalmic division of trigeminal n:<br>• Lacrimal branch<br>• Frontal branch<br>• Nasociliary branch<br>3 cranial nerves innervating the extraocular muscles of the eye:<br>• Oculomotor n.<br>• Trochlear n.<br>• Abducens n.<br>Superior ophthalmic v. (drains into cavernous sinus)<br>Inferior ophthalmic v. (on occasion—when present, drains into cavernous sinus) |
| Inferior orbital fissure | Between the:<br>• Greater wing of the sphenoid, and<br>• Maxilla and orbital portion of the palatine bones | Infraorbital n. (branch of maxillary division of trigeminal)<br>Infraorbital a. (branch of maxillary a.)<br>Infraorbital v. (drains into pterygoid plexus)<br>Zygomatic n. (branch of maxillary division of trigeminal)<br>Branch of inferior ophthalmic v. that connects to the pterygoid plexus (when present) |
| Supraorbital foramen (sometimes occurs as a notch) | Frontal | Supraorbital n. (branch of ophthalmic division of trigeminal)<br>Supraorbital a. (branch of ophthalmic a.)<br>Supraorbital v. (drains into angular v.) |
| Infraorbital groove and canal | Maxilla | Infraorbital n. (branch of maxillary division of trigeminal)<br>Infraorbital a. (branch of maxillary a.)<br>Infraorbital v. (drains into pterygoid plexus) |
| Zygomatic foramen (1or 2 openings) | Zygomatic | Zygomaticotemporal n. (branch of maxillary division of trigeminal)<br>Zygomaticofacial n. (branch of maxillary division of trigeminal) |
| Nasolacrimal canal | Lacrimal | Nasolacrimal duct |
| Anterior ethmoidal foramen | Between the:<br>• Frontal and<br>• Ethmoid | Anterior ethmoidal n. (branch of ophthalmic division of trigeminal)<br>Anterior ethmoidal a. (branch of ophthalmic a.)<br>Anterior ethmoidal v. (drains into superior ophthalmic v.) |
| Posterior ethmoidal foramen | Between the:<br>• Frontal and<br>• Ethmoid | Posterior ethmoidal n. (branch of ophthalmic division of trigeminal)<br>Posterior ethmoidal a. (branch of ophthalmic a.)<br>Posterior ethmoidal v. (drains into superior ophthalmic v.) |

BONES CREATING THE ORBITAL MARGIN
- Frontal
- Zygomatic
- Maxilla

| WALLS OF THE ORBIT | |
|---|---|
| Superior | Frontal (orbital plate) <br> Lesser wing of the sphenoid |
| Inferior | Maxilla <br> Zygomatic <br> Palatine (orbital process) |
| Medial | Ethmoid (lamina papyracea) <br> Lacrimal <br> Sphenoid <br> Maxilla |
| Lateral | Zygomatic <br> Greater wing of the sphenoid |

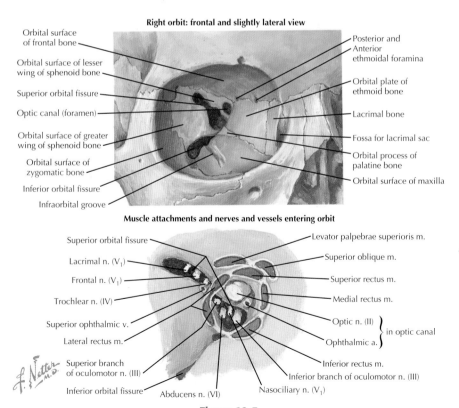

**Right orbit: frontal and slightly lateral view**

Orbital surface of frontal bone

Orbital surface of lesser wing of sphenoid bone

Superior orbital fissure

Optic canal (foramen)

Orbital surface of greater wing of sphenoid bone

Orbital surface of zygomatic bone

Inferior orbital fissure

Infraorbital groove

Posterior and Anterior ethmoidal foramina

Orbital plate of ethmoid bone

Lacrimal bone

Fossa for lacrimal sac

Orbital process of palatine bone

Orbital surface of maxilla

**Muscle attachments and nerves and vessels entering orbit**

Superior orbital fissure

Lacrimal n. (V₁)

Frontal n. (V₁)

Trochlear n. (IV)

Superior ophthalmic v.

Lateral rectus m.

Superior branch of oculomotor n. (III)

Inferior orbital fissure

Abducens n. (VI)

Levator palpebrae superioris m.

Superior oblique m.

Superior rectus m.

Medial rectus m.

Optic n. (II)

Ophthalmic a.

} in optic canal

Inferior rectus m.

Inferior branch of oculomotor n. (III)

Nasociliary n. (V₁)

**Figure 19-3**

- *Eye*: a spherical globe with a diameter of approximately 2.5 cm that lies in the orbit's anterior portion
- Surrounded by a thin capsule called the fascia bulbi (Tenon's capsule):
  - Provides support
  - Allows for movement
- Composed of 3 coats:
  - Sclera
  - Uveal tract
  - Retina
- Divided into an anterior and a posterior segment:

## ANTERIOR SEGMENT

- Filled with aqueous humor
- Separated into anterior and posterior chambers by the iris
- Contains aqueous humor secreted by the ciliary body and drained through a trabeculated network eventually into the superior ophthalmic vein
- Intraocular pressure is measured in the anterior segment, normally 10 to 20 mm Hg

## POSTERIOR SEGMENT

- Filled with vitreous fluid
- Called the vitreous cavity

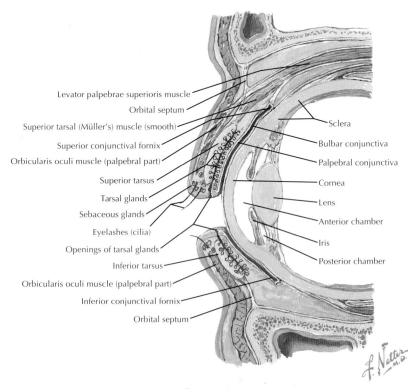

Levator palpebrae superioris muscle
Orbital septum
Superior tarsal (Müller's) muscle (smooth)
Superior conjunctival fornix
Orbicularis oculi muscle (palpebral part)
Superior tarsus
Tarsal glands
Sebaceous glands
Eyelashes (cilia)
Openings of tarsal glands
Inferior tarsus
Orbicularis oculi muscle (palpebral part)
Inferior conjunctival fornix
Orbital septum

Sclera
Bulbar conjunctiva
Palpebral conjunctiva
Cornea
Lens
Anterior chamber
Iris
Posterior chamber

**Figure 19-4**

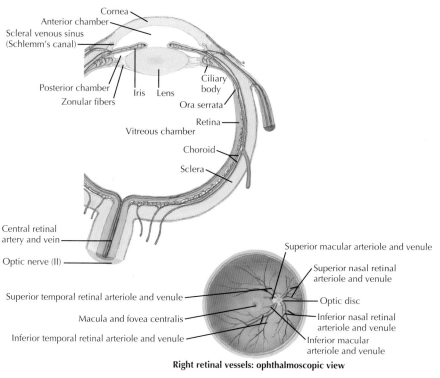

Cornea
Anterior chamber
Scleral venous sinus
(Schlemm's canal)
Posterior chamber
Iris    Lens
Zonular fibers
Ciliary
body
Ora serrata
Retina
Vitreous chamber
Choroid
Sclera
Central retinal
artery and vein
Optic nerve (II)

Superior macular arteriole and venule
Superior nasal retinal
arteriole and venule
Superior temporal retinal arteriole and venule
Optic disc
Inferior nasal retinal
arteriole and venule
Macula and fovea centralis
Inferior temporal retinal arteriole and venule
Inferior macular
arteriole and venule

**Right retinal vessels: ophthalmoscopic view**

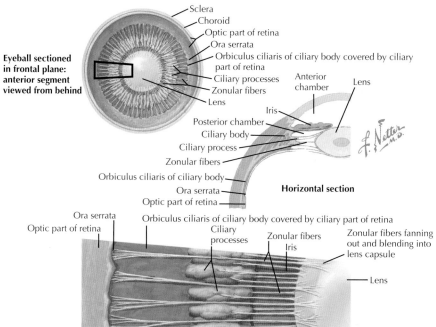

Sclera
Choroid
Optic part of retina
Ora serrata
Orbiculus ciliaris of ciliary body covered by ciliary
part of retina
Ciliary processes
Zonular fibers
Lens

**Eyeball sectioned
in frontal plane:
anterior segment
viewed from behind**

Anterior
chamber
Lens

Iris
Posterior chamber
Ciliary body
Ciliary process
Zonular fibers
Orbiculus ciliaris of ciliary body
Ora serrata
Optic part of retina

**Horizontal section**

Ora serrata
Optic part of retina
Orbiculus ciliaris of ciliary body covered by ciliary part of retina
Ciliary
processes
Zonular fibers
Iris
Zonular fibers fanning
out and blending into
lens capsule
Lens

**Enlargement of segment outlined in top illustration (semischematic)**

**Figure 19-5**

## SCLERA

- The outermost layer, very fibrous
- White along the periphery, except for the anterior portion–the cornea, which is transparent

## UVEAL TRACT

- Composed of choroid layer, ciliary body, and iris

*Choroid*
- The pigmented vascular layer between the sclera and the retina
- Extends posteriorly from the region of the optic nerve anteriorly, where it is continuous with the ciliary body near the ora serrata (anterior margin of the retina)

*Ciliary Body*
- Located between the choroid and the iris
- Ring-shaped; has a series of transparent fibers that form the suspensory ligament of the lens
- Within it is the ciliary muscle, which changes the shape of the lens

*Iris*
- A thin disclike structure with a central opening–the pupil
- Separates the aqueous humor into the anterior chamber (anterior to the iris) and the posterior chamber (between the iris and the lens)
- Contains the sphincter and dilator pupillae muscles, which change the pupil's shape in response to light

## LENS

- Located posterior to the iris
- A transparent biconcave structure responsible for focusing
- Connected to the ciliary body by the suspensory ligaments

## RETINA

- The innermost coat of the eye
- Thin and highly vascular
- 3 areas located on the retina's posterior portion:
  - Optic disc
  - Macula lutea
  - Fovea centralis

*Optic Disc*
- Area where the optic nerve enters the retina is called the "blind spot"
- Retina's central artery enters the eye through the optic disc and divides into superior and inferior branches

*Macula Lutea and Fovea Centralis*
- Macula lutea—lateral to the optic disc
- A depressed, yellow-appearing area that contains the fovea centralis in its center
- Fovea Centralis—area of highest visual acuity and contains high concentration of cone photoreceptors

| ASSOCIATED EXTRINSIC MUSCLE OF THE ORBIT | | | | | |
|---|---|---|---|---|---|
| **Muscle** | **Origin** | **Insertion** | **Actions** | **Nerve** | **Comment** |
| Levator palpebrae superioris | Sphenoid (Lesser wing) | Skin of the upper eyelid | Raises the upper eyelid | Superior division of the oculomotor<br><br>Sympathetic fibers to the superior tarsal muscle (smooth muscle) | Opposed by the palpebral part of the orbicularis oculi m.<br><br>There are smooth muscle fibers that insert into the superior tarsal plate and are innervated by sympathetic fibers<br><br>Lesions of the sympathetics will lead to a ptosis, or drooping of the upper eyelid |

| EXTRINSIC MUSCLES OF THE EYE | | | | | |
|---|---|---|---|---|---|
| **Muscle** | **Origin** | **Insertion** | **Action(s) on Eye** | **Nerve** | **Comment** |
| Superior rectus | Common tendinous ring on sphenoid | Superior sclera | Elevation<br>Adduction<br>Intorsion | Superior division of the oculomotor | A check ligament attaches it to the levator palpebrae superioris m. to help elevate the upper eyelid |
| Inferior rectus | | Inferior sclera | Depression<br>Adduction<br>Extorsion | Inferior division of the oculomotor | A check ligament attaches it to the inferior tarsal plate to help depress the lower eyelid |
| Medial rectus | | Medial sclera | Adduction | | The most medial of the extraocular muscles |
| Lateral rectus | | Lateral sclera | Abduction | Abducens | Impaired in abducens n. palsy |
| Superior oblique | Body of the sphenoid | Superior portion of the posterolateral sclera | Depression<br>Abduction<br>Intorsion | Trochlear | Tendon passes through the trochlea, a fibrocartilaginous pulley |
| Inferior oblique | Maxilla (lateral to the lacrimal groove) | Inferior portion of the posterolateral sclera | Elevation<br>Abduction<br>Extorsion | Inferior division of the oculomotor | Only extraocular muscle that attaches to the maxilla |

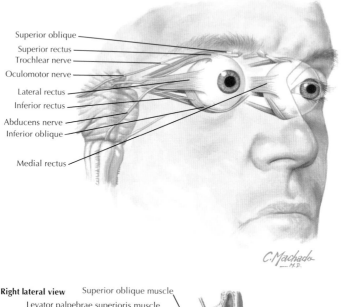

Superior oblique
Superior rectus
Trochlear nerve
Oculomotor nerve
Lateral rectus
Inferior rectus
Abducens nerve
Inferior oblique

Medial rectus

*C.Machado*
—*M.D.*

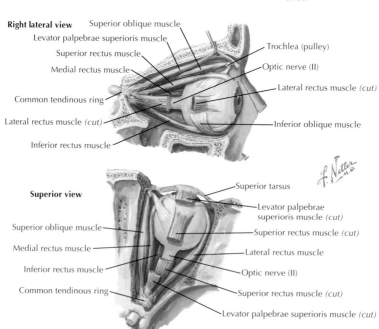

**Right lateral view**
Superior oblique muscle
Levator palpebrae superioris muscle
Superior rectus muscle
Medial rectus muscle
Trochlea (pulley)
Optic nerve (II)
Lateral rectus muscle *(cut)*
Common tendinous ring
Lateral rectus muscle *(cut)*
Inferior oblique muscle
Inferior rectus muscle

*f. Netter*
*M.D.*

**Superior view**
Superior tarsus
Levator palpebrae superioris muscle *(cut)*
Superior oblique muscle
Superior rectus muscle *(cut)*
Medial rectus muscle
Lateral rectus muscle
Inferior rectus muscle
Optic nerve (II)
Common tendinous ring
Superior rectus muscle *(cut)*
Levator palpebrae superioris muscle *(cut)*

**Figure 19-6**

Innervation and action of extrinsic eye muscles: anterior view

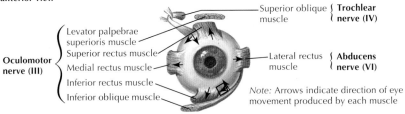

Oculomotor nerve (III)
- Levator palpebrae superioris muscle
- Superior rectus muscle
- Medial rectus muscle
- Inferior rectus muscle
- Inferior oblique muscle

Superior oblique muscle { **Trochlear nerve (IV)**

Lateral rectus muscle { **Abducens nerve (VI)**

*Note:* Arrows indicate direction of eye movement produced by each muscle

Frontal section

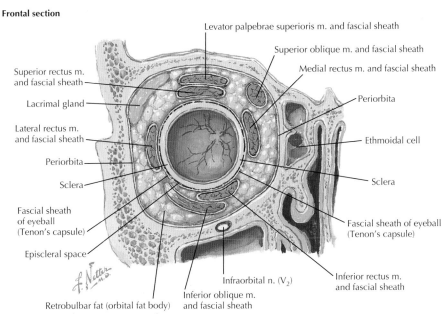

Levator palpebrae superioris m. and fascial sheath

Superior oblique m. and fascial sheath

Medial rectus m. and fascial sheath

Superior rectus m. and fascial sheath

Lacrimal gland

Lateral rectus m. and fascial sheath

Periorbita

Sclera

Fascial sheath of eyeball (Tenon's capsule)

Episcleral space

Periorbita

Ethmoidal cell

Sclera

Fascial sheath of eyeball (Tenon's capsule)

Infraorbital n. (V₂)

Inferior rectus m. and fascial sheath

Retrobulbar fat (orbital fat body)

Inferior oblique m. and fascial sheath

**Figure 19-7**

## Nerve Supply

| ORBITAL INNERVATION | |
|---|---|
| **Orbital Innervation** | **Description** |
| Sensory | **2 Major Types** <br> Vision (special somatic afferent, or SSA) via the optic n. <br> General sensation (general somatic afferent, or GSA) via the ophthalmic (and some maxillary) division of the trigeminal n. |
| Motor | **2 Major Types** <br> Motor to the extraocular muscles (general somatic efferent, or GSE) via the oculomotor, trochlear, and abducens nn. <br> Autonomics to the intrinsic muscles of the eye (general visceral efferent, or GVE) via: <br> • Parasympathetics associated with the ciliary ganglion <br> • Sympathetics associated with the superior cervical ganglion |
| Cranial nn. | 5 cranial nerves provide innervation to the orbit: <br> • Optic—vision <br> • Oculomotor—extraocular motor and autonomics to the intrinsic muscles of the eye <br> • Trochlear—extraocular motor <br> • Trigeminal—general sensation <br> • Abducens—extraocular motor |

**Eyeball**

**Section through retina**

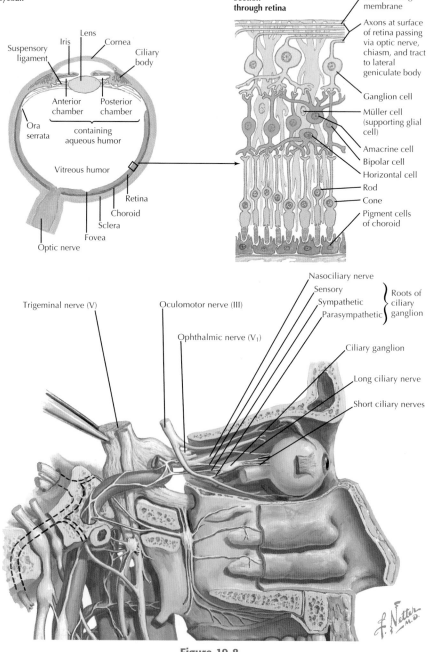

Inner limiting membrane

Axons at surface of retina passing via optic nerve, chiasm, and tract to lateral geniculate body

Ganglion cell

Müller cell (supporting glial cell)

Amacrine cell

Bipolar cell

Horizontal cell

Rod

Cone

Pigment cells of choroid

Lens

Iris

Cornea

Suspensory ligament

Ciliary body

Anterior chamber

Posterior chamber

Ora serrata

containing aqueous humor

Vitreous humor

Retina

Choroid

Sclera

Fovea

Optic nerve

Nasociliary nerve

Sensory

Sympathetic

Parasympathetic

Roots of ciliary ganglion

Trigeminal nerve (V)

Oculomotor nerve (III)

Ophthalmic nerve (V$_1$)

Ciliary ganglion

Long ciliary nerve

Short ciliary nerves

**Figure 19-8**

## OPTIC NERVE (VISION)

- About 25 mm in length, allows for eye movement via the extraocular muscles
- Covered by an outer layer of dura mater and an inner layer of arachnoid, which attach anteriorly to the eye, where the optic n. enters the sclera, and posteriorly, where it merges with the periosteum lining the orbit at the optic foramen
- Central a. of the retina enters the optic n. posterior to the bulb of the eye

*Course*

- Axons from the ganglionic cells of the retina comprise the optic n. and come together at the optic disc
- They leave the eye and travel as the optic n. posteriorly and medially through the orbit
- Posteriorly, the optic n. passes through the optic foramen to enter the cranial cavity
- The 2 optic nn. meet at the optic chiasm, located superior to the hypophyseal fossa
- Optic chiasm gives rise to the optic tracts, which terminate in the lateral geniculate nucleus of the thalamus before giving rise to the optic radiations that terminate in the occipital lobes

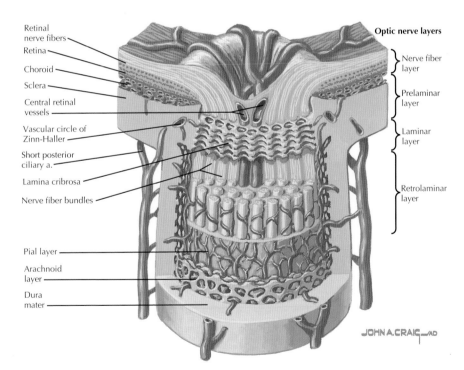

**Figure 19-9**

| GENERAL SENSATION | | |
|---|---|---|
| Ophthalmic Division of the Trigeminal Nerve | | |

- This division, being a branch of the trigeminal n., is sensory in function
- Arises from the main nerve in the middle cranial fossa
- Passes anterior on the lateral wall of the cavernous sinus immediately inferior to the oculomotor and trochlear nn., but superior to the maxillary division of the trigeminal
- Before entering the orbit, it gives rise to a small tentorial branch
- Immediately before entering the orbit, through the superior orbital fissure, it divides into 3 major branches: lacrimal, frontal, and nasociliary nn.

| Nerve | Source | Course |
|---|---|---|
| Lacrimal | Ophthalmic division of the trigeminal n. | Smallest branch of the ophthalmic division of the trigeminal n. |
| | | Passes anteriorly to enter the orbit through the superior orbital fissure |
| | | In the orbit, it travels on the superior border of the lateral rectus m. with the lacrimal a. |
| | | Before reaching the lacrimal gland, it communicates with the zygomatic branch of the maxillary division of the trigeminal to receive autonomic nervous fibers |
| | | Enters the lacrimal gland and supplies it and the conjunctiva before piercing the orbital septum to supply the skin of the upper eyelid |
| Frontal | | Largest branch of the ophthalmic division of the trigeminal n. |
| | | Passes anteriorly to enter the orbit through the superior orbital fissure |
| | | In the orbit it passes anteriorly between the periosteum of the orbit and the levator palpebrae superioris m. |
| | | About halfway in the orbit, it divides into its 2 terminal nerves:<br>• supraorbital n.<br>• supratrochlear n. |
| *Supraorbital* | Frontal n. (from the ophthalmic division of the trigeminal n.) | Passes between the levator palpebrae superioris m. and the periosteum of the orbit |
| | | Continues anteriorly to the supraorbital foramen (notch) |
| | | At the level of the supraorbital margin, it sends nerve supply to the frontal sinus and ascends superiorly along the scalp |
| | | Divides into medial and lateral branches, which travel up to the vertex of the scalp |
| *Supratrochlear* | | Once the supratrochlear a. joins it within the orbit, it continues to pass anteriorly toward the trochlear |
| | | In the trochlear region, it often supplies the frontal sinus before exiting the orbit |
| | | Ascends along the scalp, at 1st deep to the musculature in the region before piercing them to reach the cutaneous innervation along the scalp |
| Nasociliary | Ophthalmic division of the trigeminal n. | Passes anteriorly to enter the orbit through the superior orbital fissure |
| | | Enters the orbit lateral to the optic n. |
| | | Travels across the optic n. anteriorly and medially to lie between the medial rectus and the superior oblique mm. along the medial wall of the orbit |
| | | All along its path, it gives rise to other nerves, including the sensory root of the ciliary ganglion, and the long ciliary and posterior ethmoidal nn., until terminating into the anterior ethmoidal and infratrochlear nn. near the anterior ethmoidal foramen |
| *Sensory root of the ciliary ganglion* | Nasociliary n. | Travels anteriorly on the lateral side of the optic n. to enter the ciliary ganglion |
| | | Carries general sensory fibers, which are distributed by the short ciliary nn. |
| *Short ciliary* | Ciliary ganglion | Arises from the ciliary ganglion to travel to the posterior surface of the eye |
| | | Supplies the sensory fibers to the eye and helps carry the postganglionic parasympathetic fibers to the sphincter pupillae and the ciliary muscle |

| Nerve | Source | Course |
|-------|--------|--------|
| Long ciliary | Nasociliary n. | There are 2 to 4 branches that travel anteriorly to enter the posterior part of the sclera of the eye |
| Posterior ethmoidal | | Travels deep to the superior oblique m. to pass through the posterior ethmoidal foramen |
| | | Supplies the sphenoid sinus and the posterior ethmoidal sinus |
| Anterior ethmoidal | | Arises on the medial wall of the orbit |
| | | Enters the anterior ethmoidal foramen and travels through the canal to enter the anterior cranial fossa |
| | | Supplies the anterior and middle ethmoidal sinuses before entering and supplying the nasal cavity |
| | | Terminates as the external nasal n. on the face |
| Infratrochlear | | 1 of the terminal branches of the nasociliary n. |
| | | Passes anteriorly on the superior border of the medial rectus m. |
| | | Passes inferior to the trochlea toward the medial angle of the eye |
| | | Supplies the skin of the eyelids and bridge of the nose, the conjunctiva, and all of the lacrimal structures |

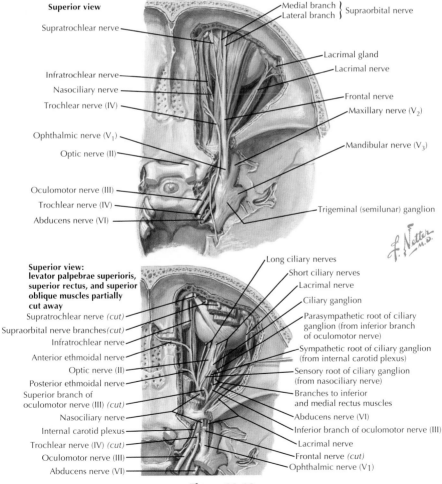

**Figure 19-10**

| GENERAL SENSATION | | |
| --- | --- | --- |
| Maxillary Division of the Trigeminal Nerve | | |

- Travels along the lateral wall of the cavernous sinus
- Before exiting the middle cranial fossa, it gives off a meningeal branch that innervates the dura mater
- Passes from the middle cranial fossa into the pterygopalatine fossa via the foramen rotundum
- Within the pterygopalatine fossa, it gives rise to *4 branches*: posterior superior alveolar n., zygomatic n., ganglionic branches, and infraorbital n.
- The zygomatic and infraorbital continue within the orbit

| Nerve | Source | Course |
| --- | --- | --- |
| Zygomatic | Maxillary division of the trigeminal n. | Enters the orbit via the inferior orbital fissure |
| | | Within the orbit, it divides into the zygomaticotemporal and zygomaticofacial branches, which exit the orbit along the lateral wall via 1 or 2 zygomatic foramina |
| Infraorbital | | Considered the continuation of the maxillary division of the trigeminal n. |
| | | Passes through the inferior orbital fissure to enter the orbit |
| | | Passes anteriorly through the infraorbital groove and infraorbital canal and exits onto the face via the infraorbital foramen |
| | | Within the infraorbital canal, it gives rise to the anterior superior alveolar and middle superior alveolar nn. |
| | | Once the infraorbital n. exits onto the face, it divides into 3 terminal branches: |
| | | • Inferior palpebral—supplies the skin of the lower eyelid and conjunctiva |
| | | • Nasal—supplies the skin of the ala of the nose |
| | | • Superior labial—supplies the skin of the upper lip |

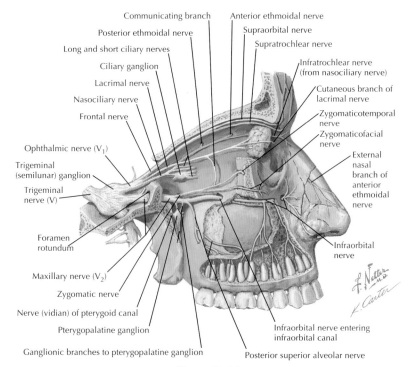

Figure 19-11

| GENERAL MOTOR | | |
|---|---|---|
| **Nerve** | **Source** | **Course** |
| Oculomotor (cranial n. III) | Ventral surface of the midbrain | Innervates 4 of the extraocular muscles—superior rectus, inferior rectus, medial rectus, and inferior oblique mm.—as well as the levator palpebrae superioris m. |
| | | Also provides parasympathetic innervation to the intrinsic muscles of the eye |
| | | Passes anterior on the lateral wall of the cavernous sinus immediately superior to the trochlear n. |
| | | Immediately before entering the orbit, it divides into superior and inferior divisions; both enter the orbit through the superior orbital fissure |
| Superior division of the oculomotor | Oculomotor | Enters the orbit via the superior orbital fissure |
| | | Travels superior to the optic n. to enter the inferior border of the superior rectus m. |
| | | Passes through the superior rectus to give rise to a branch that enters the inferior surface of the levator palpebrae superioris m. |
| Inferior division of the oculomotor | | Enters the orbit via the superior orbital fissure |
| | | Immediately divides into 3 muscular branches that enter: |
| | | • The lateral surface of the medial rectus |
| | | • The superior surface of the inferior oblique |
| | | • The superior surface of the inferior rectus |
| | | Gives rise to the parasympathetic root of the ciliary ganglion |
| Trochlear (cranial n. IV) | Dorsal surface of the midbrain | Innervates the superior oblique |
| | | Passes anterior on the lateral wall of the cavernous sinus immediately inferior to the oculomotor n. |
| | | Enters the orbit via the superior orbital fissure and immediately enters the superior oblique to innervate it |
| Abducens (cranial n. VI) | Ventral surface of the pons | Travels anteriorly within the cavernous sinus beside the internal carotid a. |
| | | Enters the orbit via the superior orbital fissure |
| | | Travels anteriorly to enter the medial surface of the lateral rectus to innervate it |

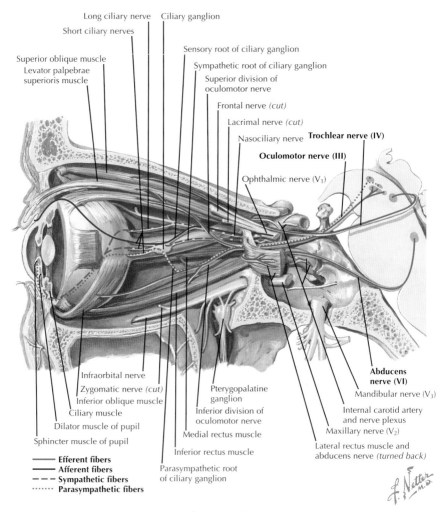

Long ciliary nerve   Ciliary ganglion
Short ciliary nerves
Sensory root of ciliary ganglion
Superior oblique muscle
Levator palpebrae
superioris muscle
Sympathetic root of ciliary ganglion
Superior division of
oculomotor nerve
Frontal nerve *(cut)*
Lacrimal nerve *(cut)*
Nasociliary nerve   **Trochlear nerve (IV)**
**Oculomotor nerve (III)**
Ophthalmic nerve (V$_1$)

Infraorbital nerve
Zygomatic nerve *(cut)*
Inferior oblique muscle
Ciliary muscle
Dilator muscle of pupil
Sphincter muscle of pupil
Pterygopalatine
ganglion
Inferior division of
oculomotor nerve
Medial rectus muscle
Inferior rectus muscle
Parasympathetic root
of ciliary ganglion

**Abducens
nerve (VI)**
Mandibular nerve (V$_3$)
Internal carotid artery
and nerve plexus
Maxillary nerve (V$_2$)
Lateral rectus muscle and
abducens nerve *(turned back)*

———— **Efferent fibers**
———— **Afferent fibers**
– – – **Sympathetic fibers**
· · · · · **Parasympathetic fibers**

**Figure 19-12**

| PARASYMPATHETICS OF THE EYE | | | |
|---|---|---|---|
| **Type of Neuron** | **Location of Cell Body** | **Characteristics of Cell Body** | **Course of the Neuron** |
| Preganglionic neuron | Edinger-Westphal nucleus | A collection of nerve cell bodies located in the midbrain | Arise from the Edinger-Westphal nucleus in the midbrain from the oculomotor n. <br><br> Oculomotor n. passes anteriorly on the lateral wall of the cavernous sinus immediately superior to the trochlear n. <br><br> Immediately before entering the orbit, the nerve divides into the superior and inferior divisions <br><br> Both the superior and inferior divisions of the oculomotor enter the orbit through the superior orbital fissure <br><br> Preganglionic parasympathetic fibers travel in the inferior division <br><br> A small parasympathetic root passes from the inferior division of the oculomotor to the ciliary ganglion, carrying the preganglionic parasympathetic fibers |
| Postganglionic neuron | Ciliary ganglion | Located anterior to the optic foramen between the optic n. and the lateral rectus <br><br> *3 roots connect to the ciliary ganglion:* <br> • Sensory root from the ophthalmic division of the trigeminal, which carries general sensation fibers to the eye via the short ciliary nn. <br> • Parasympathetic root from the inferior division of the oculomotor, carrying preganglionic parasympathetic fibers to the ganglion <br> • Sympathetic root that arises from the postganglionic sympathetic fibers, which were carried by the internal carotid a. <br><br> The short ciliary nn. usually number about 8 <br><br> Short ciliary nn. arise from the ciliary ganglion to enter the posterior portion of the eye <br><br> Fibers from all 3 roots pass through the ciliary ganglion and short ciliary nn. to enter the eye <br><br> Only the parasympathetic fibers synapse in the ciliary ganglion | Arise in the ciliary ganglion, following a synapse with the preganglionic parasympathetic fibers <br><br> Travel through the short ciliary nn. to enter the eye's posterior portion <br><br> Innervate: <br> • sphincter pupillae m. <br> • ciliary m. |

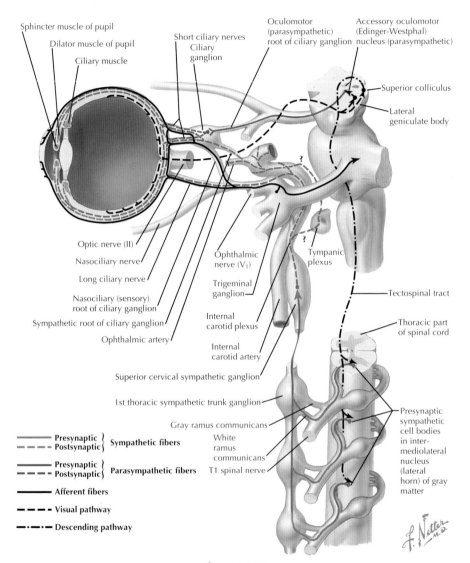

Sphincter muscle of pupil

Dilator muscle of pupil

Ciliary muscle

Short ciliary nerves
Ciliary ganglion

Oculomotor (parasympathetic) root of ciliary ganglion

Accessory oculomotor (Edinger-Westphal) nucleus (parasympathetic)

Superior colliculus

Lateral geniculate body

Optic nerve (II)

Nasociliary nerve

Long ciliary nerve

Nasociliary (sensory) root of ciliary ganglion

Sympathetic root of ciliary ganglion

Ophthalmic artery

Ophthalmic nerve (V₁)

Trigeminal ganglion

Internal carotid plexus

Internal carotid artery

Superior cervical sympathetic ganglion

1st thoracic sympathetic trunk ganglion

Gray ramus communicans

Tympanic plexus

Tectospinal tract

Thoracic part of spinal cord

Presynaptic sympathetic cell bodies in inter-mediolateral nucleus (lateral horn) of gray matter

White ramus communicans

T1 spinal nerve

——— Presynaptic }
– – – – Postsynaptic } Sympathetic fibers

——— Presynaptic }
– – – – Postsynaptic } Parasympathetic fibers

——— Afferent fibers

– – – – Visual pathway

–·–·– Descending pathway

**Figure 19-13**

| ANATOMIC PATHWAY FOR SYMPATHETICS OF THE EYE | | | |
|---|---|---|---|
| **Type of Neuron** | **Name of Cell Body** | **Characteristics of Cell Body** | **Course of the Neuron** |
| Preganglionic neuron | Intermediolateral horn nucleus | Collection of nerve cell bodies located in the lateral horn nucleus of the spinal cord between spinal segments T1 and T3 (and possibly T4) | Arise from the intermediolateral horn nuclei from T1 to T3 (or T4) Travel through the ventral root of the spinal cord to the spinal n. Enter the sympathetic chain via a white ramus communicans Once in the sympathetic chain, the preganglionic fibers for the eye will ascend and synapse with postganglionic fibers in the superior cervical ganglion |
| Postganglionic neuron | Superior cervical ganglion | Collection of nerve cell bodies located in the superior cervical ganglion, which is located at the base of the skull | Arise in the superior cervical ganglion Postganglionic fibers will follow the internal carotid a. on the internal carotid plexus As the internal carotid a. nears the orbit, the postganglionic fibers branch from the internal carotid plexus and follow various structures that connect to the eye, such as the ophthalmic a. and its branches, and the long ciliary nn. that arise from the ophthalmic division of the trigeminal n. In the eye, the postganglionic fibers innervate: • dilator pupillae m. |

| ARTERIAL SUPPLY | | |
|---|---|---|
| **Artery** | **Source** | **Course** |
| Ophthalmic | Internal carotid a. | Enters the orbit through the optic foramen immediately inferior and lateral to the optic n. |
| | | Crosses the optic n. to reach the medial part of the orbit |
| | | While in the orbit, the artery gives rise to a series of arteries that supply the orbit and associated structures |
| | | The terminal aa. of the ophthalmic a. anastomose along the scalp and face with the superficial temporal, facial, and infraorbital branches of the maxillary a. |
| *Lacrimal* | Ophthalmic a. | Arises near the optic foramen |
| | | 1 of the ophthalmic's largest branches |
| | | Follows the lacrimal n. along the superior border of the lateral rectus m. of the eye to reach and supply the lacrimal gland |
| | | Gives rise to a series of terminal branches, such as the lateral palpebral, that supply the eyelids and conjunctiva |
| | | Gives rise to a zygomatic branch that then gives rise to the zygomaticotemporal and zygomaticofacial aa. |
| | | Supply those regions of the face |
| *Supratrochlear* | | It exits the orbit at the medial angle accompanied by supratrochlear n. |
| | | Ascends on the scalp, anastomosing with the supraorbital a. and supratrochlear a. from the opposite side |
| *Supraorbital* | | Branches from the ophthalmic a. as it passes the optic n. |
| | | Passes on the medial side of the levator palpebrae superioris and superior rectus mm. to join the supraorbital n. |
| | | Passes through the supraorbital foramen (notch) and ascends superiorly along the scalp |
| | | Anastomoses with the supratrochlear a. and superficial temporal a. |
| *Anterior ethmoidal* | | Travels with the nerve through the anterior ethmoidal canal to supply the anterior and middle ethmoidal sinuses |
| | | Continues to give rise to a meningeal branch and nasal branches that supply the lateral wall and septum of the nose |
| | | Then gives rise to the terminal external nasal branch that supplies the external nose |
| • *External nasal* | A terminal branch of the anterior ethmoidal a. | Supplies the area along the external nose at the junction between the nasal bone and the lateral nasal cartilage |
| *Posterior ethmoidal* | Ophthalmic a. | Travels through the posterior ethmoidal canal to supply the posterior ethmoidal sinus |
| | | Gives rise to meningeal and nasal branches that anastomose with branches of the sphenopalatine |
| *Medial palpebral (superior and inferior)* | Ophthalmic a. of the internal carotid a. | Arise near the trochlea and exit the orbit to pass along the upper and lower eyelids |
| | | These arteries anastomose with the other arteries supplying the face in the region |
| *Dorsal nasal (infratrochlear)* | 1 of the ophthalmic a.'s terminal branches | Exits the orbit along the superomedial border along with the infratrochlear n. |
| | | Supplies the area along the bridge of the nose |
| *Muscular* | Ophthalmic a. from the internal carotid a. | Supply the extraocular muscles of the orbit |

| ARTERIAL SUPPLY | | |
|---|---|---|
| **Artery** | **Source** | **Course** |
| *Anterior ciliary* | Muscular branches from the ophthalmic a. | Pass anteriorly to the anterior surface of the eye following the tendons of the extraocular muscles |
| *Short posterior ciliary* | Ophthalmic a. from the internal carotid a. | Usually 6 to 10 arise<br><br>Travel anteriorly around the optic n. to enter the posterior portion of the eye |
| *Long posterior ciliary* | | Usually 2 arise<br><br>Travel anteriorly to enter the posterior portion of the eye near the optic n. |
| *Central a. of the retina* | | Branches from the ophthalmic a. early on its entrance into the orbit<br><br>Follows the optic n. and enters the nerve about halfway into the orbit<br><br>Supplies the retina |
| Maxillary | 1 of 2 terminal branches of the external carotid a. | Gives rise to a series of branches<br><br>Only the infraorbital branch supplies the orbit |
| *Infraorbital* | Maxillary a. | Once the infraorbital exits the infraorbital foramen, the inferior palpebral a. supplies the lower eyelid<br><br>Supplies some muscles along the floor of the orbit near the inferior orbital canal |

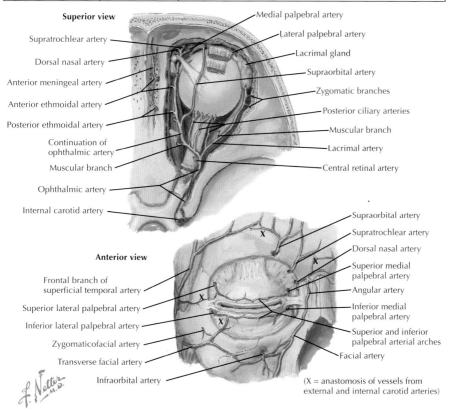

**Figure 19-14**

| VENOUS DRAINAGE | |
|---|---|
| **Vein** | **Course** |
| Superficial Veins | |
| Supraorbital | Begins on the forehead, where it communicates with the superficial temporal v. |
| | Passes inferiorly superficial to the frontalis m. and joins the supratrochlear v. at the medial angle of the orbit to form the angular v. |
| Supratrochlear | Begins on the forehead, where it communicates with the superficial temporal v. |
| | Passes inferiorly along the forehead, parallel with the vein of the opposite side |
| | At the medial angle of the orbit, the supratrochlear joins the supraorbital v. to form the angular v. |
| Angular | Forms from the confluence of the supraorbital and supratrochlear vv. along the medial part of the eye |
| | Travels along the lateral aspect of the nose to become the facial v. |
| Facial | Begins as the angular v. |
| | Passes inferiorly along the side of the nose, receiving the lateral nasal v. |
| | Continues posteroinferiorly across the angle of the mouth to the cheek receiving the superior and inferior labial vv. |
| | While passing toward the mandible, the deep facial v. connects to the pterygoid plexus |
| | In the submandibular triangle the facial v. joins the anterior branch of the retromandibular to form the common facial v. |
| | The facial v. has no valves that can allow blood to backflow |
| Deep Veins | |
| Cavernous sinus | A reticulated venous structure located on the lateral aspect of the body of the sphenoid bone |
| | Drain posteriorly into the superior and inferior petrosal sinuses |
| | Receives blood from the superior and inferior ophthalmic vv. |
| | Oculomotor and trochlear nn. and ophthalmic and maxillary divisions of the trigeminal n. lie along the lateral wall of the sinus |
| | Abducens n. and internal carotid a. lie in the sinus |
| Pterygoid plexus | An extensive network of veins that parallels the 2nd and 3rd parts of the maxillary a. |
| | Receives branches that correspond to the same branches of the maxillary a. |
| | Tributaries to the pterygoid plexus eventually converge to form a short maxillary v. |
| | Communicates with the cavernous sinus, pharyngeal venous plexus, facial v. via the deep facial v., and ophthalmic vv. |
| Communicating Veins | |
| Superior ophthalmic | Receives blood from the roof of the orbit and the scalp |
| | Travels posteriorly to communicate with the cavernous sinus |
| Inferior ophthalmic | Receives blood from the floor of the orbit |
| | Often splits into 2 branches |
| | 1 branch travels posteriorly with the infraorbital v. that passes through the inferior orbital fissure to communicate with the pterygoid plexus |
| | The other branch travels posteriorly to communicate directly with the superior ophthalmic v. in the superior orbital fissure, or it will pass through the fissure to communicate with the cavernous sinus |
| Infraorbital | Receives blood from the midface via the lower eyelid, lateral side of the nose, and the upper lip |
| | Eventually communicates with the pterygoid plexus of veins |

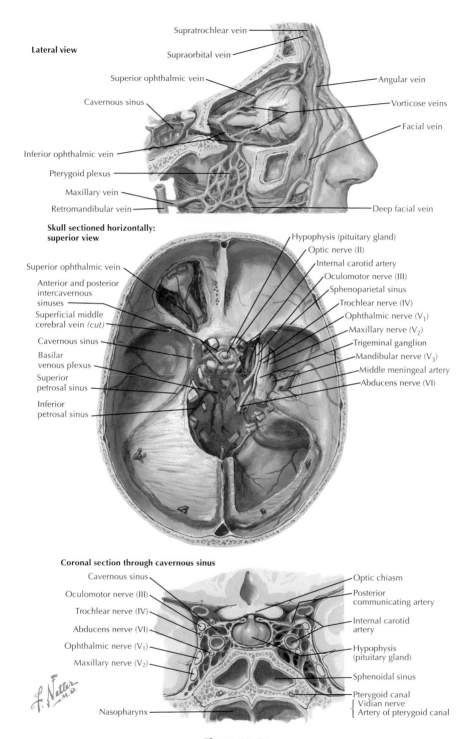

**Lateral view**

Supratrochlear vein

Supraorbital vein

Superior ophthalmic vein

Cavernous sinus

Inferior ophthalmic vein

Pterygoid plexus

Maxillary vein

Retromandibular vein

Angular vein

Vorticose veins

Facial vein

Deep facial vein

**Skull sectioned horizontally: superior view**

Superior ophthalmic vein

Anterior and posterior intercavernous sinuses

Superficial middle cerebral vein *(cut)*

Cavernous sinus

Basilar venous plexus

Superior petrosal sinus

Inferior petrosal sinus

Hypophysis (pituitary gland)

Optic nerve (II)

Internal carotid artery

Oculomotor nerve (III)

Sphenoparietal sinus

Trochlear nerve (IV)

Ophthalmic nerve (V$_1$)

Maxillary nerve (V$_2$)

Trigeminal ganglion

Mandibular nerve (V$_3$)

Middle meningeal artery

Abducens nerve (VI)

**Coronal section through cavernous sinus**

Cavernous sinus

Oculomotor nerve (III)

Trochlear nerve (IV)

Abducens nerve (VI)

Ophthalmic nerve (V$_1$)

Maxillary nerve (V$_2$)

Nasopharynx

Optic chiasm

Posterior communicating artery

Internal carotid artery

Hypophysis (pituitary gland)

Sphenoidal sinus

Pterygoid canal
{ Vidian nerve
{ Artery of pterygoid canal

**Figure 19-15**

| OVERVIEW | |
|---|---|
| **Structure/Function** | **Description** |
| Lacrimal apparatus | Composed of:<br>• Lacrimal gland<br>• Lacrimal canaliculi<br>• Lacrimal sac<br>• Nasolacrimal duct<br>Secretes and drains all tears |
| Lacrimal gland | Located in the anterolateral part of the orbit<br>Secretes serous fluid<br>Divided into 2 parts by the lateral tendon of the levator palpebrae superioris m. |
| Tear formation and absorption | Tears coat the external surface of the eye to prevent drying, act as a lubricant, and contain bactericidal enzymes<br>With blinking, tears are carried across the eye to collect near the medial canthus<br>Tears enter through the lacrimal puncta into the lacrimal canaliculi<br>Lacrimal canaliculi carry the tears to the lacrimal sac<br>Lacrimal sac carries the tears inferiorly through the nasolacrimal duct, which terminates in the inferior meatus |

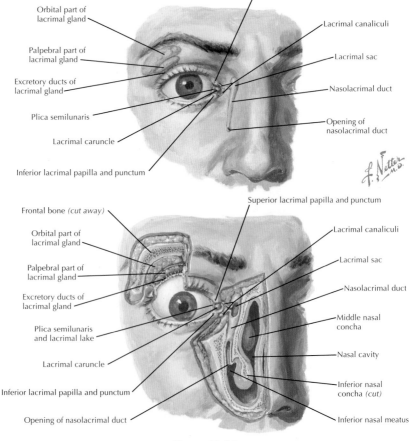

**Figure 19-16**

| PARASYMPATHETICS OF THE LACRIMAL GLAND | | | |
|---|---|---|---|
| **Type of Neuron** | **Name of Cell Body** | **Characteristics of Cell Body** | **Course of the Neuron** |
| Preganglionic neuron | Superior salivatory nucleus | A collection of nerve cell bodies located in the pons<br><br>Travel through the nervus intermedius of the facial n. into the internal acoustic meatus<br><br>In the facial canal, the facial n. gives rise to 2 *parasympathetic branches*:<br>• Greater petrosal n.<br>• Chorda tympani n | Lacrimal gland uses the greater petrosal n.<br>**Greater Petrosal Nerve**<br>Exits along the hiatus for the greater petrosal n. toward the foramen lacerum, where it joins the deep petrosal n. (sympathetics) to form the nerve of the pterygoid canal (vidian n.)<br>Vidian n. passes through the pterygoid canal and enters the pterygopalatine fossa, where it joins with the pterygopalatine ganglion |
| Postganglionic neuron | Pterygopalatine ganglion | A collection of nerve cell bodies located in the pterygopalatine fossa<br><br>Postganglionic parasympathetic fibers that arise in the pterygopalatine ganglion are distributed to the ophthalmic and maxillary divisions of the trigeminal n. to the:<br>• Lacrimal gland<br>• Nasal glands<br>• Palatine glands<br>• Pharyngeal glands<br>• Paranasal sinus glands | Lacrimal gland uses the ophthalmic and maxillary divisions<br>**Ophthalmic and Maxillary Division Distribution**<br>Postganglionic fibers travel along the zygomatic branch of the maxillary division for a short distance to enter the orbit<br>A short communicating branch joins the lacrimal n. of the ophthalmic division of the trigeminal n.<br>These fibers innervate:<br>• Lacrimal gland to cause the secretion of tears |

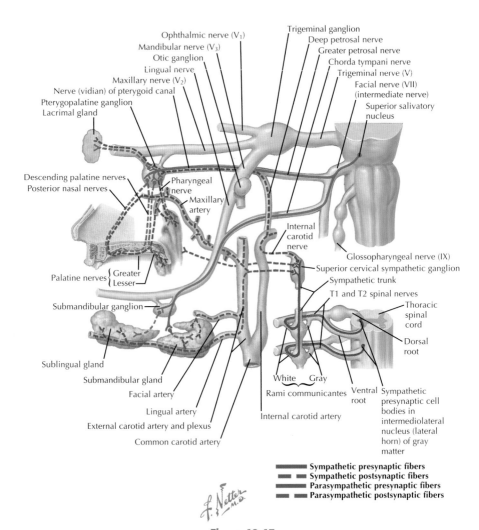

Ophthalmic nerve (V₁)
Mandibular nerve (V₃)
Otic ganglion
Lingual nerve
Maxillary nerve (V₂)
Nerve (vidian) of pterygoid canal
Pterygopalatine ganglion
Lacrimal gland

Trigeminal ganglion
Deep petrosal nerve
Greater petrosal nerve
Chorda tympani nerve
Trigeminal nerve (V)
Facial nerve (VII)
(intermediate nerve)
Superior salivatory
nucleus

Descending palatine nerves
Posterior nasal nerves
Pharyngeal
nerve
Maxillary
artery

Internal
carotid
nerve

Glossopharyngeal nerve (IX)
Superior cervical sympathetic ganglion
Sympathetic trunk
T1 and T2 spinal nerves
Thoracic
spinal
cord
Dorsal
root

Palatine nerves { Greater
Lesser

Submandibular ganglion

Sublingual gland
Submandibular gland
Facial artery
Lingual artery
External carotid artery and plexus
Common carotid artery

White    Gray
Rami communicantes  Ventral
root

Internal carotid artery

Sympathetic
presynaptic cell
bodies in
intermediolateral
nucleus (lateral
horn) of gray
matter

━━━━ Sympathetic presynaptic fibers
━ ━ ━ Sympathetic postsynaptic fibers
━━━━ Parasympathetic presynaptic fibers
━ ━ ━ Parasympathetic postsynaptic fibers

**Figure 19-17**

- *Extraocular muscle testing* examines the function of each of the 6 extraocular muscles
- While sitting upright (or standing), the patient fixates the gaze upon an object held 12 to 6 inches in front of the eyes
- The object is moved up and down and from side to side in an H-shaped pattern, while the head is kept still, to test the 6 cardinal positions of gaze
- Disorders of movement may be due to deficits in the extraocular muscles, nerves, or areas of the brain that control the muscles

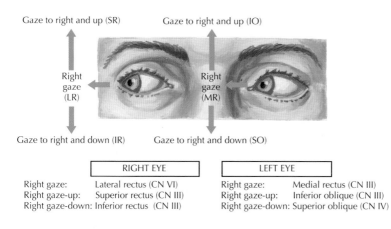

Gaze to right and up (SR)      Gaze to right and up (IO)

Right gaze (LR)      Right gaze (MR)

Gaze to right and down (IR)      Gaze to right and down (SO)

| RIGHT EYE | | LEFT EYE | |
| --- | --- | --- | --- |
| Right gaze: | Lateral rectus (CN VI) | Right gaze: | Medial rectus (CN III) |
| Right gaze-up: | Superior rectus (CN III) | Right gaze-up: | Inferior oblique (CN III) |
| Right gaze-down: | Inferior rectus (CN III) | Right gaze-down: | Superior oblique (CN IV) |

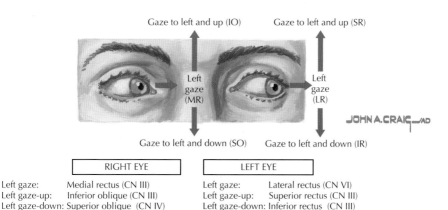

Gaze to left and up (IO)      Gaze to left and up (SR)

Left gaze (MR)      Left gaze (LR)

JOHN A.CRAIG—AD

Gaze to left and down (SO)      Gaze to left and down (IR)

| RIGHT EYE | | LEFT EYE | |
| --- | --- | --- | --- |
| Left gaze: | Medial rectus (CN III) | Left gaze: | Lateral rectus (CN VI) |
| Left gaze-up: | Inferior oblique (CN III) | Left gaze-up: | Superior rectus (CN III) |
| Left gaze-down: | Superior oblique (CN IV) | Left gaze-down: | Inferior rectus (CN III) |

**Figure 19-18**

- Because of the close proximity of the oculomotor, trochlear, and abducens nerves to blood vessels supplying the brain, *aneurysms* along these vessels may lead to a paralysis of the muscles that they innervate
- Commonly affected vessels include the basilar, posterior cerebral, and posterior communicating arteries

## NEUROMUSCULAR DISORDERS

### Abducens Palsy
- Affected eye turns medially
- May be 1st manifestation of intracavernous carotid aneurysm
- Pain above eye or on side of face may be secondary to trigeminal (V) nerve involvement

### Oculomotor Palsy
- Ptosis; eye turns laterally and inferiorly; pupil dilated
- Common finding with cerebral aneurysms, especially carotid–posterior communicating artery aneurysms

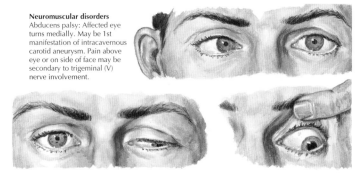

**Neuromuscular disorders**
Abducens palsy: Affected eye turns medially. May be 1st manifestation of intracavernous carotid aneurysm. Pain above eye or on side of face may be secondary to trigeminal (V) nerve involvement.

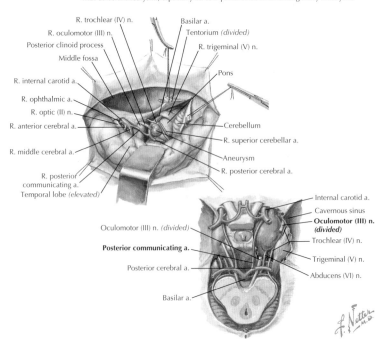

Oculomotor palsy: Ptosis, eye turns laterally and inferiorly, pupil dilated; common finding with cerebral aneurysms, especially carotid–posterior communicating artery aneurysms

**Figure 19-19**

- *Glaucoma*: damage to the optic nerve often due to increased intraocular pressure

## OPEN ANGLE GLAUCOMA

- The most common form
- Gradual and can result in gradual loss of vision
- Intraocular pressure elevates owing to insufficient drainage within the eye's canal system, located in the angle of the anterior chamber of the anterior segment
- Various medications are successful in treating this form

## CLOSED ANGLE GLAUCOMA

- Result of an anatomic blockage of the canal system at the angle of the anterior chamber of the anterior segment

*Example*: When the iris opens the pupil very wide with consequent closure of the angle, intraocular pressure can rise quickly if blockage occurs as an abrupt event

**Early**
Right eye, nasal side

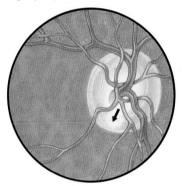

Funduscopy: notching of contour of physiologic cup in optic disc with slight focal pallor in area of notching; occurs almost invariably in superotemporal or inferotemporal (as shown) quadrants

**Minimally advanced**
Right eye, nasal side

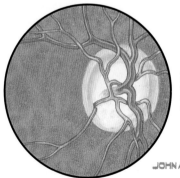

Funduscopy: increased notching of rim of cup; thinning of rim of cup (enlargement of cup); deepening of cup; lamina cribrosa visible in deepest areas.

JOHN A.CRAIG—AD

**Figure 19-20**

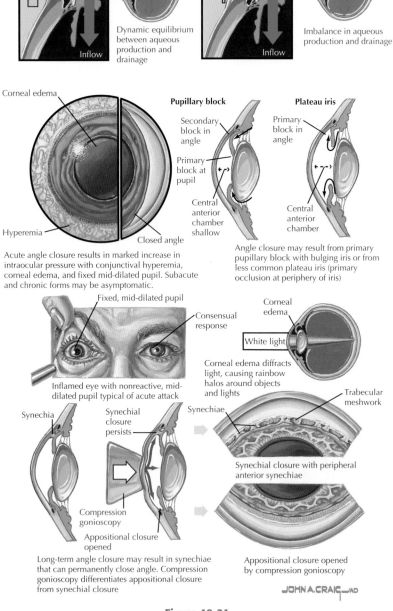

Normal

Outflow

Inflow

Dynamic equilibrium
between aqueous
production and
drainage

Increased

Outflow

Inflow

Imbalance in aqueous
production and drainage

Corneal edema

Hyperemia

Closed angle

Acute angle closure results in marked increase in
intraocular pressure with conjunctival hyperemia,
corneal edema, and fixed mid-dilated pupil. Subacute
and chronic forms may be asymptomatic.

**Pupillary block**

Secondary
block in
angle

Primary
block at
pupil

Central
anterior
chamber
shallow

**Plateau iris**

Primary
block in
angle

Central
anterior
chamber

Angle closure may result from primary
pupillary block with bulging iris or from
less common plateau iris (primary
occlusion at periphery of iris)

Fixed, mid-dilated pupil

Consensual
response

Inflamed eye with nonreactive, mid-
dilated pupil typical of acute attack

Corneal
edema

White light

Corneal edema diffracts
light, causing rainbow
halos around objects
and lights

Trabecular
meshwork

Synechiae

Synechial closure with peripheral
anterior synechiae

Synechia

Synechial
closure
persists

Compression
gonioscopy

Appositional closure
opened

Long-term angle closure may result in synechiae
that can permanently close angle. Compression
gonioscopy differentiates appositional closure
from synechial closure

Appositional closure opened
by compression gonioscopy

JOHN A.CRAIG—AD

**Figure 19-21**

- *Diabetic retinopathy*: pathologic changes to the retina resulting from damage to the blood vessels in the retina due to diabetes
- Can occur in all people with diabetes (types 1 and 2)

PATHOPHYSIOLOGY

- As the retinal blood vessels become damaged, they leak fluid into the eye
- If the fluid accumulates around the macula lutea (which contains the largest amount of cones for acute vision), macula edema occurs in which visual loss is noted
- As the permeability of the vessels worsens, lipoprotein is deposited, leading to formation of hard exudates within the retina
- As new blood vessels form, they are fragile and bleed, allowing blood to enter the eye, helping to cloud and destroy the retina

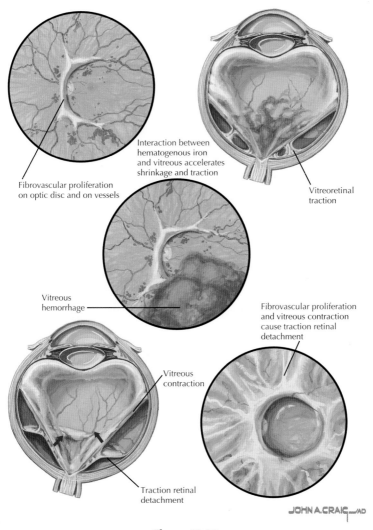

Interaction between hematogenous iron and vitreous accelerates shrinkage and traction

Fibrovascular proliferation on optic disc and on vessels

Vitreoretinal traction

Vitreous hemorrhage

Fibrovascular proliferation and vitreous contraction cause traction retinal detachment

Vitreous contraction

Traction retinal detachment

JOHN A. CRAIG—AD

**Figure 19-22**

- A series of refractive disorders of the eye that cause blurring of the image on the retina

## TYPES

*Myopia*
- Image is focused anterior to the retina
- Commonly referred to as nearsightedness

*Hyperopia*
- Image is focused posterior to the retina
- Commonly referred to as farsightedness

*Astigmatism*
- A nonspherical eye allows the parts of the image to focus at multiple locations, rather than in a single area

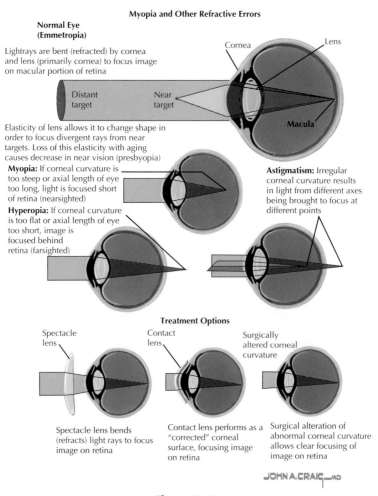

**Myopia and Other Refractive Errors**

**Normal Eye (Emmetropia)**

Lightrays are bent (refracted) by cornea and lens (primarily cornea) to focus image on macular portion of retina

Cornea

Lens

Distant target

Near target

Macula

Elasticity of lens allows it to change shape in order to focus divergent rays from near targets. Loss of this elasticity with aging causes decrease in near vision (presbyopia)

**Myopia:** If corneal curvature is too steep or axial length of eye too long, light is focused short of retina (nearsighted)

**Hyperopia:** If corneal curvature is too flat or axial length of eye too short, image is focused behind retina (farsighted)

**Astigmatism:** Irregular corneal curvature results in light from different axes being brought to focus at different points

**Treatment Options**

Spectacle lens

Contact lens

Surgically altered corneal curvature

Spectacle lens bends (refracts) light rays to focus image on retina

Contact lens performs as a "corrected" corneal surface, focusing image on retina

Surgical alteration of abnormal corneal curvature allows clear focusing of image on retina

JOHN A.CRAIG—AD

**Figure 19-23**

# AUTONOMICS OF THE HEAD AND NECK

- The autonomic nervous system (ANS) has control over the functions of many organ systems and tissues
- Provides innervation to:
  - Cardiac muscle
  - Smooth muscle
  - Glands
- Also provides innervation to the organs of the immune system and metabolic organs (mainly through the sympathetics)
- The hypothalamus exerts control over the ANS and helps the body maintain homeostasis
- The ANS uses a 2-neuron chain system:
  - Preganglionic neurons—the cell bodies are located in the central nervous system (CNS) (i.e., the brain and spinal cord), and their myelinated axons pass out to the autonomic ganglia
  - Postganglionic neurons—the cell bodies are located in the autonomic ganglia, which are outside of the CNS, and their unmyelinated axons travel to the effector organ
- The ANS is divided into 2 parts:
  - Parasympathetic—the portion responsible for preserving and restoring energy
  - Sympathetic—the portion responsible for preparing the body for emergency situations
- Organs typically receive dual innervation, which has an antagonistic action, although there are some notable exceptions, such as the arrector pili muscles (which are sympathetic only) and the male sexual response (erection is parasympathetic, ejaculation is sympathetic)
- Acetylcholine and norepinephrine are the 2 major neurotransmitters used in synapses of the ANS

## Sympathetic Nervous System

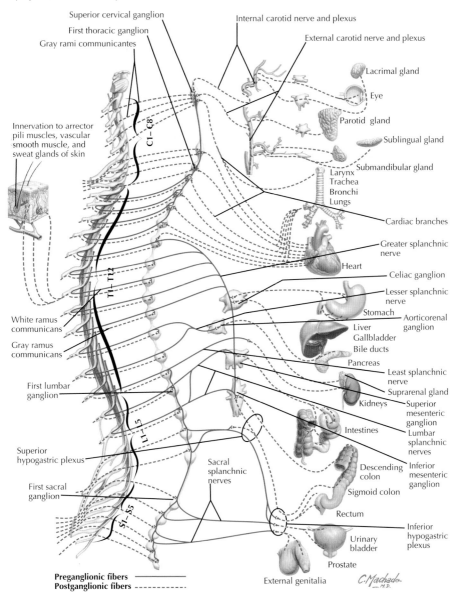

Superior cervical ganglion

First thoracic ganglion

Gray rami communicantes

Internal carotid nerve and plexus

External carotid nerve and plexus

Lacrimal gland

Eye

Parotid gland

Sublingual gland

Innervation to arrector pili muscles, vascular smooth muscle, and sweat glands of skin

Submandibular gland

Larynx
Trachea
Bronchi
Lungs

Cardiac branches

Greater splanchnic nerve

Heart

Celiac ganglion

Lesser splanchnic nerve

Stomach

Aorticorenal ganglion

White ramus communicans

Liver
Gallbladder
Bile ducts

Gray ramus communicans

Pancreas

Least splanchnic nerve

Suprarenal gland

First lumbar ganglion

Kidneys

Superior mesenteric ganglion

Intestines

Lumbar splanchnic nerves

Superior hypogastric plexus

Sacral splanchnic nerves

Descending colon

Inferior mesenteric ganglion

First sacral ganglion

Sigmoid colon

Rectum

Inferior hypogastric plexus

Urinary bladder

C1–C8

T1–T12

L1–L5

S1–S5

Prostate

Preganglionic fibers ──────

Postganglionic fibers ----------

External genitalia

C.Machado
—M.D.

**Figure 20-1**

**Parasympathetic Nervous System**

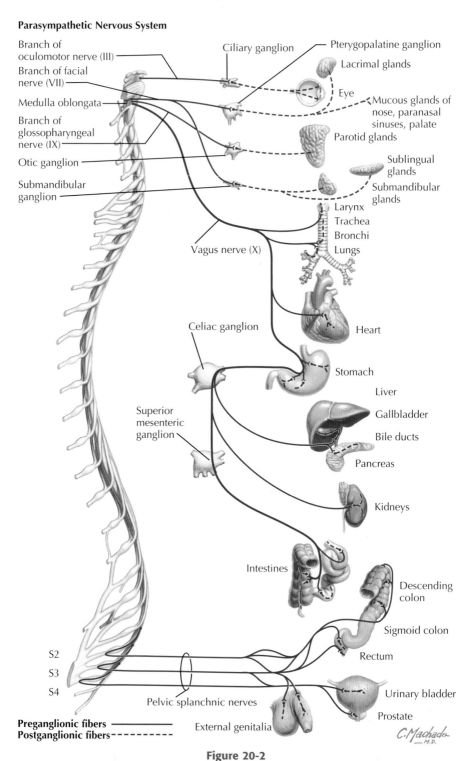

**Figure 20-2**

| DIVISIONS OF THE AUTONOMIC NERVOUS SYSTEM | |
|---|---|
| **Parasympathetic** | **Sympathetic** |
| Referred to as craniosacral fibers | Referred to as thoracolumbar fibers |
| Arise from:<br>• Cranial nerves III, VII, IX, and X<br>• Sacral fibers 2 to 4 | Arise from:<br>• Thoracic fibers 1 to 12<br>• Lumbar fibers 1 to 2/3 |
| Preganglionic fibers are myelinated and travel from the CNS to their autonomic ganglia (located near their respective effector organ in the head and neck), utilizing acetylcholine as the neurotransmitter at the synapse with the nicotinic receptor | Preganglionic fibers are myelinated and travel from the CNS to their autonomic ganglia (located in the sympathetic chain for the head and neck), utilizing acetylcholine as the neurotransmitter at the synapse with the nicotinic receptor |
| Postganglionic fibers are unmyelinated and travel from the autonomic ganglia to the effector organ, utilizing acetylcholine as the neurotransmitter at the synapse with the muscarinic receptor | Postganglionic fibers are unmyelinated and travel from the autonomic ganglia to the effector organ, typically utilizing norepinephrine* as the neurotransmitter at the synapse with the $\alpha$ or $\beta$ receptor |

*Main exception to this is in the adrenal gland, where chromaffin cells secrete epinephrine and norepinephrine into the blood.

| FUNCTIONS OF THE AUTONOMIC NERVOUS SYSTEM | |
|---|---|
| **Parasympathetic** | **Sympathetic** |
| Responsible for preserving and restoring energy | Responsible for preparing the body for emergency situations |
| Discharges focally, not as a complete system | Discharges as a complete system |
| Activated in response to the specific body function that needs to be adjusted (peristalsis, pupillary accommodation) | Activated in response to stressful situations (helps to increase cardiac output, get blood to muscles, and decrease blood flow to the skin and viscera) |

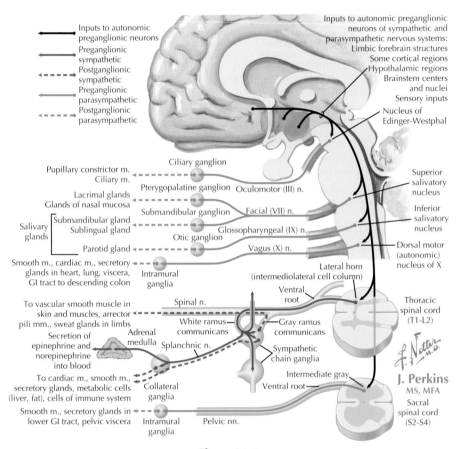

Inputs to autonomic preganglionic neurons

Preganglionic sympathetic

Postganglionic sympathetic

Preganglionic parasympathetic

Postganglionic parasympathetic

Inputs to autonomic preganglionic neurons of sympathetic and parasympathetic nervous systems:
Limbic forebrain structures
Some cortical regions
Hypothalamic regions
Brainstem centers and nuclei
Sensory inputs

Nucleus of Edinger-Westphal

Ciliary ganglion

Pupillary constrictor m.
Ciliary m.

Pterygopalatine ganglion Oculomotor (III) n.

Lacrimal glands
Glands of nasal mucosa

Submandibular ganglion Facial (VII) n.

Submandibular gland
Sublingual gland
Salivary glands
Glossopharyngeal (IX) n.
Otic ganglion

Parotid gland Vagus (X) n.

Smooth m., cardiac m., secretory glands in heart, lung, viscera, GI tract to descending colon
Intramural ganglia

Superior salivatory nucleus

Inferior salivatory nucleus

Dorsal motor (autonomic) nucleus of X

Lateral horn (intermediolateral cell column)

Ventral root

To vascular smooth muscle in skin and muscles, arrector pili mm., sweat glands in limbs

Spinal n.

White ramus communicans

Gray ramus communicans

Adrenal medulla

Secretion of epinephrine and norepinephrine into blood

Splanchnic n.

Sympathetic chain ganglia

To cardiac m., smooth m., secretory glands, metabolic cells (liver, fat), cells of immune system
Collateral ganglia

Intermediate gray

Ventral root

Smooth m., secretory glands in lower GI tract, pelvic viscera
Intramural ganglia

Pelvic nn.

Thoracic spinal cord (T1-L2)

J. Perkins
MS, MFA

Sacral spinal cord (S2-S4)

**Figure 20-3**

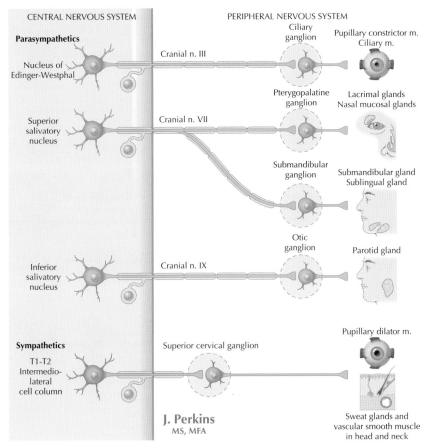

**Figure 20-4**

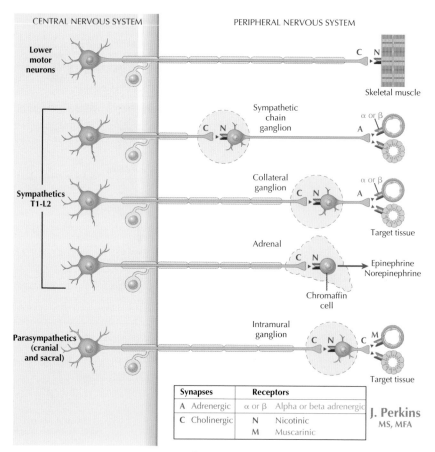

CENTRAL NERVOUS SYSTEM

PERIPHERAL NERVOUS SYSTEM

Lower motor neurons

C N

Skeletal muscle

Sympathetic chain ganglion

C N

α or β

A

Sympathetics T1-L2

Collateral ganglion

C N

α or β

A

Target tissue

Adrenal

C N

Epinephrine
Norepinephrine

Chromaffin cell

Parasympathetics (cranial and sacral)

Intramural ganglion

C N

C M

Target tissue

| Synapses | | Receptors | |
|---|---|---|---|
| A | Adrenergic | α or β | Alpha or beta adrenergic |
| C | Cholinergic | N | Nicotinic |
| | | M | Muscarinic |

J. Perkins
MS, MFA

**Figure 20-5**

| Type of Neuron | Name of Cell Body | Characteristics of Cell Body | Course of Neuron |
|---|---|---|---|
| Preganglionic fibers | Intermediolateral horn nucleus | Collection of nerve cell bodies located in the lateral horn nucleus of the spinal cord between spinal segments T1 and T3 (and possibly T4) | Fibers arise from the intermediolateral horn nuclei from T1 to T3 (or T4)<br><br>Travel through the ventral root of the spinal cord to the spinal n.<br><br>Enter the sympathetic chain via a white ramus communicans<br><br>Once in the sympathetic chain, the preganglionic fibers will ascend and synapse with postganglionic fibers in the various sympathetic chain ganglia<br><br>A majority of the preganglionic fibers will synapse with postganglionic fibers in the superior cervical ganglion, located at the base of the skull |
| Postganglionic fibers | Superior cervical ganglion* (this is where a majority of postganglionic sympathetic fibers to the head and neck begin) | Collection of nerve cell bodies located in the sympathetic chain<br><br>The location of the nerve cell body for a majority of the postganglionic neurons to the head and neck is the superior cervical ganglion<br><br>The locations of the cell bodies for other postganglionic sympathetics include the middle and inferior cervical ganglia | Postganglionic fibers arise in their respective sympathetic chain ganglia (e.g., superior cervical, middle cervical, inferior cervical ganglia)<br><br>Some of the postganglionic fibers that travel to the periphery (e.g., skin of the neck, blood vessels) will rejoin the spinal nerves in the cervical region via a gray ramus communicans, to be distributed along the path of the peripheral nerves following the path with blood vessels<br><br>A majority of the postganglionic fibers join the major blood vessels of the head (namely, the internal carotid a. and the external carotid a. and its branches) to follow the vessel until reaching their final effector organ (e.g., dilator pupillae m. of the eye) |

*Location of the cell body for the postganglionic is variable and depends on the course of this neuron.

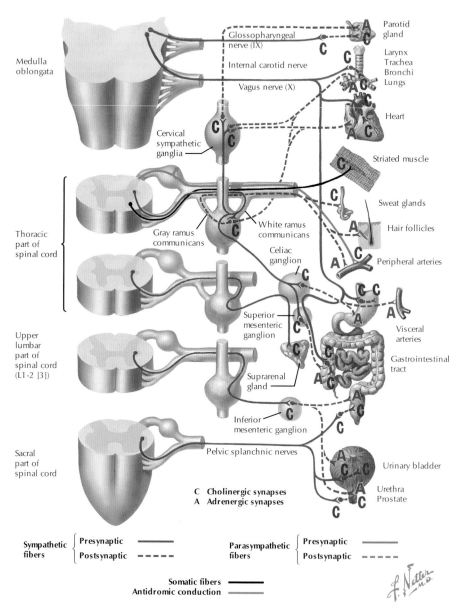

Medulla
oblongata

Glossopharyngeal
nerve (IX)

Internal carotid nerve

Vagus nerve (X)

Parotid
gland

Larynx
Trachea
Bronchi
Lungs

Heart

Cervical
sympathetic
ganglia

Striated muscle

Sweat glands

Hair follicles

Peripheral arteries

Thoracic
part of
spinal cord

Gray ramus
communicans

White ramus
communicans

Celiac
ganglion

Superior
mesenteric
ganglion

Visceral
arteries

Gastrointestinal
tract

Upper
lumbar
part of
spinal cord
(L1-2 [3])

Suprarenal
gland

Inferior
mesenteric ganglion

Sacral
part of
spinal cord

Pelvic splanchnic nerves

Urinary bladder

Urethra
Prostate

C  Cholinergic synapses
A  Adrenergic synapses

Sympathetic
fibers
{ Presynaptic ————
  Postsynaptic - - - - -

Parasympathetic
fibers
{ Presynaptic ————
  Postsynaptic - - - - -

Somatic fibers ————
Antidromic conduction ————

**Figure 20-6**

| ANATOMIC PATHWAY FOR PARASYMPATHETICS OF THE EYE | | | |
|---|---|---|---|
| **Type of Neuron** | **Name of Cell Body** | **Characteristics of Cell Body** | **Course of Neuron** |
| Preganglionic neuron | Edinger-Westphal nucleus | A collection of nerve cell bodies located in the midbrain<br><br>The Edinger-Westphal nucleus is found medial to the oculomotor nucleus and lateral to the cerebral aqueduct | Fibers arise from the Edinger-Westphal nucleus in the midbrain from the oculomotor n.<br><br>Oculomotor n. passes anteriorly on the lateral wall of the cavernous sinus immediately superior to the trochlear n.<br><br>Immediately before entering the orbit, the nerve divides into superior and inferior divisions of the oculomotor<br><br>Both the superior and the inferior divisions of the oculomotor enter the orbit through the superior orbital fissure<br><br>Preganglionic parasympathetic fibers travel in the inferior division<br><br>A small parasympathetic root passes from the inferior division of the oculomotor to the ciliary ganglion, carrying the preganglionic parasympathetic fibers |
| Postganglionic neuron | Ciliary ganglion | Located anterior to the optic foramen between the optic n. and the lateral rectus m.<br><br>*3 roots* connect to the ciliary ganglion:<br>• Sensory root from the ophthalmic division of the trigeminal n., which carries general sensation fibers to the eye via the short ciliary n.<br>• Parasympathetic root from the inferior division of the oculomotor n., carrying preganglionic parasympathetic fibers to the ganglion<br>• Sympathetic root, which arises from the postganglionic sympathetic fibers that were carried by the internal carotid a.<br><br>The short ciliary nn., usually numbering about 8 total, arise from the ciliary ganglion to enter the posterior portion of the eye<br><br>Fibers from all 3 roots pass through the ciliary ganglion and short ciliary nn. to enter the eye<br><br>Only the parasympathetic fibers synapse in the ciliary ganglion | Fibers arise in the ciliary ganglion following a synapse with the preganglionic parasympathetic fibers<br><br>Travel through the short ciliary nn. to enter the eye's posterior portion<br><br>Innervate the:<br>• Sphincter pupillae m.—constricts the pupil<br>• Ciliary m.—changes the shape of the lens during accommodation |

| ANATOMIC PATHWAY FOR SYMPATHETICS OF THE EYE | | | |
| --- | --- | --- | --- |
| **Type of Neuron** | **Name of Cell Body** | **Characteristics of Cell Body** | **Course of Neuron** |
| Preganglionic neuron | Intermediolateral horn nucleus | Collection of nerve cell bodies located in the lateral horn nucleus of the spinal cord between spinal segments T1 and T3 (and possibly T4) | Fibers arise from the intermediolateral horn nuclei from T1 to T3 (or T4)<br><br>Travel through the ventral root of the spinal cord to the spinal n.<br><br>Enter the sympathetic chain via a white ramus communicans<br><br>Once in the sympathetic chain, the preganglionic fibers for the eye will ascend and synapse with postganglionic fibers in the superior cervical ganglion |
| Postganglionic neuron | Superior cervical ganglion | Collection of nerve cell bodies located in the superior cervical ganglion, which is located at the base of the skull | Fibers arise in the superior cervical ganglion<br><br>Postganglionic fibers will form the internal carotid nerve, which travels along the internal carotid a., forming the internal carotid plexus<br><br>As the internal carotid a. nears the orbit, the postganglionic fibers branch from the internal carotid plexus and follow various structures that connect to the eye, such as the ophthalmic a. and its branches, the long ciliary nn. that arise from the ophthalmic division of the trigeminal n., and the short ciliary nn. after traveling through the sympathetic root that communicates with the ciliary ganglion.<br><br>In the eye, the postganglionic fibers innervate the eye's dilator pupillae m. |

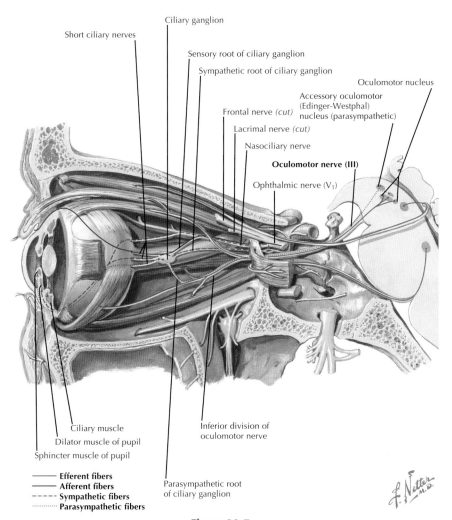

Ciliary ganglion

Short ciliary nerves

Sensory root of ciliary ganglion

Sympathetic root of ciliary ganglion

Oculomotor nucleus

Accessory oculomotor
(Edinger-Westphal)
nucleus (parasympathetic)

Frontal nerve *(cut)*

Lacrimal nerve *(cut)*

Nasociliary nerve

**Oculomotor nerve (III)**

Ophthalmic nerve (V₁)

Ciliary muscle
Dilator muscle of pupil
Sphincter muscle of pupil

Inferior division of
oculomotor nerve

——— **Efferent fibers**
——— **Afferent fibers**
----- **Sympathetic fibers**
·········· **Parasympathetic fibers**

Parasympathetic root
of ciliary ganglion

**Figure 20-7**

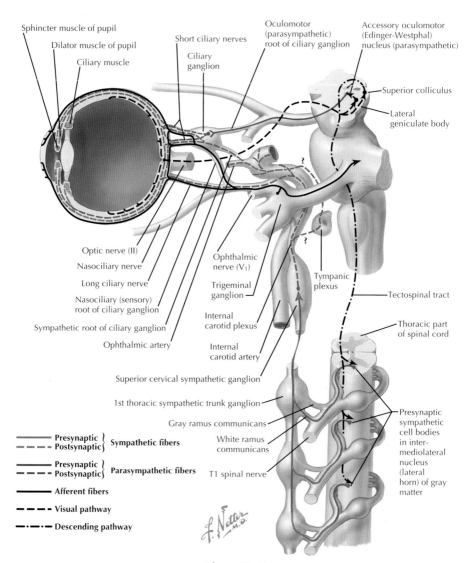

Sphincter muscle of pupil

Dilator muscle of pupil

Ciliary muscle

Short ciliary nerves

Ciliary ganglion

Oculomotor (parasympathetic) root of ciliary ganglion

Accessory oculomotor (Edinger-Westphal) nucleus (parasympathetic)

Superior colliculus

Lateral geniculate body

Optic nerve (II)

Nasociliary nerve

Long ciliary nerve

Nasociliary (sensory) root of ciliary ganglion

Sympathetic root of ciliary ganglion

Ophthalmic artery

Ophthalmic nerve (V₁)

Trigeminal ganglion

Internal carotid plexus

Internal carotid artery

Tympanic plexus

Tectospinal tract

Thoracic part of spinal cord

Superior cervical sympathetic ganglion

1st thoracic sympathetic trunk ganglion

Gray ramus communicans

White ramus communicans

T1 spinal nerve

Presynaptic sympathetic cell bodies in inter- mediolateral nucleus (lateral horn) of gray matter

——— Presynaptic ⎫
- - - Postsynaptic ⎬ **Sympathetic fibers**

——— Presynaptic ⎫
- - - Postsynaptic ⎬ **Parasympathetic fibers**

——— **Afferent fibers**

- - - **Visual pathway**

—·—· **Descending pathway**

**Figure 20-8**

| | | ANATOMIC PATHWAY FOR PARASYMPATHETICS OF THE LACRIMAL, NASAL, PALATINE, PHARYNGEAL, SUBMANDIBULAR, AND SUBLINGUAL GLANDS | |
|---|---|---|---|
| **Type of Neuron** | **Name of Cell Body** | **Characteristics of Cell Body** | **Course of Neuron** |
| Preganglionic neuron | Superior salivatory nucleus | A collection of nerve cell bodies located in the pons<br><br>Travel through the nervus intermedius of the facial n. into the internal acoustic meatus<br><br>In the facial canal, the facial n. gives rise to 2 parasympathetic branches:<br>• Greater petrosal n.<br>• Chorda tympani n. | **Greater Petrosal Nerve**<br>Exits along the hiatus for the greater petrosal n. toward the foramen lacerum, where it joins the deep petrosal n. (sympathetics) to form the nerve of the pterygoid canal (vidian n.)<br>Vidian n. passes through the pterygoid canal and enters the pterygopalatine fossa, where it joins with the pterygopalatine ganglion<br>**Chorda Tympani Nerve**<br>Exits the petrotympanic fissure to enter the infratemporal fossa, where it joins the lingual n.<br>Preganglionic fibers travel with the lingual n. into the floor of the oral cavity, where it joins with the submandibular ganglion |
| Postganglionic neuron | Pterygopalatine ganglion | A collection of nerve cell bodies located in the pterygopalatine fossa<br><br>Postganglionic parasympathetic fibers that arise in the pterygopalatine ganglion are distributed to the ophthalmic and maxillary divisions of the trigeminal n. to the:<br>• Lacrimal gland<br>• Nasal glands<br>• Palatine glands<br>• Pharyngeal glands<br>• Paranasal sinus glands | **Ophthalmic and Maxillary Division Distribution**<br>Postganglionic fibers travel along the zygomatic branch of the maxillary division for a short distance to enter the orbit<br>A short communicating branch joins the lacrimal n. of the ophthalmic division of the trigeminal n.<br>These fibers innervate:<br>• Lacrimal gland to cause the secretion of tears<br>**Maxillary Division Distribution**<br>Postganglionic fibers travel along the maxillary division of the trigeminal n. to be distributed along its branches that are located in the nasal cavity, oral cavity, and pharynx (e.g., nasopalatine, greater palatine)<br>These fibers innervate:<br>• Nasal glands<br>• Palatine glands<br>• Pharyngeal glands<br>• Paranasal sinus glands |
| | Submandibular ganglion | A collection of nerve cell bodies that is located in the oral cavity<br><br>It is suspended from the lingual n. at the posterior border of the mylohyoid m. immediately superior to the deep portion of the submandibular gland | Postganglionic parasympathetic fibers arise in the submandibular ganglion and are distributed to the:<br>• Submandibular gland<br>• Sublingual gland |

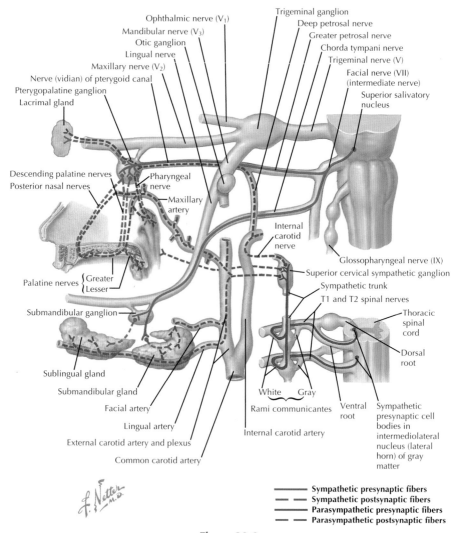

Ophthalmic nerve (V₁)
Mandibular nerve (V₃)
Otic ganglion
Lingual nerve
Maxillary nerve (V₂)
Nerve (vidian) of pterygoid canal
Pterygopalatine ganglion
Lacrimal gland

Trigeminal ganglion
Deep petrosal nerve
Greater petrosal nerve
Chorda tympani nerve
Trigeminal nerve (V)
Facial nerve (VII) (intermediate nerve)
Superior salivatory nucleus

Descending palatine nerves
Posterior nasal nerves
Pharyngeal nerve
Maxillary artery

Internal carotid nerve

Glossopharyngeal nerve (IX)
Superior cervical sympathetic ganglion
Sympathetic trunk
T1 and T2 spinal nerves

Palatine nerves { Greater
Lesser }

Submandibular ganglion

Sublingual gland

Submandibular gland

Facial artery

Lingual artery

External carotid artery and plexus

Common carotid artery

White    Gray
Rami communicantes

Internal carotid artery

Ventral root

Thoracic spinal cord

Dorsal root

Sympathetic presynaptic cell bodies in intermediolateral nucleus (lateral horn) of gray matter

————— Sympathetic presynaptic fibers
— — — Sympathetic postsynaptic fibers
————— Parasympathetic presynaptic fibers
— — — Parasympathetic postsynaptic fibers

**Figure 20-9**

| ANATOMIC PATHWAY FOR SYMPATHETICS OF THE LACRIMAL, NASAL, PALATINE, PHARYNGEAL, SUBMANDIBULAR, AND SUBLINGUAL GLANDS | | | |
|---|---|---|---|
| **Type of Neuron** | **Name of Cell Body** | **Characteristics of Cell Body** | **Course of Neuron** |
| Preganglionic neuron | Intermediolateral horn nucleus | Collection of nerve cell bodies located in the lateral horn nucleus of the spinal cord between spinal segments T1 and T3 (and possibly T4) | Fibers arise from the intermediolateral horn nuclei from T1 to T3 (or T4)<br><br>Travel through the ventral root of the spinal cord to the spinal nerve<br><br>Enter the sympathetic chain via a white ramus communicans<br><br>Once in the sympathetic chain, the preganglionic fibers for the eye will ascend and synapse with postganglionic fibers in the superior cervical ganglion |
| Postganglionic neuron | Superior cervical ganglion | Collection of nerve cell bodies located in the superior cervical ganglion, which is located at the base of the skull<br><br>Postganglionic sympathetic fibers follow the internal carotid or external carotid a. to pass near their respective effector organs:<br>• Nasal cavity<br>• Paranasal sinuses<br>• Palate<br>• Lacrimal gland<br>• Submandibular gland<br>• Sublingual gland | **Nasal Cavity, Paranasal Sinuses, and Palate**<br>• Postganglionic sympathetic fibers follow both the *internal* and *external carotid* aa.<br>• Postganglionic fibers will form the internal carotid nerve, which travels along the internal carotid a. forming the internal carotid plexus<br>• Postganglionic sympathetic fibers from the internal carotid plexus branch in the region of the foramen lacerum to form the deep petrosal n.<br>• The deep petrosal n. joins the greater petrosal n. (parasympathetics) to form the nerve of the pterygoid canal (vidian n.)<br>• Postganglionic sympathetic fibers travel along the branches of the maxillary division of the trigeminal n. associated with the pterygopalatine ganglion to be distributed along its branches in the nasal cavity, paranasal sinuses, and palate<br>• Postganglionic sympathetic fibers from the external carotid branch and follow the maxillary a.<br>• These fibers travel along the branches of the maxillary a. to be distributed along the nasal cavity, paranasal sinuses, and palate<br>**Lacrimal Gland**<br>• Postganglionic sympathetic fibers follow the internal carotid a.<br>• Postganglionic sympathetic fibers from the internal carotid plexus branch off in the region of the foramen lacerum to form the deep petrosal nerve<br>• The deep petrosal n. joins the greater petrosal n. (parasympathetics) to form the nerve of the pterygoid canal (vidian n.)<br>• Postganglionic fibers travel along the zygomatic branch of the maxillary division for a short distance to enter the orbit<br>• A short communicating branch joins the lacrimal n. of the ophthalmic division of the trigeminal n.<br>• These fibers are distributed to the lacrimal gland<br>**Submandibular and Sublingual Glands**<br>• Postganglionic sympathetic fibers follow the external carotid a.<br>• Postganglionic sympathetic fibers branch off the external carotid to follow the arteries that supply the submandibular and sublingual glands |

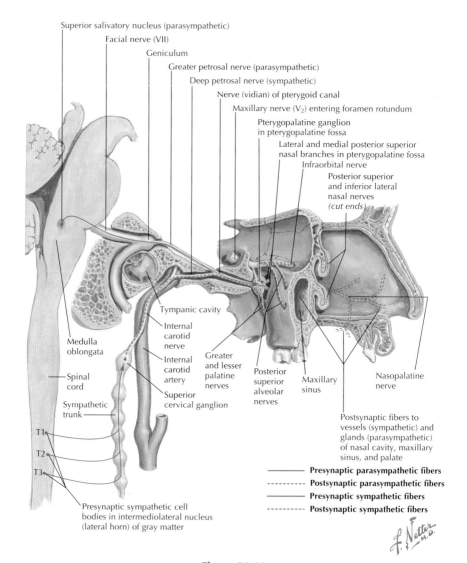

Superior salivatory nucleus (parasympathetic)

Facial nerve (VII)

Geniculum

Greater petrosal nerve (parasympathetic)

Deep petrosal nerve (sympathetic)

Nerve (vidian) of pterygoid canal

Maxillary nerve (V₂) entering foramen rotundum

Pterygopalatine ganglion in pterygopalatine fossa

Lateral and medial posterior superior nasal branches in pterygopalatine fossa

Infraorbital nerve

Posterior superior and inferior lateral nasal nerves (cut ends)

Tympanic cavity

Internal carotid nerve

Medulla oblongata

Internal carotid artery

Greater and lesser palatine nerves

Posterior superior alveolar nerves

Maxillary sinus

Nasopalatine nerve

Spinal cord

Superior cervical ganglion

Sympathetic trunk

T1

T2

T3

Presynaptic sympathetic cell bodies in intermediolateral nucleus (lateral horn) of gray matter

Postsynaptic fibers to vessels (sympathetic) and glands (parasympathetic) of nasal cavity, maxillary sinus, and palate

————— Presynaptic parasympathetic fibers
- - - - - Postsynaptic parasympathetic fibers
————— Presynaptic sympathetic fibers
- - - - - Postsynaptic sympathetic fibers

**Figure 20-10**

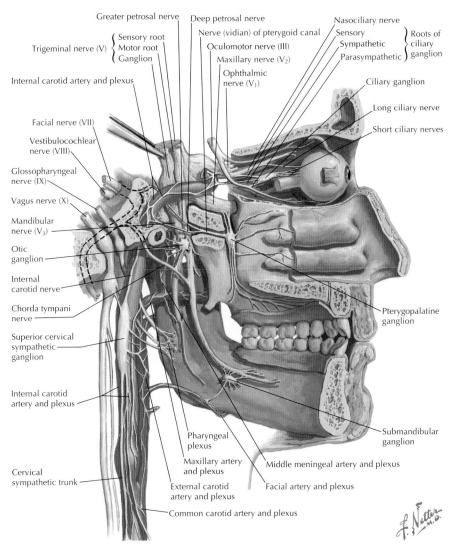

Greater petrosal nerve

Deep petrosal nerve

Nasociliary nerve

Trigeminal nerve (V) { Sensory root / Motor root / Ganglion

Nerve (vidian) of pterygoid canal

Oculomotor nerve (III)

Maxillary nerve (V₂)

Sensory } Roots of
Sympathetic } ciliary
Parasympathetic } ganglion

Ophthalmic
nerve (V₁)

Internal carotid artery and plexus

Ciliary ganglion

Long ciliary nerve

Facial nerve (VII)

Short ciliary nerves

Vestibulocochlear
nerve (VIII)

Glossopharyngeal
nerve (IX)

Vagus nerve (X)

Mandibular
nerve (V₃)

Otic
ganglion

Internal
carotid nerve

Chorda tympani
nerve

Pterygopalatine
ganglion

Superior cervical
sympathetic
ganglion

Internal carotid
artery and plexus

Submandibular
ganglion

Pharyngeal
plexus

Maxillary artery
and plexus

Middle meningeal artery and plexus

Cervical
sympathetic trunk

External carotid
artery and plexus

Facial artery and plexus

Common carotid artery and plexus

**Figure 20-11**

| ANATOMIC PATHWAY FOR PARASYMPATHETICS OF THE PAROTID GLAND | | | |
|---|---|---|---|
| **Type of Neuron** | **Name of Cell Body** | **Characteristics of Cell Body** | **Course of Neuron** |
| Preganglionic neuron | Inferior salivatory nucleus | A collection of nerve cell bodies located in the medulla | Preganglionic parasympathetic fibers arise from the inferior salivatory nucleus in the medulla<br><br>Travel through the glossopharyngeal n. and exit the jugular foramen<br><br>Gives rise to the tympanic branch of IX, which reenters the skull via the tympanic canaliculus<br><br>The tympanic branch of IX forms the tympanic plexus along the promontory of the ear<br><br>The plexus re-forms as the lesser petrosal n., which typically exits the foramen ovale to enter the infratemporal fossa<br><br>Lesser petrosal n. joins the otic ganglion |
| Postganglionic neuron | Otic ganglion | A collection of nerve cell bodies located inferior to the foramen ovale medial to the mandibular division of the trigeminal n. | Postganglionic parasympathetic fibers arise in the otic ganglion<br><br>These fibers travel to the auriculotemporal branch of the trigeminal n.<br><br>Auriculotemporal n. travels to the parotid gland<br><br>Postganglionic parasympathetic fibers innervate the:<br>• Parotid gland |
| ANATOMIC PATHWAY FOR SYMPATHETICS OF THE PAROTID GLAND | | | |
| **Type of Neuron** | **Name of Cell Body** | **Characteristics of the Cell Body** | **Course of the Neuron** |
| Preganglionic neuron | Intermediolateral horn nucleus | Collection of nerve cell bodies located in the lateral horn nucleus of the spinal cord between spinal segments T1 and T3 (and possibly T4) | Fibers arise from the intermediolateral horn nuclei from T1 to T3 (or T4)<br><br>Travel through the ventral root of the spinal cord to the spinal n.<br><br>Enter the sympathetic chain via a white ramus communicans<br><br>Once in the sympathetic chain, the preganglionic fibers for the eye will ascend and synapse with postganglionic fibers in the superior cervical ganglion |
| Postganglionic neuron | Superior cervical ganglion | Collection of nerve cell bodies located in the superior cervical ganglion, which is located at the base of the skull | Fibers arise in the superior cervical ganglion<br><br>Postganglionic fibers will follow the external carotid a.<br><br>Branches from the external carotid a. follow the arteries that supply the parotid gland |

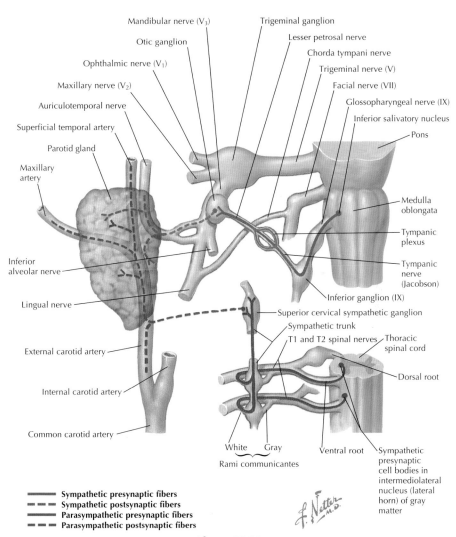

Mandibular nerve (V₃)

Otic ganglion

Ophthalmic nerve (V₁)

Maxillary nerve (V₂)

Auriculotemporal nerve

Superficial temporal artery

Parotid gland

Maxillary artery

Inferior alveolar nerve

Lingual nerve

External carotid artery

Internal carotid artery

Common carotid artery

Trigeminal ganglion

Lesser petrosal nerve

Chorda tympani nerve

Trigeminal nerve (V)

Facial nerve (VII)

Glossopharyngeal nerve (IX)

Inferior salivatory nucleus

Pons

Medulla oblongata

Tympanic plexus

Tympanic nerve (Jacobson)

Inferior ganglion (IX)

Superior cervical sympathetic ganglion

Sympathetic trunk

T1 and T2 spinal nerves

Thoracic spinal cord

Dorsal root

White / Gray

Rami communicantes

Ventral root

Sympathetic presynaptic cell bodies in intermediolateral nucleus (lateral horn) of gray matter

━━━━ Sympathetic presynaptic fibers
━ ━ ━ Sympathetic postsynaptic fibers
━━━━ Parasympathetic presynaptic fibers
━ ━ ━ Parasympathetic postsynaptic fibers

**Figure 20-12**

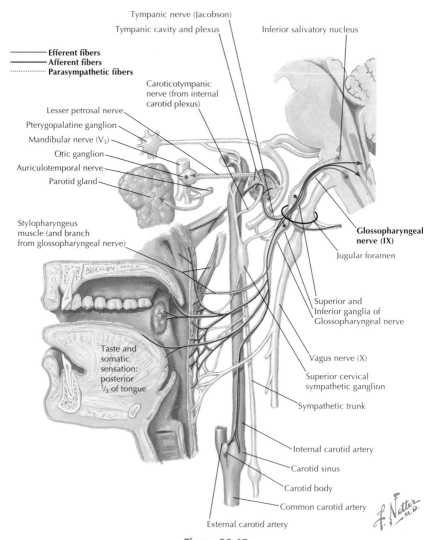

Tympanic nerve (Jacobson)

Tympanic cavity and plexus

Inferior salivatory nucleus

**Efferent fibers**
**Afferent fibers**
**Parasympathetic fibers**

Caroticotympanic nerve (from internal carotid plexus)

Lesser petrosal nerve

Pterygopalatine ganglion

Mandibular nerve (V₃)

Otic ganglion

Auriculotemporal nerve

Parotid gland

Stylopharyngeus muscle (and branch from glossopharyngeal nerve)

**Glossopharyngeal nerve (IX)**

Jugular foramen

Superior and Inferior ganglia of Glossopharyngeal nerve

Vagus nerve (X)

Superior cervical sympathetic ganglion

Sympathetic trunk

Taste and somatic sensation: posterior ⅓ of tongue

Internal carotid artery

Carotid sinus

Carotid body

Common carotid artery

External carotid artery

**Figure 20-13**

| Type of Neuron | Name of Cell Body | Characteristics of Cell Body | Course of Neuron |
|---|---|---|---|
| **ANATOMIC PATHWAY FOR PARASYMPATHETICS OF THE VAGUS NERVE\*** | | | |
| Preganglionic neuron | Dorsal motor nucleus | A collection of nerve cell bodies located in the medulla | Preganglionic fibers arise from the dorsal motor nucleus of the vagus in the medulla\*<br><br>Travel through the vagus n. and exit the jugular foramen<br><br>Various branches connect to intramural ganglia in the thorax and derivatives of both the foregut and midgut of the abdomen |
| Postganglionic neuron | Intramural ganglion | A collection of nerve cell bodies located within the walls of the individual organ | Postganglionic fibers arise in the intramural ganglia<br>These fibers travel to the various effector organs:<br>• Cardiac muscle<br>• Smooth muscle<br>• Glands |

\*The vagus n. arises in the brainstem but provides parasympathetic innervation to the thorax and greater part of the abdomen, rather than the head and neck. The sympathetics that follow the vagus n. to the thorax and greater part of the abdomen, as well as the sympathetics that follow the parasympathetic pelvic splanchnic nerves, arise from the various paravertebral and prevertebral ganglia associated with the sympathetic chain.

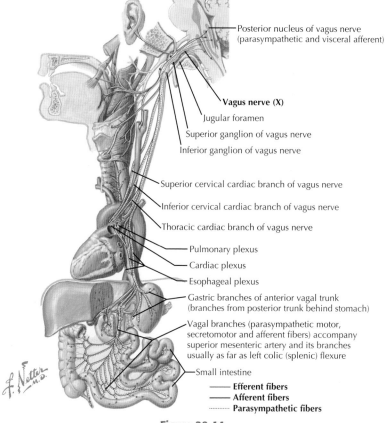

Posterior nucleus of vagus nerve (parasympathetic and visceral afferent)

Vagus nerve (X)

Jugular foramen

Superior ganglion of vagus nerve

Inferior ganglion of vagus nerve

Superior cervical cardiac branch of vagus nerve

Inferior cervical cardiac branch of vagus nerve

Thoracic cardiac branch of vagus nerve

Pulmonary plexus

Cardiac plexus

Esophageal plexus

Gastric branches of anterior vagal trunk (branches from posterior trunk behind stomach)

Vagal branches (parasympathetic motor, secretomotor and afferent fibers) accompany superior mesenteric artery and its branches usually as far as left colic (splenic) flexure

Small intestine

——— Efferent fibers
——— Afferent fibers
·········· Parasympathetic fibers

**Figure 20-14**

- Results from injury or undue stimulus to the sympathetic nerves of the head and neck
- Causes may include:
  - Stroke
  - Neck trauma
  - Carotid artery injury
  - Pancoast tumor
  - Cluster headaches
- Pharmacologic tests can help localize the affected part of the sympathetic pathway
- Treatment depends on the cause (e.g., removal of a tumor)
- Clinical manifestations include:
  - Miosis (constriction of pupil)
  - Ptosis (drooping of eyelid)
  - Anhidrosis (decreased sweating)

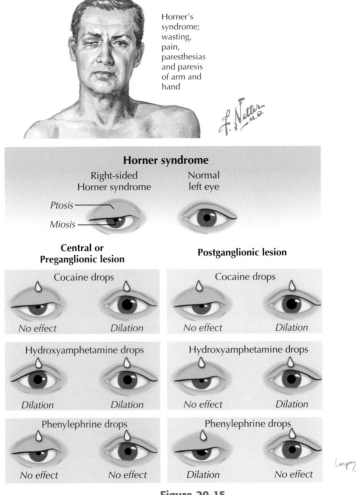

Horner's syndrome; wasting, pain, paresthesias and paresis of arm and hand

**Horner syndrome**

Right-sided Horner syndrome

Normal left eye

Ptosis

Miosis

**Central or Preganglionic lesion**

**Postganglionic lesion**

Cocaine drops

No effect — Dilation

Cocaine drops

No effect — Dilation

Hydroxyamphetamine drops

Dilation — Dilation

Hydroxyamphetamine drops

No effect — Dilation

Phenylephrine drops

No effect — No effect

Phenylephrine drops

Dilation — No effect

**Figure 20-15**

- Intraoral injections provide adequate pain control for various dental procedures
- Many techniques have been developed
- All require detailed understanding of head and neck anatomy to maximize likelihood of proper administration and to minimize complications
- Injections should not be performed in areas of infection or inflammation
- The application of topical anesthetic to the site of injection will help lessen the pain caused by insertion of the needle

## CLASSIFICATION

- *Field blocks*: Local anesthetic is placed near larger terminal nerve branches (located at the apex of the tooth) instead of by the terminal nerve endings (a field block will typically affect the area around 1 or 2 teeth—dental pulp and associated soft tissue)
- *Nerve blocks*: Local anesthetic is placed near the main nerve trunk (such as with the inferior alveolar nerve block)

## COMMON BLOCKS

- Mandibular
  - Inferior alveolar nerve
  - Long buccal nerve
  - Mental nerve
  - Gow-Gates
  - Akinosi
- Maxillary
  - Posterior superior alveolar nerve
  - Nasopalatine nerve
  - Greater palatine nerve
  - Infraorbital nerve
  - Maxillary division

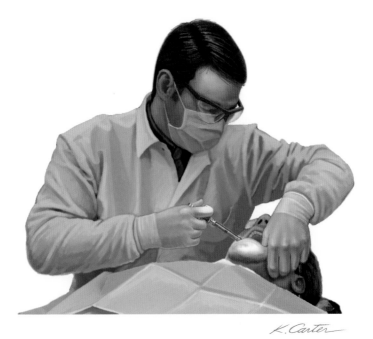

K. Carter

**Figure 21-1**

MANDIBLE: GENERAL CONSIDERATIONS AND LANDMARKS

- The strongest and largest facial bone
- Composed of 2 pieces of thick cortical bone: a lingual plate and a buccal plate
- Teeth are contained in the horseshoe-shaped body
- Ramus extends superiorly from the angle of the mandible
- The coronoid notch is the concavity on the anterior portion of the ramus used to estimate the height of the mandibular foramen, which also is located at the height of the occlusal plane

ASSOCIATED NERVES

- Inferior alveolar nerve enters the mandible at the mandibular foramen
- Lingual nerve enters the oral cavity passing against the lingual tuberosity
- Buccal nerve lies on the buccal shelf

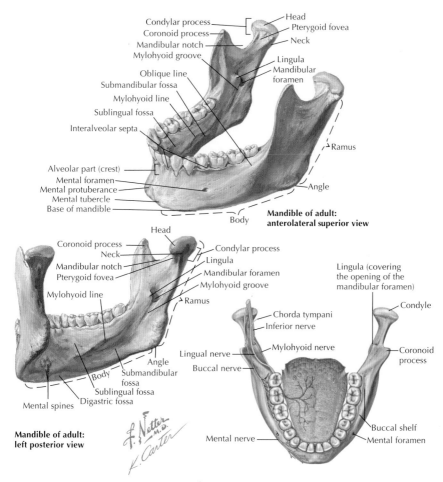

**Figure 21-2**

## OVERVIEW

- This block is important to master, because clinically acceptable mandibular anesthesia is more difficult to achieve than maxillary anesthesia owing to the thickness of the cortical bone
- Requires anesthetic deposition in the pterygomandibular space at the region of the mandibular foramen lateral to the sphenomandibular ligament
- Requires proper needle penetration and correct needle angulation in the pterygomandibular space
- Properly performed, it anesthetizes 2 nerves:
  - Inferior alveolar nerve (and its branches—the incisive and mental nerves)
  - Lingual nerve
- Areas anesthetized:
  - All mandibular teeth (inferior alveolar nerve)
  - Epithelium of the anterior 2/3 of the tongue (lingual nerve)
  - All lingual gingiva and lingual mucosa (lingual nerve)
  - All buccal gingiva and mucosa from the premolars to the midline (mental nerve)
  - Skin of the lower lip (mental nerve)

## GENERAL METHODOLOGY—STEPS

- Insert the needle into the mucosa between the deepest portion of the coronoid notch (which should represent the vertical height of the mandibular foramen) and just lateral to the pterygomandibular raphe
- Orient the needle from the contralateral premolars and advance it along the occlusal plane of the mandible
- The needle contacts the mandible after entering 20 to 25 mm (if bone is contacted immediately on penetration into the mucosa, then the temporal crest has been contacted; the needle should be reoriented to allow insertion to the proper depth)
- Withdraw the needle slightly and perform aspiration to determine whether the needle is in a blood vessel (inferior alveolar vessels)
- After obtaining a negative result on aspiration (no blood observed in the syringe), slowly inject the anesthetic into the pterygomandibular space
- If the result of aspiration is positive, readjust the needle position and perform aspiration again before injecting into the pterygomandibular space

## CONSIDERATIONS

- In *children,* the mandibular foramen is located closer to the posterior border of the mandible until more bone is added with age
- In *edentulous patients,* the alveolar bone is lost; thus, the deepest part of the coronoid notch is lower than normal, which could lead the clinician to aim the needle too low
- In *class II malocclusion,* when the mandible is hypoplastic, the mandibular foramen is typically located more inferior than the clinician may think
- In *class III malocclusion,* when the mandible is hyperplastic, the mandibular foramen is typically located more superior than the clinician may think
- A transient, dental procedure–induced *Bell's palsy* can result if the needle is placed too far posteriorly in the parotid bed and anesthetic is introduced close to the facial nerve

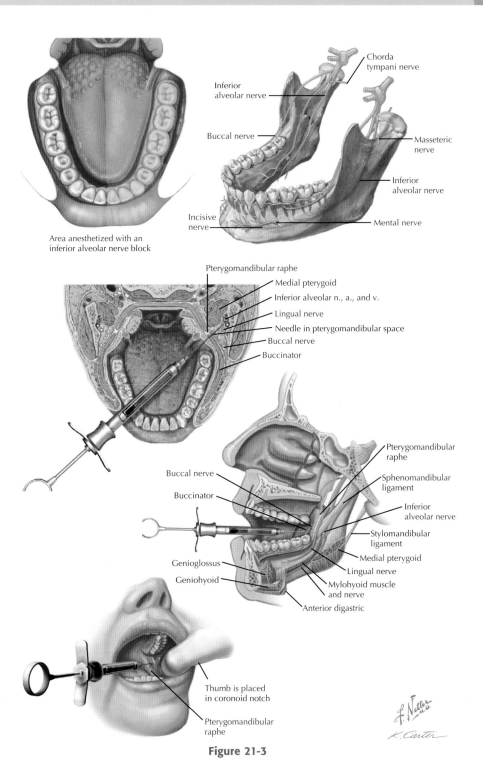

Area anesthetized with an inferior alveolar nerve block

Chorda tympani nerve

Inferior alveolar nerve

Buccal nerve

Masseteric nerve

Inferior alveolar nerve

Incisive nerve

Mental nerve

Pterygomandibular raphe

Medial pterygoid

Inferior alveolar n., a., and v.

Lingual nerve

Needle in pterygomandibular space

Buccal nerve

Buccinator

Pterygomandibular raphe

Sphenomandibular ligament

Inferior alveolar nerve

Stylomandibular ligament

Medial pterygoid

Lingual nerve

Mylohyoid muscle and nerve

Anterior digastric

Buccal nerve

Buccinator

Genioglossus

Geniohyoid

Thumb is placed in coronoid notch

Pterygomandibular raphe

**Figure 21-3**

<table>
<tr><td colspan="1"></td></tr>
</table>

**OVERVIEW**

- A branch of the mandibular division of the trigeminal nerve, the long buccal nerve is not anesthetized in an inferior alveolar injection
- This block anesthetizes all buccal gingiva opposite the mandibular molars, including the retromolar trigone

**GENERAL METHODOLOGY–STEPS**

- Insert the needle into the mucosa posterior to the last molar in the mandibular arch on the buccal side (the needle will be inserted a very short distance—about 2 mm)
- Perform aspiration; after obtaining a negative result, inject the anesthetic

**CONSIDERATIONS**

- A hematoma is rare with this block
- This injection seldom fails

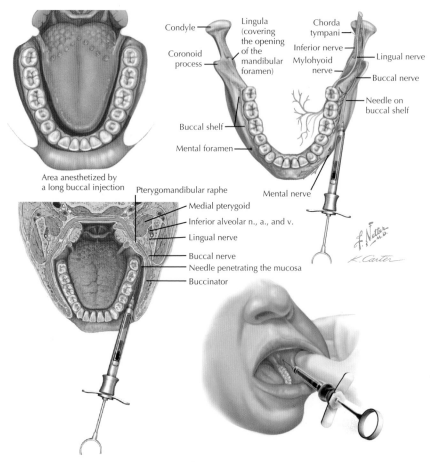

Condyle

Lingula (covering the opening of the mandibular foramen)

Coronoid process

Chorda tympani

Inferior nerve

Mylohyoid nerve

Lingual nerve

Buccal nerve

Needle on buccal shelf

Buccal shelf

Mental foramen

Area anesthetized by a long buccal injection

Pterygomandibular raphe

Mental nerve

Medial pterygoid

Inferior alveolar n., a., and v.

Lingual nerve

Buccal nerve

Needle penetrating the mucosa

Buccinator

**Figure 21-4**

### OVERVIEW

- A branch of the inferior alveolar nerve within the mandibular canal
- Areas anesthetized:
  - All buccal gingiva and mucosa from the premolars to the midline (mental nerve)
  - Skin of the lower lip (mental nerve)

### GENERAL METHODOLOGY–STEPS

- Locate the mental foramen by means of palpation
- Insert the needle into the mucosa at the mucobuccal fold at the location of the mental foramen (normally around the 2nd mandibular premolar) (the needle will be inserted a short distance in the direction of the mental foramen)
- Perform aspiration; after obtaining a negative result, slowly inject the anesthetic

### CONSIDERATIONS

- X-ray imaging can help the clinician locate the mental foramen if palpation does not do so
- This block seldom fails to achieve excellent dental anesthesia
- Often not effective for surgical procedures
- Risk of damaging the nerve if the needle drops into the mental foramen

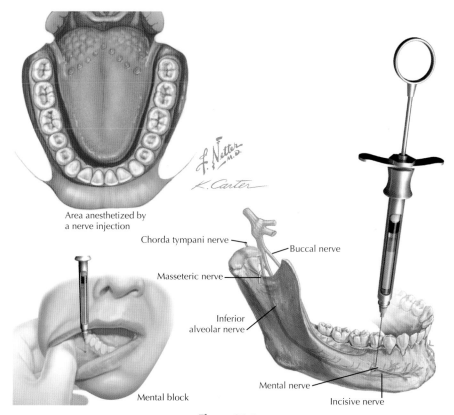

Area anesthetized by
a nerve injection

Chorda tympani nerve

Buccal nerve

Masseteric nerve

Inferior
alveolar nerve

Mental nerve

Mental block

Incisive nerve

**Figure 21-5**

| OVERVIEW |
|---|
| • A variation of the inferior alveolar nerve block, it anesthetizes the following nerves: <br>   • Inferior alveolar nerve (and its branches, the mental and incisive nerves) <br>   • Mylohyoid nerve <br>   • Lingual nerve <br>   • Long buccal nerve <br>   • Auriculotemporal nerve <br> • Low positive aspiration rate relative to that for the standard inferior alveolar nerve block injection <br> • When the injection is properly administered, the needle contacts the neck of the mandibular condyle <br> • Areas anesthetized: <br>   • All mandibular teeth (inferior alveolar nerve) <br>   • Epithelium of the anterior 2/3 of the tongue (lingual nerve) <br>   • All lingual gingiva and lingual mucosa (lingual nerve) <br>   • All buccal gingiva and mucosa (long buccal and mental nerves) <br>   • Skin of the lower lip (mental nerve) <br>   • Skin along the temple, anterior to the ear, and posterior part of the cheek (auriculotemporal and buccal nerves) |

| GENERAL METHODOLOGY–STEPS |
|---|
| • The mouth is opened as wide as possible <br> • Insert the needle high into the mucosa at the level of the 2nd maxillary molar just distal to the mesiolingual cusp <br> • Use the intertragic notch as an extraoral landmark to help reach the neck of the mandibular condyle <br> • Advance the needle in a plane from the corner of the mouth to the intertragic notch from the contralateral premolars (this position varies in accordance with individual flare of the mandible) until it contacts the condylar neck <br> • Withdraw the needle slightly and perform aspiration to observe whether the needle is in a blood vessel <br> • After obtaining a negative result on aspiration, slowly inject the anesthetic <br> • Have the patient keep the mouth open for a few minutes after injection to allow the anesthetic to diffuse around the nerves |

| CONSIDERATIONS |
|---|
| • Useful for multiple procedures on mandibular teeth and buccal soft tissue <br> • Few complications <br> • Works well for a bifid inferior alveolar nerve |

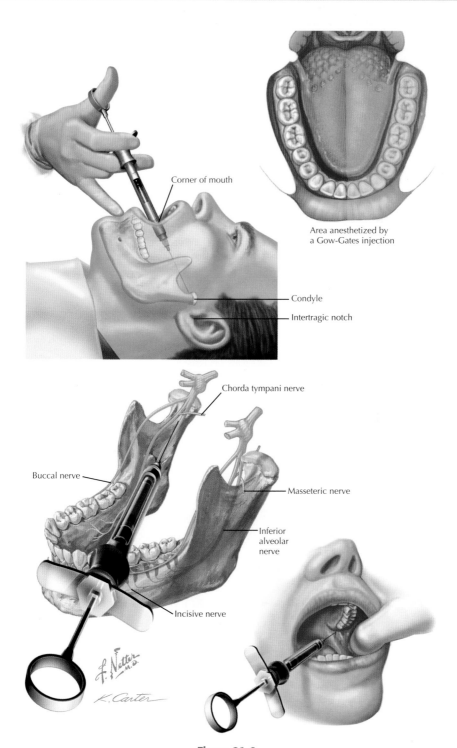

Corner of mouth

Area anesthetized by
a Gow-Gates injection

Condyle

Intertragic notch

Chorda tympani nerve

Buccal nerve

Masseteric nerve

Inferior
alveolar
nerve

Incisive nerve

**Figure 21-6**

| OVERVIEW |
|---|
| • A closed-mouth approach for the mandibular nerve block, it anesthetizes the following nerves:<br>  • Inferior alveolar nerve (and its branches, the mental and incisive nerves)<br>  • Mylohyoid nerve<br>  • Lingual nerve<br>• Useful when mandibular depression (opening) is limited, such as with trismus<br>• Considered a "blind" injection<br>• Areas anesthetized:<br>  • All mandibular teeth (inferior alveolar nerve)<br>  • Epithelium of the anterior 2/3 of the tongue (lingual nerve)<br>  • All lingual gingiva and lingual mucosa (lingual nerve)<br>  • All buccal gingiva and mucosa from the premolars to the midline (mental nerve)<br>  • Skin of the lower lip (mental nerve) |

| GENERAL METHODOLOGY–STEPS |
|---|
| • Have the patient close the mouth<br>• Insert the needle into the mucosa between the medial border of the mandibular ramus and the maxillary tuberosity at the level of the cervical margin of the maxillary molars<br>• Advance the needle parallel to the maxillary occlusal plane<br>• Once the needle is advanced approximately 23 to 25 mm, it should be located in the middle of the pterygomandibular space near the inferior alveolar and lingual nerves (*Note:* no bone will be contacted)<br>• After a negative result on aspiration, slowly inject the anesthetic |

| CONSIDERATIONS |
|---|
| • Often used in patients with a *limited ability to open the mouth* and when intraoral landmarks for a standard inferior alveolar nerve block are difficult to view<br>• A transient, dental procedure–induced *Bell's palsy* can result if the needle is placed too far posteriorly in the parotid bed and anesthetic is introduced close to the facial nerve<br>• Good for patients with a *strong gag reflex* or macroglossia |

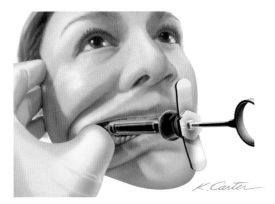

**Figure 21-7**

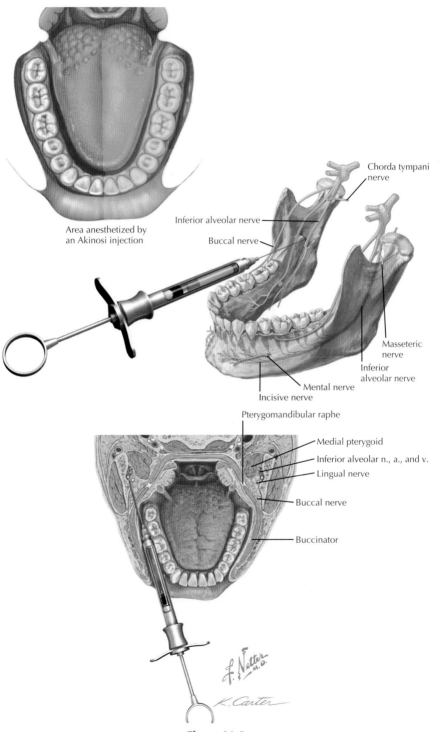

Area anesthetized by
an Akinosi injection

Chorda tympani
nerve

Inferior alveolar nerve

Buccal nerve

Masseteric
nerve

Inferior
alveolar nerve

Mental nerve

Incisive nerve

Pterygomandibular raphe

Medial pterygoid

Inferior alveolar n., a., and v.

Lingual nerve

Buccal nerve

Buccinator

**Figure 21-8**

MAXILLA: GENERAL CONSIDERATIONS

- 1 of the largest facial bones
- Porous bone, which aids in achieving anesthesia of the maxillary teeth

TEETH

- Contained in the alveolar bone
- Maxillary teeth are supplied by the anterior, middle, and posterior superior alveolar nerves (in some patients, the middle superior alveolar nerve may not be present)

HARD PALATE

- Composed of the palatal process of the maxilla and the horizontal plate of the palatine
- Supplied by the nasopalatine and greater palatine nerves

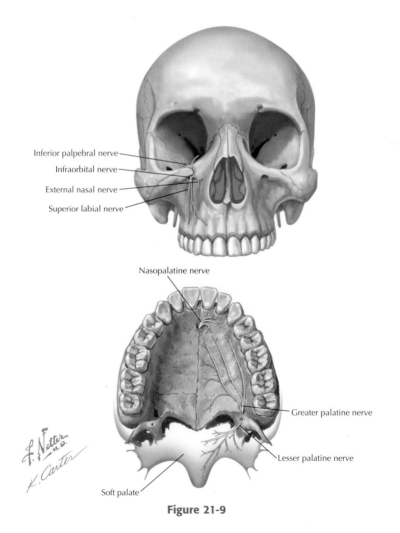

Inferior palpebral nerve

Infraorbital nerve

External nasal nerve

Superior labial nerve

Nasopalatine nerve

Greater palatine nerve

Lesser palatine nerve

Soft palate

**Figure 21-9**

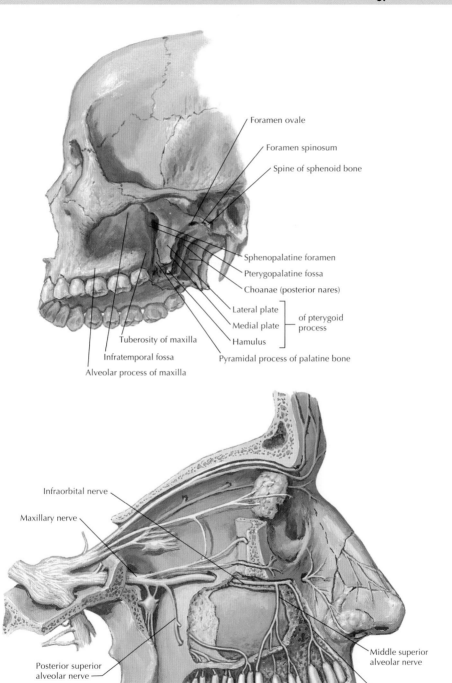

Foramen ovale

Foramen spinosum

Spine of sphenoid bone

Sphenopalatine foramen

Pterygopalatine fossa

Choanae (posterior nares)

Lateral plate

Medial plate

Hamulus

of pterygoid process

Pyramidal process of palatine bone

Tuberosity of maxilla

Infratemporal fossa

Alveolar process of maxilla

Infraorbital nerve

Maxillary nerve

Posterior superior alveolar nerve

Middle superior alveolar nerve

Anterior superior alveolar nerve

**Figure 21-10**

| OVERVIEW |
|---|
| • A frequently used block<br>• The injection is in the infratemporal fossa<br>• Areas anesthetized:<br>  • All maxillary molars, with the possible exception of the mesiobuccal root of the 1st maxillary molar<br>  • Buccal gingiva opposite the teeth |
| **GENERAL METHODOLOGY–STEPS** |
| • With the mouth open, the patient is instructed to deviate the mandible toward the same side as the injection, to produce more work space for the clinician<br>• Insert the needle into the mucosa at the mucobuccal fold just superior to the maxillary 2nd molar, between the medial border of the ramus of the mandible and the maxillary tuberosity<br>  • In a single motion, the needle needs to be advanced approximately 15 mm in the following x-y-z plane at the same time, to reach the posterior superior alveolar nerve along the posterior surface of the maxilla:<br>  • Medially at a 45-degree angle to the maxillary occlusal plane<br>  • Superiorly at a 45-degree angle to the maxillary occlusal plane<br>  • Posteriorly at a 45-degree angle to the maxillary occlusal plane<br>• Perform aspiration owing to the close proximity of the pterygoid plexus<br>• After obtaining a negative result on aspiration, slowly inject the anesthetic |
| **CONSIDERATIONS** |
| • Significant potential for formation of a hematoma involving the pterygoid plexus<br>• Short needles are preferred, to reduce the risk of hematoma<br>• Frequent occurrence of a positive result on aspiration |

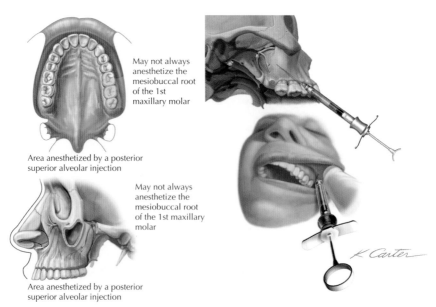

May not always anesthetize the mesiobuccal root of the 1st maxillary molar

Area anesthetized by a posterior superior alveolar injection

May not always anesthetize the mesiobuccal root of the 1st maxillary molar

Area anesthetized by a posterior superior alveolar injection

K Carter

**Figure 21-11**

| OVERVIEW |
| --- |

- Considered the most painful of dental injections
- Because of the sensitivity of the area, pressure anesthesia (e.g., using a cotton swab applicator) is helpful at the site of injection
- Areas anesthetized:
  - The area's palatal gingiva and mucosa from the maxillary canine on the right to the maxillary canine on the left side of the maxilla
  - Both the right and left nasopalatine nerves, because they exit onto the hard palate in close proximity
- Oral mucosa in this region is tightly adherent to the hard palate; thus deposition of anesthetic in the area has less space to diffuse

| GENERAL METHODOLOGY–STEPS |
| --- |

- Use a cotton swab applicator to apply pressure to the injection site
- Insert the needle into the palatal mucosa lateral to the incisive papilla
- Deposit a small amount of anesthetic to help lessen the trauma; the vasoconstrictor norepinephrine then causes the area's soft tissue to blanch
- Advance the needle until it contacts the hard palate
- Withdraw the needle slightly and perform aspiration
- After obtaining a negative result on aspiration, very slowly inject the anesthetic

| CONSIDERATIONS |
| --- |

- Pressure anesthesia is beneficial to help lessen the pain
- Because the tissue is so dense and is attached to the bone, this block requires a slow injection
- For surgical procedures, the nasopalatine nerve block often does not provide profound palatal anesthesia, so the initial injection should be followed by infiltration of the palatal gingiva of the surgical site for best effect

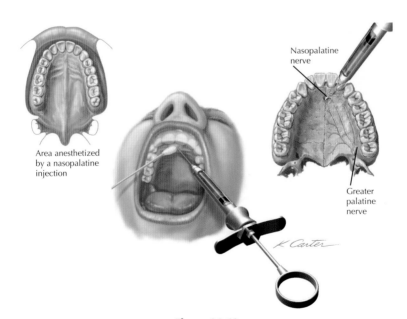

**Figure 21-12**

## OVERVIEW

- Another commonly used block to anesthetize areas of the hard palate
- Not as traumatic for the patient as the nasopalatine nerve block
- Because of the sensitivity of the area, pressure anesthesia (e.g., using a cotton swab applicator) is helpful at the site of injection
- Areas anesthetized:
  - Palatal gingiva and mucosa in the area from the maxillary 1st premolar (anteriorly) to the posterior portion of the hard palate to the midline

## GENERAL METHODOLOGY–STEPS

- Locate the greater palatine foramen by using a cotton swab applicator to press down on the tissue in the region of the 1st maxillary molar, moving posteriorly until the swab dips into the tissue (usually posterior to the 2nd maxillary molar)
- Use a cotton swab applicator to apply pressure to the injection site
- Insert the needle and inject a small amount of anesthetic to lessen patient discomfort; the tissue of the area will begin to blanch from the effects of the anesthetic agent
- Advance the needle until it contacts the hard palate
- Withdraw the needle slightly and perform aspiration
- After obtaining a negative result on aspiration, slowly inject the anesthetic

## CONSIDERATIONS

- The clinician should be able to feel the needle contact bone; otherwise, the needle could be too posterior in the soft palate
- For surgical procedures, the greater palatine nerve block often does not provide profound palatal anesthesia, so the initial injection should be followed by infiltration of the palatal gingiva of the surgical site for best effect

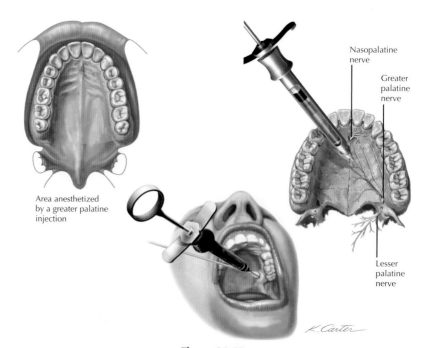

Area anesthetized by a greater palatine injection

Nasopalatine nerve

Greater palatine nerve

Lesser palatine nerve

K. Carter

**Figure 21-13**

| OVERVIEW |
| --- |
| • The middle superior alveolar nerve is reported to be present in about 30% of all people |
| • Areas anesthetized: |
|   • All maxillary premolars and possibly the mesiobuccal root of the 1st maxillary molar |
|   • Buccal gingiva opposite the teeth |

| GENERAL METHODOLOGY–STEPS |
| --- |
| • Insert the needle into the mucosa at the mucobuccal fold just superior to the area of the maxillary 2nd premolar |
| • Advance the needle until the tip is superior to the apex of the maxillary 2nd premolar for maximum anesthesia |
| • After obtaining a negative result on aspiration, slowly inject the anesthetic |

| CONSIDERATIONS |
| --- |
| • Local infiltrations are a common substitute for this block |
| • This area is somewhat avascular, and hematoma formation is rare |

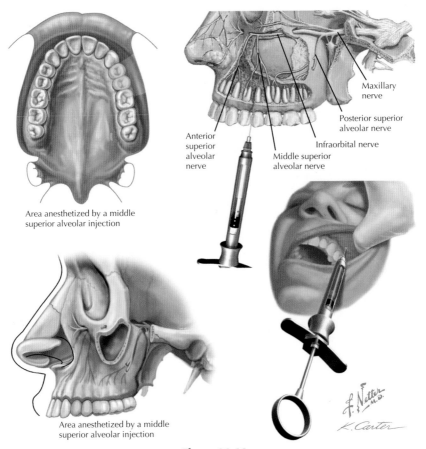

Area anesthetized by a middle superior alveolar injection

Maxillary nerve

Posterior superior alveolar nerve

Anterior superior alveolar nerve

Infraorbital nerve

Middle superior alveolar nerve

Area anesthetized by a middle superior alveolar injection

**Figure 21-14**

| OVERVIEW |
| --- |
| • Less frequently used because of associated risk of injury to the patient's eye<br>• This block anesthetizes the following nerves:<br>  • Anterior superior alveolar nerve<br>  • Middle superior alveolar nerve (when present)<br>  • Infraorbital nerve<br>• Areas anesthetized:<br>  • All maxillary teeth from the central incisor to the premolars, with the possible inclusion of the mesiobuccal root of the 1st maxillary molar<br>  • Buccal gingiva opposite these teeth<br>  • Lateral aspect of nose, lower eyelid, and upper lip |

| GENERAL METHODOLOGY–STEPS |
| --- |
| • Locate the infraorbital foramen by means of palpation<br>• Insert the needle into the mucosa at the mucobuccal fold in the area superior to the 1st maxillary premolar<br>• Advance the needle parallel to the long axis of the tooth until it contacts the bone of the infraorbital foramen<br>• After obtaining a negative result on aspiration, slowly inject the anesthetic |

| CONSIDERATIONS |
| --- |
| • No significant potential for a hematoma<br>• Useful when pulpal anesthesia cannot be achieved in a local infiltration because of dense bone or when anesthesia is required on multiple teeth that would require more than 1 injection<br>• Also useful for dealing with infected teeth/abscess |

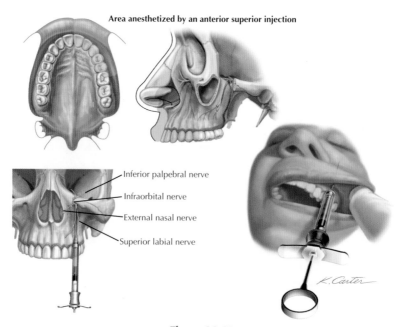

Area anesthetized by an anterior superior injection

Inferior palpebral nerve
Infraorbital nerve
External nasal nerve
Superior labial nerve

K. Carter

**Figure 21-15**

| OVERVIEW |
|---|

- An excellent technique to achieve hemimaxillary anesthesia
- Anesthetizes all of the branches of the maxillary division of the trigeminal nerve
- Useful in extensive quadrant procedures and surgery
- With blocking of the entire division, the following nerves are anesthetized:
  - Posterior superior alveolar nerve
  - Middle superior alveolar nerve
  - Anterior superior alveolar nerve
  - Nasopalatine nerve
  - Greater palatine nerve
  - Infraorbital nerve
- Areas anesthetized:
  - All maxillary teeth
  - All buccal gingiva
  - All palatal gingiva and mucosa
  - Lateral aspect of nose, lower eyelid, and upper lip

| GENERAL METHODOLOGY–STEPS |
|---|

- **Goal:** to deposit the anesthetic in the pterygopalatine fossa using its eventual connection with the greater palatine foramen
- Locate the greater palatine foramen by using a cotton swab applicator to press in the region of the 1st maxillary molar, moving posteriorly until the swab dips into the tissue (usually posterior to the 2nd maxillary molar)
- Use a cotton swab applicator to apply pressure to the injection site
- Insert the needle into the mucosa and inject a small amount of anesthetic to lessen patient discomfort; the tissue will begin to blanch as a result of effects of the anesthetic agent
- Insert the needle further and locate the greater palatine foramen with the needle
- Once the foramen is located, insert the needle and advance it approximately 28 to 30 mm; at this location, the needle should be in the pterygopalatine fossa
- During the passage, if any bony resistance is met, the needle may be rotated to aid insertion (*Note:* under NO circumstances should the needle be forced)
- After obtaining a negative result on aspiration, slowly inject the anesthetic

| CONSIDERATIONS |
|---|

- The needle should NEVER be forced into the greater palatine foramen, because occasionally the canal is not vertical, so that forced entry will fracture the bone
- Because the orbit is located superior to the pterygopalatine fossa, if the needle is placed too far superiorly, the anesthetic can be deposited in this region, affecting the eye
- Because the palatine vessels also are contents of the canal, care must be taken to prevent hematoma
- Also useful for dealing with infected teeth/abscess

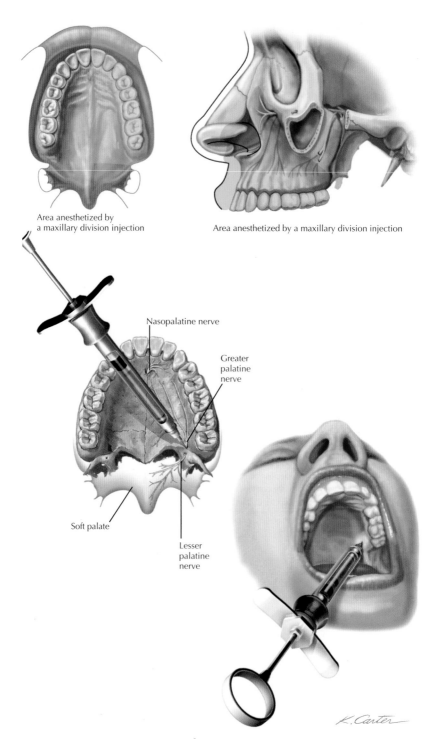

Area anesthetized by
a maxillary division injection

Area anesthetized by a maxillary division injection

Nasopalatine nerve

Greater
palatine
nerve

Soft palate

Lesser
palatine
nerve

**Figure 21-16**

- Achieving adequate pulpal anesthesia in the mandible can be challenging for a variety of reasons
- As a result, a series of supplemental injection techniques are available for use when standard techniques have failed
- Additionally, there are occasions in which mandibular molars in opposite quadrants require treatment, and performing an inferior alveolar nerve block in both quadrants would produce profound soft tissue sensory anesthesia, which the patient would find very uncomfortable
- There are 4 supplemental injections in common use:
  - Periodontal ligament (PDL) injection—excellent for pulpal anesthesia of the mandible on specific teeth
  - Intraseptal injection—useful for periodontal surgery
  - Intraosseous injection—requires a hole in the interseptal bone, so many clinicians prefer specialized delivery systems for this technique
  - Intrapulpal injection—useful for endodontic treatment, but painful on initiation of the injection
- Only the PDL injection is discussed in this chapter, because of its overall ease of use and application in general dentistry

| OVERVIEW |
|---|
| • The PDL injection allows the clinician to achieve pulpal anesthesia of a single tooth |
| • An excellent choice when treatment of specific teeth in both mandibular quadrants is required |
| • Less soft tissue anesthesia is present |
| • Can use traditional syringe or special syringes |
| • Areas anesthetized: |
|   • Pulpal and apical tissue |
|   • Soft tissue and bone of injection site |

| GENERAL METHODOLOGY–STEPS |
|---|
| • Insert the needle interproximally along the vertical axis of the tooth |
| • Because each root needs to be anesthetized, the needle can be inserted: |
|   • *Single-root tooth*–on mesial OR distal root |
|   • *Multi-root tooth*–on mesial AND distal roots |
| • Advance the needle until the tip is at the level of the gingival sulcus–the needle will resist further insertion |
| • Very slowly inject the anesthetic |

| CONSIDERATIONS |
|---|
| • The root of each tooth must be anesthetized |
| • There is no positive aspiration with this injection |
| • Difficult to reach 2nd and 3rd mandibular molars with this technique |

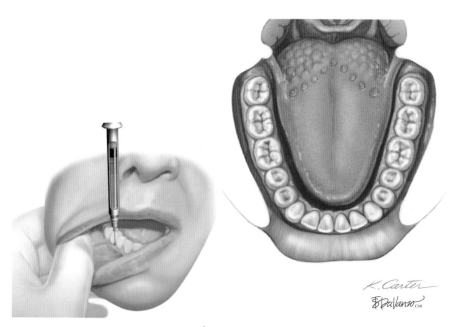

**Figure 21-17**

# CHAPTER 22

# INTRODUCTION TO THE UPPER LIMB, BACK, THORAX, AND ABDOMEN

UPPER LIMB

- The upper limb is the region of the body composed of the:
  - Pectoral girdle
  - Brachium (arm)
  - Antebrachium (forearm)
  - Carpus, metacarpus, phalanges (wrist and hand)
- It is a very mobile structure that allows manipulation of objects
- All motor and sensory innervation is derived from the brachial plexus, which arises from the ventral rami of C5 to T1
- It is a frequent site of traumatic injury

BACK AND THORAX

- The thoracic cavity is divided into:
  - 2 pleural cavities
  - Mediastinum

ANTEROLATERAL ABDOMINAL WALL

- Layers of the anterolateral abdominal wall:
  - Skin
  - Superficial fascia
    - Fatty superficial layer (Camper's)
    - Membranous superficial layer (Scarpa's)
  - External oblique
  - Internal oblique
  - Transversus abdominis
  - Transversalis fascia
  - Extraperitoneal fat
  - Parietal peritoneum

ABDOMEN

- Part of the trunk that lies between the thorax and the pelvis, containing:
  - Peritoneal cavity
  - Gastrointestinal (GI) organs
  - Liver and biliary system
  - Adrenal glands
  - Pancreas
  - Kidneys and upper part of ureters
  - Nerves and blood vessels
- Divided into body planes:
  - Xiphisternal—T9
  - Transpyloric—L1
  - Subcostal—L3
  - Supracristal—L4
  - Transtubercular—L5
  - Interspinous—S2

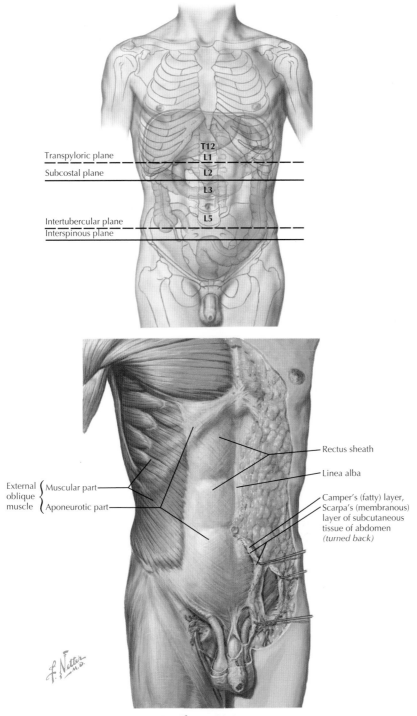

Transpyloric plane

Subcostal plane

Intertubercular plane
Interspinous plane

T12
L1
L2
L3
L5

External oblique muscle { Muscular part
Aponeurotic part

Rectus sheath

Linea alba

Camper's (fatty) layer,
Scarpa's (membranous)
layer of subcutaneous
tissue of abdomen
*(turned back)*

**Figure 22-1**

| BONES OF THE PECTORAL GIRDLE |
|---|
| Clavicle |

- Is convex anteriorly at the sternal end (medial 2/3) and concave anteriorly at the acromial end (lateral 1/3)
- Provides for the attachment of 4 muscles:
  - Pectoralis major
  - Deltoid
  - Trapezius
  - Sternocleidomastoid
- Transmits force from the upper limb to the axial skeleton
- Is paired
- Is frequently fractured

| Scapula |
|---|

- Is flat and triangular in shape
- Is paired
- Has numerous parts:
  - Costal surface—provides attachment for subscapularis
  - Spine—provides attachment for trapezius and deltoid
  - Acromion—provides attachment for trapezius and deltoid and articulates with clavicle
  - Glenoid cavity—articulates with the head of the humerus
  - Supraglenoid tubercle—provides attachment for the long head of the biceps brachii
  - Infraglenoid tubercle—provides attachment for the long head of the triceps brachii
  - Scapular notch—is crossed superiorly by the transverse scapular ligament; suprascapular n. passes inferior to ligament while suprascapular vv. pass superior to ligament
  - Coracoid process—provides attachment for pectoralis minor, short head of biceps brachii, and coracobrachialis

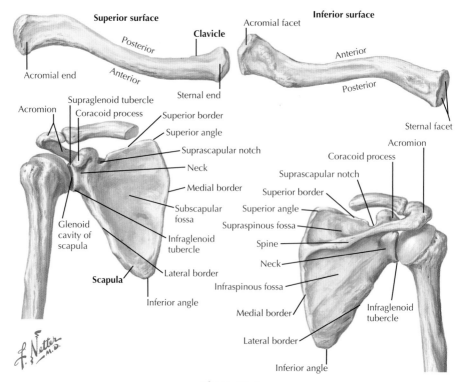

**Figure 22-2**

| BONES OF THE UPPER LIMB |
|---|

### Humerus

- Articulates with the scapula, ulna, and radius
- Longest bone of the upper limb
- Has 8 centers of ossification
- Has 16 major parts:
  - Head—smooth surface that articulates with the glenoid cavity of the scapula
  - Anatomic neck—oblique passing groove that provides attachment for the articular capsule
  - Greater tubercle—provides attachment for 3 rotator cuff muscles: supraspinatus, infraspinatus, and teres minor
  - Lesser tubercle—provides attachment for 1 rotator cuff muscle: subscapularis
  - Intertubercular groove—between greater and lesser tubercles; long head of the biceps brachii located in groove
  - Surgical neck—axillary nerve and posterior humeral circumflex a. and v. lie in contact with medial portion of surgical neck
  - Radial groove—posterior surface of humerus where radial n. and profunda brachii a. and v. are located
  - Deltoid tuberosity—provides attachment of deltoid
  - Capitulum—rounded distal end of the lateral humerus that provides articulation with the radius (head)
  - Trochlea—pulley-shaped distal end of the medial humerus that provides articulation with the ulna (trochlear notch)
  - Olecranon fossa—depression on posterior humerus superior to trochlea; provides area for olecranon process of ulna to occupy during extension of antebrachium
  - Coronoid fossa—depression on anterior humerus superior to trochlea that provides area for coronoid process to occupy during flexion of antebrachium
  - Radial fossa—depression on anterior humerus superior to capitulum that provides area for radius (head) during flexion of antebrachium
  - Supracondylar ridges—sharp elevations of bone on lateral portion of distal humerus that provides attachment of brachial fascia
  - Medial epicondyle—elevation at distal part of medial supracondylar ridge; ulnar n. and superior ulnar collateral a. and v. are located posterior
  - Lateral epicondyle—elevation at distal part of lateral supracondylar ridge

### Radius

- Articulates with capitulum of humerus superiorly
- Articulates with scaphoid and lunate inferiorly
- Is shorter than ulna
- Is frequently fractured at distal end (Colles' fracture)
- Has 3 major anatomic structures:
  - Head—proximal end of radius; provides articulation with capitulum of humerus
  - Radial tuberosity—provides attachment for biceps brachii
  - Styloid process—provides attachment for brachioradialis

### Ulna

- Articulates with trochlea of humerus
- Has 6 major anatomic structures:
  - Olecranon—proximal portion of ulna; provides attachment for triceps brachii
  - Coronoid process—provides attachment for brachialis
  - Trochlear notch—depression for articulation with trochlea of humerus
  - Radial notch—depressed area for radius (head)
  - Head—distal portion of ulna
  - Styloid process—projects posterior and medial

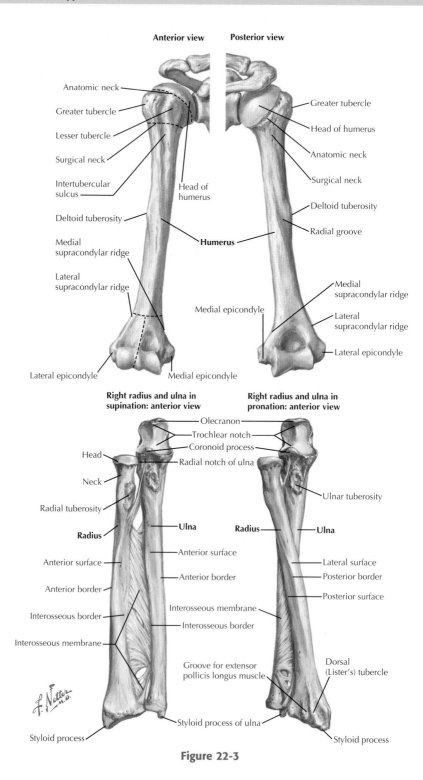

**Anterior view**    **Posterior view**

Anatomic neck
Greater tubercle
Lesser tubercle
Surgical neck
Intertubercular sulcus
Deltoid tuberosity
Medial supracondylar ridge
Lateral supracondylar ridge
Lateral epicondyle

Head of humerus
**Humerus**
Medial epicondyle
Medial epicondyle

Greater tubercle
Head of humerus
Anatomic neck
Surgical neck
Deltoid tuberosity
Radial groove
Medial supracondylar ridge
Lateral supracondylar ridge
Lateral epicondyle

**Right radius and ulna in supination: anterior view**

**Right radius and ulna in pronation: anterior view**

Olecranon
Trochlear notch
Coronoid process
Radial notch of ulna

Head
Neck
Radial tuberosity
**Radius**
Anterior surface
Anterior border
Interosseous border
Interosseous membrane

**Ulna**
Anterior surface
Anterior border
Interosseous membrane
Interosseous border

Groove for extensor pollicis longus muscle
Styloid process
Styloid process of ulna

**Radius**
**Ulna**
Ulnar tuberosity
Lateral surface
Posterior border
Posterior surface
Dorsal (Lister's) tubercle
Styloid process

**Figure 22-3**

**BONES OF THE CARPUS, METACARPUS, AND PHALANGES**

- The wrist (carpus) comprises 2 rows of small bones:
  - *Proximal* row (lateral to medial):
    - Scaphoid—frequently fractured
    - Lunate
    - Triquetrum
    - Pisiform
  - *Distal* row (lateral to medial):
    - Trapezium
    - Trapezoid
    - Capitate
    - Hamate
- There are 5 metacarpal bones that articulate with the distal row of carpal bones
- There are 14 phalanges
  - Fingers 2–5 have a total of 3 phalanges per digit (1 proximal, 1 middle, 1 distal)
  - Finger 1 (thumb) has a total of 2 phalanges (1 proximal and 1 distal)

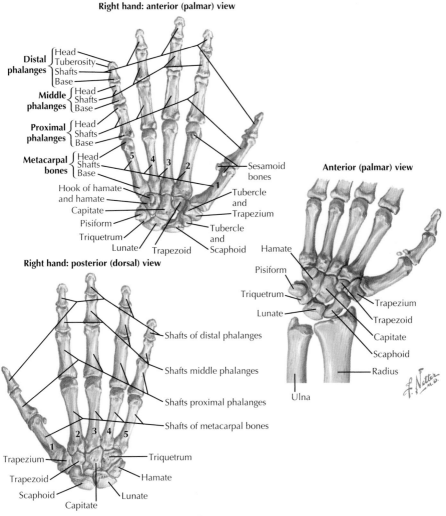

Right hand: anterior (palmar) view

Right hand: posterior (dorsal) view

Anterior (palmar) view

**Figure 22-4**

## BONES OF BACK

### Overview

- Vertebral column includes 33 vertebrae:
  - 7 cervical
  - 12 thoracic
  - 5 lumbar
  - 5 sacral—fuse to form sacrum
  - 4 coccygeal—fuse to form coccyx
- Functions include:
  - Support of body weight
  - Maintenance of posture
  - Allowing locomotion
  - Protection of spinal cord and spinal roots
- Important vertebral levels:
  - T2—suprasternal
  - T3—spine of scapula
  - T7—inferior angle of the scapula
  - T9—xiphoid process
  - L1—transpyloric plane
  - L3—subcostal plane
  - L4—supracristal plane
  - L5—transtubercular plane
  - S2—interspinous plane

### Parts of the Typical Vertebra

- Body
- Vertebral arch
- Pedicles
- Superior and inferior articulating facets
- Transverse process
- Lamina
- Spinous process
- Superior and inferior vertebral notches
- Intervertebral foramen

| Types of Vertebra | Characteristics |
|---|---|
| Cervical | 7 in number (C1–C7)<br>C1 is the atlas (has no body or spinous process)<br>C2 is the axis (has dens)<br>C3–C6 have small bodies and spinous processes<br>C7 has long spinous process |
| Thoracic | 12 in number (T1–T12)<br>Costal facets on body and transverse process<br>Long spinous processes<br>Heart-shaped body |
| Lumbar | 5 in number (L1–L5)<br>Thick body<br>No costal facets |
| Sacral | 5 in number (S1–S5)<br>Fused to form sacrum<br>4 pairs of sacral foramina<br>Sacral hiatus |
| Coccygeal | 3–5 in number (typically 4)<br>Fused to form coccyx<br>Mainly provides muscle and ligament attachment |

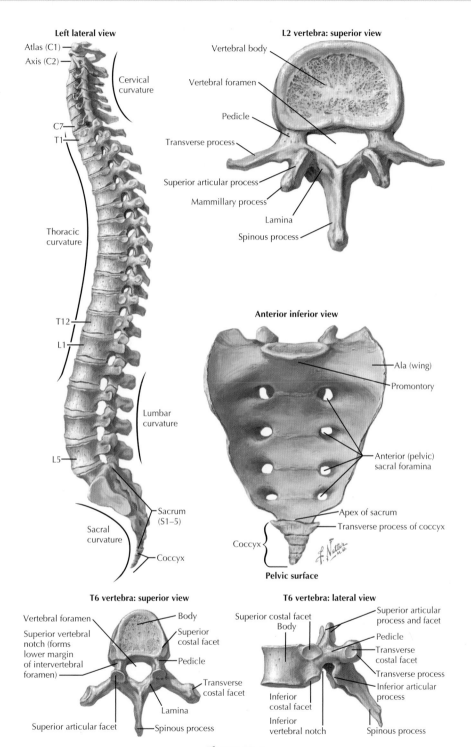

**Left lateral view**

Atlas (C1)
Axis (C2)
Cervical curvature
C7
T1
Thoracic curvature
T12
L1
Lumbar curvature
L5
Sacrum (S1–5)
Sacral curvature
Coccyx

**L2 vertebra: superior view**

Vertebral body
Vertebral foramen
Pedicle
Transverse process
Superior articular process
Mammillary process
Lamina
Spinous process

**Anterior inferior view**

Ala (wing)
Promontory
Anterior (pelvic) sacral foramina
Apex of sacrum
Transverse process of coccyx
Coccyx
**Pelvic surface**

**T6 vertebra: superior view**

Vertebral foramen
Body
Superior vertebral notch (forms lower margin of intervertebral foramen)
Superior costal facet
Pedicle
Transverse costal facet
Lamina
Spinous process
Superior articular facet

**T6 vertebra: lateral view**

Superior costal facet
Body
Superior articular process and facet
Pedicle
Transverse costal facet
Transverse process
Inferior articular process
Inferior costal facet
Inferior vertebral notch
Spinous process

**Figure 22-5**

INTRODUCTION TO THE UPPER LIMB, BACK, THORAX, AND ABDOMEN **597**

| BONES OF THORAX | | |
|---|---|---|
| Overview | | |

- Landmarks include:
  - Midclavicular line—vertical line passing through the midpoint of the clavicle
  - Midaxillary line—vertical line passing through the midpoint of the axilla
  - Scapular line—vertical line passing through the inferior angle of scapula
  - Suprasternal notch—T2
  - Sternal angle—T4
- The thoracic apertures:
  - *Superior thoracic aperture*
    - Boundaries
      - Body of T1 vertebra
      - 1st pair of ribs and cartilages
      - Manubrium (superior portion)
    - Major contents
      - Trachea
      - Esophagus
      - Great vessels and nerves
      - Thoracic duct
      - Lungs
  - *Inferior thoracic aperture*
    - Boundaries
      - Body of T12 vertebra
      - 12th pair of ribs
      - Costal margins
      - Xiphoid process

| Sternum | | |
|---|---|---|
| **Parts** | **Characteristics** | |
| Manubrium | Superior part of sternum<br>Quadrangular in shape<br>Superior border is known as jugular notch or suprasternal notch (vertebral level T2)<br>Articulates with:<br>• Clavicle<br>• 1st costal cartilage<br>• 2nd costal cartilage<br>• Body of sternum | |
| Body | Longest part of sternum<br>Articulates with 2nd through 7th ribs<br>Articulates with:<br>• Manubrium at manubriosternal joint (vertebral level T4)<br>• Xiphoid process (vertebral level T9) | |
| Xiphoid process | Cartilaginous process, which ossifies | |

| Ribs | | |
|---|---|---|
| **Type** | **Characteristics** | |
| Vertebrosternal | Ribs 1–7<br>Known as "true ribs" because they articulate with the sternum through the costal cartilage<br>Articulate with the sternum through the costal cartilage | |
| Vertebrochondral | Ribs 8–10<br>Known as "false ribs" because they do not possess a direct articulation to the sternum<br>These ribs articulate to a common cartilaginous connection to the sternum | |
| Vertebral | Ribs 11 and 12<br>Most commonly known as "floating ribs"<br>They also are "false ribs" because they do not possess a direct articulation to the sternum<br>Do not articulate with the sternum and end in the posterior abdominal wall | |

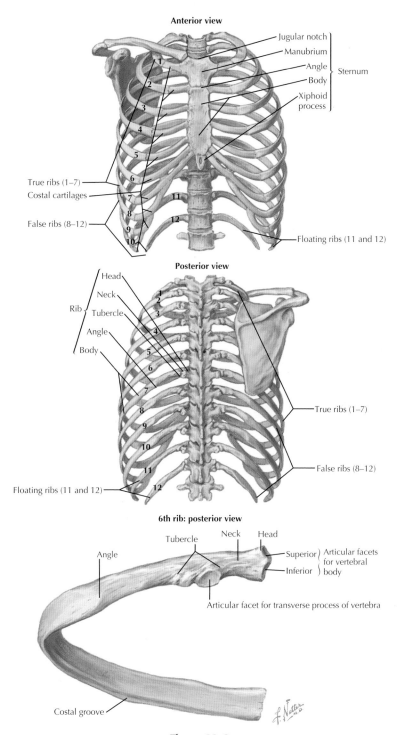

**Anterior view**

Jugular notch
Manubrium
Angle
Body
Xiphoid process

Sternum

1
2
3
4
5
6
7
8
9
10
11
12

True ribs (1–7)
Costal cartilages
False ribs (8–12)
Floating ribs (11 and 12)

**Posterior view**

Head
Neck
Tubercle
Angle
Body

Rib

1
2
3
4
5
6
7
8
9
10
11
12

True ribs (1–7)
False ribs (8–12)
Floating ribs (11 and 12)

**6th rib: posterior view**

Tubercle
Neck
Head
Angle

Superior
Inferior

Articular facets for vertebral body

Articular facet for transverse process of vertebra

Costal groove

**Figure 22-6**

| BONES OF ABDOMEN AND PELVIS | |
|---|---|
| Overview | |

- The 5 lumbar vertebra are in the abdomen
- Bones of the pelvis comprised of 3 structures:
  - Sacrum
  - Coccyx
  - Os coxae (hip bone)
    - Ilium
    - Ischium
    - Pubis
- The pelvis is the inferior portion of abdomen providing a connection of the spinal column to the femur
- Multiple functions:
  - Bear weight
  - Allow locomotion
  - Maintain posture
  - Provide for muscle and ligament attachment
- Has a pelvic cavity that is divided by the pelvic brim into:
  - False pelvis—superior to pelvic brim and contains inferior portion of abdominal cavity
  - True pelvis—inferior to pelvic brim and contains the:
    - Bladder
    - Terminal colon and rectum
    - Some reproductive and accessory reproductive organs:
      - Prostate
      - Seminal vesicles
      - Vas deferens
      - Uterus with uterine tubes and ovary
      - Vagina

| Os Coxae | |
|---|---|
| **Part** | **Characteristics** |
| Ilium | Largest part of the hip bone<br>Comprises the:<br>• Ala (wing)<br>• Body<br>Provides muscle and ligament attachments |
| Ischium | Most posterior and inferior portion of the hip bone<br>Comprise the:<br>• Body<br>• Superior ischial ramus<br>• Inferior ischial ramus<br>Provides muscle and ligament attachments |
| Pubis | Most anterior portion of the hip bone<br>Comprises the:<br>• Superior pubic ramus<br>• Inferior pubic ramus<br>Provides muscle and ligament attachment<br>Right and left hip bones articulate at the pubic symphysis |

**Anterior view**

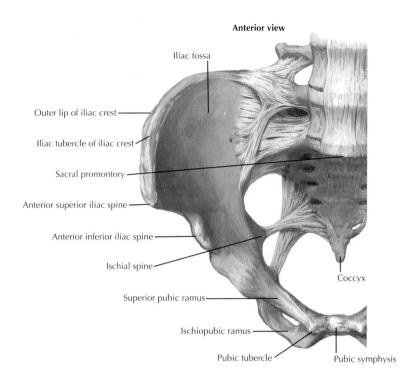

Iliac fossa

Outer lip of iliac crest

Iliac tubercle of iliac crest

Sacral promontory

Anterior superior iliac spine

Anterior inferior iliac spine

Ischial spine

Superior pubic ramus

Ischiopubic ramus

Pubic tubercle

Coccyx

Pubic symphysis

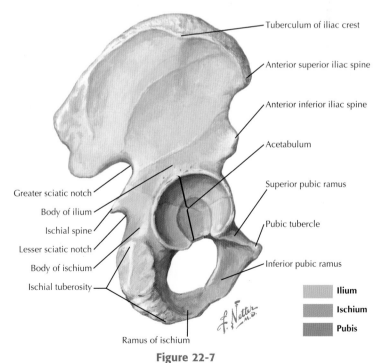

Tuberculum of iliac crest

Anterior superior iliac spine

Anterior inferior iliac spine

Acetabulum

Superior pubic ramus

Pubic tubercle

Inferior pubic ramus

Greater sciatic notch

Body of ilium

Ischial spine

Lesser sciatic notch

Body of ischium

Ischial tuberosity

Ramus of ischium

Ilium

Ischium

Pubis

**Figure 22-7**

| MUSCLES OF PECTORAL REGION | | | | |
|---|---|---|---|---|
| **Muscle** | **Origin** | **Insertion** | **Action(s)** | **Nerve Supply** |
| Pectoralis major | Clavicular head<br>• Clavicle (medial 1/2)<br>Sternocostal head<br>• Anterior surface of sternum<br>• Upper 6 costal cartilages | Lateral lip of intertubercular groove | Flexion of humerus<br>Adduction of humerus<br>Medial rotation of humerus | Medial pectoral n.<br>Lateral pectoral n. |
| Pectoralis minor | Ribs 3–5 | Coracoid process | Protraction of scapula<br>Aids in stabilization of scapula | Medial pectoral n. |
| Serratus anterior | Ribs 1–8 | Medial border of scapula | Protraction of scapula<br>Rotates the scapula<br>Aids in stabilization of the scapula | Long thoracic n. |
| Subclavius | 1st rib and 1st costal cartilage | Inferior surface of clavicle | Aids in depressing lateral part of clavicle | Subclavius n. |

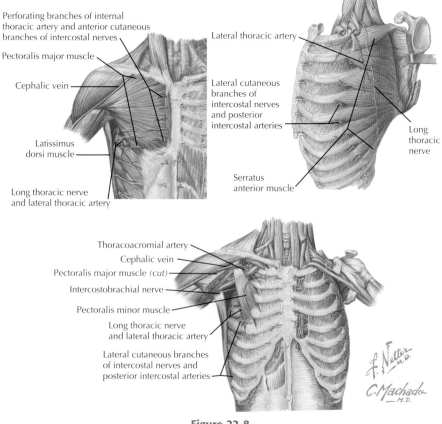

Perforating branches of internal thoracic artery and anterior cutaneous branches of intercostal nerves

Pectoralis major muscle

Cephalic vein

Latissimus dorsi muscle

Long thoracic nerve and lateral thoracic artery

Lateral thoracic artery

Lateral cutaneous branches of intercostal nerves and posterior intercostal arteries

Serratus anterior muscle

Long thoracic nerve

Thoracoacromial artery

Cephalic vein

Pectoralis major muscle *(cut)*

Intercostobrachial nerve

Pectoralis minor muscle

Long thoracic nerve and lateral thoracic artery

Lateral cutaneous branches of intercostal nerves and posterior intercostal arteries

**Figure 22-8**

| MUSCLES OF SHOULDER | | | | |
|---|---|---|---|---|
| **Muscle** | **Origin** | **Insertion** | **Actions** | **Nerve Supply** |
| Deltoid | • Lateral 1/3 of clavicle<br>• Acromion<br>• Spine of scapula | Deltoid tuberosity | Abduction of humerus<br><br>Anterior fibers aid in flexion of humerus and medial rotation of humerus<br><br>Posterior fibers aid in extension of humerus and lateral rotation of humerus | Axillary n. |
| Teres major | Inferior angle of posterior scapula | Medial lip of intertubercular groove | Adduction of humerus<br>Medial rotation of humerus | Lower subscapular n. |
| Supraspinatus | Supraspinous fossa | Greater tubercle (superior facet) | Abduction of humerus (1st 10–15 degrees)<br>Aids in holding humerus in glenoid cavity | Suprascapular n. |
| Infraspinatus | Infraspinous fossa | Greater tubercle (middle facet) | Lateral rotation of humerus<br>Aids in holding humerus in glenoid cavity<br>Aids in adduction | Suprascapular n. |
| Teres minor | Lateral border of scapula | Greater tubercle (inferior facet) | Lateral rotation of humerus<br>Aids in holding humerus in glenoid cavity<br>Aids in adduction | Axillary n. |
| Subscapularis | Subscapular fossa | Lesser tubercle | Medial rotation of humerus<br>Aids in holding humerus in glenoid cavity<br>Aids in adduction | Upper subscapular n.<br>Lower subscapular n. |

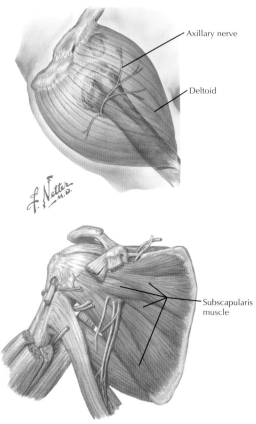

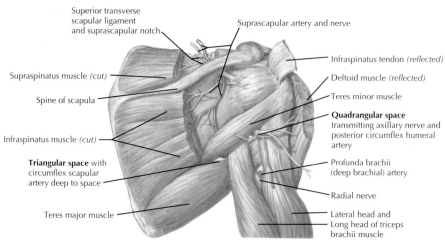

Superior transverse
scapular ligament
and suprascapular notch

Suprascapular artery and nerve

Infraspinatus tendon *(reflected)*

Supraspinatus muscle *(cut)*

Deltoid muscle *(reflected)*

Spine of scapula

Teres minor muscle

**Quadrangular space**
transmitting axillary nerve and
posterior circumflex humeral
artery

Infraspinatus muscle *(cut)*

**Triangular space** with
circumflex scapular
artery deep to space

Profunda brachii
(deep brachial) artery

Radial nerve

Teres major muscle

Lateral head and
Long head of triceps
brachii muscle

Axillary nerve

Deltoid

Subscapularis
muscle

**Figure 22-9**

| MUSCLES OF BRACHIUM | | | | |
|---|---|---|---|---|
| Flexor Compartment | | | | |
| **Muscle** | **Origin** | **Insertion** | **Action(s)** | **Nerve Supply** |
| Biceps brachii | Long head <br>• Supraglenoid tubercle <br>Short head <br>• Coracoid process | Radial tuberosity of radius | Flexion of antebrachium <br>Supination of antebrachium <br>Aids in flexion of brachium | Musculocutaneous n. |
| Brachialis | Anterior surface of distal portion of humerus | • Coronoid process of ulna <br>• Ulnar tuberosity | Flexion of antebrachium | Musculocutaneous n. |
| Coracobrachialis | Coracoid process | Middle 1/3 of medial humerus | Flexion of brachium <br>Adduction of brachium | Musculocutaneous n. |
| Extensor Compartment | | | | |
| Triceps brachii | Long head <br>• Infraglenoid tubercle <br>Lateral head <br>• Superior to radial groove <br>Medial head <br>• Inferior to radial groove | Olecranon of ulna | Extension of antebrachium <br>Long head aids in slight adduction of brachium | Radial n. |
| Anconeus | Lateral epicondyle of humerus | Olecranon of ulna | Extension of antebrachium | Radial n. |

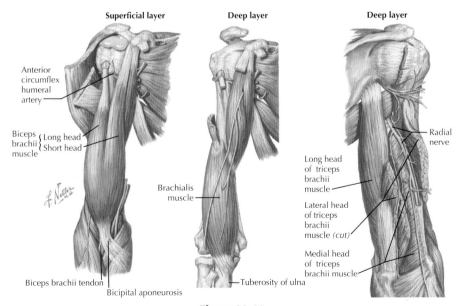

**Figure 22-10**

| MUSCLES OF FLEXOR SURFACE OF ANTEBRACHIUM | | | | |
|---|---|---|---|---|
| Superficial Group | | | | |
| **Muscle** | **Origin** | **Insertion** | **Action(s)** | **Nerve Supply** |
| Pronator teres | Medial epicondyle of humerus<br>Coronoid process of ulna | Lateral surface of radius (middle portion) | Pronation of antebrachium<br>Weak flexion of antebrachium | Median n. |
| Flexor carpi radialis | Medial epicondyle of humerus | Base of 2nd and 3rd metacarpal | Flexion of antebrachium (little)<br>Flexion of wrist<br>Abduction of wrist | Median n. |
| Palmaris longus | Medial epicondyle of humerus | Palmar aponeurosis | Weak flexion of antebrachium<br>Flexion of wrist | Median n. |
| Flexor carpi ulnaris | Medial epicondyle of humerus<br>Posterior ulna | Pisiform<br>Hamate (hook)<br>Base of 5th metacarpal | Weak flexion of antebrachium<br>Flexion of wrist<br>Adducton of wrist | Ulnar n. |
| Intermediate Group | | | | |
| Flexor digitorum superficialis | Medial epicondyle of humerus<br>Coronoid process<br>Radius (oblique line) | Middle phalanges of digits 2–5 | Weak flexion of antebrachium<br>Flexion of hand<br>Flexion of proximal interphalangeal joints of digits 2–5 | Median n. |
| Deep Group | | | | |
| Flexor digitorum profundus | Anterior and medial surface of ulna<br>Interosseous membrane | Base of distal phalanges of digits 2–5 | Flexion of hand<br>Flexion of distal interphalangeal joints of digits 2–5 | Anterior interosseous of the median n. (lateral 1/2)<br>Ulnar n. (medial 1/2) |
| Flexor pollicis longus | Anterior surface of radius<br>Interosseous membrane | Base of distal phalanx of thumb | Flexion of thumb | Anterior interosseous of the median n. |
| Pronator quadratus | Anterior surface of distal ulna | Anterior surface of distal radius | Pronation of antebrachium | Anterior interosseous of the median n. |

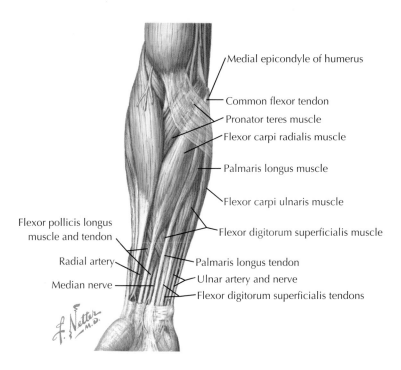

Medial epicondyle of humerus

Common flexor tendon

Pronator teres muscle

Flexor carpi radialis muscle

Palmaris longus muscle

Flexor carpi ulnaris muscle

Flexor pollicis longus
muscle and tendon

Flexor digitorum superficialis muscle

Radial artery

Palmaris longus tendon

Median nerve

Ulnar artery and nerve

Flexor digitorum superficialis tendons

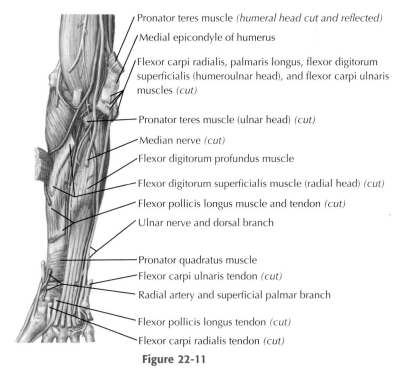

Pronator teres muscle *(humeral head cut and reflected)*

Medial epicondyle of humerus

Flexor carpi radialis, palmaris longus, flexor digitorum superficialis (humeroulnar head), and flexor carpi ulnaris muscles *(cut)*

Pronator teres muscle (ulnar head) *(cut)*

Median nerve *(cut)*

Flexor digitorum profundus muscle

Flexor digitorum superficialis muscle (radial head) *(cut)*

Flexor pollicis longus muscle and tendon *(cut)*

Ulnar nerve and dorsal branch

Pronator quadratus muscle

Flexor carpi ulnaris tendon *(cut)*

Radial artery and superficial palmar branch

Flexor pollicis longus tendon *(cut)*

Flexor carpi radialis tendon *(cut)*

**Figure 22-11**

INTRODUCTION TO THE UPPER LIMB, BACK, THORAX, AND ABDOMEN **607**

| MUSCLES OF EXTENSOR SURFACE OF ANTEBRACHIUM | | | | |
|---|---|---|---|---|
| **Muscle** | **Origin** | **Insertion** | **Action(s)** | **Nerve Supply** |
| Brachiora-dialis | Lateral supracondylar ridge of humerus | Styloid process of distal radius | Flexion of antebrachium | Radial n. |
| Extensor carpi radialis longus | Lateral epicondyle of humerus | Base of 2nd metacarpal | Extension of wrist Abduction of wrist Weakly aids in flexion of forearm | Radial n. |
| Extensor carpi radialis brevis | | Base of 3rd metacarpal | Extension of wrist Abduction of wrist Weakly aids in flexion of forearm | Deep radial n. |
| Extensor digitorum | | Joints extensor expansion of digits 2–5 | Extension of wrist Extension of digits 2–5 | Posterior interosseous n. from the radial n. |
| Extensor digiti minimi | | Joins extensor expansion of the extensor digitorum tendon of proximal phalanx 5th digit | Extension of 5th digit (little finger) | Posterior interosseous n. from the radial n. |
| Extensor carpi ulnaris | Lateral epicondyle of humerus Posterior ulna | Base of 5th metacarpal | Extension of wrist Adduction of wrist | Posterior interosseous n. from the radial n. |
| Supinator | Lateral epicondyle of humerus Ulna | Radial tubercle Oblique line of radius | Supination | Deep radial n. |
| Extensor indicis | Posterior ulna Interosseous membrane | Joins extensor expansion of the extensor digitorum of index finger (2nd digit) | Extension of index finger (2nd digit) | Posterior interosseous n. from the radial n. |
| Abductor pollicis longus | Lateral posterior ulna Interosseous membrane Posterior radius | Base of 1st metacarpal (lateral side) | Abducts 1st digit Adducts wrist | Posterior interosseous n. from the radial n. |
| Extensor pollicis longus | Posterior ulna Interosseous membrane | Base of distal phalanx of 1st digit | Extension of distal phalanx of 1st digit Helps extend and abduct wrist | Posterior interosseous n. from the radial n. |
| Extensor pollicis brevis | Posterior ulna Interosseous membrane Posterior radius | Base of proximal phalanx of 1st digit | Extend and abduct 1st digit | Posterior interosseous n. from the radial n. |

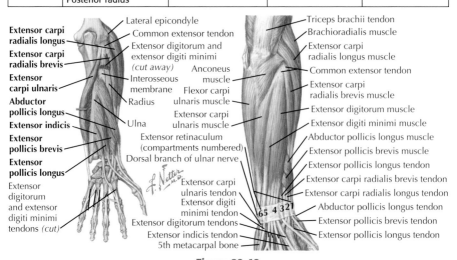

Figure 22-12

| MUSCLES OF THE HAND | | | | |
|---|---|---|---|---|
| **Muscle(s)** | **Origin** | **Insertion** | **Action(s)** | **Nerve Supply** |
| Abductor pollicis brevis | Flexor retinaculum<br>Tubercle of scaphoid<br>Tubercle of trapezium | Base of proximal phalanx of thumb (radial side) | Abduction of thumb<br>Aids in opposition of thumb<br>Aids in extension of thumb | Recurrent branch of median n. |
| Opponens pollicis | Flexor retinaculum<br>Tubercle of trapezium | 1st metacarpal (radial side) | Opposition of thumb | |
| Flexor pollicis brevis | | Base of proximal phalanx of thumb (radial side) | Flexion of thumb at metacarpo-phalangeal joint | |
| Abductor digiti minimi | Flexor retinaculum<br>Pisiform | Base of proximal phalanx of 5th digit | Abduction of 5th digit (little finger) | Deep branch of ulnar n. |
| Opponens digiti minimi | Flexor retinaculum<br>Hamulus of hamate | Shaft of 5th metacarpal | Flexion of 5th metacarpal<br>Laterally rotate 5th metacarpal | |
| Flexor digiti minimi brevis | Flexor retinaculum<br>Hamulus of hamate | Base of proximal phalanx of 5th digit | Flexion of metacarpo-phalangeal joint of 5th digit | |
| Palmaris brevis | Flexor retinaculum<br>Palmar aponeurosis | Skin of palm | Raises hypothenar eminence | Superficial branch of ulnar n. |
| Adductor pollicis<br>• Oblique head<br>• Transverse head | • Capitate, 2nd and 3rd metacarpals<br>• Shaft of 3rd metacarpal | Base of proximal phalanx of thumb | Adduction of thumb | Deep branch of ulnar n. |
| Lumbrical<br>• *1st and 2nd are unipennate*<br>• *3rd and 4th are bipennate* | *1st and 2nd*—radial side of flexor digitorum profundus tendons of middle index and fingers<br>*3rd*—side of flexor digitorum profundus tendons of middle and ring fingers<br>*4th*—side of flexor digitorum profundus tendons of ring and little fingers | Extensor expansion | Flexion of proximal phalanx<br>Extension of middle and distal phalanges | • Median n. for 1st and 2nd lumbricals<br>• Deep branch of ulnar n. for 3rd and 4th lumbricals |
| Dorsal interosseous (bipennate) | *1st*—radial side of 2nd metacarpal; ulnar side of 1st metacarpal<br>*2nd*—radial side of 3rd metacarpal; ulnar side of 2nd metacarpal<br>*3rd*—radial side of 4th metacarpal; ulnar side of 3rd metacarpal<br>*4th*—radial side of 5th metacarpal; ulnar side of 4th metacarpal | *1st*—radial side of 2nd proximal phalanx; extensor expansion<br>*2nd*—radial side of 3rd proximal phalanx; extensor expansion<br>*3rd*—ulnar side of 3rd proximal phalanx; expansion extensor<br>*4th*—ulnar side of 4th proximal phalanx; extensor expansion | Abduction of fingers from the middle finger<br>Aid in flexion of metacarpo-phalangeal joint<br>Aid in extension of interphalangeal joints | Deep branch of ulnar n. |
| Palmar interosseous (unipennate) | *1st*—ulnar side of 2nd metacarpal<br>*2nd*—radial side of 4th metacarpal<br>*3rd*—radial side of 5th metacarpal | *1st*—ulnar side of proximal phalanx of 2nd digit<br>*2nd*—radial side of proximal phalanx of 4th digit<br>*3rd*—radial side of proximal phalanx of 5th digit | Adduction of fingers toward the middle finger<br>Aid in flexion of metacarpo-phalangeal joint<br>Aid in extension of interphalangeal joints | |

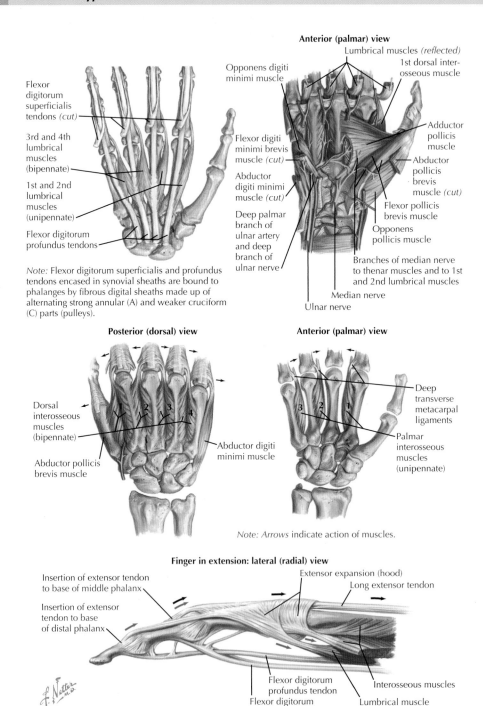

**Anterior (palmar) view**

Flexor digitorum superficialis tendons *(cut)*

3rd and 4th lumbrical muscles (bipennate)

1st and 2nd lumbrical muscles (unipennate)

Flexor digitorum profundus tendons

*Note:* Flexor digitorum superficialis and profundus tendons encased in synovial sheaths are bound to phalanges by fibrous digital sheaths made up of alternating strong annular (A) and weaker cruciform (C) parts (pulleys).

Lumbrical muscles *(reflected)*

Opponens digiti minimi muscle

1st dorsal interosseous muscle

Flexor digiti minimi brevis muscle *(cut)*

Abductor digiti minimi muscle *(cut)*

Deep palmar branch of ulnar artery and deep branch of ulnar nerve

Adductor pollicis muscle

Abductor pollicis brevis muscle *(cut)*

Flexor pollicis brevis muscle

Opponens pollicis muscle

Branches of median nerve to thenar muscles and to 1st and 2nd lumbrical muscles

Median nerve

Ulnar nerve

**Posterior (dorsal) view**

Dorsal interosseous muscles (bipennate)

Abductor pollicis brevis muscle

Abductor digiti minimi muscle

**Anterior (palmar) view**

Deep transverse metacarpal ligaments

Palmar interosseous muscles (unipennate)

*Note: Arrows* indicate action of muscles.

**Finger in extension: lateral (radial) view**

Insertion of extensor tendon to base of middle phalanx

Insertion of extensor tendon to base of distal phalanx

Extensor expansion (hood)

Long extensor tendon

Flexor digitorum profundus tendon

Flexor digitorum superficialis tendon

Interosseous muscles

Lumbrical muscle

*Note: Black arrows* indicate pull of long extensor tendon; *red arrows* indicate pull of interosseous and lumbrical muscles.

**Figure 22-13**

| OVERVIEW OF MUSCLES OF BACK | | |
|---|---|---|
| Extrinsic | Superficial | Connect upper limb to trunk |
| | Intermediate | Superficial respiratory muscles such as serratus posterior |
| Intrinsic | Superficial | Splenius muscles |
| | Intermediate | • Spinalis<br>  • Spinalis thoracis<br>  • Spinalis cervicis<br>  • Spinalis capitis<br>• Longissimus<br>  • Longissimus thoracis<br>  • Longissimus cervicis<br>  • Longissimus capitis<br>• Iliocostalis<br>  • Iliocostalis lumborum<br>  • Iliocostalis thoracis<br>  • Iliocostalis cervicis |
| | Deep<br>(transversospinal) | • Semispinalis<br>  • Semispinalis thoracis<br>  • Semispinalis cervicis<br>  • Semispinalis capitis<br>• Multifidus<br>• Rotatores (long and short) |
| Others | • Interspinales<br>• Intertransversarii | |

| MAJOR EXTRINSIC MUSCLES OF THE BACK | | | | |
|---|---|---|---|---|
| **Muscle** | **Origin** | **Insertion** | **Action(s)** | **Nerve Supply** |
| Trapezius | External occipital protuberance, ligamentum nuchae, spinous processes of C7-T12 | Lateral 1/3 of clavicle, acromion, and spine of scapula | Elevates pectoral girdle<br>Retracts pectoral girdle<br>Depresses pectoral girdle<br>Rotates scapula | Spinal accessory n. |
| Latissimus dorsi | Spinous processes of T7–12, thoracolumbar fascia, iliac crest, inferior 3–4 ribs | Floor of intertubercular groove | Extends humerus<br>Adducts humerus<br>Medial rotates humerus | Thoracodorsal n. |
| Levator scapulae | Transverse processes of C1–4 | Superior angle of scapula | Elevates scapula | Dorsal scapular n. |
| Rhomboid major | Spinous processes of T2–5 | Medial border of scapula below the spine of the scapula | Retracts scapula<br>Helps rotate scapula | |
| Rhomboid minor | Ligamentum nuchae, spinous processes of C7–T1 | Medial border at the level of the spine of the scapula | Retracts scapula<br>Helps rotate scapula | |

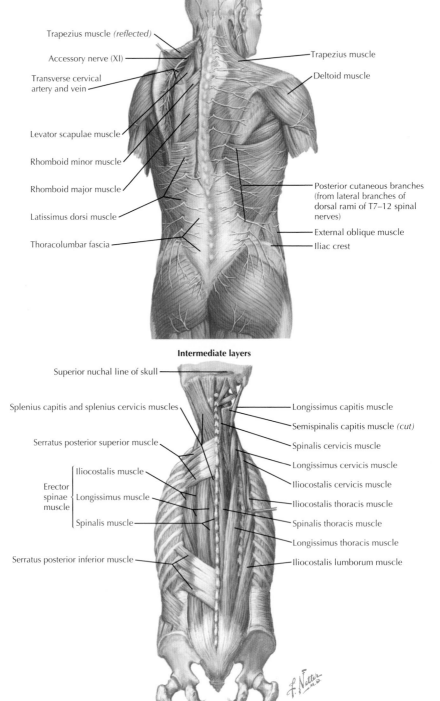

**Intermediate layers**

Trapezius muscle *(reflected)*

Accessory nerve (XI)

Transverse cervical artery and vein

Levator scapulae muscle

Rhomboid minor muscle

Rhomboid major muscle

Latissimus dorsi muscle

Thoracolumbar fascia

Trapezius muscle

Deltoid muscle

Posterior cutaneous branches (from lateral branches of dorsal rami of T7–12 spinal nerves)

External oblique muscle

Iliac crest

Superior nuchal line of skull

Splenius capitis and splenius cervicis muscles

Serratus posterior superior muscle

Erector spinae muscle
- Iliocostalis muscle
- Longissimus muscle
- Spinalis muscle

Serratus posterior inferior muscle

Longissimus capitis muscle

Semispinalis capitis muscle *(cut)*

Spinalis cervicis muscle

Longissimus cervicis muscle

Iliocostalis cervicis muscle

Iliocostalis thoracis muscle

Spinalis thoracis muscle

Longissimus thoracis muscle

Iliocostalis lumborum muscle

**Figure 22-14**

| Muscle(s) | Origin | Insertion | Action(s) | Nerve Supply |
|---|---|---|---|---|
| External intercostals | Inferior border of ribs | Upper border of ribs | Extend from tubercles to angles of ribs and aid in respiration by elevating ribs for inspiration | Intercostal n. in intercostal space |
| Internal intercostals | Inferior border of ribs | Upper border of ribs | Extend from sternum to cartilages and aid in respiration by depressing ribs for exhalation | Intercostal n. in intercostal space |
| Transversus thoracis | Posterior body of sternum and xiphoid | Inferior border of costal cartilages of ribs 2–6 | Depresses ribs | Intercostal n. in intercostal space |
| Innermost intercostal | Inferior border of ribs | Upper border of ribs | Aids in respiration by depressing ribs for exhalation | Intercostal n. in intercostal space |
| Subcostal | Near angle of rib in lower thorax | 2 or 3 ribs inferior | Helps raise ribs | Intercostal n. in intercostal space |

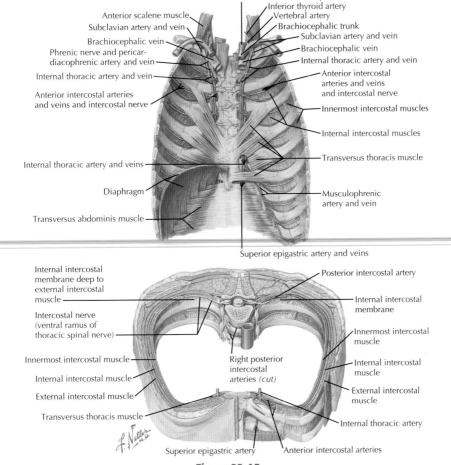

**Figure 22-15**

| Muscle | Origin | Insertion | Action(s) | Nerve Supply |
|--------|--------|-----------|-----------|--------------|
| External oblique | Ribs 5–12 | Muscular<br>• Anterior 1/2 of iliac crest<br>Aponeurotic<br>• Xiphoid process<br>• Linea alba<br>• Pubic symphysis, crest, and tubercle<br>• Anterior superior iliac spine | Compresses abdomen<br>Flexes abdomen<br>Rotates trunk to contralateral side | Ventral rami of T7–12 |
| Internal oblique | Thoracolumbar fascia, anterior 2/3 of iliac crest, lateral 2/3 of inguinal ligament | Muscular<br>• Ribs 10–12<br>Aponeurotic<br>• Above arcuate line—splits to form rectus sheath<br>• Anterior rectus sheath<br>• Posterior rectus sheath<br>• Below arcuate line<br>• Forms conjoint tendon<br>• Anterior rectus sheath | Compresses abdomen<br>Flexes abdomen<br>Rotates trunk to ipsilateral side | Ventral rami of T7–L1 |
| Transversus abdominis | Thoracolumbar fascia, anterior 2/3 of iliac crest, lateral 1/3 of inguinal ligament, lower 6 costal cartilages | Aponeurotic<br>*Above arcuate line:*<br>• Forms posterior rectus sheath<br>*Below arcuate line:*<br>• Forms conjoint tendon<br>• Anterior rectus sheath | Compresses abdomen | |
| Rectus abdominis | Pubic symphysis, crest and tubercle | Costal cartilages of ribs 5, 6, and 7 | Compresses abdomen<br>Flexes abdomen | Ventral rami of T7–T12 |
| Diaphragm | Sternal portion<br>• Xiphoid process<br>Costal portion<br>• Costal cartilages and ribs 7–12<br>Lumbar portion<br>• Lateral arcuate ligament<br>• Medial arcuate ligament<br>• Crura<br>• Right crus—L1–3<br>• Left crus—L1 and 2 | Central tendon | Contraction causes central tendon to depress, creating a negative pressure in the thoracic cavity, thus causing inhalation | Phrenic n. (C3–5) |
| Psoas major | Transverse processes of L1–5<br>Sides of bodies of T12–L5 | Lesser trochanter of femur | Flexes femur<br>Aids in flexing spine<br>Aids in lateral flexion | Ventral rami of L2 and L3 |
| Iliacus | Iliac fossa | Lesser trochanter of femur | Flexes femur | Femoral n. |
| Quadratus lumborum | Iliac crest | 12th rib<br>Transverse processes of L1–4 | Lateral flexion | Ventral rami of T12–L4 |

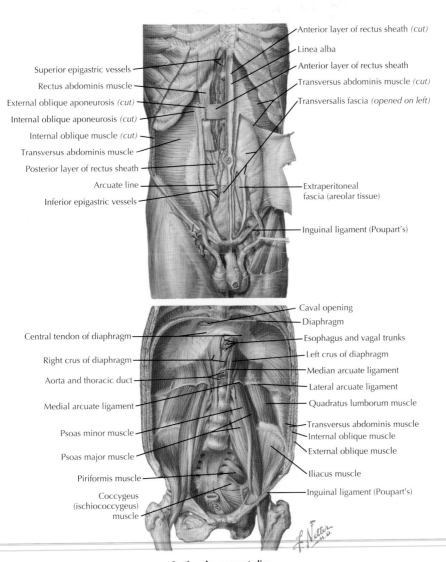

Anterior layer of rectus sheath *(cut)*

Linea alba

Anterior layer of rectus sheath

Transversus abdominis muscle *(cut)*

Transversalis fascia *(opened on left)*

Superior epigastric vessels

Rectus abdominis muscle

External oblique aponeurosis *(cut)*

Internal oblique aponeurosis *(cut)*

Internal oblique muscle *(cut)*

Transversus abdominis muscle

Posterior layer of rectus sheath

Arcuate line

Inferior epigastric vessels

Extraperitoneal fascia (areolar tissue)

Inguinal ligament (Poupart's)

Caval opening

Diaphragm

Esophagus and vagal trunks

Central tendon of diaphragm

Right crus of diaphragm

Aorta and thoracic duct

Medial arcuate ligament

Psoas minor muscle

Psoas major muscle

Piriformis muscle

Coccygeus (ischiococcygeus) muscle

Left crus of diaphragm

Median arcuate ligament

Lateral arcuate ligament

Quadratus lumborum muscle

Transversus abdominis muscle

Internal oblique muscle

External oblique muscle

Iliacus muscle

Inguinal ligament (Poupart's)

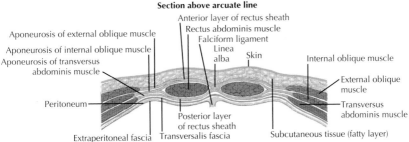

**Section above arcuate line**

Anterior layer of rectus sheath

Rectus abdominis muscle

Falciform ligament

Linea alba

Skin

Aponeurosis of external oblique muscle

Aponeurosis of internal oblique muscle

Aponeurosis of transversus abdominis muscle

Peritoneum

Extraperitoneal fascia

Transversalis fascia

Posterior layer of rectus sheath

Internal oblique muscle

External oblique muscle

Transversus abdominis muscle

Subcutaneous tissue (fatty layer)

Aponeurosis of internal oblique muscle splits to form anterior and posterior layers of rectus sheath. Aponeurosis of external oblique muscle joins anterior layer of sheath; aponeurosis of transversus abdominis muscle joins posterior layer. Anterior and posterior layers of rectus sheath unite medially to form linea alba.

**Figure 22-16**

- There are 2 pleural cavities
- The contents of each cavity consist of a 2-layered pleural sac that secretes a thin layer of serous fluid
  - Visceral layer—lines the lung and fissures
  - Parietal layer—lines the wall of the cavity
    - Costal—lines the cavity along the ribs
    - Mediastinal—lines the cavity along the mediastinum
    - Diaphragmatic—lines the cavity along the diaphragm
    - Cervical (cupula)—lines the cavity forming a dome in the ribs opposite the apex of the lung
- Pleural reflections—abrupt lines where the parietal pleura folds back or changes direction
  - Vertebral (posterior)—where costal pleura is continuous with the mediastinal pleura at the vertebral column
  - Costal (inferior)—where costal pleura is continuous with diaphragmatic pleura
  - Sternal (anterior)—here costal pleura is continuous with the mediastinal pleura posterior to sternum
- Boundaries
  - Anterior midline—6th rib (right), 4th rib (left)
  - Midclavicular line—8th rib
  - Midaxillary line—10th rib
  - Scapular line—12th rib
- Inferior border of lungs in quiet respiration
  - Anterior midline—6th rib (right), 4th rib (left)
  - Midclavicular line—6th rib
  - Midaxillary line—8th rib
  - Scapular line—10th rib
- Pleural recesses—potential spaces in the pleural cavity where parts of the parietal pleura contact one another during quiet respiration
  - Costomediastinal—potential space where costal and mediastinal pleurae come together
  - Costodiaphragmatic—potential space where costal and diaphragmatic pleurae come together
- Pulmonary ligament—a fold created where the mediastinal pleural layers at the root of the lung come together and extend inferiorly

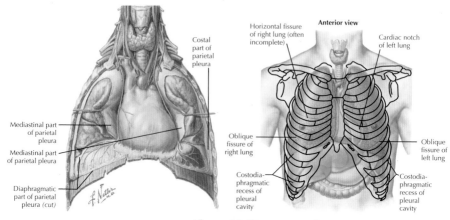

**Figure 22-17**

| Surface anatomy | • Apex—extends 1 inch into neck<br>• Base—concave area that is located on the convexity of the diaphragm<br>• Costal—large convex area that conforms to the thoracic cavity<br>• Mediastinal—area in contact with the mediastinal pleura<br>• Hilus—area where the structures that make the root of the lung enter and exit |
|---|---|
| Lobes | • Right lung<br>  • Superior<br>  • Middle<br>  • Inferior<br>• Left lung<br>  • Superior<br>  • Inferior |
| Air conduction system | • Primary bronchus—travels to lung<br>  • Right bronchus—more vertical, wider in diameter, shorter<br>  • Left bronchus—less vertical, narrower in diameter, longer<br>• Secondary bronchus—travels to lobes<br>• Tertiary bronchus—travels to bronchopulmonary segment |
| Fissures | • Oblique<br>  • Right lung—separates superior and middle lobes from inferior lobe<br>  • Left lung—separates superior and inferior lobes<br>• Horizontal—between superior and middle lobes of right lung beginning at oblique fissure and paralleling the 4th rib anteriorly |
| Borders | • Anterior<br>• Posterior<br>• Inferior |
| Structures located on the root of the lung | • Pulmonary vv.<br>• Bronchus<br>• Bronchial vv.<br>• Pulmonary plexus<br>• Lymphatics |

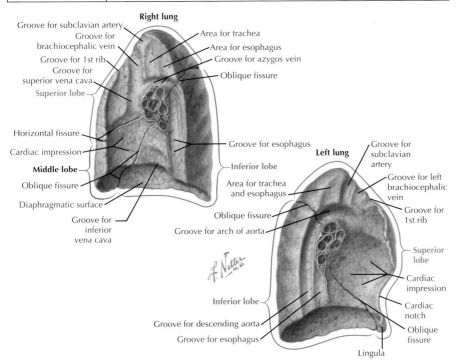

**Figure 22-18**

INTRODUCTION TO THE UPPER LIMB, BACK, THORAX, AND ABDOMEN  **617**

- Region in the middle of the thorax between the 2 pleural sacs
- Subdivided into superior and inferior

| SUPERIOR MEDIASTINUM | |
| --- | --- |
| Borders include: <br> • Superior-Superior thoracic aperture <br> • Inferior-Horizontal plane at level of sternal angle (T4) <br> • Anterior-Manubrium <br> • Posterior-Bodies of T1–T4 vertebra <br> • Lateral-Pleura | |
| Major Contents | |
| Vessels | • Superior vena cava <br> • Brachiocephalic vv. <br> • Arch of the aorta: brachiocephalic a., left common carotid a., left subclavian a. <br> • Thoracic duct |
| Nerves | • Phrenic n. <br> • Vagus n. <br> • Left recurrent laryngeal n. <br> • Plexus: <br>   • Cardiac plexus branches (parasympathetic and sympathetic branches) <br>   • Pulmonary plexus branches (parasympathetic and sympathetic branches) |
| Viscera | • Esophagus <br> • Trachea <br> • Thymus (remnants) |

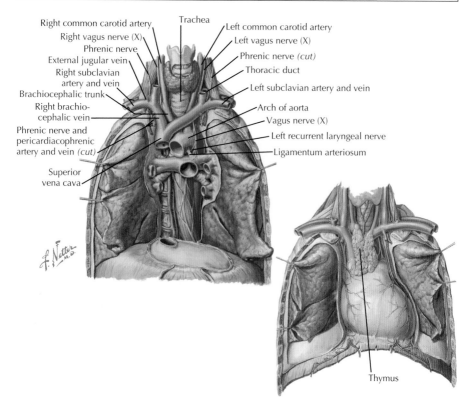

**Figure 22-19**

| INFERIOR MEDIASTINUM | |
|---|---|
| **Anterior Mediastinum** | |
| Borders | • From lower border of superior mediastinum (T4) to diaphragm (T9)<br>• Body of sternum and transversus thoracis to fibrous pericardium |
| Contents | • No major structures<br>• Remnants of the thymus<br>• Lymph nodes |
| **Middle Mediastinum** | |
| Borders | • From lower border of superior mediastinum (T4) to diaphragm (T9/T10)<br>• Anterior and posterior borders are the fibrous pericardium |
| Contents | • Heart and pericardium<br>• Vessels (roots of the great vessels):<br>  • Ascending aorta<br>  • Pulmonary trunk (with origins of pulmonary arteries)<br>  • Superior vena cava<br>  • Pericardiacophrenic vv.<br>• Phrenic |
| **Posterior Mediastinum** | |
| Borders | • Lower border of superior mediastinum (T4) to diaphragm (T12)<br>• Fibrous pericardium to vertebral column |
| Contents | • Esophagus<br>• Thoracic aorta (and branches):<br>  • Posterior intercostal aa.<br>  • Bronchial aa.<br>  • Esophageal aa.<br>• Azygos venous system<br>• Hemiazygos and accessory hemiazygos<br>• Thoracic duct<br>• Cisterna chyli<br>• Vagus<br>• Esophageal plexus<br>• Sympathetic trunk<br>  • Greater splanchnic n. (T5–9)<br>  • Lesser splanchnic n. (T10–11)<br>  • Least splanchnic n. (T12) |

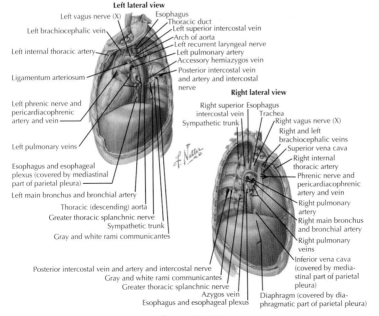

**Figure 22-20**

INTRODUCTION TO THE UPPER LIMB, BACK, THORAX, AND ABDOMEN **619**

| PERICARDIUM |
|---|
| • A double-walled fibroserous sac that encloses the heart and the roots of the great vessels |
| • Subdivided into: |
|   • Fibrous pericardium—outer layer |
|   • Serous pericardium—secretes serous fluid |
|     • Parietal pericardium—lines wall of pericardium |
|     • Visceral pericardium—lines the heart |

| SURFACES OF THE HEART | |
|---|---|
| Inferior or diaphragmatic surface | • Shape—concave<br>• Position—lower border of T8, T9<br>• Formed by:<br>  • Largely left ventricle, some right ventricle |
| Posterior surface | • Shape—quadrilateral<br>• Position—opposite 5th to 8th thoracic vertebrae<br>• Formed by:<br>  • Largely left atrium, some right atrium |
| Anterior or sternocostal surface | • Shape—flattened<br>• Position—posterior to sternum and costal cartilages 3–6<br>• Formed by:<br>  • Atrial region—largely right atrium and left auricle<br>  • Ventricular region—largely right ventricle, some left ventricle |
| Right surface | • Shape—convex<br>• Position—just lateral to the right border of the sternum<br>• Formed by:<br>  • Right atrium |
| Left surface | • Shape—convex<br>• Position—1/2 inch to left of manubriosternal junction to apex<br>• Formed by:<br>  • Largely left ventricle, some left auricle |

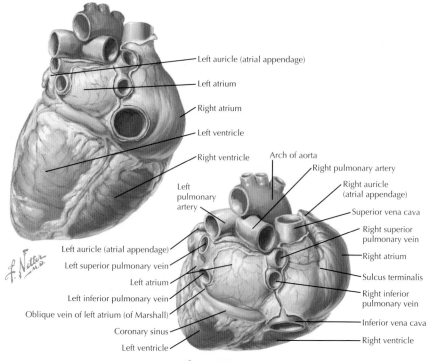

Left auricle (atrial appendage)

Left atrium

Right atrium

Left ventricle

Right ventricle

Arch of aorta

Right pulmonary artery

Left pulmonary artery

Right auricle (atrial appendage)

Superior vena cava

Right superior pulmonary vein

Right atrium

Sulcus terminalis

Right inferior pulmonary vein

Inferior vena cava

Right ventricle

Left auricle (atrial appendage)

Left superior pulmonary vein

Left atrium

Left inferior pulmonary vein

Oblique vein of left atrium (of Marshall)

Coronary sinus

Left ventricle

**Figure 22-21**

| CHAMBERS OF THE HEART | |
|---|---|
| Right atrium | • Pectinate muscle<br>• Fossa ovalis<br>• Coronary sinus opening<br>• Superior and inferior vena cava opening<br>• Valves of the coronary sinus and inferior vena cava |
| Right ventricle | • Leaflets of the tricuspid valve<br>• Trabeculae carneae<br>• Papillary muscles (anterior, posterior, and septal)<br>• Chordae tendineae<br>• Septomarginal trabeculae<br>• Conus arteriosus (infundibulum) |
| Left atrium | • Pectinate muscle in the auricle |
| Left ventricle | • Leaflets of the bicuspid (mitral) valve<br>• Trabeculae carneae<br>• Papillary muscles (anterior and posterior)<br>• Chordae tendineae<br>• Membranous part of the interventricular septum |
| VALVES OF THE HEART | |
| • Atrioventricular—close during systole to prevent the backflow of blood into the atrium<br>   • Tricuspid—between right atrium and right ventricle<br>   • Bicuspid (mitral)—between left atrium and left ventricle<br>• Semilunar—close during diastole to prevent the backflow of blood into the ventricles<br>   • Pulmonary—between pulmonary artery and right ventricle<br>   • Aortic—between aorta and left ventricle | |

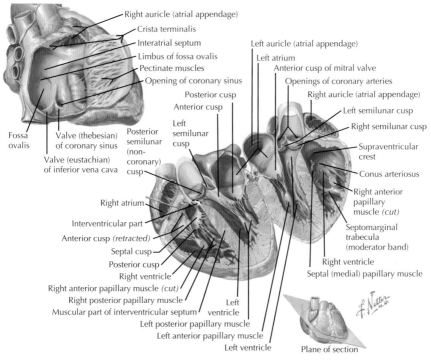

**Figure 22-22**

INTRODUCTION TO THE UPPER LIMB, BACK, THORAX, AND ABDOMEN **621**

| CORONARY CIRCULATION OF THE HEART | |
|---|---|
| Arterial supply | • Right coronary<br> • Major branches include:<br>  • Conus a.<br>  • Marginal<br>  • Sinus nodal a.<br>  • Posterior interventricular a.<br>  • Atrioventricular nodal a.<br> • Left coronary<br> • Major branches include:<br>  • Anterior interventricular a.<br>  • Diagonal a.<br>  • Circumflex a.<br>  • Marginal a. |
| Venous supply | • Cardiac veins<br> • Coronary sinus<br>  • Great cardiac v.<br>  • Middle cardiac v.<br>  • Posterior vein of the left ventricle<br>  • Oblique vein of the left atrium<br>  • Small cardiac v.<br>  • Anterior cardiac v.<br> • Venae cordis minimae |

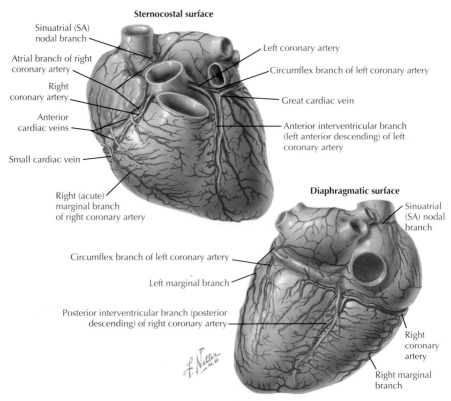

Sternocostal surface

Sinuatrial (SA) nodal branch

Atrial branch of right coronary artery

Right coronary artery

Anterior cardiac veins

Small cardiac vein

Right (acute) marginal branch of right coronary artery

Left coronary artery

Circumflex branch of left coronary artery

Great cardiac vein

Anterior interventricular branch (left anterior descending) of left coronary artery

Diaphragmatic surface

Circumflex branch of left coronary artery

Left marginal branch

Posterior interventricular branch (posterior descending) of right coronary artery

Sinuatrial (SA) nodal branch

Right coronary artery

Right marginal branch

**Figure 22-23**

- Part of the foregut
- There are 4 anatomic parts of the stomach:
  - Cardia—where esophagus enters the stomach
  - Fundus—created by the superior portion of the greater curvature
  - Body—primary central area
  - Pylorus—inferior portion that continues to narrow until reaching the pyloric sphincter
- The mucosal lining of the stomach has raised elevations known as *gastric rugae*
- There are 2 major curvatures:
  - Greater curvature—provides attachment for some remnants of the dorsal mesogastrium:
    - Gastrophrenic
    - Gastrosplenic
    - Greater omentum
  - Lesser curvature—provides attachment for remnants of the ventral mesogastrium:
    - Lesser omentum
      - Hepatogastric portion (hepatoduodenal portion does not attach to the stomach)
- There are 2 sphincters associated with the stomach:
  - Esophageal—not an anatomic sphincter
  - Pyloric—has a thick muscular sphincter
- Receives extensive autonomic nerve supply
- Is supplied by branches of the celiac artery
- Releases pepsin and hydrochloric acid to aid in digestion

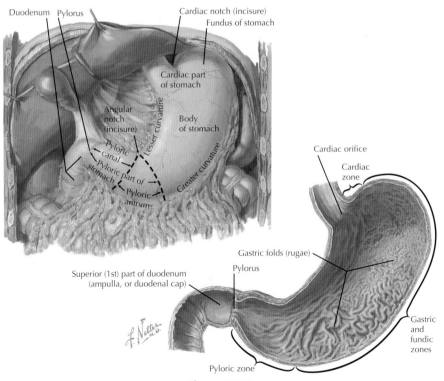

**Figure 22-24**

- Is the 1st of the 3 parts of the small intestine:
  - Duodenum
  - Jejunum
  - Ileum
- Part of the foregut and midgut
- There are 4 anatomic parts of the duodenum:
  - 1st part—intraperitoneal, part of foregut
  - 2nd part—retroperitoneal, part of foregut
    - Minor duodenal papilla—where accessory pancreatic duct (if present) drains
    - Major duodenal papilla—where pancreas, liver, and gallbladder drain
  - 3rd part—retroperitoneal, part of midgut
  - 4th part—retroperitoneal, part of midgut
- The mucosal lining of the duodenum has raised elevations known as *plicae circulares*
- Receives extensive autonomic nerve supply
- Is supplied by branches of the celiac and superior mesenteric arteries
- Is the portion of the small intestine where the majority of chemical digestion occurs
- A major histologic feature is the presence of mucus-secreting glands—Brunner's glands

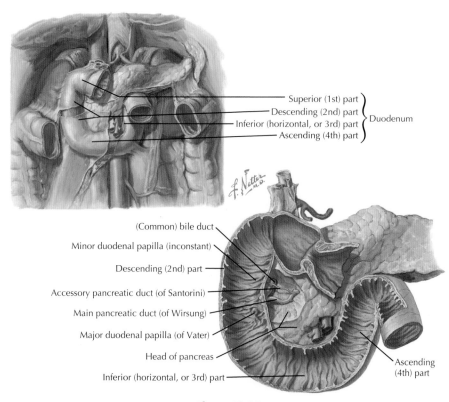

**Figure 22-25**

- Are the final 2 of the 3 parts of the small intestine:
  - Duodenum
  - Jejunum
  - Ileum
- Part of the midgut
- Intraperitoneal
- Suspended by the mesentery proper
- The mucosal lining has raised elevations known as *plicae circulares*
- Receive extensive autonomic nerve supply
- Supplied by branches of the superior mesenteric artery

### JEJUNUM

- Is about 7 to 8 feet in length
- Has scattered lymphatic nodules and very few Brunner's glands
- Has prominent plicae circulares
- Vascular supply has large prominent arterial arcades terminating with long vasa recta

### ILEUM

- Is about 6 to 12 feet in length
- Has extensive Peyer's patches (lymphatic nodules)
- Has fewer plicae circulares than the jejunum
- Vascular supply has large smaller layers of arterial arcades terminating with short, compact vasa recta
- Ends in the large intestine at the ileocecal valve
- Is the embryologic connection to the umbilicus via the vitelline duct; a Meckel's diverticulum is a remnant of the duct in the adult

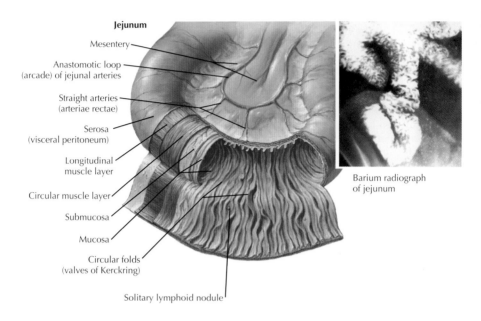

**Jejunum**

Mesentery

Anastomotic loop (arcade) of jejunal arteries

Straight arteries (arteriae rectae)

Serosa (visceral peritoneum)

Longitudinal muscle layer

Circular muscle layer

Submucosa

Mucosa

Circular folds (valves of Kerckring)

Solitary lymphoid nodule

Barium radiograph of jejunum

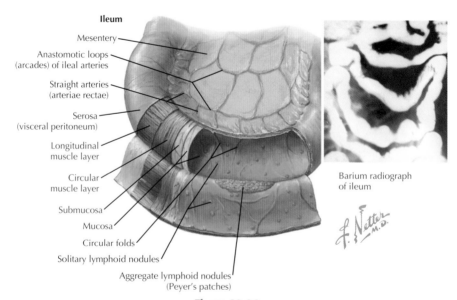

**Ileum**

Mesentery

Anastomotic loops (arcades) of ileal arteries

Straight arteries (arteriae rectae)

Serosa (visceral peritoneum)

Longitudinal muscle layer

Circular muscle layer

Submucosa

Mucosa

Circular folds

Solitary lymphoid nodules

Aggregate lymphoid nodules (Peyer's patches)

Barium radiograph of ileum

**Figure 22-26**

- Is divided into:
  - Cecum with appendix
  - Ascending colon
  - Transverse colon
  - Descending colon
  - Sigmoid colon
  - Rectum
- Has the following characteristic features:
  - Taeniae coli—3 separate bands of longitudinal muscle
  - Haustra—pouch-like appearance caused by the contraction of the taeniae coli
  - Epiploic appendages—small pouches of fat along the peritoneum
- Part of the midgut and hindgut
- Is intraperitoneal and retroperitoneal
- The mucosal lining has raised elevations known as *plicae semilunares*
- Receives extensive autonomic nerve supply
- Is supplied by branches of the superior mesenteric and inferior mesenteric arteries
- Major function is the absorption of water from the indigestible waste and expulsion from the body

## CECUM

- Is intraperitoneal
- Connects ileum to the large intestine at the ileocecal valve
- Blind pouch
- Appendix is a small (typically around 4 inches) blind tubular intraperitoneal structure connected to the cecum

## ASCENDING COLON

- Is retroperitoneal
- Begins at ileocecal valve and ascends
- Makes a colic impression on the liver and makes a sharp turn to the left side of the body, known as the right colic (hepatic) flexure, before continuing as the transverse colon

## TRANSVERSE COLON

- Is intraperitoneal, suspended by the transverse mesocolon
- Longest portion of the large intestine
- At the area of the spleen, makes a sharp turn to travel inferiorly, known as the left colic (splenic) flexure, before continuing as the descending colon

## DESCENDING COLON

- Is retroperitoneal
- Descends until it ends at the sigmoid colon
- Terminal portion of the descending colon is often called the iliac colon because it lies in the iliac fossa
- Typically is smaller in diameter than the ascending colon

## SIGMOID COLON

- Is intraperitoneal, suspended by the sigmoid mesocolon
- Begins at the level of the pelvic brim
- Travels toward the midline, where it ends at the rectum

## RECTUM

- Begins as intraperitoneal, but is retroperitoneal until it passes through the pelvic floor
- Is about 4 to 5 inches in length
- Does not have taeniae coli, because the separate bands merge to form a complete band of longitudinal muscle at the rectum
- Ends at the anus

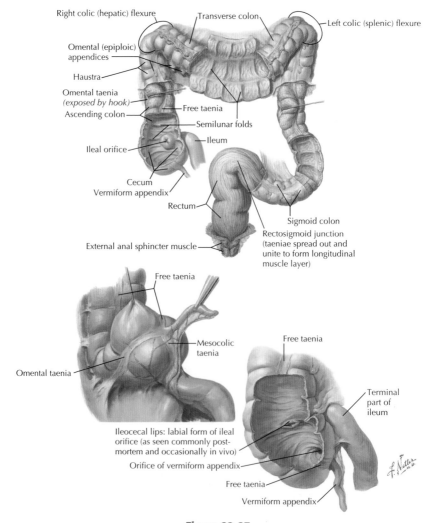

**Figure 22-27**

- Large, multifunctional organ, with roles including:
  - Detoxification
  - Glycogen storage
  - Production of hormones
  - Synthesis of plasma proteins
  - Production of bile
- Divided into 4 anatomic lobes:
  - Right—largest lobe
  - Caudate—located between fissure for the ligamentum venosum and the inferior vena cava
  - Quadrate—located between fissure for the ligamentum teres hepatis (round ligament of the liver) and the gallbladder
  - Left—flattened lobe
- Is further subdivided into functional segments based on the vascular supply
- Is completely covered by visceral peritoneum except an area where the liver connects with the diaphragm, known as the *bare area*
- The porta hepatis is the central portion of the liver, where the following structures enter and exit:
  - Hepatic portal vein—provides 75% of the blood to the liver
  - Proper hepatic artery—provides 25% of the blood to the liver
  - Common bile duct
- Is intraperitoneal
- Is supplied by branches of the celiac artery
- All remnants of the ventral mesentery attach to the liver:
  - Falciform ligament
  - Coronary ligament
  - Triangular ligament
  - Lesser omentum
    - Hepatogastric ligament
    - Hepatoduodenal ligament
- The liver is subject to development of numerous pathologic conditions, including:
  - Hepatitis
  - Cirrhosis
  - Cancer

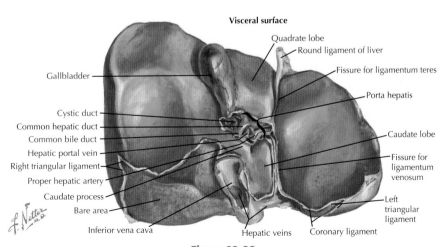

**Visceral surface**

Quadrate lobe
Round ligament of liver
Fissure for ligamentum teres
Gallbladder
Porta hepatis
Cystic duct
Common hepatic duct
Common bile duct
Caudate lobe
Hepatic portal vein
Right triangular ligament
Fissure for ligamentum venosum
Proper hepatic artery
Caudate process
Left triangular ligament
Bare area
Inferior vena cava
Hepatic veins
Coronary ligament

**Figure 22-28**

- The pancreas functions as 2 types of glands:
  - Endocrine—islets of Langerhans producing hormones
  - Exocrine—compound tubuloalveolar pancreatic acini producing digestive enzymes
- Comprises 4 major parts:
  - Head—located in the C or curve formed by the duodenum; is retroperitoneal
    - Uncinate process—an extension of the head crossed by the superior mesenteric veins
  - Neck—constricted portion of pancreas connecting the head to the body; is retroperitoneal
  - Body—largest part of the pancreas separated from the stomach by the omental bursa; is retroperitoneal
  - Tail—extends into the lienorenal ligament with the splenic veins to the spleen
- Is part of the foregut
- Develops as 2 separate outgrowths from the 2nd part of the duodenum:
  - Ventral pancreatic bud—an outgrowth of the hepatic bud
    - Develops into the head and neck of the pancreas
  - Dorsal pancreatic bud—a direct outgrowth of the 2nd part of the duodenum
    - Develops into the body and tail of the pancreas
- Drains into the 2nd part of the duodenum
  - Main pancreatic duct—drains into the major duodenal papilla by joining the common bile duct, forming the hepatopancreatic ampulla
  - Accessory pancreatic duct—drains into the minor duodenal papilla (if present and patent)
- Is supplied by branches of the celiac and superior mesenteric arteries
- Receives extensive autonomic nerve supply

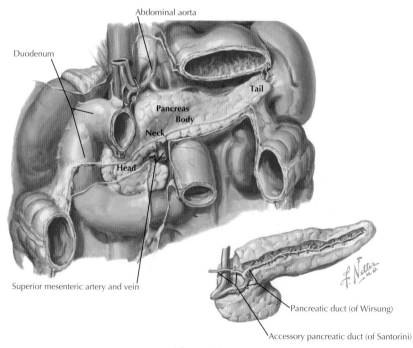

**Figure 22-29**

## GALLBLADDER

- Small intraperitoneal organ
- Is part of the foregut
- Stores and concentrates bile, which emulsifies fat during digestion
- Is located in a fossa on the liver where the linea semilunaris attaches to the rib cage at the 9th costal cartilage
- Divided into 3 parts:
  - Fundus
  - Body
  - Neck
- Is supplied by branches of the celiac artery
- Receives extensive autonomic nerve supply

## DUCT SYSTEM

- The cystic duct joins the common hepatic duct to form the common bile duct
- The common bile duct joins the main pancreatic duct within the substance of the pancreas to form the hepatopancreatic ampulla, which passes through the wall of the 2nd part of the duodenum into the major duodenal papilla

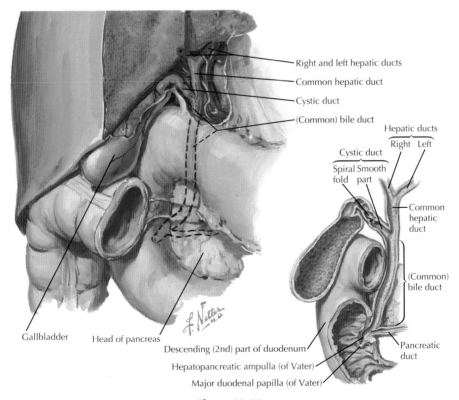

**Figure 22-30**

- A lymphatic organ on the left side of the body divided into:
  - Red pulp
  - White pulp
- Is intraperitoneal
- Major functions include:
  - Storage of red blood cells
  - Filtration of red blood cells
  - Removal of old red blood cells
  - Storage of monocytes
- Is not a derivative of the foregut, although it receives its arterial supply from branches of the celiac artery
- Is located between the 9th and 11th ribs, paralleling the 10th rib
- Has contact with 4 organs:
  - Stomach
  - Large intestine
  - Left kidney
  - Tail of pancreas
- Is suspended by dorsal mesentery of the foregut:
  - Lienorenal—contains tail of the pancreas and splenic veins
  - Gastrosplenic—contains short gastric and left gastroepiploic veins

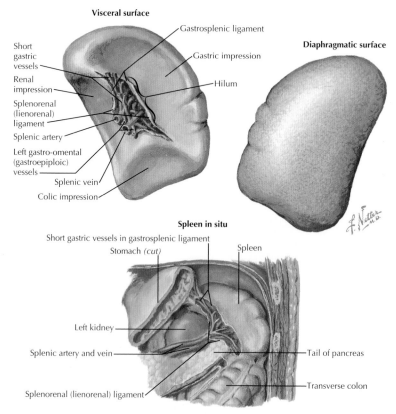

Figure 22-31

## KIDNEY

- Paired organs
- Is retroperitoneal
- Has multiple functions, with roles including:
  - Filtration of blood
  - Regulation of electrolytes
  - Regulation of blood pressure
  - Production of hormones
- Nephron is the functional unit
- Located between T12 and L3, with hilum at L1
- Left kidney is slightly larger than the right kidney
- Right kidney is slightly inferior to the left kidney owing to presence of the liver
- Surrounded by a tough capsule
- Divided into:
  - Cortex
  - Medulla
- Receives arterial supply from renal veins
- Receives extensive autonomic nerve supply

## URETER

- Is retroperitoneal
- Carries urine from kidney to the bladder
- Begins at hilum, or L1, and travels inferior to the bladder
- Common sites of kidney stones include:
  - Uteropelvic junction
  - Crossing iliac veins on pelvis
  - Junction with bladder

## SUPRARENAL GLAND

- Also known as *adrenal gland*
- Paired glands of endocrine type
- Divided into:
  - Cortex—responsible for production of mineralocorticoids, glucocorticoids, and androgens
  - Medulla—responsible for catecholamines via sympathetic response ("flight or flight")
- Receives threefold arterial supply:
  - Superior suprarenal—from inferior phrenic artery
  - Middle suprarenal—from aorta
  - Inferior suprarenal—from renal artery

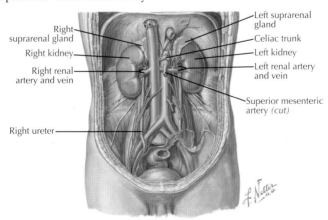

Right suprarenal gland
Right kidney
Right renal artery and vein
Right ureter
Left suprarenal gland
Celiac trunk
Left kidney
Left renal artery and vein
Superior mesenteric artery (cut)

**Figure 22-32**

- Bladder
- Prostate
- Seminal vesicle
- Ductus deferens
- Rectum

**Paramedian (sagittal) dissection**

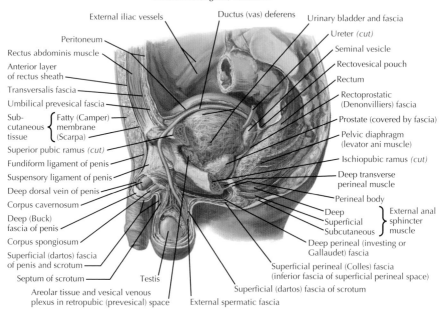

External iliac vessels
Ductus (vas) deferens
Urinary bladder and fascia
Peritoneum
Ureter *(cut)*
Rectus abdominis muscle
Seminal vesicle
Anterior layer of rectus sheath
Rectovesical pouch
Transversalis fascia
Rectum
Umbilical prevesical fascia
Rectoprostatic (Denonvilliers) fascia
Subcutaneous tissue { Fatty (Camper) membrane / (Scarpa) }
Prostate (covered by fascia)
Superior pubic ramus *(cut)*
Pelvic diaphragm (levator ani muscle)
Fundiform ligament of penis
Ischiopubic ramus *(cut)*
Suspensory ligament of penis
Deep transverse perineal muscle
Deep dorsal vein of penis
Perineal body
Corpus cavernosum
Deep / Superficial / Subcutaneous } External anal sphincter muscle
Deep (Buck) fascia of penis
Corpus spongiosum
Deep perineal (investing or Gallaudet) fascia
Superficial (dartos) fascia of penis and scrotum
Septum of scrotum
Testis
Superficial perineal (Colles) fascia (inferior fascia of superficial perineal space)
Areolar tissue and vesical venous plexus in retropubic (prevesical) space
External spermatic fascia
Superficial (dartos) fascia of scrotum

**Median (sagittal) section**

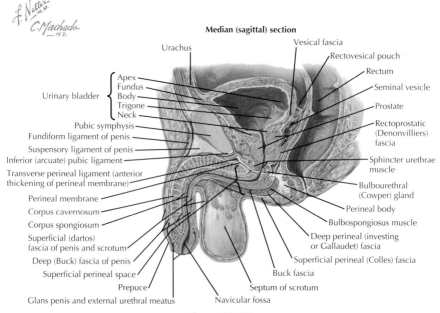

Urachus
Vesical fascia
Rectovesical pouch
Rectum
Apex
Seminal vesicle
Fundus
Urinary bladder { Body
Prostate
Trigone
Neck
Rectoprostatic (Denonvilliers) fascia
Pubic symphysis
Fundiform ligament of penis
Suspensory ligament of penis
Sphincter urethrae muscle
Inferior (arcuate) pubic ligament
Transverse perineal ligament (anterior thickening of perineal membrane)
Bulbourethral (Cowper) gland
Perineal membrane
Perineal body
Corpus cavernosum
Bulbospongiosus muscle
Corpus spongiosum
Deep perineal (investing or Gallaudet) fascia
Superficial (dartos) fascia of penis and scrotum
Superficial perineal (Colles) fascia
Deep (Buck) fascia of penis
Buck fascia
Superficial perineal space
Prepuce
Septum of scrotum
Glans penis and external urethral meatus
Navicular fossa

**Figure 22-33**

- Bladder
- Uterus (and uterine tube) and vagina
- Ovary
- Rectum

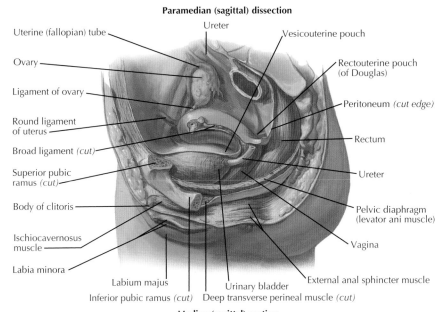

**Paramedian (sagittal) dissection**

Uterine (fallopian) tube
Ovary
Ligament of ovary
Round ligament of uterus
Broad ligament *(cut)*
Superior pubic ramus *(cut)*
Body of clitoris
Ischiocavernosus muscle
Labia minora
Labium majus
Inferior pubic ramus *(cut)*

Ureter
Vesicouterine pouch
Rectouterine pouch (of Douglas)
Peritoneum *(cut edge)*
Rectum
Ureter
Pelvic diaphragm (levator ani muscle)
Vagina
External anal sphincter muscle
Urinary bladder
Deep transverse perineal muscle *(cut)*

**Median (sagittal) section**

Suspensory ligament of ovary
Uterine (fallopian) tube
Ovary
External iliac vessels
Ligament of ovary
Body of uterus
Round ligament of uterus (ligamentum teres)
Fundus of uterus
Urinary bladder
Pubic symphysis
Urethra
Sphincter urethrae
Crus of clitoris
Deep dorsal vein of clitoris
Labium majus
External urethral orifice
Labium minus
Vaginal orifice
Superficial transverse perineal muscle

Sacral promontory
Ureter
Vesicouterine pouch
Uterosacral ligament
Rectouterine pouch (of Douglas)
Cervix of uterus
Posterior part of vaginal fornix
Anterior part of vaginal fornix
Rectum
Vagina
Levator ani muscle
Anal canal
External anal sphincter muscle
Anus
Perineal membrane
Deep transverse perineal muscle

**Figure 22-34**

ARTERIAL SUPPLY OF THE AXILLA

- Axillary artery—divided into 3 parts based on its relationship to the pectoralis minor:
- 1st part
  - Superior thoracic—supplies 1st 2 intercostal spaces
- 2nd part
  - Thoracoacromial
    - *Pectoral*
    - *Acromial*
    - *Deltoid*—accompanies cephalic vein
    - *Clavicular*
  - Lateral thoracic—follows inferior border of pectoralis minor to thorax
- 3rd part
  - Subscapular
    - *Scapular circumflex*—located in triangular space
    - *Thoracodorsal*—passes with thoracodorsal nerve to latissimus dorsi
  - Posterior humeral circumflex—travels in quadrangular space with axillary nerve
  - Anterior humeral circumflex

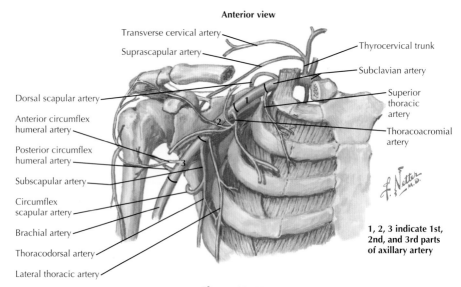

**Anterior view**

Transverse cervical artery

Suprascapular artery

Thyrocervical trunk

Subclavian artery

Dorsal scapular artery

Superior thoracic artery

Anterior circumflex humeral artery

Thoracoacromial artery

Posterior circumflex humeral artery

Subscapular artery

Circumflex scapular artery

Brachial artery

Thoracodorsal artery

Lateral thoracic artery

**1, 2, 3 indicate 1st, 2nd, and 3rd parts of axillary artery**

**Figure 22-35**

## ARTERIAL SUPPLY OF THE BRACHIUM

- Brachial artery—begins at inferior border of teres major
  - Profunda brachii
    - *Middle collateral*
    - *Radial collateral*
  - Supraduodenal ulnar collateral—passes with ulnar nerve posterior to medial epicondyle
  - Inferior ulnar collateral
  - Muscular branches

## ARTERIAL SUPPLY OF THE ANTEBRACHIUM

- Brachial artery—divides into:
  - Radial
    - *Radial recurrent*
    - *Palmar carpal branch*
    - *Superficial palmar branch*
  - Ulnar
    - *Anterior ulnar recurrent*
    - *Posterior ulnar recurrent*
    - *Common interosseous*
    - *Palmar carpal branch*

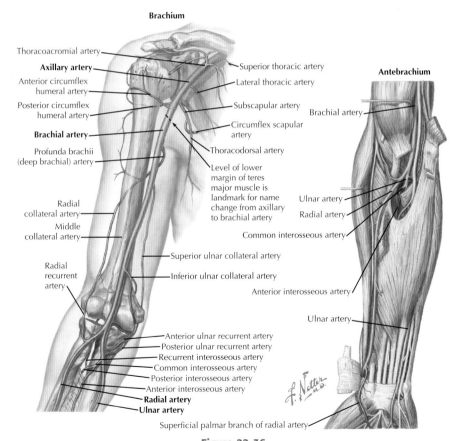

**Brachium**

Thoracoacromial artery

**Axillary artery**

Anterior circumflex humeral artery

Posterior circumflex humeral artery

**Brachial artery**

Profunda brachii (deep brachial) artery

Radial collateral artery

Middle collateral artery

Radial recurrent artery

Superior thoracic artery

Lateral thoracic artery

Subscapular artery

Circumflex scapular artery

Thoracodorsal artery

Level of lower margin of teres major muscle is landmark for name change from axillary to brachial artery

Superior ulnar collateral artery

Inferior ulnar collateral artery

Anterior ulnar recurrent artery
Posterior ulnar recurrent artery
Recurrent interosseous artery
Common interosseous artery
Posterior interosseous artery
Anterior interosseous artery
**Radial artery**
**Ulnar artery**

**Antebrachium**

Brachial artery

Ulnar artery

Radial artery

Common interosseous artery

Anterior interosseous artery

Ulnar artery

Superficial palmar branch of radial artery

**Figure 22-36**

## CARPUS, METACARPUS, AND PHALANGES

*Ulnar*
- Dorsal carpal branch
- Deep branch of the ulnar
- Palmar carpal branch
- Superficial palmar arch
  - Common palmar digital
  - Proper palmar digital

*Radial*
- Princeps pollicis
- Radialis indicis
- Deep palmar arch

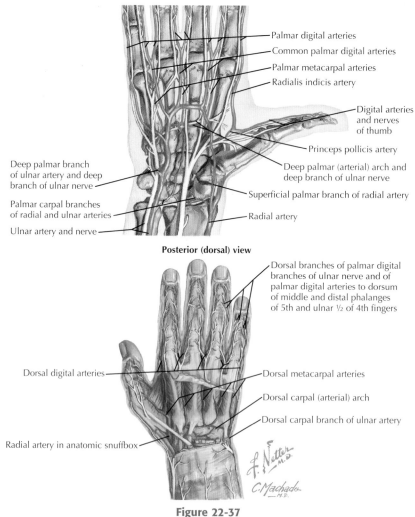

Palmar digital arteries

Common palmar digital arteries

Palmar metacarpal arteries

Radialis indicis artery

Digital arteries and nerves of thumb

Princeps pollicis artery

Deep palmar branch of ulnar artery and deep branch of ulnar nerve

Deep palmar (arterial) arch and deep branch of ulnar nerve

Palmar carpal branches of radial and ulnar arteries

Superficial palmar branch of radial artery

Ulnar artery and nerve

Radial artery

**Posterior (dorsal) view**

Dorsal branches of palmar digital branches of ulnar nerve and of palmar digital arteries to dorsum of middle and distal phalanges of 5th and ulnar ½ of 4th fingers

Dorsal digital arteries

Dorsal metacarpal arteries

Dorsal carpal (arterial) arch

Dorsal carpal branch of ulnar artery

Radial artery in anatomic snuffbox

**Figure 22-37**

VEINS

2 types of veins:
- Superficial—lie in superficial fascia
  - Cephalic
  - Basilic
- Deep (have either):
  - Single similar-sized vein following the artery of the upper limb (e.g., subclavian vein or axillary vein)
  - Vena comitans—accompanying vein
    - A pairing of veins with both surrounding the artery
    - Typically, any veins that are distal to the axillary vein is a vena comitans (e.g., brachial veins, ulnar veins, and radial veins), which are paired around the artery of the same name

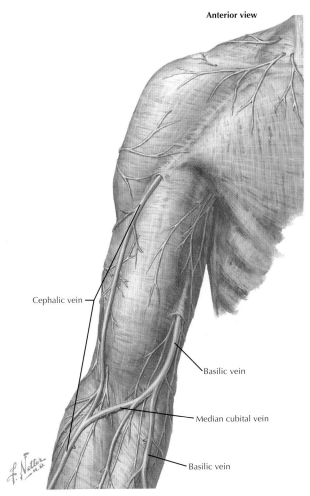

**Anterior view**

Cephalic vein

Basilic vein

Median cubital vein

Basilic vein

**Figure 22-38**

ARTERIAL SUPPLY OF THE THORAX

*Thoracic Wall*
- Internal thoracic—arises from subclavian artery
  - Pericardiacophrenic (does not supply wall)
  - Terminates as:
    - Musculophrenic
    - Superior epigastric
- Intercostal arteries
  - Posterior intercostal
    - 2 (Costocervical trunk)
    - 9 (Thoracic aorta)
    - 1 Subcostal (thoracic aorta)
  - Anterior intercostal
    - 6 (Internal thoracic)
    - 3 (Musculophrenic)

*Visceral Contents*
- Esophagus (in Thorax)
  - Esophageal (thoracic aorta)
- Lungs
  - Bronchial
  - Right (3rd posterior intercostal artery)
  - 2 left (thoracic aorta)
- Diaphragm
  - Superior phrenic (thoracic aorta)
  - Pericardiacophrenic (internal thoracic)
  - Musculophrenic (internal thoracic)
  - Inferior phrenic (abdominal aorta)

VEINS

- Azygos system
  - Posterior intercostal veins
  - Esophageal veins
  - Bronchial veins
  - Right side of thorax
    - *Right supreme intercostal vein*
    - *Right superior intercostal vein*
  - Left side of thorax
    - *Left supreme intercostal vein*
    - *Left superior intercostal vein*
    - *Accessory hemiazygos vein*
    - *Hemiazygos vein*

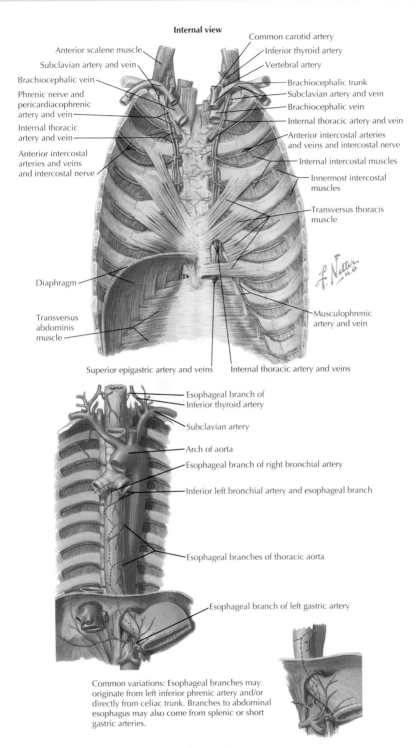

**Internal view**

Anterior scalene muscle

Subclavian artery and vein

Brachiocephalic vein

Phrenic nerve and pericardiacophrenic artery and vein

Internal thoracic artery and vein

Anterior intercostal arteries and veins and intercostal nerve

Common carotid artery

Inferior thyroid artery

Vertebral artery

Brachiocephalic trunk

Subclavian artery and vein

Brachiocephalic vein

Internal thoracic artery and vein

Anterior intercostal arteries and veins and intercostal nerve

Internal intercostal muscles

Innermost intercostal muscles

Transversus thoracis muscle

Diaphragm

Transversus abdominis muscle

Musculophrenic artery and vein

Superior epigastric artery and veins

Internal thoracic artery and veins

Esophageal branch of Inferior thyroid artery

Subclavian artery

Arch of aorta

Esophageal branch of right bronchial artery

Inferior left bronchial artery and esophageal branch

Esophageal branches of thoracic aorta

Esophageal branch of left gastric artery

Common variations: Esophageal branches may originate from left inferior phrenic artery and/or directly from celiac trunk. Branches to abdominal esophagus may also come from splenic or short gastric arteries.

**Figure 22-39**

INTRODUCTION TO THE UPPER LIMB, BACK, THORAX, AND ABDOMEN **641**

UNPAIRED VISCERAL ARTERIES

| CELIAC ARTERY (ARTERY OF THE FOREGUT)–ARISES AT T12 |
|---|
| • Left gastric<br>• Common hepatic<br> • Proper hepatic<br>  • Right gastric<br>  • Left hepatic<br>  • Right hepatic<br>   • Cystic<br>• Gastroduodenal<br> • Supraduodenal<br> • Right gastroepiploic<br> • Anterior and posterior superior pancreaticoduodenal<br>• Splenic<br> • Pancreatic branches<br> • Short gastric<br> • Left gastroepiploic |

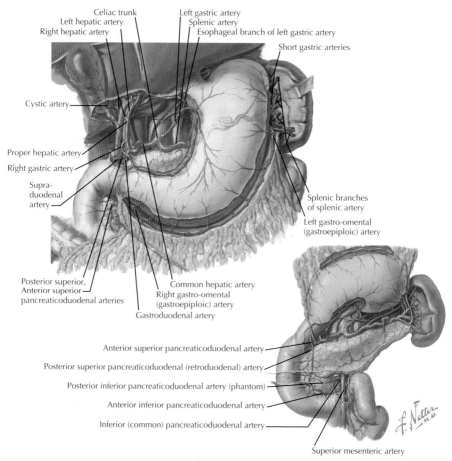

**Figure 22-40**

| SUPERIOR MESENTERIC ARTERY (ARTERY OF THE MIDGUT)–ARISES AT L1 |
| --- |

- Anterior and posterior inferior pancreaticoduodenal
- Jejunal mesenteric
  - Arterial arcades and vasa recta
- Ileal mesenteric
  - Arterial arcades and vasa recta
- Ileocolic
  - Appendicular
- Right colic
- Middle colic

| INFERIOR MESENTERIC ARTERY (ARTERY OF THE HINDGUT)–ARISES AT L3 |
| --- |

- Left colic
- Sigmoid
- Superior rectal

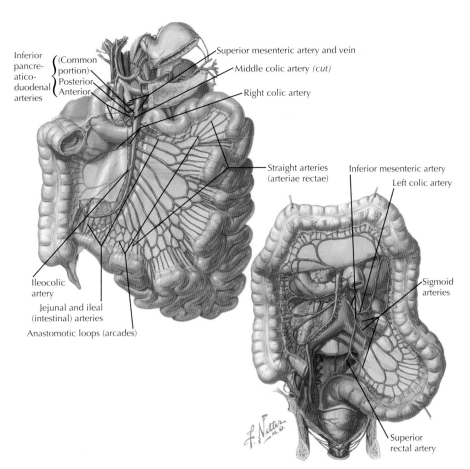

**Figure 22-41**

PAIRED VISCERAL AND PARIETAL ARTERIES

- Paired visceral branches—paired branches supplying organs
  - Renal—arises at L2
  - Gonadal—arises between L2 and L3
    - Testicular
    - Ovarian
  - Suprarenal
    - Superior—arises from the inferior phrenic
    - Middle—arises from the aorta
    - Inferior—arises from the renal
- Paired parietal (body wall) branches—paired branches supplying the wall
  - Inferior phrenic
  - Lumbar—4 arise from the aorta

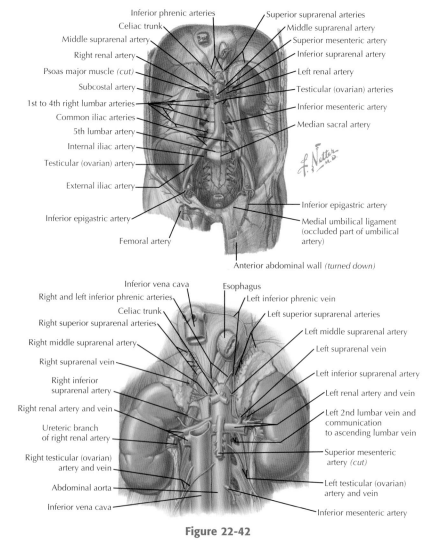

**Figure 22-42**

VENOUS SUPPLY OF THE VISCERA

- Veins that drain the abdominal viscera closely follow the celiac, superior mesenteric, and inferior mesenteric arteries
- These veins eventually drain into the hepatic portal vein, which passes into the liver, allowing it to clear the blood of any wastes and to store nutrients
- The hepatic portal vein is formed by the:
  - Superior mesenteric vein
  - Splenic vein
- After passing through the liver, the blood returns into the systemic system via hepatic veins into the inferior vena cava
- Because the veins in this region lack valves, they take the path of least resistance
- If there is an obstruction in the path of the hepatic portal vein, the blood will attempt to return toward the heart by bypassing the block and using the anastomosis between the portal system and the systemic system (vena cava)
- There are 4 major collaterals between the portal and systemic systems:
  - Esophageal
  - Paraumbilical
  - Rectal
  - Retroperitoneal

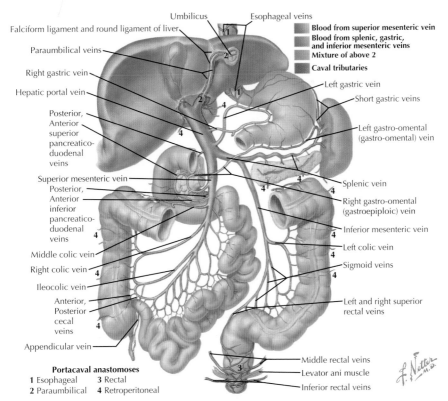

Falciform ligament and round ligament of liver

Paraumbilical veins

Right gastric vein

Hepatic portal vein

Posterior, Anterior superior pancreatico-duodenal veins

Superior mesenteric vein

Posterior, Anterior inferior pancreatico-duodenal veins

Middle colic vein

Right colic vein

Ileocolic vein

Anterior, Posterior cecal veins

Appendicular vein

Umbilicus

Esophageal veins

Blood from superior mesenteric vein
Blood from splenic, gastric, and inferior mesenteric veins
Mixture of above 2
Caval tributaries

Left gastric vein

Short gastric veins

Left gastro-omental (gastro-omental) vein

Splenic vein

Right gastro-omental (gastroepiploic) vein

Inferior mesenteric vein

Left colic vein

Sigmoid veins

Left and right superior rectal veins

Middle rectal veins

Levator ani muscle

Inferior rectal veins

**Portacaval anastomoses**
1 Esophageal    3 Rectal
2 Paraumbilical    4 Retroperitoneal

**Figure 22-43**

HEPATIC PORTAL VEIN

- Minor direct tributaries include:
  - Cystic vein
  - Right gastric vein
  - Left gastric vein
    - Esophageal veins
  - Posterior superior pancreaticoduodenal vein
- Major tributaries include:
  - Superior mesenteric vein
    - Right gastroepiploic vein
      - Anterior superior pancreaticoduodenal vein
      - Anterior inferior pancreaticoduodenal vein
    - Posterior inferior pancreaticoduodenal vein
    - Middle colic vein
    - Jejunal mesenteric veins
      - Venous anastomotic loops
      - Vasa recta
    - Ileal mesenteric veins
      - Venous anastomotic loops
      - Vasa recta
    - Ileocolic vein
    - Right colic vein
  - Splenic vein
    - Pancreatic branches
    - Short gastric vein
    - Left gastroepiploic vein
    - Inferior mesenteric—sometimes joins to form hepatic portal vein
      - Left colic vein
      - Sigmoid veins
      - Superior rectal vein

VENOUS SUPPLY OF THE POSTERIOR ABDOMINAL WALL

- Veins of the posterior abdominal wall drain into the inferior vena cava
- Tributaries include:
  - Hepatic veins
    - Right hepatic vein
    - Middle hepatic vein
    - Left hepatic vein
  - Inferior phrenic vein
  - Suprarenal vein
  - Renal vein
    - Left gonadal vein
      - Testicular
      - Ovarian
    - Right gonadal vein
      - Testicular
      - Ovarian
  - Subcostal vein
  - Lumbar veins

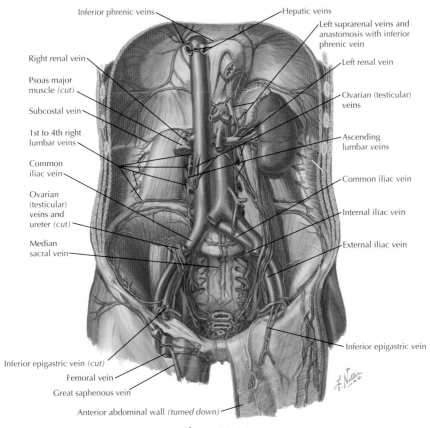

**Figure 22-44**

ARTERIAL SUPPLY OF THE PELVIS

- External iliac
  - Inferior epigastric
  - Deep circumflex iliac
- Internal iliac
  - Posterior division
    - Iliolumbar
    - Lateral sacral
    - Superior gluteal
  - Anterior division
    - Umbilical
      - Superior vesical
    - Obturator
    - Uterine (in female)
    - Vaginal (in female)
    - Inferior vesical
    - Middle rectal
    - Internal pudendal
    - Inferior gluteal

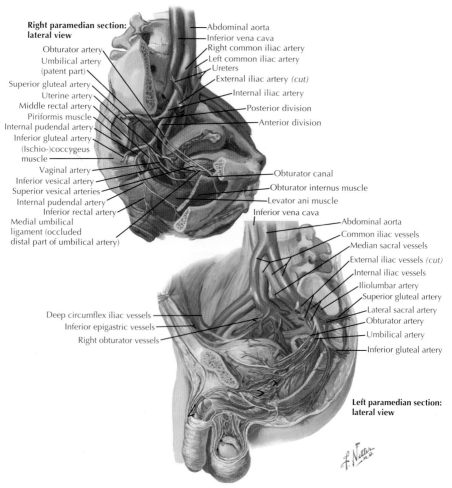

**Figure 22-45**

- Alternating joining and branching of nerves to reorganize the terminal branches, with contributions from multiple spinal cord levels
- Origin from ventral rami of 5th to 8th cervical and 1st thoracic spinal nerves
- General organization is:
  - 5 ventral rami
  - 3 trunks
  - 6 divisions
  - 3 cords
  - 6 branches
- Nerves to muscles on ventral and dorsal surfaces of upper limb are derived from anterior and posterior divisions, respectively
- Location and arterial relations:
  - Rami and trunks—posterior triangle of neck; subclavian artery
  - Divisions—behind clavicle; subclavian artery and 1st part of axillary artery
  - Cords—axilla; 2nd part of axillary artery
  - Branches—axilla; 3rd part of axillary artery
- Key landmark of M formed by medial and lateral cords and terminal branches

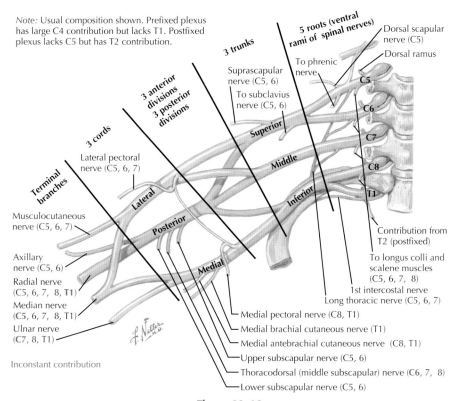

*Note:* Usual composition shown. Prefixed plexus has large C4 contribution but lacks T1. Postfixed plexus lacks C5 but has T2 contribution.

**Figure 22-46**

| BRACHIAL PLEXUS | | |
|---|---|---|
| **Nerve** | **Source** | **Comments** |
| Dorsal scapular (C5) | Ventral rami | Passes posteriorly to lie along the medial border of the scapula<br>Innervates the:<br>• Levator scapulae<br>• Rhomboid major<br>• Rhomboid minor |
| Long thoracic (C5, C6, C7) | Ventral rami | Passes inferiorly along the serratus anterior<br>Innervates the serratus anterior |
| Muscular branches | Ventral rami | Supplies the scalenes and longus colli |
| Subclavius (C5, C6) | Upper trunk | Innervates the subclavius |
| Suprascapular (C5, C6) | Upper trunk | Innervates the:<br>• Supraspinatus<br>• Infraspinatus |
| Lateral pectoral (C5, C6, C7) | Lateral cord | Innervates the clavicular head of the pectoralis major |
| Musculocutaneous (C5, C6, C7) | Lateral cord | Passes into the coracobrachialis to enter the flexor compartment of the brachium<br>After passing through the coracobrachialis, it travels distally in the brachium between the biceps brachii and the brachialis<br>Innervates the:<br>• Coracobrachialis<br>• Biceps brachii<br>• Brachialis<br>Terminates as the lateral cutaneous nerve of the antebrachium upon exiting the distal compartment |
| Median (C5, C6, C7) from lateral head (C8, T1) from medial head | Lateral and medial cord | **Brachium:**<br>Has no motor or sensory branches in the arm<br>**Antebrachium:**<br>No sensory branches in antebrachium<br>Innervates:<br>• Pronator teres<br>• Flexor carpi radialis longus<br>• Palmaris longus<br>• Flexor digitorum superficialis<br>Has 1 major motor branch innervating the deep flexor muscles:<br>• Flexor pollicis longus<br>• Flexor digitorum profundus<br>• Pronator quadratus<br>**Carpus, Metacarpus, and Phalanges:**<br>*Sensory branches*:<br>• Palmar cutaneous branch—lateral portion of palm<br>• Common palmar digital branches—lateral portion of palm<br>• Proper palmar digital branches—palmar surface of 1st, 2nd, and 3rd digits and lateral 1/2 of 4th digit<br>*Motor branches*:<br>Recurrent branch of median n.<br>• Opponens pollicis<br>• Abductor pollicis brevis<br>• Flexor pollicis brevis<br>Motor branches to 1st and 2nd lumbricals |
| Medial brachial cutaneous (T1) | Medial cord | Provides sensory innervation to the medial aspect of the superior portion of the brachium |

*Continued on next page*

| BRACHIAL PLEXUS—cont'd | | |
|---|---|---|
| **Nerve** | **Source** | **Comments** |
| Medial antebrachial cutaneous (C8, T1) | Medial cord | Provides sensory innervation to the medial aspect of the inferior portion of the brachium |
| Medial pectoral (C8, T1) | Medial cord | Innervates:<br>• Pectoralis minor<br>• Sternal head of pectoralis major |
| Ulnar (C7, C8, T1) | Medial cord | **Brachium:**<br>Has no motor or sensory branches in the arm<br>**Antebrachium:**<br>Has no sensory branches in the antebrachium<br>Innervates:<br>• Flexor carpi ulnaris<br>• Flexor digitorum profundus (medial 1/2)<br>**Carpus, Metacarpus, and Phalanges:**<br>*Sensory branches*:<br>• Dorsal cutaneous n.—posterior surface of medial portion of manus<br>• Dorsal digital branches—dorsal aspect of 5th digit and medial 1/2 of 4th digit<br>• Palmar cutaneous n.—medial aspect of palm<br>• Common palmar cutaneous branches—distal portion of medial aspect of palm<br>• Proper palmar digital branches—palmar surface of 5th digit and medial 1/2 of 4th digit<br>*Motor branches*:<br>Superficial ulnar n.<br>• Palmaris brevis<br>Deep ulnar n.<br>• Abductor digiti minimi<br>• Flexor digiti minimi brevis<br>• Opponens digiti minimi<br>• Adductor pollicis<br>• Dorsal interosseous<br>• Palmar interosseous<br>• 3rd and 4th lumbrical |
| Upper subscapular (C5, C6) | Posterior cord | Innervates the upper portion of the subscapularis |
| Thoracodorsal (C6, C7, C8) | Posterior cord | Innervates the latissimus dorsi |
| Lower subscapular (C5, C6) | Posterior cord | Innervates:<br>• Lower portion of the subscapularis<br>• Teres major |
| Axillary (C5, C6) | Posterior cord | Innervates:<br>• Deltoid<br>• Teres minor<br>Has a sensory branch on the lateral aspect of the superior portion of the brachium:<br>• Superior lateral cutaneous branch |

INTRODUCTION TO THE UPPER LIMB, BACK, THORAX, AND ABDOMEN **651**

| BRACHIAL PLEXUS | | |
|---|---|---|
| **Nerve** | **Source** | **Comments** |
| Radial (C5, C6, C7, C8, T1) | Posterior cord | **Brachium:**<br>Innervates the:<br>• Triceps brachii<br>• Anconeus<br>Has 2 sensory branches:<br>• Inferior lateral cutaneous n.—sensory on lateral aspect of inferior brachium<br>• Posterior cutaneous n.—sensory on posterior surface of brachium<br>**Antebrachium:**<br>Has 1 sensory branch:<br>• Posterior cutaneous n. of the antebrachium<br>Innervates the:<br>• Brachioradialis<br>• Extensor carpi radialis longus<br>Divides into:<br>• Superficial radial n. (sensory in manus)<br>• Deep radial n. (motor in antebrachium)<br>Deep radial innervates:<br>• Extensor carpi radialis brevis<br>• Supinator<br>Deep radial passes through the supinator to the posterior surface, becoming the posterior interosseus<br>The posterior interosseus innervates:<br>• Extensor digitorum<br>• Extensor carpi ulnaris<br>• Extensor indicis<br>• Extensor digiti minimi<br>• Extensor pollicis longus<br>• Abductor pollicis longus<br>• Extensor pollicis brevis<br>**Carpus, Metacarpus, and Phalanges:**<br>Sensory branches:<br>• Superficial radial nerve—dorsal aspect of manus<br>• Dorsal digital branches—dorsal aspect of 1st digit<br>There are no motor branches in the manus |

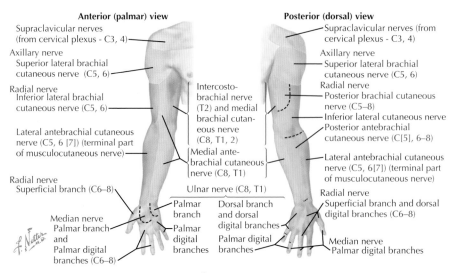

**Anterior (palmar) view**

Supraclavicular nerves (from cervical plexus - C3, 4)

Axillary nerve
Superior lateral brachial cutaneous nerve (C5, 6)

Radial nerve
Inferior lateral brachial cutaneous nerve (C5, 6)

Lateral antebrachial cutaneous nerve (C5, 6 [7]) (terminal part of musculocutaneous nerve)

Radial nerve
Superficial branch (C6–8)

Median nerve
Palmar branch and Palmar digital branches (C6–8)

Intercostobrachial nerve (T2) and medial brachial cutaneous nerve (C8, T1, 2)

Medial antebrachial cutaneous nerve (C8, T1)

Ulnar nerve (C8, T1)
Palmar branch
Palmar digital branches

Dorsal branch and dorsal digital branches
Palmar digital branches

**Posterior (dorsal) view**

Supraclavicular nerves (from cervical plexus - C3, 4)

Axillary nerve
Superior lateral brachial cutaneous nerve (C5, 6)

Radial nerve
Posterior brachial cutaneous nerve (C5–8)
Inferior lateral cutaneous nerve
Posterior antebrachial cutaneous nerve (C[5], 6–8)

Lateral antebrachial cutaneous nerve (C5, 6[7]) (terminal part of musculocutaneous nerve)

Radial nerve
Superficial branch and dorsal digital branches (C6–8)

Median nerve
Palmar digital branches

**Figure 22-47**

NERVES

- Subcostal—T12
- Iliohypogastric—L1
- Ilioinguinal—L1
- Lateral femoral cutaneous nerve—L2, L3
  - Genitofemoral—L1, L2
  - Genital branch—cremaster
  - Femoral branch—sensory on thigh
- Femoral—L2, L3, L4
- Obturator—L2, L3, L4

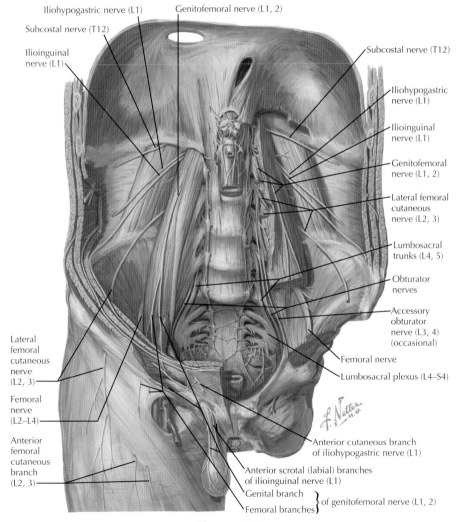

Iliohypogastric nerve (L1)
Genitofemoral nerve (L1, 2)
Subcostal nerve (T12)
Ilioinguinal nerve (L1)
Subcostal nerve (T12)
Iliohypogastric nerve (L1)
Ilioinguinal nerve (L1)
Genitofemoral nerve (L1, 2)
Lateral femoral cutaneous nerve (L2, 3)
Lumbosacral trunks (L4, 5)
Obturator nerves
Accessory obturator nerve (L3, 4) (occasional)
Femoral nerve
Lumbosacral plexus (L4–S4)
Lateral femoral cutaneous nerve (L2, 3)
Femoral nerve (L2–L4)
Anterior femoral cutaneous branch (L2, 3)
Anterior cutaneous branch of iliohypogastric nerve (L1)
Anterior scrotal (labial) branches of ilioinguinal nerve (L1)
Genital branch
Femoral branches } of genitofemoral nerve (L1, 2)

**Figure 22-48**

- The lymphatic system is a major part of the body's immune system that functions to:
  - Collect, filter, and return excess interstitial fluid to the venous system
  - Absorb fat and fat-soluble vitamins (from the villi of the small intestine)
  - Help defend against microorganisms

## PARTS OF THE LYMPHATIC SYSTEM

*Lymph*
- Lymph is a clear fluid that comes from excess tissue fluid
- Fluids pass out of capillaries at the arterial end and bathe cells
- Osmotic pressure aids in the return of the fluid into the venous end of the capillary
- Excess interstitial fluid (containing waste and microorganisms such as bacteria) enters the lymphatic capillaries and is now called lymph
- The lymph is then filtered through lymph nodes and returned to the venous system
- Lymph contains plentiful lymphocytes and other white blood cells
- Lymph from the villi of the small intestine also absorbs fat and fat-soluble vitamins
- The absorbed fat makes the lymph from this area have a milky color, and it is now called chyle

*Lymphatic Vessels*
- Lymphatic vessels carry lymph in only 1 direction—away from the tissues
- Lymphatic capillaries are located throughout the tissue spaces within the cardiovascular capillary beds
- Lymphatic capillaries are composed of overlapping endothelial cells, which form a 1-way valve allowing the excess interstitial tissue fluid to enter the lymphatic capillary, but not lymph, which then must travel in the vessel away from the tissue

*Lymph Nodes*
- Lymphatic vessels are connected to lymph nodes and filter the lymph
- Because lymphatic vessels are 1-way, lymph enters the lymph node through afferent lymph vessels, where it is filtered
- In addition to its filtration function, the lymph node has a rich supply of lymphocytes and other white blood cells that help provide an immune response to (foreign) microorganisms

*Lymphatic Ducts*
- Lymphatic vessels continue to take lymph toward the heart to join the venous system at an area of low pressure
- There are 2 connections into the venous system at the junction of the internal jugular vein and the subclavian vein:
  - Right lymphatic duct—carries lymph from right arm, right thorax, and right side of head
  - Thoracic duct—carries lymph from remainder of the body

*Tonsils*
- Tonsils are lymphatic tissue that are associated with the immune functions that defend the body
- Tonsils are part of the mucosa-associated lymphatic tissue (MALT) system of lymphoid tissue
- There are 4 sets of tonsils, together known as Waldeyer's ring, located in the nasopharynx and oropharynx that guard against foreign microorganisms:
  - Pharyngeal tonsils (adenoids)
  - Tubal tonsils (very small, located at entrance of auditory tube in nasopharynx)
  - Palatine tonsils (between palatoglossal and palatopharyngeal folds)
  - Lingual tonsils (on posterior 1/3 of the tongue)

**OTHER LYMPHOID ORGANS**
- Thymus
- Spleen

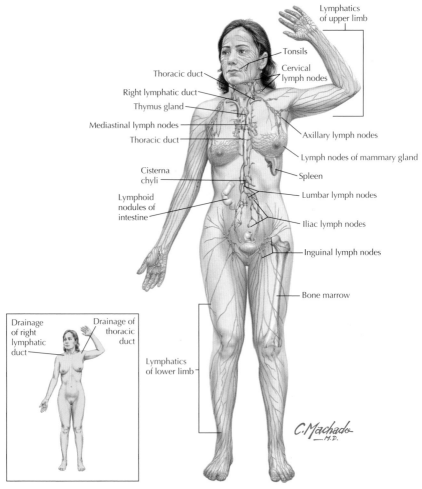

**Figure A-1**

- There are multiple ways to classify lymphatics of the head and neck; one way is to divide lymph nodes into:
  - Superficial nodes
  - Deep nodes
- This classification results in 4 types of lymph nodes:
  - Superficial lymph nodes of the head
  - Deep lymph nodes of the head
  - Superficial lymph nodes of the neck
  - Deep lymph nodes of the neck
    - Upper deep cervical
    - Lower deep cervical
- After being filtered by lymph nodes (primary node), the lymph will connect to another lymph node and be filtered again (secondary node)
- Eventually, all lymph will drain into the inferior group of deep cervical lymph nodes where they join the jugular lymph trunks, which eventually create the right lymphatic duct (on the right side) and the thoracic duct (on the left side), which empties into the venous system at the junction of the internal jugular vein and the brachiocephalic vein

| SUPERFICIAL LYMPH NODES OF THE HEAD | | |
|---|---|---|
| **Node** | **Location** | **Structure(s) Drained** |
| Facial | Along cheek | Superficial face<br>Cheek |
| Parotid (superficial nodes) | Along superficial lobe of parotid gland and anterior to the ear | Upper parts of face<br>Lateral parts of face<br>Anterior scalp<br>Lateral scalp<br>External ear (anterior portion) |
| Mastoid | Along mastoid process superficial to the attachment of the sternocleidomastoid | Lateral scalp<br>External ear (posterior portion) |
| Occipital | Along the apex of the posterior triangle where the trapezius and sternocleidomastoid converge near the superior nuchal line | Posterior scalp<br>Upper neck |
| Submental | Between anterior bellies of the digastric in Submental triangle | Tip of tongue<br>Medial portion of inferior lip<br>Mandibular incisors and associated gingiva<br>Anterior floor of the mouth<br>Chin |
| Submandibular | Inferior to mandible between anterior and posterior digastrics in the Submandibular triangle | Superior lip<br>Lateral portion of lower lip<br>Cheek<br>Hard palate<br>Soft palate<br>Teeth and associated gingiva (except mandibular incisors)<br>Tongue (anterior 2/3—except the tip and central 1/3)<br>Floor of the mouth<br>Sublingual gland<br>Submandibular gland<br>Nose and nasal vestibule<br>Nasal cavity (anterior portion)<br>Medial eyelids<br>Frontal sinus<br>Anterior and middle ethmoid sinus<br>Maxillary sinus<br>Submental nodes |

| SUPERFICIAL LYMPH NODES OF THE NECK | | |
|---|---|---|
| **Node** | **Location** | **Structure(s) Drained** |
| Posterior cervical nodes | Along external jugular vein | Skin of angle of mandible<br>External ear (inferior portion)<br>Parotid region |
| Anterior cervical nodes | Along pretracheal fascia with anterior triangle | Skin of anterior neck inferior to the hyoid |
| DEEP LYMPH NODES OF THE HEAD | | |
| **Node** | **Location** | **Structure(s) Drained** |
| Parotid (deep) | Deep in parotid gland | Tympanic cavity<br>Parotid gland<br>Auditory tube<br>External acoustic meatus (portion) |
| Retropharyngeal | Posterior to superior constrictor at the base of the skull immediately anterior to the atlas | Sphenoid sinus<br>Posterior ethmoid sinus<br>Nasal cavity (majority)<br>Soft palate<br>Nasopharynx<br>Auditory tube<br>Oropharynx<br>Pharyngeal tonsils<br>Tubal tonsils |
| DEEP LYMPH NODES OF THE NECK | | |
| **Node** | **Location** | **Structure(s) Drained** |
| Upper deep cervical nodes | Along superior portion of the internal jugular vein superior to the omohyoid | Occipital nodes<br>Mastoid nodes<br>Parotid nodes (superficial and deep)<br>Submandibular nodes<br>Superficial cervical nodes<br>Retropharyngeal nodes<br>Palatine tonsil |
| Jugulodigastric node (subset of upper deep cervical nodes) | Along lower portion of the internal jugular vein | Tongue (posterior 1/3)<br>Palatine tonsil<br>Occasionally mandibular molars |
| Juxtavisceral nodes (includes: Prelaryngeal Pretracheal Paratracheal) | Midline nodes located along anatomic area for which they are named | Larynx<br>Thyroid gland<br>Trachea<br>Esophagus |
| Inferior deep cervical nodes | Along inferior portion of internal jugular vein near the intermediate tendon of the omohyoid | Upper deep cervical nodes<br>Jugulodigastric nodes<br>Tongue (anterior 2/3—except tip and lateral margin)<br>Superficial cervical nodes<br>Transverse cervical nodes |

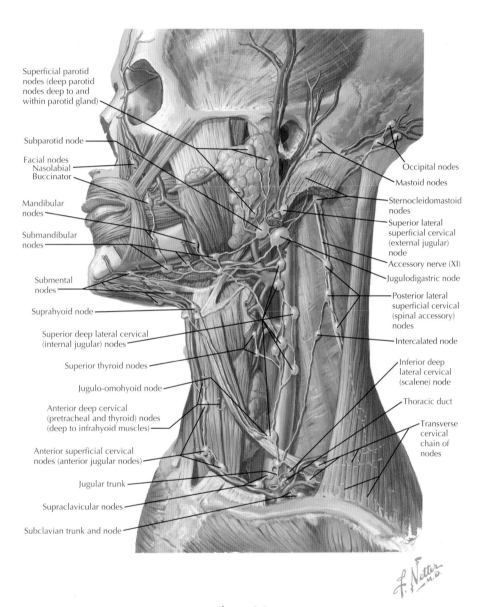

Superficial parotid nodes (deep parotid nodes deep to and within parotid gland)

Subparotid node

Facial nodes
Nasolabial
Buccinator

Mandibular nodes

Submandibular nodes

Submental nodes

Suprahyoid node

Superior deep lateral cervical (internal jugular) nodes

Superior thyroid nodes

Jugulo-omohyoid node

Anterior deep cervical (pretracheal and thyroid) nodes (deep to infrahyoid muscles)

Anterior superficial cervical nodes (anterior jugular nodes)

Jugular trunk

Supraclavicular nodes

Subclavian trunk and node

Occipital nodes

Mastoid nodes

Sternocleidomastoid nodes

Superior lateral superficial cervical (external jugular) node

Accessory nerve (XI)

Jugulodigastric node

Posterior lateral superficial cervical (spinal accessory) nodes

Intercalated node

Inferior deep lateral cervical (scalene) node

Thoracic duct

Transverse cervical chain of nodes

Figure A-2

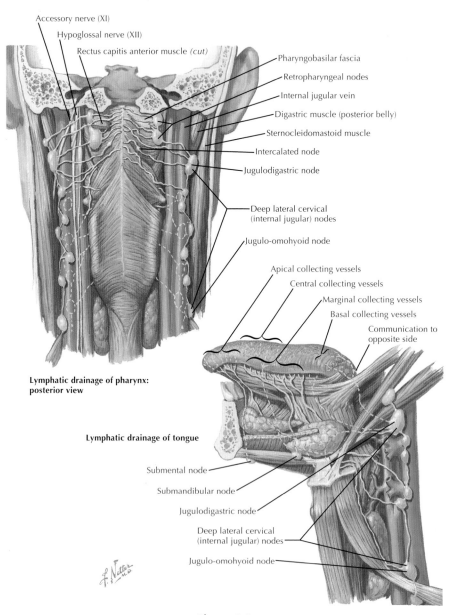

Accessory nerve (XI)

Hypoglossal nerve (XII)

Rectus capitis anterior muscle *(cut)*

Pharyngobasilar fascia

Retropharyngeal nodes

Internal jugular vein

Digastric muscle (posterior belly)

Sternocleidomastoid muscle

Intercalated node

Jugulodigastric node

Deep lateral cervical (internal jugular) nodes

Jugulo-omohyoid node

Apical collecting vessels

Central collecting vessels

Marginal collecting vessels

Basal collecting vessels

Communication to opposite side

**Lymphatic drainage of pharynx: posterior view**

**Lymphatic drainage of tongue**

Submental node

Submandibular node

Jugulodigastric node

Deep lateral cervical (internal jugular) nodes

Jugulo-omohyoid node

**Figure A-3**

# QUESTIONS AND ANSWERS

## CHAPTER 1  DEVELOPMENT OF THE HEAD AND NECK

1. All of the following are structures derived from neural crest *except*:
   A. Incus
   B. Anterior ligament of the malleus
   C. Thyroid cartilage
   D. Lesser cornu of the hyoid
   E. Styloid process

2. What adult structure arises from the 1st pharyngeal pouch?
   A. Tympanic cavity
   B. Thymus
   C. Superior parathyroid gland
   D. Ultimobranchial body
   E. Tonsillar fossa

3. All of the following cranial nerves provide general somatic afferent (GSA) fibers to the epithelium of the tongue *except*:
   A. Glossopharyngeal
   B. Facial
   C. Vagus
   D. Trigeminal
   E. C and D

## CHAPTER 2  OSTEOLOGY

4. The ophthalmic artery passes through the:
   A. Optic canal
   B. Inferior orbital fissure
   C. Superior orbital fissure
   D. Condylar canal
   E. Sphenopalatine foramen

5. The anterior tympanic artery passes through the:
   A. Tympanic canaliculus
   B. Jugular foramen
   C. Hiatus for the greater petrosal nerve
   D. Foramen ovale
   E. Petrotympanic fissure

6. A horizontal fracture of the midface extending from the lateral margin of the piriform aperture to the pterygoid plates superior to the apices of the teeth is termed:
   A. Le Fort I
   B. Le Fort II
   C. Le Fort III
   D. Jefferson
   E. Hangman's

ANSWERS

6 A
5 E
4 A
3 B
2 A
1 C

## CHAPTER 3 BASIC NEUROANATOMY AND CRANIAL NERVES

7. Which of the following is a collection of nerve cell bodies located in the peripheral nervous system?
   A. Superior salivatory nucleus
   B. Oculomotor nucleus
   C. Tractus solitarius
   D. Trigeminal ganglion
   E. Trigeminothalamic tract

8. Which of the following is responsible for proprioception of the trigeminal nerve?
   A. Principal sensory nucleus of V
   B. Motor nucleus of V
   C. Spinal nucleus of V
   D. Nucleus ambiguus
   E. Mesencephalic nucleus of V

9. Which of the following functional columns is responsible for innervating branchial arch muscles?
   A. GSE
   B. SVE
   C. GVE
   D. SSA
   E. SVA

## CHAPTER 4 THE NECK

10. Which of the following muscles is a boundary for the carotid and submandibular triangles?
    A. Anterior digastric
    B. Posterior digastric
    C. Superior belly of the omohyoid
    D. Inferior belly of the omohyoid
    E. Sternocleidomastoid

11. Which of the following muscles is innervated by the ventral rami of C1?
    A. Anterior digastric
    B. Stylohyoid
    C. Mylohyoid
    D. Thyrohyoid
    E. Hyoglossus

12. Which vessel is the origin of the submental artery?
    A. Lingual
    B. Facial
    C. Maxillary
    D. Superior laryngeal
    E. Ascending pharyngeal

13. All of the following cross the sternocleidomastoid *except*:
    A. External jugular vein
    B. Great auricular nerve
    C. Investing layer of deep cervical fascia
    D. Suprascapular nerve
    E. Transverse cervical nerve

ANSWERS

13 D
12 B
11 D
10 B
9 B
8 E
7 D

## CHAPTER 5  SCALP AND MUSCLES OF FACIAL EXPRESSION

14. All of the following statements regarding facial anatomy are correct *except*:
    A. The skin is attached to the underlying bone by retaining ligaments which are in constant locations on the face
    B. The superficial fascia of the face has varying amounts of adipose tissue
    C. The superficial muscular aponeurotic system (SMAS) is deep to the superficial fascia and provides a surgical plane for surgery of the face
    D. The muscles of facial expression are also called mimetic muscles
    E. There is deep fascia along the face

15. Which of the following muscles depresses the corners of the mouth in an inferior and lateral direction?
    A. Depressor labii inferioris
    B. Mentalis
    C. Depressor anguli oris
    D. Risorius
    E. Orbicularis oris

16. Which of the following muscles does *not* connect the superficial veins of the face to the deep veins of the face in the "danger area of the face"?
    A. Superior ophthalmic vein
    B. Deep facial vein
    C. Transverse facial vein
    D. Infraorbital vein
    E. Inferior ophthalmic vein

17. Which branch(es) of the facial nerve is/are responsible for innervating the orbicularis oculi?
    A. Temporal only
    B. Zygomatic only
    C. Temporal and zygomatic
    D. Buccal only
    E. Zygomatic and buccal

## CHAPTER 6  PAROTID FOSSA AND GLAND

18. All of the following statements concerning the parotid gland are correct *except*:
    A. The parotid gland receives parasympathetic innervation from the glossopharyngeal nerve
    B. The parotid gland enters the oral cavity opposite the 2nd maxillary premolar
    C. The deep lobe lies adjacent to the lateral pharyngeal space
    D. About 75% of the parotid gland is retromandibular
    E. Most tumors of the parotid gland are benign

19. The common facial vein is formed by the joining of which 2 veins?
    A. Posterior division of the retromandibular vein and the posterior auricular veins
    B. Anterior and posterior divisions of the retromandibular vein
    C. Anterior division of the retromandibular vein and the facial vein
    D. Superficial temporal and transverse facial veins
    E. Superficial temporal and maxillary veins

20. All of the following statements concerning the parotid gland are correct *except*:
    A. The parotid gland is the largest salivary gland
    B. The parotid gland is responsible for 80% of the saliva formed by the salivary glands
    C. The parotid gland is entirely serous in secretion
    D. The external carotid artery passes within the substance of the parotid gland
    E. The retromandibular vein passes within the substance of the parotid gland

## CHAPTER 7 TEMPORAL AND INFRATEMPORAL FOSSAE

21. The auriculotemporal nerve wraps around which artery?
    A. Posterior deep temporal artery
    B. Inferior alveolar artery
    C. Middle meningeal artery
    D. Masseteric artery
    E. Anterior tympanic artery

22. Which of the following arteries located in the infratemporal fossa arises from the 3rd part of the maxillary artery?
    A. Posterior superior alveolar artery
    B. Middle meningeal artery
    C. Descending palatine artery
    D. Artery of the pterygoid canal
    E. Buccal artery

23. All of the following are branches of the posterior division of the trigeminal nerve within the infratemporal fossa *except*:
    A. Auriculotemporal nerve
    B. Mylohyoid nerve
    C. Lingual nerve
    D. Inferior alveolar nerve
    E. Masseteric nerve

## CHAPTER 8 MUSCLES OF MASTICATION

24. The parotid duct crosses superficial to the:
    A. Temporalis
    B. Masseter
    C. Medial pterygoid
    D. Tensor veli palatini
    E. Lateral pterygoid

25. Which muscle attaches along the medial surface of the ramus and angle of the mandible?
    A. Lateral pterygoid
    B. Temporalis
    C. Tensor veli palatini
    D. Medial pterygoid
    E. Masseter

## CHAPTER 9 TEMPOROMANDIBULAR JOINT

26. The anterior boundary of the glenoid fossa is the:
    A. Articular eminence
    B. Postglenoid tubercle
    C. Tympanic plate
    D. Petrotympanic fissure
    E. Squamotympanic fissure

27. Which of the following sensory nerves of the temporomandibular joint arise from the posterior division of the trigeminal nerve?
    A. Posterior deep temporal nerve
    B. Anterior deep temporal nerve
    C. Lingual nerve
    D. Auriculotemporal nerve
    E. Masseteric nerve

ANSWERS

27 D
26 A
25 D
24 B
23 B
22 A
21 C

28. Which ligament attaches to the lingula?
    A. Stylomandibular ligament
    B. Temporomandibular ligament
    C. Sphenomandibular ligament
    D. Medial collateral ligament
    E. Lateral collateral ligament

## CHAPTER 10  PTERYGOPALATINE FOSSA

29. All of the following have a direct communication with the pterygopalatine fossa via an opening on the fossa *except*:
    A. Infratemporal fossa
    B. Oral cavity
    C. Middle cranial fossa
    D. Nasopharynx
    E. Temporal fossa

30. The inferior orbital fissure communicates the pterygopalatine fossa with the:
    A. Middle cranial fossa
    B. Orbit
    C. Infratemporal fossa
    D. Nasal cavity
    E. Nasopharynx

## CHAPTER 11  NOSE AND NASAL CAVITY

31. All of the following arteries contribute to Kiesselbach's plexus *except*:
    A. Sphenopalatine
    B. Greater palatine
    C. Posterior ethmoid
    D. Anterior ethmoid
    E. Septal branch from the superior labial artery

32. The sphenopalatine foramen communicates the nasal cavity with the:
    A. Middle cranial fossa
    B. Pterygopalatine fossa
    C. Infratemporal fossa
    D. Oropharynx
    E. Maxillary sinus

## CHAPTER 12  PARANASAL SINUSES

33. The nasolacrimal duct drains into the:
    A. Sphenoethmoid recess
    B. Superior meatus
    C. Middle meatus
    D. Hiatus semilunaris
    E. Inferior meatus

34. Which paranasal sinus is most prone to sinusitis?
    A. Anterior ethmoid
    B. Posterior ethmoid
    C. Maxillary
    D. Frontal
    E. Sphenoid

ANSWERS

34 C
33 E
32 B
31 C
30 B
29 E
28 C

## CHAPTER 13   ORAL CAVITY

35. The depressed area located between the base of the nose and the vermilion border of the upper lip is known as the:
    A. Philtrum
    B. Vestibule
    C. Labial commissure
    D. Retromolar region
    E. Mucobuccal fold

36. What structure drains into the sublingual papilla?
    A. Sublingual gland
    B. Parotid gland
    C. Buccal gland
    D. Palatal gland
    E. Submandibular gland

## CHAPTER 14   TONGUE

37. The taste buds innervated by the glossopharyngeal nerve are associated with which papilla?
    A. Submandibular
    B. Foliate
    C. Fungiform
    D. Filiform
    E. Circumvallate

38. What structure lies deep to the hyoglossus?
    A. Lingual nerve
    B. Lingual artery
    C. Hypoglossal nerve
    D. Submandibular duct
    E. Sublingual gland

## CHAPTER 15   PHARYNX

39. The superior boundary of the oropharynx is the:
    A. Epiglottis
    B. Palatoglossal fold
    C. Palatopharyngeal fold
    D. Nasopharynx
    E. Oropharynx

40. The anterior boundary of the oropharynx is the:
    A. Palatoglossal fold
    B. Palatopharyngeal fold
    C. Epiglottis
    D. Inferior border of the cricoid
    E. Soft palate

## CHAPTER 16   LARYNX

41. The depression in the mucosa between the pharyngeal portion of the tongue and the anterior border of the epiglottis is known as the:
    A. Piriform recess
    B. Pharyngeal recess
    C. Vallecula
    D. Vestibule
    E. Tonsillar sinus

ANSWERS

41  C
40  A
39  D
38  B
37  E
36  E
35  A

42. The mucosa covering the posterior surface of the epiglottis is:
    A. Pseudostratified columnar epithelium with cilia
    B. Stratified squamous epithelium
    C. Stratified squamous nonkeratinized epithelium
    D. Simple columnar epithelium
    E. Simple squamous epithelium

## CHAPTER 17  CERVICAL FASCIA

43. The superior boundary of the canine fascial space is the:
    A. Levator anguli oris
    B. Levator labii superioris
    C. Zygomaticus major
    D. Nasalis
    E. Procerus

## CHAPTER 18  EAR

44. The roof of the middle ear is the:
    A. Tympanic canaliculus
    B. Auditory tube
    C. Facial canal
    D. Tegmen tympani
    E. Mastoid antrum

## CHAPTER 19  EYE AND ORBIT

45. The pigmented vascular layer between the sclera and the retina is the:
    A. Choroid
    B. Ciliary body
    C. Iris
    D. Aqueous humor
    E. Posterior chamber

## CHAPTER 20  AUTONOMICS OF THE HEAD AND NECK

46. All of the following cranial nerves are responsible for parasympathetic activity *except*:
    A. Oculomotor
    B. Trigeminal
    C. Facial
    D. Glossopharyngeal
    E. Vagus

47. The greater petrosal nerve contains:
    A. Preganglionic parasympathetic fibers
    B. Postganglionic parasympathetic fibers
    C. Preganglionic sympathetic fibers
    D. Postganglionic sympathetic fibers
    E. Taste fibers to the anterior 2/3 of the tongue

## CHAPTER 21  INTRAORAL INJECTIONS

48. All of the following areas are anesthetized in a maxillary division block *except*:
    A. All maxillary teeth
    B. All maxillary buccal gingiva
    C. All maxillary palatal gingiva
    D. Upper lip
    E. Lower lip

ANSWERS

48 E
47 A
46 B
45 A
44 D
43 B
42 A

## CHAPTER 22   INTRODUCTION TO THE UPPER LIMB, BACK, THORAX, AND ABDOMEN

49. The layer of parietal pleura that lines the cavity along the ribs is the:
    A. Cervical
    B. Costal
    C. Diaphragmatic
    D. Mediastinal
    E. Visceral

50. The septomarginal trabeculae is located in the:
    A. Right atrium
    B. Right ventricle
    C. Left atrium
    D. Left ventricle
    E. Fossa ovalis

Page numbers followed by "*f*" indicate figures.